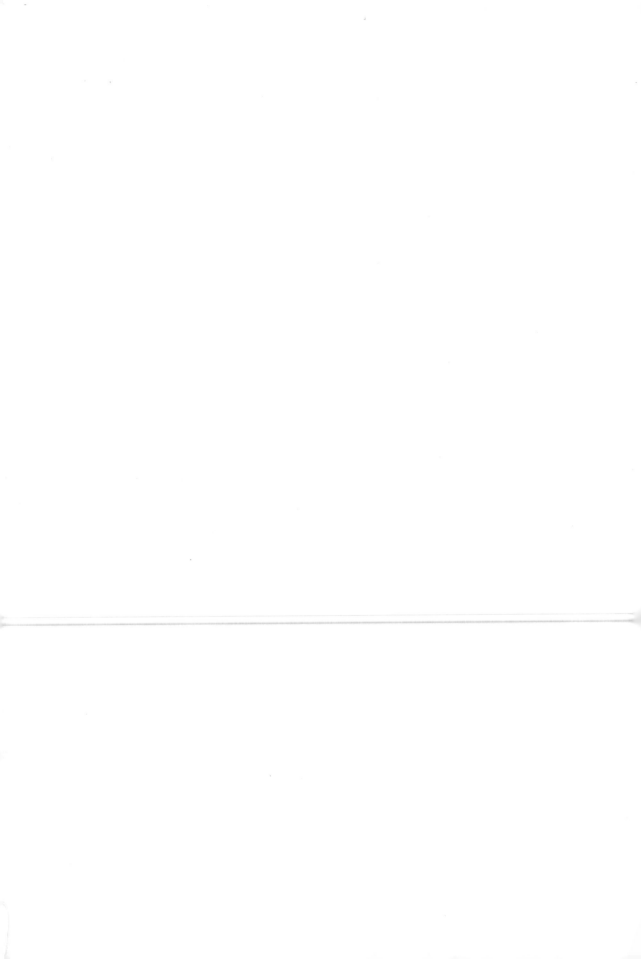

Measurement in Nursing and Health Research

Third Edition

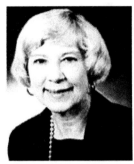

Carolyn F. Waltz, PhD, RN, FAAN, is Professor and Director of International Activities at the University of Maryland School of Nursing. She received her BSN and MS degrees in nursing from the University of Maryland and her doctorate in education with specialization in research, evaluation, and measurement from the University of Delaware. Dr. Waltz is an internationally recognized expert in the development of outcomes evaluation in clinical and educational settings. She has published extensively including award winning books and articles on research, measurement, nursing outcomes, program development and evaluation. She has provided numerous outcomes evaluations, consultations, presentations, and workshops to varied health care audiences nationally and internationally and is widely acknowledged as a pioneer in outcomes evaluation and research.

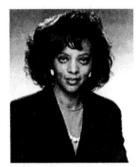

Ora Lea Strickland, PhD, RN, FAAN, is Professor in the Nell Hodgson Woodruff School of Nursing at Emory University in Atlanta, Georgia. She earned a doctoral degree in child development and family relations from the University of North Carolina, Greensboro; a master's degree in maternal and child health nursing from Boston University, Massachusetts; and a bachelor's degree in nursing from North Carolina Agricultural and Technical State University, Greensboro. She is the founder and senior editor of the *Journal of Nursing Measurement*. As an internationally known specialist in nursing research, measurement, evaluation, maternal and child health and parenting, Dr. Strickland has published widely in professional journals and books, and is called upon as a consultant by health care agencies, universities, government agencies, and community organizations. She has presented more than 200 lectures, speeches, and workshops, and her research has been featured in newspapers and magazines, as well as on radio and television.

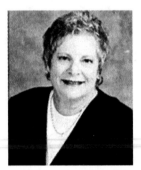

Elizabeth R. Lenz, PhD, RN, FAAN, is Professor and Dean of the Ohio State University College of Nursing in Columbus, Ohio. From 1996–2001 she was the Associate Dean for Research and Doctoral Studies and the Anna C. Maxwell Professor of Nursing Research at the Columbia University School of Nursing in New York City. She has also held faculty positions at Boston College; Georgetown University; and the University of Maryland where she was the founding director of the PhD program and Associate Dean for Graduate Studies and Research. At the Pennsylvania State University she served as Professor of Nursing and Director of the Center for Nursing Research at Penn State's Milton S. Hershey Medical Center. Dr. Lenz received the Bachelor of Science in Nursing from DePauw University, Master of Science from Boston College, and Doctor of Philosophy with a major in sociology from the University of Delaware.

Dr. Lenz is an internationally-known expert on doctoral nursing education, and currently chairs the AACN Task Force on the Clinical Nursing Doctorate. She is known for her theoretical work in the areas of social support, information-seeking, middle-range theories in nursing science, and the conceptual basis for measurement. She coauthored the *Theory of Unpleasant Symptoms*. She has received research funding from multiple governmental and foundation sources, authored over 80 articles and book chapters, and served as an editor of *Scholarly Inquiry for Nursing Practice: An International Journal* between 1997 and 2001.

Measurement in Nursing and Health Research

Third Edition

Carolyn Feher Waltz, PhD, RN, FAAN
Ora Lea Strickland, PhD, RN, FAAN
Elizabeth R. Lenz, PhD, RN, FAAN

 Springer Publishing Company

Springer Publishing Company, Inc.
11 West 42nd Street
New York, NY 10036

Acquisitions Editor: Ruth Chasek
Production Editor: Sara Yoo
Cover design by Joanne Honigman

05 06 07 08 09 / 5 4 3 2 1

Library of Congress Cataloging-in-Publication Data

Waltz, Carolyn Feher.
    Measurement in nursing and health research / Carolyn Feher Waltz, Ora L. Strickland, Elizabeth R. Lenz, authors. — 3rd ed.
        p. ; cm.
    Rev. ed. of: Measurement in nursing research / Carolyn Feher Waltz, Ora L. Strickland, Elizabeth R. Lenz, 2nd ed. 1991.
    Includes bibliographical references and index.
    ISBN 0-8261-2635-9
    1. Nursing—Research—Methodology. 2. Medical care—Research-Methodology.
    [DNLM: 1. Nursing Research—Nurses' Instruction. 2. Health Services Research—Nurses' Instruction. 3. Research Design—Nurses' Instruction. WY 20.5 W24lm 2005] I. Strickland, Ora. II. Lenz, Elizabeth R., 1943– III. Waltz, Carolyn Feher. Measurement in nursing research. IV. Title.

RT81.5.W36 2005
610.73'072—dc22

                                                                                    2004023629

Printed in the United States of America by Integrated Book Technology.

Contents

Part IV   Special Issues

Contributors

Theresa L. Dremsa, Lt.Col., USAF NC, PhD
Nurse Researcher
Clinical Research Squadron
Wilford Hall Medical Center
Lackland AFB, Texas

Susan K. Frazier, PhD, RN
Associate Professor
Ohio State University
College of Nursing
Columbus, Ohio

Judith E. Hupcey, EdD, RN, CRNP
Associate Professor
Pennsylvania State University
School of Nursing
College of Health and Human Development
Associate Professor of Humanities College
    of Medicine
Hershey, Pennsylvania

Louise S. Jenkins, PhD, RN
Associate Professor
University of Maryland
School of Nursing
Baltimore, Maryland

Meg Johantgen, PhD, RN
Associate Professor
University of Maryland
School of Nursing
Baltimore, Maryland

Karen L. Soeken, PhD
Professor
University of Maryland
School of Nursing
Baltimore, Maryland

Nola Stair, MBA
Instructional Design Technologist
University of Maryland
School of Nursing
Baltimore, Maryland

Kathleen S. Stone, PhD, RN, FAAN
Professor
Ohio State University
College of Nursing
Columbus, Ohio

Preface

The third edition of this text was written in response to the numerous requests from satisfied readers who valued it as a textbook for research and measurement courses. It has been a significant resource for those conducting their own research and seeking to understand the significance of others' research in order to decide whether or not to use results as evidence for their practice. While nurses remain the primary audience for this book, we found that a significant number of readers were health professionals from a variety of disciplines. This was not surprising given the significant increase in interdisciplinary research and collaboration since the last edition was published. To reflect this fact we have added content and examples throughout to accommodate the needs and interests of this broader audience and have included "health research" in the title.

The intent, as with earlier editions, is to present a pragmatic account of the process involved in designing, testing, and/or selecting instruments, methods, and procedures for measuring variables in clinical, educational, and research settings. Topics included in this edition were selected on the basis of our own and our readers' experiences in teaching measurement to nurses and other health professionals, as well as our own and our readers' involvement in constructing and employing measurement principles and practices in a variety of nursing and health care situations. This selection process, we believe, has resulted in a third edition that includes the "best" of the measurement content, strategies, and procedures presented in the first two editions, and offers additional content, strategies, and procedures with direct applicability for nurses and health professionals in a variety of roles, including those of student, educator,

clinician, researcher, administrator, and consultant. Thus, this book should serve as a valuable resource for readers who seek basic or advanced content, to develop their skill in measurement.

Since the second edition of this book was published, there have been incredible advances in the science of nursing and health care, and the importance given to employing sound measurement principles and practices has increased markedly, as has the sophistication of nurses and health professionals who conduct and/or employ research results. For this reason, this edition seeks to meet the needs of a large and diversified audience ranging from neophytes to those who are more advanced in their knowledge and experience in measurement. We do not assume that most readers have an extensive background in measurement or statistics. Rather, we begin our discussion of content assuming little background in these areas and subsequently develop, explain in detail, and illustrate by example the concepts and principles that are operationally important to the content presented. In this manner, it is possible for the less sophisticated reader to develop the level of knowledge necessary to understand the content that is included for the benefit of the more advanced reader, such as item response theory, confirmatory factor analysis, triangulation, and the multitrait-multimethod approach to item development.

The focus, as in previous editions, is increasing the reader's ability to employ measures that are operationalized within the context of theories and conceptual frameworks, derived from sound measurement principles and practices, and adequately tested for reliability and validity using appropriate methods and procedures. More attention is given in this edition to qualitative data collection and analysis, physiologic measures, nonclassical measurement approaches such as item-response theory, and more advanced procedures for investigating validity such as confirmatory factor analysis. Step-by-step approaches for developing and testing norm-referenced and criterion-referenced measurement tools and procedures are presented, and a chapter on instrumentation and data collection methods has been added that focuses on the essential considerations to be made in selecting an instrumentation method and the specific steps to be undertaken in constructing and testing the resulting instrument.

Also since the second edition was published, the measurement issues to be addressed in nursing and health research have increased in number and complexity. For this reason, consideration of measurement issues has been expanded to include issues related to implementation of HIPAA requirements; selection and use of existing databases, large data sets, and secondary data analysis; internet data collection; and making sense of findings from the use of multiple measures, including triangulation and other strategies for combining qualitative and quantitative methodologies. Of particular note is the addition of appendices on measurement resources which provide useful sources of information including journals, instrument compendia and resource books, internet sites, computer software, and existing databases.

Throughout the book we provide additional reference sources for readers who desire to pursue further the topics presented. References have been selected for materials that are readily available in most libraries, and whenever possible, comprehensive summaries of literature in an area of significant interest are cited rather than a myriad of individual books and articles.

We thank the many of you who requested this book and sincerely hope that it proves to be worth the wait.

CAROLYN F. WALTZ, PHD, RN, FAAN
ORA LEA STRICKLAND, PHD, RN, FAAN
ELIZABETH R. LENZ, PHD, RN, FAAN

Acknowledgment

The authors extend sincere appreciation to Sandra A. Murphy, Administrative Assistant in the School of Nursing at the University of Maryland, who graciously contributed her time and effort to ensure the completion of this book. Her commitment, perseverance, outstanding organizational ability, and many talents were valuable assets to us during the preparation of this manuscript. Sandy, thank you very much.

Part I

Basic Principles of Measurement

I

An Introduction to Measurement

In this chapter, we discuss terms and ideas essential to understanding the content of subsequent chapters and present an overview of the types of measures that are most often used.

THEORY-BASED MEASURES

A *theory* is defined as "a set of interrelated constructs, definitions, and propositions that present a systematic view of phenomena by specifying relations among variables, with the purpose of explaining and predicting the phenomena" (Kerlinger, 1973, p. 9). A *theoretical rationale,* according to LoBiondo-Wood and Haber (1994), "provides a road map or context for examining problems, and developing and testing hypotheses. It gives meaning to the problem and study findings by summarizing existing knowledge in the field of inquiry and identifying linkages among concepts" (p. 157). *Conceptual models,* they note, provide a context for constructing theories that deal with phenomena of concern to a discipline and help define how it is different from other disciplines.

Various authors have defined and analyzed concepts in numerous ways (Glaser & Strauss, 1967; Orem, 1995; Leonard & George, 1995; Meleis, 1997; Allegood & Marriner-Tomey, 2002; George, 2002; Renpenning & Taylor, 2003). Simply defined, a *concept* is a thought, notion, or idea. It is an abstraction. For example, nursing concepts are thoughts, notions, or ideas about nursing or nursing practice. Thus, concepts define the content of interest in measuring phenomena. *Phenomena* are observable facts or events. To render concepts measurable it is necessary to translate them into phenomena. When one operationalizes a concept, one translates an abstract concept into concrete observable events or phenomena. For example, the concept of "attitude" is frequently operationalized as a tendency to respond in a consistent manner to a certain category of stimuli (Campbell, 1963). If the stimulus is a 17-item questionnaire regarding children's concerns about health care, such as the Child Medical Fear Scale developed by Broome and Mobley (2003, pp. 196–206), in which the child indicates whether he or she was "not at all," "a little," or "a lot" afraid of selected experiences associated with health care described in the items, and the subject responds "a lot" to the majority of the 17 items, one would infer from the responses that the child's attitude or fearfulness of the experiences associated with health care was high.

Variables are quantities that may assume different values; they are changeable. The process whereby one decides how to measure a variable is referred to as *instrumentation,* that is, the process of selecting or developing tools and methods appropriate for measuring an attribute or characteristic of interest. In the example above, the 17-item questionnaire was a form of instrumentation selected to measure attitudes of children toward the medical experience. Instrumentation is a component of the measurement process. *Measurement* is defined as the process of assigning numbers to objects to represent the kind and/or amount of attributes or characteristics possessed by those objects. This definition of measurement includes what has traditionally been referred to as *qualitative measurement* (i.e., assigning objects to categories that represent the kind of characteristic possessed and that are mutually exclusive and exhaustive) as well as *quantitative measurement* (i.e., assigning objects to categories that represent the amount of a characteristic possessed).

The utilization of a conceptual framework to systematically guide the measurement process increases the likelihood that concepts and variables universally salient to nursing and health care practice will be identified and explicated. That is, when measurement concerns emanate from an empirical rather than a conceptual point of view, there is higher probability of investigating and measuring these variables from an esoteric or limited perspective that overlooks important dimensions of the variables that should be measured.

Concepts of interest to nurses and other health professionals are usually difficult to operationalize, that is, to render measurable. This is explained in part by the fact that nurses and other health professionals deal with a multiplicity of complex variables in diverse settings, employing a myriad of roles as they collaborate with a variety of others to attain their own and others' goals. Hence, the dilemma that they are apt to encounter in measuring concepts is twofold: first, the significant variables to be measured must somehow be isolated; and second, very ambiguous and abstract notions must be reduced to a set of concrete behavioral indicators. What tools, therefore, are available to nurses and other health care professionals who must begin to grapple with this dilemma?

Because of the challenge to provide services of broadening scope and diversity in order to keep pace with the rapidly changing and volatile health care scene coupled with severe shortages in nursing and other health care disciplines, a great deal of controversy and confusion has ensued regarding which functions should be included within the realm of each of the practice disciplines and which information should be shared. For nursing, this is evidenced by the proliferation of definitions and models for nursing practice evident in the literature. Although, for the most part, the definitions of nursing advanced in the literature remain ambiguous and global, in each view the major focus for nursing practice can be placed on a continuum ranging from direct to indirect involvement in patient care. *Direct* nursing practice involves the continuous, ongoing provision of direct services to patients and clients (e.g., the primary care nurse practitioner provides

direct nursing services). *Indirect* nursing practice is usually characterized by activities on behalf of the patient, that is, working with or through others who are directly responsible for the provision of direct services to patients and clients. Nursing education, administration, and health policy activities exemplify indirect nursing practice. This scheme for categorizing nursing practice has utility for the nurse who is attempting to operationalize nursing concepts.

More specifically, the first task is to identify a definition of nursing that is consistent with the nurses' own views and beliefs about nursing practice. Similarly, although the extent to which available conceptual frameworks and models for nursing practice have been refined and tested varies, their very existence affords nurses a rich opportunity to select a conceptual framework to guide them in systematically identifying and further explicating concepts and variables germane to nursing and nursing practice concerns within their primary focus. The problems, settings, roles, and purposeful activities undertaken by nurses will differ, depending upon whether their primary focus is direct or indirect nursing practice. Furthermore, the goals for, and outcomes likely to result from, the application of direct and indirect nursing processes will vary. Although there will be differences among each of these categories of practice, there will also be commonalities in process and outcomes within each focus. Therefore, if nurses consider their measurement concerns within the context of their primary focus, delimit the processes and outcomes that characterize that practice, and then search for behavioral indicators within the primary focus that extend beyond their immediate setting (i.e., that are common across settings similar to their own), they are apt to reduce the abstract concepts emanating from their conceptual framework to behavioral indicators with more universal acceptance than those likely to result from a more esoteric approach. In this manner, nurses will ultimately make a contribution to the profession by accruing information to add to the body of knowledge about nursing, the specific definition and conceptual framework employed, and its utility as a guide for operationalizing nursing and nursing practice concerns. It should be noted that when nurses whose measurement concerns emanate from their ongoing practice fail to step back and rethink the problem from a conceptual point of view, they also have a high probability of investigating and measuring their variables from a limited perspective that overlooks important dimensions of the variables that should be measured.

In nursing and the health professions where the concern is with the measurement of process variables, which are dynamic, as well as outcome variables, which are usually static, and in which results of the measurement are likely to be applied to the solution of significant problems across practice settings, two characteristics of measurement—reliability and validity—become of utmost importance. First, tools and methods selected or developed for measuring a variable of interest must demonstrate evidence for reliability and validity. *Reliability* in this case refers to the consistency with which a tool or method assigns scores to subjects. *Validity* refers to the determination of whether or not a tool or method is useful for the purpose for which it is intended, that is, measures what it purports to measure. Second, in addition to the concern with instrument reliability and validity, attention needs to be given to the reliability and validity of the measurement process per se. To increase the probability that the measurement process will yield reliable and valid information, it is necessary whenever possible to employ multiple tools or methods to measure any given variable (all of which have demonstrated evidence for instrument reliability and validity) and to obtain information about any given variable from a number of different perspectives or sources. Measurement reliability and validity is thus largely a function of a well-designed and well-executed measurement process. For this reason, the intent of this book is to provide the reader with a sound background in the theories, principles, and practices of measurement and instrumentation that are germane to the measurement of concepts in nursing and the health professions.

Examples of theory-based measures can be found in Bramadat and Drieger (1993); Kempen, Miedema, Ormel, and Molenar (1996); and Fry (2001).

MEASUREMENT FRAMEWORKS

Just as it is important to identify and employ a conceptual framework for determining what is to be measured and delineating how it will be operationalized, it is important to identify and employ a measurement framework to guide the design and interpretation of the measurement per se. The two major frameworks for measurement are the norm-referenced and the criterion-referenced approaches.

A *norm-referenced approach* is employed when the interest is in evaluating the performance of a subject relative to the performance of other subjects in some well-defined comparison or norm group. The Stress of Discharge Assessment Tool (SDAT-2) developed by Toth (2003, pp. 99–109) is an example of a 60-item, norm-referenced measure of the stress experienced by patients at hospital discharge and in the early recovery period at home following acute myocardial infarction. Scores on each item in the SDAT-2 range from 1 to 5 points, depending on the patient's degree of agreement with the item. A high score indicates high stress for that item, and a low score indicates low stress. The total possible score ranges from 60 to 300 points, and its value for a given subject takes on meaning when it is considered in light of the scores obtained by other patients who responded to the same tool.

Similarly, the results of the application of physiologic measures such as blood pressure readings are often interpreted on the basis of readings (usually ranges of values) considered normal for some well-defined comparison group (e.g., black males over 40 years of age with no significant health problems). It should be noted that the terms "norm-referenced" and "standardized" are not synonymous. Standardized tests are one type of norm-referenced measure; there are other types as well. A *standardized test,* unlike most other norm-referenced measures, is designed by experts for wide use and has prescribed content, well-defined procedures for administration and scoring, and established norms. The Graduate Record Examination (Stein & Green, 1970), the National League for Nursing Achievement Test Battery (Waltz, 1988), and nurse practitioner certification examinations such as the Neonatal Intensive Care Nursing Examination (Perez-Woods, Burns, & Chase, 1989) are examples of standardized measures.

A key feature of a norm-referenced measure is variance. The task when using a norm-referenced measure is to construct a tool or method that measures a specific characteristic in such a way that it maximally discriminates among subjects possessing differing amounts of that characteristic, that is, spreads people out along the possible ranges of scores. For example, if the characteristic to be measured is knowledge of human sexuality content, then test items are designed to differentiate between individuals with varying levels of knowledge of the content. The goal is to obtain scores in such a manner that the result is a few high scores, most scores in the middle range, and a few low scores. If this goal is achieved, the resulting distribution of scores on the measure should look much like a normal curve. Figure 1.1 illustrates the distribution of scores that one would expect to result from the employment of the hypothetical 5-item, norm-referenced measure of human sexuality content.

The sole purpose of a *criterion-referenced measure* is to determine whether or not a subject has acquired a predetermined set of target behaviors. The task in this case is to specify the important target behaviors precisely and to construct a test or measure that discriminates between those subjects who have and those who have not acquired the target behaviors. How well a subject's performance compares with the performance of others is irrelevant when a criterion-referenced framework is employed. Criterion-referenced measures are particularly useful in the clinical area when the concern is with the measurement of process and outcome variables. For example, a criterion-referenced measure of process would require that one identify standards for the patient care intervention and then compare subjects' clinical performance with the standards for performance (i.e., predetermined target behaviors) rather than compare subjects' performance with that of other subjects, all of whom may not meet the standards. Similarly, when a criterion-referenced measure is employed to measure patient outcomes, a given patient's status is determined by comparing his or her performance with a set of predetermined criteria (e.g., ECG normal, diastolic pressure below 80, other vital signs stable for 4 hours post-op) or target behaviors (e.g., requests for pain medication have ceased by 2 days post-op, desire to return to normal activities is verbalized by third day post-op) rather than by comparing his or her performance with that of other patients.

King's (2003, pp. 3–20) Measure of Goal Attainment Tool is an example of a criterion-referenced measure of functional abilities and goal attainment behaviors. This tool was constructed to assess individuals' physical abilities to perform activities of daily living and the behavioral response of individuals to the performance of these activities. Goal attainment was defined as mutual goal setting by nurse and patient, and assessment of goal attainment. Each of these areas comprises three components: (1) personal hygiene, (2) movement, and (3) human interaction. Essential tasks in performing actions related to each of these areas are reflected in items contained on the tool. Percentage scores are determined to evaluate the independence or dependence of subjects related to the essential tasks. Thus, the individual's performance, as reflected by the score, is interpreted on the basis of his or her ability to perform the essential tasks and is not related to the evaluation of the performance of others using the same tool.

One would expect the distribution of scores resulting from a 5-item, criterion-referenced measure to look like the one illustrated in Figure 1.2. It should be noted that not only does the distribution of scores

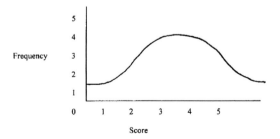

FIGURE 1.1   Normal distribution of scores on a 5-item, norm-referenced test.

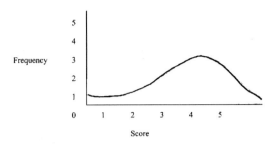

FIGURE 1.2 Skewed distribution of scores on a 5-item, criterion-referenced test.

resulting from a criterion-referenced measure have less variance or spread than that resulting from a norm-referenced measure, but it also is skewed in shape. In a *skewed distribution,* scores tend to cluster at one end of the scale; in the example in Figure 1.2, the high end. A more detailed discussion of score spread (variance) and distribution shape (normal and skewed) is presented in chapter 3.

Because the design, scoring, interpretation, reliability, and validity testing for norm-referenced and criterion-referenced measures differ, it is important to decide which of the two measurement frameworks will be employed prior to the conduct of any other steps in the measurement process.

TYPES OF MEASURES

Once the conceptual basis for the measure and the measurement framework have been determined, attention turns to the selection of the specific type of measure to be employed. Semantics is often a problem for newcomers to the field of measurement. Many different terms are employed to label like measures. For this reason, it is important to consider some of the classification schemes and terms that are used to label the different types of measures.

In addition to being categorized as either norm-referenced or criterion-referenced, approaches to measurement are also usually referred to as qualitative or quantitative in nature. Whether the approach is qualitative, quantitative, or a combination of both will largely be a function of the measurement problem, the conceptual basis guiding the determi-

nation of what is to be measured, and the nature of the variables to be measured.

When a *qualitative* approach to measurement is employed, objects are assigned to mutually exclusive and exhaustive categories that represent the kind of characteristic possessed by the object. Qualitative measurement methods are usually indicated when the theoretical orientation for the measurement derives from phenomenology, existentialism, symbolic interactionism, or ethnomethodology (Chenitz & Swanson, 1986, p. 3). Knafl (1989) suggests that within nursing, ethnography, phenomenology, and grounded theory appear to be the dominant approaches. The major goal of qualitative methods is to document and interpret as fully as possible the whole of what is being measured from the frame of reference of the subjects involved (Filstead, 1974; Duffy, 1987; Diekelman, 1992; Girot, 1993). Hinds and Young (1987) note that qualitative methods usually attempt to describe processes and thus tend to be measures of dynamic and changing phenomena. While the measurement strategies and techniques employed across the qualitative theoretical perspectives may differ somewhat, the types of measures employed are often the same and are also employed when quantitative approaches are used. Qualitative measurement methodologies generally include content analysis of documents; reviews of the literature and of findings from studies to identify common themes; participant and nonparticipant observations; interviews or focus groups that may be structured or nonstructured, but are usually open ended; and open-ended questionnaires. Qualitative data collection and analysis procedures are discussed in chapter 8.

Quantitative measurement assigns objects to categories that represent the amount of a characteristic possessed by the object. Quantitative methods emphasize the search for facts and causes of human behavior through objective, observable, and quantifiable data (Duffy, 1987). Hinds and Young (1987) suggest that quantitative approaches provide outcome data and information on the representativeness of the studied sample and thus tend to be measures of more stable phenomena. Specific types of methods employed with quantitative approaches include the variety of types of measures discussed in later sections of this chapter.

Single studies of a problem using qualitative or quantitative methods rarely involve full exploration of the problem area (Bergstrom, 1989), and together the two approaches to measurement provide information regarding the internal and external validity of the studies or measurement processes (Vedich & Shapiro, 1955; Campbell & Fiske, 1959; Webb, Campbell, Schwartz, & Sechrest, 1966). Thus, to develop an adequate and useful repertoire of measurement principles and practices, one needs to understand when and how to use both qualitative and quantitative approaches to measurement, as well as how they can be combined as measurement methodologies.

Stainbeck and Stainbeck (1984) note that qualitative and quantitative approaches, because they derive from different perspectives, have several inherent differences that should be understood prior to considering how the two methods can complement each other in the measurement of nursing phenomena. Major differences noted by them include the following:

1. When quantitative approaches are employed, the goal is to arrive at an understanding of a phenomenon from the outsider's perspective by maintaining a detached, objective view that hypothetically is unbiased. The perspective, on the other hand, when qualitative approaches are employed is that of an insider and the goal is to obtain information by talking to and/or observing subjects who have experienced firsthand the phenomena under scrutiny.

2. Quantitative methods focus on the accumulation of facts and causes of behavior assuming that facts gathered do not change, while qualitative methods are concerned with the changing, dynamic nature of reality.

3. When quantitative approaches are used, the situation is structured by identifying and isolating specific variables for measurement and by employing specific measurement tools and methods to collect information on these variables. In

contrast, qualitative approaches attempt to gain a complete or holistic view of what is being measured by using a wide array of data including documents, records, photographs, observations, interviews, case histories, and even quantitative data.

4. Usually highly structured procedures, designed to verify or disprove predetermined hypotheses, are employed with quantitative approaches. Flexibility is kept to a minimum in an attempt to minimize bias. Procedures used with qualitative approaches, on the other hand, are usually flexible, exploratory, and discovery oriented.

5. Quantitative approaches yield objective data that are typically expressed in numbers, while qualitative approaches focus on subjective data that are typically expressed or reported through language.

6. Quantitative data are usually collected under controlled conditions, while qualitative data are usually collected within the context of their natural occurrence.

7. In both approaches reliability and validity are valued. In the quantitative approach there is a heavy emphasis on reliability, that is, data that are consistent, stable, and replicable. Qualitative approaches, while recognizing that reliability is a necessary prerequisite for validity, tend to concentrate on validity, that is, data that are representative of a true and full picture of the phenomenon that is investigated (pp. 130–131).

Over time, more researchers have come to value using both approaches and have begun to recognize the value of integrating qualitative and quantitative approaches within the context of a given study. It should be noted that the integration of qualitative and quantitative approaches is not simply mixing methods, but rather requires one to assume that the two approaches are complementary and that the primacy of the paradigmatic assumptions underlying one or the other approach can be eliminated as unproductive (Haase & Myers, 1988). Triangulation, discussed in more detail in chapter 25, is one methodological strategy for combining qualitative and quantitative approaches. In *triangulation,* multiple data sources, collection techniques, theories, and investigators are employed to assess the phenomenon of interest (Madey, 1982; Mitchell, 1986; Fielding & Fielding, 1986). Examples of the use of triangulation for combining qualitative and quantitative approaches can be found in Breitnauer, Ayres, and Knafl (1993), Floyd (1993), Corey (1993), and Mason (1993).

In addition to being categorized as norm-referenced or criterion-referenced, qualitative or quantitative, measuring tools and methods may be classified by (1) what they seek to measure, (2) the manner in which responses are obtained and scored, (3) the type of subject performance they seek to measure, or (4) who constructs them.

What Is Measured

In nursing and the health professions, there is usually interest in measuring cognition, affect, and psychomotor skills and/or physical functioning. *Cognitive* measures assess the subject's knowledge or achievement in a specific content area. Indicators of cognitive behavior usually are obtained as follows:

1. Achievement tests (objective and essay) that measure the extent to which cognitive objectives have been attained.
2. Self-evaluation measures designed to determine subjects' perceptions of the extent to which cognitive objectives have been met.
3. Rating scales and checklists for judging the specific attributes of products produced in conjunction with or as a result of an experience.
4. Sentence-completion exercises designed to categorize the types of responses and enumerate their frequencies relative to specific criteria.
5. Interviews to determine the frequencies and levels of satisfactory responses to formal and informal questions raised in a face-to-face setting.
6. Peer utilization surveys to ascertain the frequency of selection or assignment to leadership or resource roles.
7. Questionnaires employed to determine the frequency of responses to items in an objective format or number of responses to categorized dimensions developed from the content analysis of answers to open-ended questions.
8. Anecdotal records and critical incidents to ascertain the frequency of behaviors judged to be highly desirable or undesirable.
9. Review of records, reports, and other written materials (e.g., articles, autobiographical data, awards, citations, honors) to determine the numbers and types of accomplishments of subjects.

The number of cognitive measures employed far exceed the number of other types of measures. Specifically, written multiple-choice tests are the most often used, perhaps because they are the most objective of the various cognitive measures and the most reliable, and because they have the greatest utility in measuring all types of knowledge. Multiple-choice tests are further discussed in chapters 4 and 17. Examples of cognitive measures can be found in Smith (1991), Grant et al. (1999), Story (2001), and Arnold (2001). It should be noted that cognitive measures are not limited to paper and pencil tests and that a variety of other approaches exist including computer-based testing and simulations that are discussed in chapter 23.

Affective measures seek to determine interests, values, and attitudes. *Interests* are conceptualized as preferences for particular activities. Examples of statements relating to interests are:

- I prefer community-based nursing practice to practice in the hospital setting.
- I like to work with student nurses as they give care to patients.
- I prefer teaching responsibilities to administrative responsibilities.
- I would enjoy having one day a week to devote to giving direct care to patients in addition to my teaching responsibilities.

Values concern preferences for life goals and ways of life, in contrast to interests, which concern preferences for particular activities. Examples of statements relating to values are:

- I consider it important to have people respect nursing as a profession.
- A nurse's duty to her patient comes before duty to the community.
- Service to others is more important to me than personal ambition.
- I would rather be a teacher than an administrator.

Attitudes concern feelings about particular social objects, that is, physical objects, types of people, particular persons, or social institutions. Examples of statements relating to attitudes are:

- Nursing as a profession is a constructive force in determining health policy today.
- Continuing education for nurses should be mandatory for relicensing.
- Humanistic care is a right of all patients.
- All nurses should be patient advocates.

The feature that distinguishes attitudes from interests and values is that attitudes always concern a particular target or object. In contrast, interests and values concern numerous activities: specific activities in measures of interest and very broad categories of activities in measures of value.

It is extremely difficult to preserve the conceptual differences among interests, values, and attitudes when actually constructing measures of affect. Thus, for the purpose of rendering them measurable, they are all subsumed under the rubric of *acquired behavioral dispositions* (Campbell, 1963) and are defined as tendencies to respond in a consistent manner to a certain category of stimuli. For example, when patients are asked to respond to a questionnaire to indicate their satisfaction with the quality of care received, one is interested in measuring their tendency to consistently respond that they are satisfied or dissatisfied, given a set of questions that ask them about the care they received (the stimuli).

Self-report measures are the most direct approach to the determination of affect. In this type of measure subjects are asked directly what their attitudes, interests, or values are. For example, subjects might be given a list of favorable and unfavorable statements regarding antagonistic patients and asked to agree or disagree with each. Such a self-report inventory is referred to as an attitude scale. Other indicators of affective behaviors include, but are not limited to:

1. Sentence-completion exercises designed to obtain ratings of the psychological appropriateness of an individual's responses relative to specific criteria
2. Interviews
3. Questionnaires
4. Semantic differential, Q-sort, and other self-concept perception devices
5. Physiologic measures
6. Projective techniques, for example, role playing or picture interpretation
7. Observational techniques and behavioral tests, including measures of congruence between what is reported and how an individual actually behaves in a specific situation
8. Anecdotal records and critical incidents

From the empirical evidence concerning the validity of different approaches, it appears that self-report offers the most valid approach currently available. For this reason, at present, most measures of affect are based on self-report and usually employ one of two types of scales: a summated rating scale or a semantic differential scale.

A *scale* is a measuring tool or method composed of:

1. A stem, which is a statement relating to attitudes or an attitudinal object to be rated by the respondent
2. A series of scale steps
3. Anchors that define the scale steps

Figure 1.3 presents examples of the components of a scale.

There are different types of anchors that can be employed: numbers, percentages, degrees of agreement/disagreement, adjectives (e.g., worthless/valuable), actual behavior, and

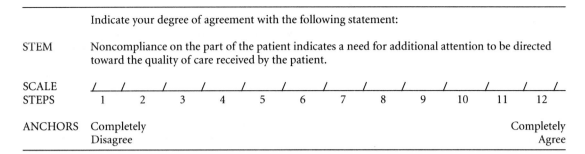

	Indicate your degree of agreement with the following statement:
STEM	Noncompliance on the part of the patient indicates a need for additional attention to be directed toward the quality of care received by the patient.
SCALE STEPS	/ / / / / / / / / / / / 1 2 3 4 5 6 7 8 9 10 11 12
ANCHORS	Completely Disagree ... Completely Agree

FIGURE 1.3   The components of a scale.

products (e.g., samples of nursing care plans to be rated 1 to 6). Usually numerical anchors are preferred because:

1. If the meaning of each step on the scale is specified at the beginning of the rating form, as is usually the case, numbers provide an effective means of coordinating those definitions with rating scales.
2. Numbers on scales constantly remind subjects of the meanings of scale steps.
3. Numbers facilitate the analysis of data, for example, inputting ratings for computer analysis (Nunnally, 1967; Nunnally & Bernstein, 1994).

Summated Rating Scale

A summated rating scale contains a set of scales, all of which are considered approximately equal in attitude or value loading. The subjects respond with varying degrees of intensity on a scale ranging between extremes such as agree/disagree, like/dislike, or accept/reject. The scores of all scales in the set are summed or summed and averaged to yield an individual's attitude score. An example of a summated rating scale is given in Figure 1.4.

Summated rating scales are easy to construct, are usually reliable, and are flexible in that they may be adapted for the measurement of many different kinds of attitudes. Nunnally (1967) and Nunnally and Bernstein (1994) suggest that the reliability of summated scales is a direct function of the number of items. When there are a reasonable number (e.g., 20) items on the scale, fewer scale steps for individual scales are required for a high degree of reliability. When there are fewer items, more scale steps for indi-

vidual scales are required for reliability. In most cases, 10 to 15 items using 5 or 6 steps are sufficient. Individual scales on summated attitude scales tend to correlate substantially with each other, because it is fairly easy for the constructor to devise items that obviously relate to each other and for subjects to see the common core of meaning in the items. Additional information regarding summated attitude scales can be found in Edwards (1957), Shaw and Wright (1967), Nunnally (1967), or Nunnally and Bernstein (1994).

Semantic Differential Scales

The semantic differential is a method for measuring the meaning of concepts that was developed by Osgood, Suci, and Tannenbaum (1957). The semantic differential has three components: (1) the concept to be rated in terms of its attitudinal properties, (2) bipolar adjectives that anchor the scale, and (3) a series of 5 to 9 scale steps (7 is the optimal number of steps suggested). Figure 1.5 presents an example of a semantic differential scale. The concept to be rated in Figure 1.5 is "noncomplying patient." Respondents are instructed to rate the concept according to how they perceive it or feel about it by placing an X along the 7-point scale anchored by the bipolar adjective pairs. The resulting scale response can be converted to numerical values and treated statistically.

Nunnally (1967) and Nunnally and Bernstein (1994) explain that the logic underlying the semantic differential stems from the recognition that, in spoken and written language, characteristics of ideas and objects are communicated largely by adjectives. It is reasonable on this basis to assume that meaning often can be

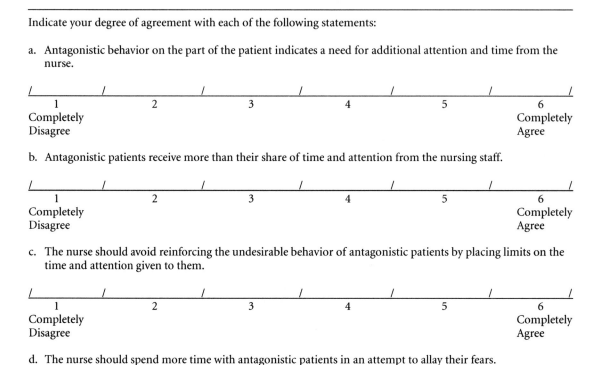

Indicate your degree of agreement with each of the following statements:

a. Antagonistic behavior on the part of the patient indicates a need for additional attention and time from the nurse.

/_____	/_____	/_____	/_____	/_____	/_____	/
1	2	3	4	5	6	
Completely Disagree					Completely Agree	

b. Antagonistic patients receive more than their share of time and attention from the nursing staff.

/_____	/_____	/_____	/_____	/_____	/_____	/
1	2	3	4	5	6	
Completely Disagree					Completely Agree	

c. The nurse should avoid reinforcing the undesirable behavior of antagonistic patients by placing limits on the time and attention given to them.

/_____	/_____	/_____	/_____	/_____	/_____	/
1	2	3	4	5	6	
Completely Disagree					Completely Agree	

d. The nurse should spend more time with antagonistic patients in an attempt to allay their fears.

/_____	/_____	/_____	/_____	/_____	/_____	/
1	2	3	4	5	6	
Completely Disagree					Completely Agree	

FIGURE 1.4   Example of a summated rating scale.

and usually is communicated by adjectives; it is also reasonable to assume that adjectives can be used to measure various facets of meaning. The semantic differential primarily measures connotative aspects of meaning, that is, what implications the object in question has for the respondents. For example, if an individual rating the concept, noncomplying patient, said, "I dislike them very much," this statement would represent a connotation or sentiment for that type of patient. The semantic differential is one of the most valid measures available for assessing the connotative aspects of meaning, particularly the evaluative connotations of objects.

Factor analytic studies of semantic differential scales have suggested that there are three major factors of meaning assessed by such scales: (1) evaluation, (2) potency, and (3) activity. Table 1.1 presents the pairs of adjectives most frequently used to define each of these factors.

Additional information regarding semantic differential scales can be obtained from Osgood, Suci, and Tannenbaum (1957) and Snider and Osgood (1969). In chapters 15 and 16 issues related to the selection and use of two additional types of scales that are being given increased attention by nurses and other health professionals—visual analog and magnitude estimation—are discussed. Affective measures are exemplified in the work of Cousins (1997), Czar and Engler (1997), Adam and Freeman (2001), and Kelly (2001).

Psychomotor measures seek to assess subjects' skill, that is, their ability to perform specific tasks or carry out specific procedures, techniques, and the like. An important consideration in the measurement of psychomotor objectives involves the manner in which the skills and materials or objects to be manipulated or coordinated are specified. Specifically, criteria for the

Rate the following concept in terms of how you feel about it at this point in time:
Noncomplying Patient

/	/	/	/	/	/	/	/
1	2	3	4	5	6	7	
Ineffective						Effective	

/	/	/	/	/	/	/	/
1	2	3	4	5	6	7	
Foolish						Wise	

/	/	/	/	/	/	/	/
1	2	3	4	5	6	7	
Weak						Strong	

/	/	/	/	/	/	/	/
1	2	3	4	5	6	7	
Useless						Useful	

/	/	/	/	/	/	/	/
1	2	3	4	5	6	7	
Bad						Good	

FIGURE 1.5   Example of a semantic differential scale.

successful manipulation of an object must be clearly and unambiguously stated at the time when objectives are made explicit. Task-analysis procedures (Gagne, 1962) are often used to accomplish this.

The most viable approach to the measurement of psychomotor skills at this time is the observation method combined with a performance checklist or rating scale. The observation method always involves some interaction between subject and observer in which the observer has an opportunity to watch the subject perform. Checklists and rating scales are often employed to record in a systematic manner behaviors and events occurring during the observation period. A checklist is most often used to note the presence or absence or the frequency of occurrence of the specified behavior, conditions, characteristics, or events. Rating scales are employed when it is desirable that the observer rate the behavior in terms of points along a continuum. Ratings may occur at predetermined intervals throughout the observation session or at the end of the observation to summarize what occurred during the observation period.

The conceptual definition of the phenomenon to be measured forms the basis for how and where the observation should occur. Qualitative conceptual perspectives generally lead to free and unstructured observations in naturalistic settings, while quantitative conceptualizations more often lead to more structured observations using guidelines and trained observers. The work of Cohn, Matias, Tronick, Connell, and Lyons (1986) provides an example of a study combining both structured, standardized observation methods and naturalistic unstructured observations of depressed mothers and their infants. The reader will find an interesting comparison and contrast between the two approaches for collecting observational data.

Unstructured or *semistructured* observations involve the collection of descriptive information that is generally analyzed in a qualitative manner. When *structured* observation is employed, it is often necessary that the nurse prepare an observation guide to structure the observation and train the observer in its use. This guide increases the probability that the crucial behaviors of concern will be considered, which

TABLE 1.1   Frequently Employed Anchors for Semantic Differential Factors

	Factor		
	Evaluation	**Potency**	**Activity**
BIPOLAR ADJECTIVES	good . . . . bad	strong . . . . .weak	active . . . . .passive
	fair . . . . unfair	large . . . . .small	quick . . . . .slow
	positive. . . . . negative	severe . . . . .lenient	tense . . . . .relaxed
	honest . . . . dishonest	hard . . . . .soft	sharp . . . . .dull
	successful . . . . unsuccessful		
	valuable . . . . worthless		

increases the reliability and validity of the method. When possible, the guide should specify when an observation begins and ends as well as what behaviors are to be observed. Frequently, time is the vehicle for accomplishing this purpose. For example, it might be specified that observation of the nurse's history taking begin when the nurse enters the room and continue for the first 5 minutes of the nurse-patient interaction. Using a more elaborate scheme, observations will begin when the nurse enters the room, and will continue for 2 minutes; then observers will rest for the next 2 minutes, rate for 2 minutes, rest for 2 minutes, and so forth, until the nurse leaves the room and the encounter ends.

No matter how structured the observation or how well trained or competent the observer, observation techniques, in order to be sound, require more than one observer. This provides an estimate of the accuracy or reliability of the observations and provides a basis for determining the degree of confidence to be placed in the data.

Three factors must be considered in the discussion of observational techniques: (1) interaction between respondents and observers, (2) whether or not respondents know they are being observed, and (3) whether or not respondents know when they will be observed. Observation is difficult because watching a situation often changes it so that the observers are no longer certain of what they are observing. This implies that a basic criterion for evaluating studies in which observation is used is the extent to which the situation observed was natural. Observations of a subject's psychomotor

skills should be accomplished with as little effect as possible on the natural situation in which the skills are normally performed. Webb, Campbell, Schwartz, and Sechrest (1966) have published a useful book full of suggestions about how measures can be collected as unobtrusively as possible.

It is necessary to weigh the value of collecting observational data over time as opposed to collecting information at one isolated point in time. Observational data collected at one time are subject to more errors of measurement and, hence, lower reliability and validity than observational data collected at multiple times. When subjects' psychomotor performance is of interest, the concern is usually with how they perform most of the time, or typically; that is, patterns of performance or consistency in performance over time becomes important. When observational data are collected at one point in time, there is greater probability that the results of the measurement will reflect more of the conditions surrounding that isolated point in time than the true abilities of the subjects to perform the tasks or behaviors. Hence, whenever possible, measures of performance should occur at more than one point in time.

Observational techniques may be direct or indirect. In *direct observation* the observer evaluates psychomotor performance by simply watching the subject perform. A limitation of this approach stems from the fact that it is both time-consuming and expensive. It is, however, an excellent technique for the assessment of behavior in conjunction with clinical performance in nursing, especially when the concern is with dynamic or process variables. Similarly, a unique strength of the observation method results from the fact that if the observer wishes to learn how a subject functions under the pressure of supervision, there is no substitute for direct observation that is known and scheduled.

Indirect methods of observation include motion picture, television, videotaping, and other devices for recording subjects' activities. The value of indirect techniques results from the opportunities they afford subjects to become involved in the evaluation of their performance as the recording is viewed jointly by the observer and respondents. Indirect observations are limited in that they are not sensitive to the tone, mood, or affect of the situation. Another limitation is that mechanical devices selectively record depending on their placement—where they are aimed by the operator—and hence, the total situation may be missed. This limitation can be turned into an advantage, however, if multiple devices are used to record all that happens before them. Examples of psychomotor measures can be found in Bujak, McMillan, Dwyer, and Hazleton (1991), DeMattes et al. (1993), Mason and Redeker (1993), Finke et al. (2001), Mims (2001), and Kostopoulos (2001). Observational methods are discussed in more detail in chapter 9.

Physiologic measures seek to quantify the level of functioning of living beings. Indicators of physiologic functioning include but are not limited to:

1. Blood pressure readings
2. Temperature readings
3. Respiratory measures
4. Metabolic readings
5. Diabetic and other screening devices
6. Readings from cardiac and other monitoring instruments
7. ECG and EEG readings
8. Results of blood tests and analyses
9. Measures of height and weight

Physical functioning can often be measured by a scientific instrument, and the results of physiologic measures usually are expressed as a quantitative scale that can be graded into finely distinguished numerical values. For example, the variable diastolic blood pressure is measured using a scientific instrument referred to as a sphygmomanometer. Its scale is in a quantitative form ranging from 0 to 300, providing a total of 300 different continuous scale points or values to which a subject can be assigned and which differentiate among the various degrees of the variable possessed by the subjects measured. Thus, on the basis of blood pressure readings, one can state that a subject with a diastolic pressure of 100 is 20 points higher than one with a diastolic pressure of 80. This 20-point difference is significant in comparing the physical status of two patients.

Well-designed and implemented physiologic measures are among the most precise methods one can employ; they yield data measured at the interval or ratio level of measurement, allow a wide range of statistical procedures to be employed in their analysis, and tend to produce results that demonstrate a high degree of reliability and validity. Examples of physiologic measures can be found in Heidenreich and Giuffre (1990), and Bridges and Woods (1993). The physiologic approach to measurement is discussed in detail in chapter 18.

How Responses are Obtained and Scored

The distinction to be considered is whether a measure is objective or subjective. It should be noted that a given method or technique is generally viewed as more or less objective or subjective; that is, one may think in terms of a continuum anchored by the terms objective and subjective, and then place a given method on the continuum, depending on whether it possesses characteristics more like those of an objective or subjective measure.

Objective measures contain items that allow subjects little if any latitude in constructing their responses and spell out criteria for scoring so clearly that scores can be assigned either by individuals who know nothing of the content or by mechanical means. Multiple-choice questions and physiologic measures are examples of the most objective methods that can be employed.

Subjective measures allow respondents considerable latitude in constructing their responses. In addition, the probability that different scorers may apply different criteria is greater. Examples of subjective measures are the essay test, open-ended interview questions, case studies, and nursing care plans. The *essay* question is a method requiring a response constructed by the subject, usually in the form of one or more sentences. The nature of the response is such that (1) no single answer or pattern of answers can be listed as correct, and (2) the quality of the response can be judged only subjectively by one skilled or informed in the subject (Stalnaker, 1951). Thus, significant features of the essay method are (1) the freedom of response allowed the respondents, (2) the fact that no single answer can be identified as correct or complete, and (3) responses must be scored by experts who themselves usually cannot classify a response as categorically right or wrong. Essay questions may require subjects to express their own thoughts on an issue of interest to the profession, outline a research design for investigating a research question, derive a mathematical proof, or explain the nature of some nursing phenomenon. Items may require only a brief response or may demand an extensive exposition.

Advocates of the essay approach argue that an important characteristic of individuals is their ability to interact effectively with other individuals in the realm of ideas. The basic tool of interaction is language, and successful individuals are those who can react appropriately to questions or problems in their field as they encounter them. It is not enough, they contend, to be able to recognize a correct fact when it is presented or to discriminate among alternatives posed by others. Successful individuals are the masters of their collection of ideas and are able to cite evidence to support a position and contribute to the advancement of ideas and constructs within their field. The only way to assess the extent to which individuals have mastered a field is to present them with questions or problems in the field and assess how they perform. Hence, they argue, the essay format provides an avenue for assessing scholarly and/or professional performances better than other available methods (Coffman, 1971).

Even so, because of their subjective nature, essay questions have inherent limitations that must be recognized and minimized if sound measurement is to result from their use. The limitations of essays and other subjective measures fall into two general categories: (1) problems related to the difficulty in achieving consistency in scoring responses and (2) problems associated with the sampling of content. Empirical evidence regarding the reliability of subjective measures suggests that different raters tend to assign different scores to the same response, a single rater tends to assign different scores to the same response on different occasions, and the differences tend to increase as the measure permits greater freedom of response (Hartog & Rhodes, 1936; Finlayson, 1951; Vernon & Millican, 1954; Pearson, 1955; Noyes, 1963). Different raters may differ as a result of a number of factors including the severity of their standards, the extent to which they distribute scores throughout the score scale, and real differences in the criteria they are applying.

Basic to problems associated with the sampling of content is the notion that each sample unit should be independent and equally likely to be chosen in the sample. In general, the greater the number of different questions, the higher the reliability of the score. The compromise to be made, however, is between the desire to increase the adequacy of the sample of content by asking many different questions and the desire to ask questions that probe deeply the subjects' understanding. Additional information regarding essay items is presented in Stalnaker (1951) and Coffman (1971). Other subjective measures are described in more detail in part III.

Type of Performance Measured

When performance is of interest, one may seek to measure typical performance or maximum performance. If the interest is in assessing subjects as they do their best (produce their highest quality work), then a *maximum performance* measure is appropriate. Such measures are indices of cognition that generally measure a set of skills a subject possesses but that differ among themselves in the specificity of their focus and the use to which scores are put. Maximum performance measures of particular interest include aptitude measures, achievement measures, and diagnostic measures.

Aptitude tests are specific measures of capacity for success and tend to focus on various general aspects of human ability (e.g., mechanical aptitude, artistic aptitude). They are often used as predictors of performance in special fields.

Achievement measures are tests of particular skills and knowledge and are more specific than aptitude tests. They usually sample a wide range of skills and are constructed by nurses and other health professionals for their own use. Commercially produced achievement measures are also available in many different content areas.

Diagnostic tests are even more specific in their focus than achievement measures, although this need not always be the case. They focus on specific skills and often employ multiple measures of particular skills. Their intent is to pinpoint specific weaknesses that might not be apparent otherwise. Once specific deficiencies are identified and remediation has taken place, one might predict that achievement, which is assumed to be dependent on these more specific skills, will improve.

If information about subjects' typical behavior (i.e., what they usually do or would do) is of interest, it is appropriate to use a *typical performance* measure. These are measures of affective behavior and usually attempt to have respondents describe the way they typically perceive themselves or their behavior. Typical performance measures usually ask the subjects for scaled responses, forced-choice responses, or criterion-keyed responses. Figure 1.6 presents examples of each of these types of responses.

Who Constructs Measures

Standardized measures are developed by specialists for wide use. Their content is set, the directions for administration (often including time limits) are clearly described, and the scoring procedure to be used is completely prescribed. Information on norms concerning scores is generally available. Examples of standardized measures employed to assess the outcomes of nursing education programs are presented in *Educational Outcomes: Assessment of Quality—A Prototype for Student Outcome Measurement in Nursing Programs* (Waltz, 1988). In chapter 7, standardized approaches to measurement are discussed in detail.

Informal tools and methods are typically constructed by nurses and other health professionals for their own use. They are not content constrained; that is, the user is free to define the content as well as administration procedures and scoring. Norms may be available for local groups but more often are not available for any group.

In summary, the measurement framework employed in a given situation will have important implications for instrument development and for what can be done with and on the basis of the resulting information. Thus, it is important to clarify at the outset the type of measurement that will yield data appropriate for the types of questions and/or hypotheses one seeks to answer. In chapters 2 through 23 attention will be focused on instrument development and testing in both the norm-referenced and criterion-referenced cases. In chapters 24 and 25 measurement issues and important considerations to be made in using the types of measures presented in this section will be addressed, and in the appendices a variety of available measurement resources will be presented.

RELIABILITY AND VALIDITY OF MEASURES

As indicated in the foregoing sections reliability and validity are essential characteristics of any measuring tool or method. Factors that may affect the degree of consistency obtained for a given measure (reliability) are: (1) the manner in which the measure is scored; (2) characteristics of the measure itself; (3) the physical and/or emotional state of the individual at measurement time; and (4) properties of the situation in which the measure is administered (e.g., the amount of noise, lighting conditions, temperature of the room).

Strictly speaking, one validates not the measurement tool or method but rather some use to which the measure is put. For example, an instrument designed to select participants who would benefit from a primary care fellowship experience must be valid for that purpose, but it would not necessarily be valid for other purposes such as measuring how well participants

Scaled response

In a scaled response situation, the respondent indicates on a scale what his/her rating or answer is to the question posed. An example is the item:

Did this course provide information that will be meaningful to you in your clinical work?
Please rate.

not at all	very little	somewhat	enough	very much
1	2	3	4	5

Forced-choice response

With a forced-choice response item, the respondent is asked to choose between two or three different alternatives, all of which may be appealing responses. The point is that one particular response is most appealing to the subject. An example of this type of item is:

A program of ongoing evaluation of patient care does not exist in the agency with which you are affiliated. You are aware of a need to evaluate the various approaches to patient care management. You would prefer to have this need met by:

1. Referring the task to someone else.
2. Supporting the activities of the professional nursing organizations that are seeking to stimulate interest and involvement in evaluation of patient care.
3. Supporting a policy change in the agency responsible for care.
4. Acting as a resource person to staff by providing them with knowledge and materials to enable them to develop such a program.
5. Becoming a member of a committee of practitioners who are developing and testing a pilot program of evaluation in conjunction with the patients for whom they deliver care.
6. Initiating the idea of such a program by providing care to a small group of clients and sharing with staff your evaluation of the various approaches you use.

Criterion-keyed response

Criterion-keyed responses depend on information previously obtained about how certain groups answered the items. If a present respondent's score looks like those from members of a certain predefined group, then he/she is classified as a member of that group. Criterion keying assumes that the criterion for membership in a particular group is having a set of responses on the measurement instrument that looks like those from the predefined group.

Example: The Minnesota Multiphasic Personality Inventory (MMPI) was originally used with hospitalized psychiatric patients and normal (i.e., nonhospitalized respondents) to construct a criterion-keyed set of questions which had some value as predictors of mental stability, that is, if a particular item was responded to differently by the two groups, it was included in the test.

FIGURE 1.6   Sample responses of typical performance measures.

master objectives at the completion of the fellowship experience.

Both reliability and validity are matters of degree rather than all-or-none properties. Measures should be assessed each time they are used to see if they are behaving as planned. New evidence may suggest modifications in an existing measure or the development of a new and better approach to measuring the attribute in question. Reliability is a necessary prerequisite for validity; that is, if a measure does not assign scores consistently, it cannot be useful for the purpose for which it is intended. Reliability is not, however, a sufficient condition for validity; that is, because a measure consistently measures

a phenomenon does not ensure that it measures the phenomenon of interest.

As stated earlier, the determination of the reliability and validity of a specific tool or method will differ depending on whether it is norm-referenced or criterion-referenced. Specific techniques for determining reliability and validity in each case are discussed in chapters 5 and 6. In either case, the reliability and validity of the measurement process itself is increased when multiple measures of the same thing are employed; that is, more than one type of instrumentation is used to answer a given question. Similarly, reliability and validity increase when the answer to a given measurement concern is elicited by collecting data from a number of difference sources using the same measurement tool or method.

REFERENCES

Adam, P. F., & Freeman, L. H. (2001). Assertive behavior inventory tools. In C. F. Waltz & L. S. Jenkins (Eds.), *Measurement of nursing outcomes* (2nd ed.), (Vol. 1, pp. 245–250). New York: Springer Publishing.

Allegood, M. R., & Marriner-Tomey, A. (1997). *Nursing theory: Utilization and application.* St. Louis: Mosby, Inc.

Arnold, J. M. (2001). Diagnostic reasoning simulations and instruments. In C. F. Waltz & L. S. Jenkins (Eds.), *Measurement of nursing outcomes* (2nd ed.), (Vol. 1, pp. 3–21). New York: Springer Publishing.

Bergstrom, N. (1989, April, 28–30). Nursing diagnosis research: Inductive and deductive approaches. In *Proceedings of Invitational Conference on Research Methods for Validating Nursing Diagnosis.* Cosponsored by the North American Nursing Diagnosis Association and Case Western University, Palm Springs, CA.

Bramadat, I. J., & Driedger, M. (1993). Satisfaction with childbirth: Theories and methods of measurement. *Birth: Issues in Prenatal Care and Education, 20*(1), 22–29.

Breitnauer, B. J., Ayres, L., & Knafl, K. A. (1993). Triangulation in qualitative research: Evaluation of completeness and confirmation purposes. *Image: Journal of Nursing Scholarship, 25*(3), 237–243.

Bridges, E. J., & Woods, S. L. (1993). Pulmonary artery pressure measurement: State of the art. *Heart and Lung: Journal of Critical Care, 22*(2), 99–111.

Broome, M. E., & Mobley, T. (2003). The child medical fears scale. In O. L. Strickland & C. DiIorio (Eds.), *Measurement of nursing outcomes* (2nd ed.), (Vol. 2, pp. 196–206). New York: Springer Publishing.

Bujak, L., McMillan, M., Dwyer, J., & Hazelton, M. (1991). Assessing comprehensive nursing performance: The objective structural clinical assessment. *Nurse Education Today, 11*(3), 179–184.

Campbell, D. T. (1963). Social attitudes and other acquired behavioral dispositions. In S. Koch (Ed.), *Psychology: A study of a science* (Vol. 6, pp. 94–172). New York: McGraw-Hill.

Campbell, D. T., & Fiske, D. W. (1959). Convergent and discriminant validation by the multitrait-multimethod matrix. *Psychological Bulletin, 56*(2), 81–105.

Chenitz, W. C., & Swanson, J. M. (1986). *From practice to groundel theory: Qualitative research in nursing.* Menlo Park, CA: Addison-Wesley.

Coffman, E. E. (1971). Essay examinations. In R. L. Thorndike (Ed.), *Educational measurement* (pp. 271–302). Washington, DC: American Council on Education.

Cohn, J. F., Matias, R., Tronick, E. Z., Cornell, D., & Lyons, R. K. (1986). Face-to-face interactions of depressed mothers and their infants. In E. Z. Tronick & T. Fields (Eds.), *New Directions for Child Development, 34,* 31–45.

Corey, J. W. (1993). Linking qualitative and quantitative methods: Integrating cultural factors into public health. *Qualitative Health Research, 3*(3), 298–318.

Cousins, S. O. (1997). Validity and reliability of self-reported health of persons aged 70 and older. *Health Care for Women International, 18*(2), 165–174.

Czar, M. L., & Engler, M. M. (1997). Perceived learning needs of patients with coronary artery disease using a questionnaire assessment tool. *Heart & Lung, 26*(2), 109–117.

DeMattes, O., Law, M., Russell, D., Pollock, N., Rosenbaum, P., & Walter, S. (1993). The reliability and validity of the quality of upper extremity skills test. *Physical and Occupational Therapy in Pediatrics, 13*(2), 1–18.

Diekelmann, N. L. (1992). Learning as listening: A Heideggerian hermeneutical analysis of the lived experiences of students and teachers in nursing. *Advances in Nursing Science, 14*(3), 72–83.

Duffy, M. E. (1987). Methodological triangulation: A vehicle for merging quantitative and qualitative research methods. *Image: Journal of Nursing Scholarship, 19*(3), 130–133.

Edwards, A. (1957). *Techniques of attitude scale construction.* New York: Appleton-Century-Crofts.

Fielding, N., & Fielding, J. (1986). *Linking data: Qualitative research methods, series 4.* Beverly Hills, CA: Sage.

Filstead, W. J. (1974). *Qualitative methodology: First-hand involvement with the social world.* Chicago: Markham.

Finke, L., Messmer, P., Spruck, M., Gilman, B., Weiner, E., & Emerson, L. A. (2001). Measuring RN students' clinical skills via computer. In C. F. Waltz & L. S. Jenkins (Eds.), *Measurement of nursing outcomes* (2nd ed.), (Vol. 1, pp. 194–198). New York: Springer Publishing.

Finlayson, D. S. (1951). The reliability of the marking of essays. *British Journal of Educational Psychology, 21,* 126–134.

Floyd, J. R. (1993). The use of across-method triangulation in the study of sleep concerns in healthy older adults. *Advances in Nursing Science, 16* (2), 70–80.

Fry, S. T. (2001). Justification of moral judgment and action tool. In C. F. Waltz & L. S. Jenkins (Eds.), *Measurement of nursing outcomes* (2nd ed.), (Vol. 1, pp. 276–281). New York: Springer Publishing.

Gagne, R. M. (1962). The acquisition of knowledge. *Psychological Review, 69,* 255–476.

George, J. B. (2002). *Nursing theories* (5th ed.). Upper Saddle River, NJ: Prentice Hall.

Girot, E. A. (1993). Assessment of competence in clinical practice: A phenomenological approach. *Journal of Advanced Nursing, 18*(1), 114–119.

Glaser, B. G., & Strauss, A.L. (1967). *The discovery of groundel theory.* Chicago: Aldine Publishing.

Grant, E., Turner, K., Daugherty, S., Li, T., Eckenfels, E., Baier, C., et al. (1999). Development of a survey of asthma knowledge, attitudes, and perceptions: The Chicago Community Asthma Survey. *Chest, 116*(4), 178–183.

Haase, J. E., & Myers, S. T. (1988). Reconciling paradigm assumptions of qualitative and quantitative research. *Western Journal of Nursing Research, 10*(2), 128–137.

Hartog, P., & Rhodes, E. C. (1936). *The marks of examiners.* New York: Macmillan.

Heidenreich, I., & Giuffre, M. (1990). Postoperative temperature measurement. *Nursing Research, 39*(3), 154–155.

Hinds, P. S., & Young, K. J. (1987). A triangulation of methods and paradigms to study nurse-given wellness care. *Nursing Research, 36*(3), 195–198.

Kelly, K. (2001). Nursing activity scale. In C. F. Waltz & L. S. Jenkins (Eds.), *Measurement of nursing outcomes* (2nd ed.), (Vol. 1, pp. 253–266). New York: Springer Publishing.

Kempen, G., Miedema, I., Ormel, J., & Molenar, W. (1996). The assessment of disability with the Gronigen Activity Restriction Scale: Conceptual framework and psychometric properties. *Social Science and Medicine, 43*(11), 1601–1610.

Kerlinger, F. N. (1973). *Foundations of behavioral research* (2nd ed.). New York: Holt, Rinehart & Winston.

King, I. M. (2003). Assessment of functional abilities and goal attainment scales: A criterion-referenced measure. In O. L. Strickland & C. Dilorio (Eds.), *Measurement of nursing outcomes* (2nd ed.), (Vol 2. pp. 3–20). New York: Springer Publishing.

Knafl, K. A. (1989). Concept development. In *Proceedings of Invitational Conference on Research Methods for Validating Nursing Diagnosis.* Palm Springs, CA: North American Nursing Diagnosis Association and Case Western University.

Kostopoulos, M. R. (2001). Performance appraisal tool. In C. F. Waltz & L. S. Jenkins (Eds.), *Measurement of nursing outcomes* (2nd ed.), (Vol. 1, pp. 79–91). New York: Springer Publishing.

Leonard, M. K., & George, J. B. (1995). In J. B. George (Ed.), *Nursing theories: The base for professional nursing practice* (4th ed., pp. 145–164). East Norwalk, CT: Appleton & Lange.

LoBiondo-Wood, G., & Haber, J. (1994). *Nursing research methods, critical appraisal, and utilization* (3rd ed.). St. Louis: CV Mosby.

Madey, D. L. (1982). Benefits of qualitative and quantitative methods in program evaluation, with illustrations. *Educational Evaluation and Policy Analysis,* (4), 223–236.

Mason, D. J., & Redeker, N. (1993). Measurement of activity. *Nursing Research, 42*(2), 87–92.

Mason, S. A. (1993). Employing quantitative and qualitative methods in one study. *British Journal of Nursing, 2*(17), 869–872.

Meleis, A. I. (1997). *Theoretical nursing: Development and progress* (3rd ed.). New York: J.B. Lippincott.

Mims, B. C. (2001). Clinical performance examination for critical care nurses. In C. F. Waltz & L. S. Jenkins (Eds.), *Measurement of nursing outcomes* (2nd ed.), (Vol. 1, pp. 102–111). New York: Springer Publishing.

Mitchell, E. S. (1986). Multiple triangulation: A methodology for nursing science. *Advances in Nursing Science, 8*(3), 10–26.

Noyes, E. S. (1963). Essay and objective tests in English. *College Board Review, 49,* 7–10.

Nunnally, J. C. (1967). *Psychometric theory.* New York: McGraw-Hill.

Nunnally, J. C., & Bernstein, I. H. (1994). *Psychometric theory* (3rd ed.). New York: McGraw-Hill.

Orem, D. E. (1995). *Nursing concepts of practice* (5th ed.). St. Louis: Mosby Year Books.

Osgood, C. E., Suci, G. J., & Tannenbaum, P. H. (1957). *The measurement of meaning.* Chicago: University of Illinois Press.

Pearson, R. (1955). The test fails as an entrance examination. In Should the general composition test be continued? *College Board Review, 25,* 209.

Perez-Woods, R. C., Burns, B., & Chase, C. I. (1989). The anatomy of NCC certification examinations: The Neonatal Intensive Care Nursing Examination. *Neonatal Network Journal of Neonatal Nursing, 7*(6), 53–59.

Renpenning, K. M., & Taylor, S. G. (Eds.) (2003). *Self-care theory in nursing: Selected papers of Dorothea Orem.* New York: Springer Publishing.

Shaw, R. E., & Wright, J. M. (1967). *Scales for the measurement of attitudes.* New York: McGraw-Hill.

Smith, M. M. (1991). Coronary Heart Disease Knowledge Test: Developing a valid and reliable tool. *Nurse Practitioner: American Journal of Primary Health Care, 16*(4), 28, 31, 35–36.

Snider, J. G., & Osgood, C. E. (Eds.). (1969). *Semantic differential technique.* Chicago: Aldine Publishing.

Stainbeck, S., & Stainbeck, N. (1984). Broadening the research perspective in education. *Exceptional Children, 50,* 400–408.

Stalnaker, J. M. (1951). The essay type of examination. In E. F. Lindquist (Ed.), *Educational measurement* (pp. 495–530). Washington, DC: American Council on Education.

Stein, R. F., & Green, E. J. (1970). The Graduate Record Examination as a predictive potential in the nursing major. *Nursing Research, 19*(1), 42–47.

Story, D. K. (2001). Measuring clinical decision making using a clinical simulation film. In C. F. Waltz & L. S. Jenkins (Eds.), *Measurement of nursing outcomes* (2nd ed.), (Vol. 1, pp. 102–111). New York: Springer Publishing.

Toth, J. C. (2003). Measuring stress after acute myocardial infarction: The stress of discharge assessment tool, Version Two (SDAT-2). In O. L. Strickland & C. Dilorio (Eds.), *Measurement of nursing outcomes* (2nd ed.), (Vol 2, pp. 99–109). New York: Springer Publishing.

Vedich, A. J., & Shapiro, F. (1955). A comparison of participant observation and survey data. *American Sociological Review, 20,* 28–33.

Vernon, P. E., & Millican, G. D. (1954). A further study of the reliability of English essays. *British Journal of Statistical Psychology, 7,* 65–74.

Waltz, C. F. (1988). *Educational outcomes: Assessment of quality—A prototype for student outcome measurement in nursing programs.* New York: National League for Nursing Publications.

Webb, E. E., Campbell, D. T., Schwartz, R. D., & Sechrest, L. (1966). *Unobtrusive measures: Nonreactive research in the social sciences.* Chicago: Rand McNally.

2

Operationalizing Nursing Concepts

Concepts are the basic building blocks of nursing knowledge, thought, and communication. In recent years, many books and articles have described approaches that can be used in analyzing and developing concepts, and have provided examples of concept analyses. These applications have called attention to the importance of a conceptual approach to measurement.

Concepts that are commonly used in nursing research and practice differ considerably in their level of maturity or clarity. According to Morse, Hupcey, Mitcham, and Lenz (1996), a mature concept is clearly defined, and has distinct characteristics and defined boundaries, so it is ready to be operationalized. On the other hand, concepts that have multiple meanings, even within a discipline, or whose meanings and boundaries are vague or variable, need further development before they can be operationalized effectively for research purposes. For example, following an analysis of the concept of trust in discipline-specific literature, Hupcey, Penrod, Morse, and Mitcham (2001) determined that the concept was immature. They identified commonalities and structural features of trust as used in the literature of several disciplines, and also identified areas in which the meaning remains unclear and needs further research and refinement. In a review of measures of the concept of health in 17 nursing studies, Reynolds (1988) found that although health was believed to hold a central position of importance, there was little agreement on its meaning. Even for a concept as prevalent and central as health, there is a need to continue to evaluate and strengthen the links between accumulated knowledge and observation. This chapter provides an orientation to concepts as a basis for measurement, and presents strategies for defining and operationalizing them.

TERMINOLOGY

A concept is a word or term that symbolizes aspects of reality that can be thought about and communicated to others. It denotes a notion or idea by naming it. Often such notions are formed from particular observations or sensory experiences, but may be constructed on the basis of more abstract experiences, such as listening or reading. The concept name is used to denote phenomena (objects, attributes, characteristics, or events) that share a combination of similar properties or characteristics that set them apart from other phenomena that do not share the properties. The concept "dog" denotes a class of animals that share certain characteristics which, when taken together, are different from those of other classes of animals. Because a concept is a symbol, it is an abstraction from observable reality and a kind of shorthand device for labeling ideas. Therefore, concepts serve as a language link between abstract thought and sensory experience.

It is often said that concepts are the basic elements, or building blocks, of scientific theories. Theories are interrelated sets of propositions or statements that provide the basis for describing, explaining, predicting, and/or controlling phenomena. Propositions, in turn, are statements that include and specify the relationship(s) between two or more concepts. A theory generally contains many concepts. A conceptual framework (or conceptual model) also contains a number of concepts. In a conceptual framework concepts are identified, defined, and linked by broad generalizations. A conceptual framework provides an orienting scheme or worldview that helps focus thinking and may provide direction for the development of specific theories (Fawcett, 1984). In short, concepts provide the basis for building the complex statements and theories that form the subject matter for the discipline.

A distinction is generally made between concepts, which are abstract, and those attributes, properties, behaviors, or objects that are perceptually accessible, directly or indirectly, through the senses. The latter are often termed "observables," even though they may not be directly observed in the ordinary sense of the word. The color of a patient's skin or the odor of discharge from a wound can be sensed directly. Such directly observable properties (e.g., color, odor) often are used to indicate more complex concepts, such as infection. Some properties of individuals require amplification or transformation devices to be made observable. For example, cardiac arrhythmias are observed indirectly through an electrocardiograph. Advances in the use of electronic data gathering devices that are easy to use in a variety of settings have increased their use in nursing research (Scisney-Matlock et al., 2000).

Observable attributes or characteristics associated with a given concept are often termed indicators of the concept, or its empirical referents. Redness and swelling are indicators of an infection. Other indicators would include pain/discomfort, increased temperature, and increased white cell count. A given observable may be an indicator for more than one concept. For example, shortness of breath could be an indicator of cardiac insufficiency, dyspnea, or anxiety. An infant's cry can be an indicator of pain, hunger, or boredom.

Behavioral concepts tend to be relatively abstract; however, they can be indicated by behaviors that can be observed. For example, the behaviors that are displayed by mother and infant before an observer can be used to indicate parenting skill. Some behaviors and characteristics are observed indirectly through responses to questions. For example, a client can report the frequency with which he or she contacted a helpline (an indicator of help-seeking), or responses to questions can be used to observe the client's level of satisfaction with a health care provider, or the likelihood of engaging in a particular risky behavior (an indicator of risk-taking).

Operationalization is the process of delineating how a concept will be measured. It involves making a concept explicit in terms of the observable indicators associated with it and/or the operations that must be carried out in order to measure it. The process of operationalization involves a mode of thinking that proceeds from the abstract to the concrete. One moves from a relatively abstract idea (the concept) to identifying the dimensions of its meaning or its attributes, the concrete observables associated with those meaning dimensions or attributes, and the way in which those observables will be measured. It is important to note that operationalization is not an arbitrary process. The operational indicators for a given concept are specified based on theoretical and empirically observed regularities. The process of operationalization will be described in greater detail in later sections of this chapter.

The term operationalization is most often used in conjunction with research. It is also an inherent part of nursing practice. If a nursing note in a patient's record states that the patient seemed anxious about his upcoming surgery because he was restless, unable to sleep, and complained about diarrhea, the nurse who wrote the note actually operationalized the concept of anxiety by suggesting several observable indicators of the condition.

Careful operationalization of concepts is an essential step in nursing research, particularly research using quantitative methods. Given a problem or question to be investigated or a theory to be tested, the researcher must identify the key ideas or concepts involved, and define and operationalize each of them before the study can be carried out. Other nursing activities require precise operationalization of concepts as well. For example, in order to develop a nursing care plan the nurse must decide what needs to be known about the patient and which observations must be made to yield the information. Specifying the observations that must be made in order to assess the functional health status of a patient with chronic obstructive pulmonary disease is an example of operationalizing that concept (Leidy, 1999). In order to render nursing assessment precise and ensure that other nurses will base their judgments on the same kinds of observations, various checklists, protocols, or guidelines may be developed. All such devices incorporate the operationalization of concepts. Other examples of activities that require precise operationalization of relatively complex concepts include evaluating the quality of nursing care, identifying patient outcomes to judge the effectiveness of a given intervention (e.g., Maas, Johnson, & Moorhead, 1996), and assessing student or employee performance in the clinical setting.

NURSING CONCEPTS

Nursing has key concepts that designate its essential subject matter. Some represent ideas that are vital to the thought and language of all nurses, regardless of the settings and specialties in which they practice. It must be noted that even though these concepts may be claimed by nursing and used frequently in nursing research and practice, the same terms may be important in other disciplines as well.

Among the concepts that are considered central to nursing and are important in all subspecialty areas are person, health, nursing, environment, care or caring, patient safety, and interaction. Other concepts represent narrower domains of knowledge, because they are of concern primarily to specific subgroups within the profession. For example, the concept "mother-infant attachment" is of interest primarily to nurses working with infants and young families, and the concept "dyspnea" is of primary interest to nurses working with cardiac or pulmonary patients. There need not be agreement that a given concept is important to nursing knowledge; however, specific concepts that emerge as most important for building nursing knowledge will generate cumulative knowledge building by clusters of researchers.

There is considerable variation among nursing concepts, since they represent a wide range of phenomena that are of interest to the profession. Some represent animate or inanimate objects (e.g., patient, crutch, needle, endorphins), whereas others represent attributes or characteristics of objects or persons (e.g., size, color, intelligence, attitudes). Some nursing concepts represent either relatively static characteristics (e.g., socio-economic status) or those that may vary considerably over time (e.g., job satisfaction, hope) but can be measured by taking a "snapshot" at a given point in time. Others represent dynamic processes that, by definition, unfold over time (e.g., socialization, interaction) and are difficult to characterize using a snapshot approach. Some concepts can be viewed both as static and dynamic; social support, for example. It can be viewed either as a commodity that is given and received and can be described at a particular point in time, or it can be viewed as an ongoing process of social interaction. Whereas some concepts refer to individuals or their properties, others represent relations between and among individuals, (e.g., subordination, exchange) or properties of collective units such as families, groups, or communities (e.g., structure, pattern). Often, individual-level concepts such as health are applied to aggregates (e.g., families, organizations, or communities). Such extension requires making some important conceptual decisions about the nature of both the property or entity and the aggregate to which it is being applied.

Table 2.1 contains examples of some concepts used in nursing research projects and specifies the ways in which each was operationalized. This table reveals that nursing concepts differ in several respects. First, they differ in their complexity; that is, the number of observable properties, characteristics, or behaviors designated by the concept name. Although the concept "perfusion" is relatively straightforward and is designated by one observable property (partial pressure of transcutaneous O_2), others such as functional health status are highly complex, in that they encompass a large number of characteristics (or behaviors) and their meanings have several dimensions. Functional health status is a very encompassing construct, of which functional performance is one dimension (Leidy, 1999); both the inclusive concept and the subconcept are measured with multi-item scales.

In general, the more complex the concept, the more difficult it is to specify its meaning, the less likely it is to be defined identically by everyone using it, and the more complex its

TABLE 2.1   Concepts and Indicators From Reports of Nursing Research

Concept	Operational Indicator(s)
Pain	Score on a Visual Analog Scale (a horizontal 100-mm line with anchors representing sensory extremes)[1]
Functional performance	Score on the Functional Performance Inventory (a 65-item scale with 6 subscales; subscale and total scores are generated)[2]
Functional health status	Score on the Inventory of Functional Status in the elderly (a 46-item self-report measure) and the Sickness Impact Profile[3]
Treatment seeking	Time in hours from onset of symptoms for the acute event to the time of admission to the emergency department (self-reported symptom onset time compared with ED admission time)[4]
Infant health	Number and length of hospitalizations, number and diagnoses of illness episodes, and number of emergency room visits in the 24 months following birth[5]
Asthma medication adherence	Number of daily uses of medication canister as measured by electronic Doser CT (a device secured to top of the medication canister that records number of puffs taken each day of use; adjusted doser data were used to control for excess usage)[6]
Perfusion	Partial pressure of transcutaneous oxygen as measured with a Novametrix 840 PrO$_2$ monitor[7]
Mother-infant interaction quality	Scores on the Nursing Child Assessment Teaching Scale (NCAT) and Mother Infant Communication Screening Scale[8]
Nurse staffing	RN proportion or skill mix: #RN hours/#all hours, where RN hours is the number of productive hours worked by RNs per patient day and all hours is the total number of productive hours worked by all nursing personnel per patient day[9]

[1]Adachi, D., Shimoda, A., & Usui, A. (2003). The relationship between parturient's position and perception of labor pain intensity. *Nursing Research, 52,* 47–57.

[2]Leidy, N. K. (1999). Psychometric properties of the Functional Performance Inventory in patients with chronic obstructive pulmonary disease. *Nursing Research, 48,* 20–28.

[3]DiMattio, M. J., & Tulman, L. (2003). A longitudinal study of functional status and correlates following coronary artery bypass graft surgery in women. *Nursing Research, 52,* 98–107.

[4]Zerwic, J. J., Ryan, C. J., deVon, H. A., & Drell, M. J. (2003) Treatment seeking for acute myocardial infarctions symptoms. *Nursing Research, 52,* 159–167.

[5]Koniak-Griffin, D., Verzemnieks, I. L., Anderson, N. L. R., Brecht, M-L, Lesser, J., Kim, S., & Turner-Pluta, C. (2003). Nurse visitation for adolescent mothers. *Nursing Research, 52,* 127–136.

[6]Bender, B., Wamboldt, F. S., O'Connor, S. L., Rand, C., Szefler, S., Milgrom, H., & Wamboldt, M. Z. (2000). Measurement of children's asthma medication adherence by self report, mother report, canister weight and Doser CT. *Annals of Allergy, Asthma & Immunology, 85,* 416–421.

[7]Wipke-Tervis, D. D., Stotts, N. A., Williams, D. A., Froelicher, E. S., & Hunt, T. K. (2001). Tissue oxygenation, perfusion, and position in patients with venous leg ulcers. *Nursing Research, 50,* 24–32.

[8]Byrne, M. W., & Keefe, M. R. (2003). Comparison of two measures of parent-child interaction. *Nursing Research, 52,* 34–41.

[9]Cho, S-H, Ketefian, S., Barkauskas, V., & Smith, D. G. (2003). The effects of nurse staffing on adverse events, mortality and medical costs. *Nursing Research, 52,* 71–79.

operationalization. The relatively complex concepts in Table 2.1 are either operationalized with several discrete observables (e.g., infant health) or by means of indices that combine several discrete observable indicators into one score (e.g., functional health status, mother-infant interaction quality). For two of the concepts (treatment-seeking and pain)—concepts that represent complex processes (treatment-seeking) or have complex psychological and physiological meaning (pain)—a single indicator is used, so the potential complexity of the concept meaning is not readily apparent to those who are not familiar with the literature.

Nursing concepts also differ in their level of abstraction, that is, in the number of inferential steps needed to translate observation into meaning. The concept "syringe" is relatively concrete, in that most of its properties are directly observable. On the other hand, the concepts in Table 2.1 are more abstract, because they cannot be observed directly and their presence or occurrence must be inferred. Concepts such as "asthma medication adherence," "social competence," and "perfusion" require the use of special devices or instruments. The concept "mother-infant interaction quality" is inferred through a combination of direct observation and the use of instruments.

Most nursing concepts are relatively abstract. As a result the multiple dimensions and characteristics included in their meaning must be specified carefully and with precision. Highly abstract concepts that are not directly observable are sometimes termed *constructs* because they are constructed of less abstract concepts that are observed directly or indirectly. Morse, Hupcey, Mitcham, and Lenz (1996) refer to such abstract concepts as behavioral concepts, in order to differentiate them from more concrete physiological or disease-state terms. Examples of constructs or behavioral concepts include quality of life, stress, coping, moral development, self-concept, anxiety, and job satisfaction. In this chapter, the term "concept" is used inclusively and refers to ideas at all levels of abstraction.

Many of the concepts that appear in Table 2.1 that express important ideas in nursing are also used as basic elements of theory in other disciplines as well. Functional status, for example, is commonly used in several disciplines, including sociology, epidemiology, social work, physical therapy, and medicine. The term "borrowed concepts" has been used to describe concepts that have a rich tradition and plentiful literature in another field, but are being used in nursing research. In reality, knowledge is not owned by a given discipline, so to call such concepts "borrowed" is probably a misnomer. Because nursing incorporates and builds on the knowledge of related sciences and the humanities, its concepts are generally not unique; however, the perspective taken by nursing and the use to which its knowledge is put helps guide the selection of concepts from other disciplines and influences the ways in which they are defined, conceptualized, and operationalized (Hupcey, Penrod, Morse, & Mitcham, 2001).

THEORETICAL AND OPERATIONAL DEFINITIONS

A theoretical definition provides meaning by defining a concept in terms of other concepts; it involves substituting one or more words for another. An operational definition provides meaning by defining a concept in terms of the observations and/or activities that measure it.

The theoretical definition of a concept generally consists of words, phrases, or sentences selected from among several alternative or possible meanings. Sometimes several meanings, each equally plausible, are included. Theoretical definitions vary considerably in complexity. In the scientific and practice literature they should be sufficiently complex to include the essential meaning of a concept as it is being used in that particular practice or research context, yet very precise and clear. The theoretical definition is the primary vehicle for communicating the meaning of a concept to the reader or listener.

Theoretical definitions may be derived from common usage, borrowed intact from a preexisting theory, or synthesized on the basis of literature and/or observation in the clinical or field setting. Ideally, the theoretical definition of a concept is consistent with its use within the discipline. In theoretical and empirical literature a theoretical definition based simply on common usage of the concept, or borrowed uncritically from another discipline, is generally inadequate because the meaning of many concepts is discipline-specific. Within the context of a given theory, a concept may either be defined within the theory itself using the concepts of the theory to construct the definition, or may be introduced into the theory without a definition as long at it has an agreed upon meaning, and can be defined relatively simply (Meleis, 1997).

The operational definition is stated in terms of the way the concept is being measured. It includes the empirical indicators of the concept and any procedures (e.g., instruments, laboratory protocols) that are being used to discern those indicators. It represents the outcome of the process of operationalization. For example, the concept functional health status was theoretically defined by DiMattio and Tulman

(2003) as "performance of activities associated with life roles" (p. 99). The operational definition of the concept was the patient's scores on two instruments: the Inventory of Functional Status in the Elderly (Paier, 1994) and the Sickness Impact Profile (Damiano, 1996). Giuliano, Scott, Brown, and Olson (2003), in a study of the impact of bed position on cardiac output, defined the latter as "the amount of blood in liters ejected from the left ventricle per minute" (p. 242). The physiological device-assisted measures used were thermodilution and the continuous cardiac output method of measuring the transfer of heat. See Table 2.2 for these and other examples of theoretical and operational definitions.

The operational definition of a concept generally refers to the way in which the concept is measured within the context of a particular study or activity. It is frequently acknowledged that a given operationalization does not completely reflect the full richness of the theoretical meaning of the concept. The operational definition usually is more restrictive and situationally specific than the theoretical definition.

Both theoretical and operational definitions are important and useful for understanding and building nursing knowledge. To define nursing concepts either exclusively in terms of their observable indicators and operations or in terms of other concepts would inhibit essential links between theory and research. Theoretical and operational definitions play complementary roles. The presence of a carefully developed theoretical definition helps guide the selection of indicators and is the basis for determining whether a given set of indicators is relevant. Indicators lend focus and clarity to, and help demonstrate the utility and validity of, theoretical ideas. An operational definition helps focus the meaning of a theoretically defined construct within a particular context, and a theoretical definition can give greater breadth of meaning than highly specific indicators. Unfortunately, investigators studying relatively commonly encountered and seemingly straightforward concepts (e.g., pain, adverse events, nurse staffing, pressure ulcer risk) often do not provide theoretical definitions, even though they describe the chosen measures in detail.

Because it may be difficult to capture all of the rich meaning of a complex concept in operational indicators, it is important not to rush prematurely toward closure in operationalizing a concept before the theoretical work to elucidate its dimensions and nuances of meaning is well advanced. Hupcey, Penrod, Morse, and Mitcham (2001) and Hupcey and Penrod (2003) noted that the nursing literature embodies many examples of uncritical use of the concept of "trust" without clear concept development. They provided an example of how techniques of concept analysis and concept development using data from the literature and sequential qualitative studies were used to advance the meaning of the concept, thereby paving the way for its use in research. The recent surge of interest in qualitative research in nursing and in concept analysis and development approaches that are grounded in both real-world observation and the literature (see Swartz-Barcott & Kim, 2000; Sadler, 2000; Hupcey & Penrod, 2003) has helped reveal the potential richness of meaning of concepts in common use and has provided considerable insight that needs to be taken into account in developing operational definitions.

OPERATIONALIZING NURSING CONCEPTS

The process of operationalizing a concept is an ongoing and cumulative process that involves several interrelated steps: (1) developing the theoretical definition; (2) specifying variables derived from the theoretical definition; (3) identifying observable indicators; (4) developing means for measuring the indicators; and (5) evaluating the adequacy of the resulting operational definition. Each of the steps represents progression from the abstract to the concrete; however, there is actually considerable interplay between steps, and one is rarely completed before the next is begun. Although there is no specific way to go about operationalizing a concept, the following is a description of the approach that we have found to be useful. Each of the major steps is considered in detail with specific strategies included. For an excellent

TABLE 2.2   Examples of Theoretical and Operational Definitions

Concept	Theoretical Definition	Operational Definition
Fatigue	"A subjective feeling of tiredness that is influenced by circadian rhythms and can vary in unpleasantness, duration, and intensity."[1]	Total score on the 22-item Piper Fatigue Scale, which has 4 dimensions: behavioral, sensory, cognitive, affective[2]
Social competence	A mother's ability "to handle her inner world" and her "ability to interact effectively with partners, family, peers and social agencies."[3] (p. 128)	Scores from a composite derived from the following instruments: the Rosenberg Self-Esteem Inventory, Perlin's Sense of Mastery Scale, CES-D, Perceived Stress Scale, Community Life Skills Scale, and the Social Skills Inventory.[3]
Cardiac output	"The amount of blood in liters ejected from the left ventricle per minute"—the product of heart rate and stroke volume.[4] (p. 242)	1) Thermodilution approach in which the difference between the temperature of solution injected into a pulmonary artery catheter and the blood in circulation in the heart, is plotted on a time-temperature curve, and 2) the continuous cardiac output method, measuring the transfer of heat from a heated filament in the pulmonary artery catheter to the blood that flows by a thermistor near the tip of the catheter.[4] (p. 243)
Parenting self-efficacy	"The parent's overall belief in his or her capability to talk with his/her adolescent about specific sex-related topics."[5] (p. 137)	Total scores on a self-efficacy scale comprised of 16 items to measure the following aspects of sex-based discussions: physiological processes, practical issues, and safer sex messages. The items are rated on a 7-point scale, and the total score is summed across all items.[5]
Maternal competence in infant care	"The mother's self-evaluation or rating of her knowledge and abilities within her role as infant care provider, as well as her evaluation of the infant's behavioral response to her interventions . . . [the definition] is specific to the infant care-provider role, it incorporates the infant's role in communicating needs for care, and it is based on the assumption that the infant's behavioral quality affects maternal competence levels."[6] (p. 100)	Scores on the Infant Care Questionnaire, comprised of 38 items to assess maternal perceptions regarding "a) maternal knowledge, confidence, and ability in infant care, and b) infant behavioral quality."[6] (p. 101) Scoring can be via total factor score or average, and a competence rating based on the factor score's falling above or below a cut score.[6] (p. 102)
Perceived health status	"The relative sense of wellness from an adolescent's perspective, based on a multidimensional conceptualization of health."[7] (p. 234)	Score on the Adolescent Health Chart, a set of 6 charts (physical fitness, emotional feelings, school work, social support, family communication, and health habits), each with a 5-choice response ranging from good to bad.[7]

TABLE 2.2   *(Continued)*

[1]Piper, B. F., Lindsey, A. M., & Dodd, M. L. (1987). Fatigue mechanisms in cancer patients: Developing nursing theory. *Oncology Nursing Forum, 14*(6), 17.

[2]Piper, B. F., Dibble, S. L., Dodd, M. L., Weiss, M. C., Slaughter, R. E., & Paul, S. M. (1998). The revised Piper Fatigue Scale: Psychometric evaluation in women with breast cancer. *Oncology Nursing Forum, 25,* 677–684.

[3]Koniak-Griffin, D., Verzemnieks, I. L., Anderson, N. L. R., Brecht, M-L, Lesser, J., Kim, S., & Turner-Pluta, C. (2003). Nurse visitation for adolescent mothers. *Nursing Research, 52,* 127–136.

[4]Giuliano, K. K., Scott, S. S., Brown, V., & Olson, M. (2003). Backrest angle and cardiac output measurement in critically ill patients. *Nursing Research, 52,* 242–248.

[5]Dilorio, C., Dudley, W. N., Wang, D. T., Wasserman, J., Eichler, M., Belcher, L., & West-Edwards, C. (2001). Measurement of parenting self-efficacy and outcome expectancy related to discussions about sex. *Journal of Nursing Measurement, 9,* 135–149.

[6]Secco, L. (2002). The Infant Care Questionnaire: Assessment of reliability and validity in a sample of healthy mothers. *Journal of Nursing Measurement, 10,* 97–110.

[7]Honig, J. (2002). Perceived health status in urban minority young adolescents. *MCN, 27,* 233–237.

example of the application of this approach, refer to Beck and Gable's (2001) description of the development and assessment of the Postpartum Depression Screening Scale.

DEVELOPING THE THEORETICAL DEFINITION

The purpose of defining a concept is to convey as clearly as possible the idea that is represented when a given term is used. Generally, when a concept is used in conversation or encountered in the literature, the user or reader has some idea, more or less precise, of the meaning assigned to the term. In order to formulate a theoretical definition for a concept that is to be used in nursing theory, research, or practice it is necessary to translate one's informal, personal working definition of the concept into a theoretical definition that is precise, understandable to others, and appropriate for the context in which the term will be used. The series of activities involved can be long and intensive. The activities include (1) developing a preliminary definition, (2) reviewing literature, (3) developing or identifying exemplars, (4) mapping the concept's meaning, and (5) stating the theoretical definition. The activities involved in developing a theoretical definition are similar to those involved in conceptualization, the act of arriving at abstract understanding of a phenomenon, but are often formalized, and culminate in a written product.

Although parallels can be drawn between conceptualization and the processes of concept analysis and development, as described in the theoretical and qualitative research literature of nursing and related disciplines (e.g., Hupcey, Morse, Lenz, & Tason, 1996; Rodgers & Knafl, 2000), some distinctions are necessary. Whereas conceptualization is an active, generational process of theoretical thinking, concept analysis is more reflexive, involving critical evaluation of conceptualization that has already occurred (Kim, 2000). It more closely resembles the inductive, integrative thinking involved in concept development. As will be shown below, the steps involved in formulating theoretical definitions generally entail both active conceptualization and analysis of preexisting conceptualizations. The recent literature that has focused on concept analysis, development, exploration, and advancement (e.g., Rodgers & Knafl, 2000; Hupcey & Penrod, 2003) has been oriented primarily toward theory-building rather than toward research applications. Therefore, the most advanced thinking about concepts and the most careful and elaborate conceptualization has often not been linked directly to operationalization. Conversely, many of the concepts that have been studied empirically have been operationalized without benefit of thoughtful conceptualization.

As a means of shortcutting the process of conceptualization one may be tempted to turn to the dictionary or a frequently cited reference and simply borrow the definition. Such shortcuts are problematic. Dictionary definitions reflect the meanings of terms as they are used in everyday language. Common sense meanings may differ from, and are much less precise than, scientific meanings, which reflect the result of systematic study and have been consensually validated by the members of a scientific community. For example, disease-oriented definitions of health derived from the biomedical model are not consistent with the basic philosophical stance or human health response model reflected in contemporary nursing thought. Although a dictionary definition can often serve as a useful early step in developing a concept (Chinn & Jacobs, 1983), it should never be a substitute for examining the scientific literature.

Use of a preexisting theoretical definition may sometimes be the most appropriate approach to defining a concept. For example if one is testing a theory in which clear theoretical definitions have been stated, they should not be altered. Likewise if theoretical development is being done within the context of a well-established theory with accepted, clearly defined concepts, it is appropriate to use the definitions without modification, assuming they convey the essential meaning. Borrowing another's theoretical definition also may be acceptable, even if the definition was developed within a different context or discipline, provided it clearly represents the meaning to be conveyed. Usually, however, its appropriateness cannot be determined until a variety of possible definitions have been explored. The activities that are undertaken to develop a theoretical definition are described below.

The Preliminary Definition

It is often useful to begin development of a theoretical definition by writing one's own definition of the concept, including key ideas and synonyms. The sources of this definition may include clinical observation and experience, or literature. Additionally, it is helpful to indicate the purpose for which the concept is being defined and operationalized. Possible purposes might include testing a particular theory, conducting research to describe a nursing phenomenon, developing and testing instruments for use in patient assessment, documenting the outcomes of nursing interventions, or identifying the defining characteristics of a new nursing diagnosis. The preliminary definition is only a

starting point for conceptualization, so should never be viewed as an end in itself.

By way of example, assume that the concept to be operationalized for research purposes is help-seeking. A preliminary definition might be stated as follows: help-seeking is the process of looking for assistance from others to solve a problem. This preliminary definition suggests that help-seeking involves a sequence of behaviors (a "process") that are interpersonal (involve "others") and are purposely undertaken by the searcher in order to achieve a goal ("solving a problem").

These preliminary activities help to set the stage for concept definition in several ways. First, they force translation of an idea into words and call attention to aspects that may be important to include in a later, more precise formulation of the definition. Second, they help to place limits or boundaries around the concept and eliminate meanings that are irrelevant to the purpose at hand. Many concepts have a wide range of possible meanings depending on the context in which they are used. For example, the concept "reaction" conveys a different sense when used in the context of chemistry or pharmacology (e.g., chemical reaction, negative reaction to a drug) than when used in the context of human behavior (e.g., psychological reaction to a stimulus event). Third, the preliminary definition helps to identify the perspective or worldview that will be used and the assumptions that will be made in defining the concept. Each discipline has a somewhat unique world view, but even within a discipline there can be many different perspectives that suggest very different definitions for a given concept. For example, within the field of sociology, some definitions of social support are based on theories of attachment and role, and others are based on exchange theories. Depending on the theoretical perspective, the respective definitions would be likely to emphasize either the need for human contact and types of support emanating from different role relationships, or the reciprocal nature of the support. One's own orientation should be recognized and compared with others' orientations in order to reveal biases or inconsistencies that should be rectified as the definition is refined.

Literature Review

Once the preliminary working definition has been written, the very essential next step is to examine the current knowledge about the concept by means of a review of relevant literature in nursing and related fields. Additionally, exemplars or cases that synthesize the meaning gleaned from the literature and exemplify the concept can serve to enhance refinement of the theoretical definition. The step of reviewing literature is consistently included in descriptions of concept analysis and development, and is a vital activity. Walker and Avant (2005) and Rodgers (2000) recommend an extensive literature review in order to generate and then validate the ultimate choice of the concept's defining attributes. Morse (2000) and Morse, Hupcey, Mitcham, and Lenz (1996) recommend conducting an exhaustive review of the literature about a concept to determine its level of maturity. "A mature concept, that is, one that can be readily adapted for research purposes, is well-defined, has distinct attributes or characteristics, delineated boundaries and well-described pre-conditions and outcomes" (Hupcey, Penrod, Morse, & Mitcham, 2001, p. 283).

The literature needs to be identified by searching bibliographic databases from a variety of disciplines, not just nursing. Frequently, literature in related disciplines is helpful in defining a concept, and sometimes the bodies of literature that can contribute to concept development and definition seem distant indeed. The information published in the literature of other disciplines should be interpreted with care, recognizing possible limitations in one's ability to understand what is written. Often it is helpful to seek input and validation of one's understanding from scholars in the parent discipline of the publication.

Choice of literature to review should be guided by the purpose for which the concept is being developed and measured, the unit(s) of analysis to which it applies (e.g., individual, group, family, community, society), and the conceptual or theoretical framework that is being used. While the review should not be overly limited in scope, choice of literature should be targeted to relevant materials. The review should include, but not be limited to, recent publications. Frequently tracing the historical evolution of a concept reveals important advances that have been made in reformulating it or adding new dimensions to its meaning (Rodgers, 2000; Broome, 2000).

A number of techniques that can be used to help construct theoretical definitions by integrating the results of the literature review information gleaned from the literature review and from case development are listed below. Usually a combination of techniques is required.

1. List all definitions of the concept (that is, the word label) from the literature that are potentially relevant. Include both explicit and implicit (suggested but not stated) definitions. Identify commonalities and differences. Elements common to the definitions of a concept are considered critical attributes. They are the elements that one would want to be sure to include in a meaningful theoretical definition, because they express the meaning of the concept and help differentiate it from others. For example, Miller and Powers (1988) identified 10 critical elements of the concept "hope" by reviewing the literature. These elements were viewed as important dimensions of the concept and included mutuality-affiliation, sense of the possible, avoidance of absolutizing, anticipation, achieving goals, psychological well-being and coping, purpose and meaning in life, freedom, reality surveillance-optimism, and mental and physical activation (pp. 6–7).

2. List synonyms and their definitions. This activity is useful in differentiating terms and identifying subtle differences in meaning.

3. List examples or instances of the concept recorded in the literature or recalled from clinical practice. Some authors recommend making up fictitious examples or cases that serve to clearly exemplify the concept (model case) or its opposite (contrary case), or a similar or related phenomenon (borderline case or related case, respectively). This strategy was suggested by Wilson (1963) and adapted by Walker and Avant (2005), Avant (2000), and Sadler (2000) and others. It is a mental exercise that can aid in clarifying the concept and its critical attributes,

has been applied with varying degrees of success by many authors of articles communicating the results of concept analyses, and remains very popular (see Hupcey, Morse, Lenz, & Tason, 1996, for examples and a critique of these approaches). Used very selectively and thoughtfully, this strategy can add richness to one's understanding of the concept itself and how it fits into a larger network of ideas; it may also help differentiate concepts that are similar, but not identical, in meaning. Made up examples and cases are generally less useful than real-world examples taken from the empirical literature or from one's own "meticulously collected observational or interview data" (Hupcey, Morse, Lenz, & Tason, 1996, p. 202). Unfortunately, many applications of the techniques have resulted in confusing analyses that add little to our understanding.

4. For complex concepts it may be desirable to identify multiple concepts that are similar or related and analyze them simultaneously. The simultaneous activity results in a richer analysis than single concept analysis. This is a complicated undertaking on which several experts (termed a consensus group) may be involved. Haase, Leidy, Coward, Britt, and Penn (2000) describe the process used to analyze the concepts of spirituality, perspective, hope, acceptance, and self-transcendence. After each concept was analyzed individually, a validity matrix was constructed, and ultimately a process model developed.

The literature review and the above techniques serve several useful purposes. They set limits and create boundaries around the meaning of a concept, help differentiate the concept from others related to it, and indicate the aspects or dimensions of meaning that should be included in the theoretical definition and ultimately in the identification of empirical indicators.

Mapping the Meaning

After having determined the critical attributes of a concept and the aspects of its meaning, it is helpful to develop a scheme for logically organizing the meaning of the concept, often termed

its meaning space or content domain. Although the mapping process can be difficult, the purpose and context for use of the concept, the theoretical framework (orienting perspective), and the literature provide helpful direction. State-of-the-science reviews of the literature surrounding a given concept, and articles addressing theoretical and methodological issues often provide guidance for concept mapping. Dijkers (1999), for example, provided a structure for the study of quality of life that included several domains (e.g., activities of daily living, symptoms, social functioning).

There are also some common distinctions that provide starting points and structures for mapping the meaning of concepts. For example, many concepts of interest to nursing—quality of life is a good example—include objective (perceivable by others) and subjective (perceivable only by the individual experiencing it) aspects (see Dijkers, 1999). Although both aspects might make up the meaning in the larger sense, one aspect might be eliminated as irrelevant for a given purpose. If the purpose of an inquiry were to determine whether an individual's perception of his or her quality of life was related to mood, objective aspects of the meaning might be less important than subjective aspects. Other common distinctions within the meaning space of concepts include differentiating stable from transitory patterns (referred to as *trait* and *state* characteristics, respectively), and the inclusion of both structural and functional patterns.

Recent research and theoretical literature contains many examples of suggested ways to organize the meaning of important nursing concepts. For example, the Middle-Range Theory of Unpleasant Symptoms (Lenz, Suppe, Gift, Pugh, & Milligan, 1995; Lenz, Pugh, Milligan, Gift, & Suppe, 1997) defines symptoms as subjectively perceived (by definition) and suggests that all symptoms can be described using common dimensions, such as intensity or severity, timing (duration and frequency), associated distress, and impact on function. Guided by a worldview that incorporates the assumption that persons are bio-psycho-social beings, Lenz and colleagues included physiological, psychological, and social/environmental aspects in mapping the meaning of and influences on the symptom experience. This assumption would result in a very different map than would a framework that addresses people as solely physiologic entities. In examining the ways in which a concept has been mapped in the literature, it is important to remember that the discipline of the author and the population and context for which the concept meaning is being mapped, influence the dimensions and aspects that are highlighted. Sources of information for concept mapping include existing literature, personal observation and experience, and previous research. Qualitative and exploratory studies of the phenomenon can provide rich information to inform the conceptualization. For example, Beck and Gable (2001), drew on Beck's multistudy program of research about postpartum depression to specify the concept domain.

Strategies that may be helpful in mapping the meaning space of a concept include the following:

1. List major elements in each major organizing scheme and identify similarities and differences. Determine whether one set of organizing elements or categories can be subsumed under another. Eliminate schemes that do not apply to the purpose at hand.
2. Construct an outline or table with major headings representing key aspects of meaning. Include under each heading elements that are subsumed or summarized. Figure 2.1 is an example of an outline depicting the process of help-seeking which was adapted from an analogous process, information-seeking. Analogous thinking can help map concept meaning (see Walker & Avant, 2005).
3. Pose questions about the concepts that derive from the theoretical framework, purpose, and/or literature reviewed. Regarding the help-seeking concept, possible questions might include: What is being sought, from whom is it being sought, how is it being sought and for what purpose, and to what extent is the purpose achieved?
4. Construct diagrams to represent the concept meaning. Venn diagrams that depict

meanings in terms of discrete, overlapping, and/or inclusive sets are particularly useful (Thigpen & Drane, 1967). Flow diagrams are often used for mapping concepts that denote processes. Highly complex diagrams may be needed to depict the meaning of some concepts, such as trust (see Hupcey, 2002). It is important that any diagram's meaning by readily discernible and essentially self-evident. Therefore, a diagram should follow standard conventions (e.g., placement of elements to reflect time-ordering or causal linkages), and all of the diagram's elements (boxes, circles, arrows, and so forth) should be translatable into words.
5. Once the general structure of the meaning map is identified (major stages or subdomains), keep a list of the possible ways in which variation can occur within the categories of the structure based on literature or observation. These lists will be useful during the process of operationalization.

Depending on the nature of the concept, the mapping may be simple, consisting of one or two words that designate aspects of the meaning, or may be highly elaborate and complex. The map is essentially a tool that organizes the meaning of the concept into a usable framework and helps to assure that critical elements are identified, included in the theoretical framework, and ultimately taken into account in measurement. A preliminary map, which provides the basis for the theoretical definition, generally becomes more precise as the concept is operationalized. For a more detailed discussion of strategies that can be used for mapping the meaning of concepts, the reader is referred to Walker and Avant (2005) and Hupcey (2002).

Stating the Theoretical Definition

The preliminary procedures to identify and organize the essential elements and dimensions of meaning denoted by a concept, pave the way for selecting or constructing the theoretical definition. Ideally, the theoretical definition includes critical attributes of the concept's meaning that

I. Stimulus
   A. Type of problem
   B. Specificity
   C. Immediacy

II. Preliminary Activities
   A. Feasibility of goal
   B. Specificity of goal

III. Decision to Seek Help
   A. Immediacy
   B. Active vs. passive

IV. Information Search
   A. Extent
   B. Duration
   C. Type of method
   D. Number of consultants
   E. Expertise of consultants

V. Information Acquisition
   A. Extent
   B. Specificity
   C. Degree of fit with goal

VI. Resource Selection
   A. Relevance of criteria to goal
   B. Specificity of criteria
   C. Number of options considered

VII. Resource Contact
   A. Success
   B. Type of resource contacted

VIII. Outcomes
   A. Success (receipt of help)
   B. Level of satisfaction with help received
   C. Continuation of search/termination of search

FIGURE 2.1   **Outline of several variable dimensions of the help-seeking process.**

differentiate it from other terms. It should orient the reader to the definer's frame of reference and help to assure that the concept will be interpreted similarly by all who read it. The process of constructing a theoretical definition from a conceptual mapping involves a process which is essentially the reverse of concept analysis. Whereas concept analysis involves breaking the concept into its component elements, the theoretical definition represents an integration and synthesis of those elements into a meaningful whole.

Although the theoretical definition is not long enough to capture the full richness of the meaning of the concept, it can communicate a great deal. For example, consider the following theoretical definition of fatigue by Piper, Lindsey, and Dodd (1987): "A subjective feeling of tiredness that is influenced by circadian rhythms and can vary in unpleasantness, duration and intensity" (p. 17). This definition tells the reader that fatigue is subjective, patterned, and varies along at least three dimensions. Another definition to consider is the following: "Help-seeking is a multistage process that an individual undertakes for the purpose of securing needed assistance from another; it has cognitive and behavioral elements." This definition denotes several essential aspects of the meaning intended by the definer: (1) help-seeking (the concept) involves both cognition and behavior carried out at the level of the individual; (2) it involves a sequence of several activities carried out over time (multistage process); (3) the sequence is carried out for a purpose; (4) it is carried out with a perceived need or goal (securing needed assistance) in mind; (5) the goal involves at least one other individual; and (6) the goal need not be achieved for the process to be carried out.

This definition depicts the meaning of the concept as a sequence of cognitive and behavioral steps initiated by a mental process (perception of need). It also helps the reader to eliminate from consideration certain phenomena that do not meet the definitional criteria. For example, random behaviors are eliminated, because they are not purposeful or goal directed. The definition would not necessarily eliminate looking for information from impersonal sources, such as books, provided the information was used to direct the seeker to a personal help provider. Looking for help in a book (e.g., looking up directions on how to remove a stain) would be eliminated, however, because the receipt of help would not meet the criterion of being interpersonal. On the basis of the definition, the reader is able to differentiate help-seeking from related concepts that denote different phenomena, for example, help finding, helping, acquiring help, and information seeking.

Theoretical definitions of relatively abstract and complex concepts are frequently supplemented with definitions for included terms and/or with statements that clarify the definition. The clarifying statements that supplement the definition help the reader reconstruct the author's map of the concept and provide the groundwork for subsequent steps in operationalizing it. Abstract theoretical definitions generally require supplementary definitions of their major components or subconcepts in order to clarify meaning and bridge the gap between language and experience. Regardless of the level of abstraction, theoretical definitions should be stated with enough generality to be applicable across a variety of real-world situations and populations.

It is not always necessary to develop a theoretical definition from scratch. Once the critical attributes have been identified and the concept's meaning mapped, an existing theoretical definition may well be appropriate for the current purpose and context. If so, it is preferable to use the existing definition in order to allow accumulation of evidence about the concept as defined. An existing definition is *not* appropriate unless it accurately and adequately represents the desired meaning or cannot be applied legitimately to nursing situations without substantially changing the meaning intended by the originator of the definition.

SPECIFYING VARIABLE ASPECTS OF A CONCEPT

Concepts of interest to nurses tend to have multiple dimensions, each of which can vary. These multiple, variable dimensions are more important in practice and research than the definition of the concept "per se". For example, nurses are less interested in whether a particular object can be classified as a needle than they are in its variable properties: its sharpness, length, diameter, curvature, and composition. This activity is closely related to the mapping procedure, but carries it a step further, in that essential parts of the meaning are expressed as characteristics that can assume different values.

A well-developed theoretical definition generally provides important clues to salient dimensions of the concept, as was illustrated in the above example of help-seeking. Dimensions of this concept can be identified from each of the key steps in the process. Possible variable dimensions would include: (1) the degree and immediacy with which assistance is required, (2) the nature of the information search carried out, including its extensiveness, duration, type of strategy(ies) used, and number of information sources consulted, (3) the extent and type of resource information obtained, (4) the type and nature of resource selected and factors taken into account in making the selection, and (5) the level of satisfaction with the assistance obtained.

Sometimes variable dimensions of a concept are not easily derived from the theoretical definition and require a return to the literature. Research reports suggest several generic variables that are applicable to many concepts. For example, most studies of expectations or beliefs reveal differences in the strength with which people hold the expectation or belief. Therefore, strength would represent a potentially salient variable for operationalizing concepts that incorporate expectation or belief. Studies of behavior often represent differences in the frequency with which the behavior is carried out, suggesting frequency to be a salient variable in behavioral research. Examining examples of a given concept and determining ways in which these examples differ can also be a way to identify its variable dimensions. For example, asking oneself about ways in which patient education programs differ can reveal several variable dimensions such as length, comprehensiveness, difficulty level, complexity, sequence of content, types of variable aspects strategies used, and types of information included.

Once possible variables are identified, the selection of those that ultimately will be included in the operationalization is determined by the purpose for which the concept is being developed and the context in which it will be used. The following are possible questions to ask when selecting variable aspects or dimensions for inclusion in an operationalization:

1. Which variables will provide the most useful information to nurses?
2. Which variables have others found to be most important in understanding the phenomenon?
3. Which variables have others found to be related to other concepts of interest or to help explain or predict occurrences of interest to nurses?
4. Which variables can be rendered observable and measurable, given our present state of knowledge and technology?

IDENTIFYING OBSERVABLE INDICATORS

The selection of observable indicators of the concept is guided by the theoretical definition, the map of the concept's meaning, and the variable dimensions that have been identified. Three examples are provided below to demonstrate the way in which the selection of indicators flows directly from the previous steps.

Example 1. Continuing the example of help-seeking, specific indicators can be identified for each of the variable dimensions. Examples of possible indicators for the information search stages and outcomes are provided in Table 2.3.

Example 2. The concept functional status is defined as "a multidimensional concept characterizing one's ability to provide for the necessities of life—those activities people do in the normal course of their lives to meet basic needs, fulfill usual roles, and maintain their health and well being" (Leidy, 1999, p. 20). Six dimensions of functional status were identified: body care, household maintenance, physical exercise, recreation, spiritual activities, and social activities. Each dimension can be represented by several behavioral indicators. For example, the body care dimension of functional health status could be indicated by the individual's ability to bathe him or herself or groom his/her hair (e.g., able without help, able with help, unable to perform). Recreation could be indicated by ability to go to entertainment venues such as movies, attend social events, or travel locally or to a remote location. A matrix could then be constructed to guide the selection of indicators. Ideally in operationalizing the concept for research purposes, several indicators would be identified for each dimension.

Example 3. The meaning of the concept, infant development, is frequently mapped as progressive change in several different aspects of functioning, such as gross motor ability, fine motor coordination, language ability, and social ability. Within these broad categories of functioning, specific behaviors have been found to emerge at different ages, and norms have been established. Indicators of infant development would therefore have to be age-specific and should represent each major category of functioning. For example, at 6 months of age the infant would be expected to display the following sample behaviors (one is given for each realm of development): (a) gross motor—plays with toes, (b) fine motor—holds cube in each hand, (c) language—babbles, (d) social—holds arms up when about to be lifted.

When selecting indicators, it is important to determine whether the concept represents an either/or phenomenon (i.e., a state or object) or one that varies. One could define pain, for example, in terms of its presence or absence, or

TABLE 2.3   Variables and Indicators for Selected Aspects of Help Seeking*

Variable	Indicator
Extent of search	Number of search activities reported by the individual, calculated as the sum of separate activities undertaken by the individual for the purpose of acquiring information about potential sources of help.
Duration of search	Number of days during which the individual reportedly engaged in information-seeking activities, i.e., interval between deciding to seek help and contacting a potential source of help.
Method of search	Designation of reported search activities as personal or impersonal, with the categories defined as follows: personal method involves use of an individual known personally to the searcher as a source of information; impersonal method involves using a nonhuman source of information or an individual not known personally to the searcher.
Number of consultants	Number of persons whom the searcher reportedly contacted for information about sources of help, calculated as the sum of individuals from whom information was sought and/or received.
Expertise of consultants	Median level of expertise of persons consulted for information, with level of expertise being designated as lay, semiprofessional, or professional with respect to the health-care system.
Receipt of help	Reported occurrence of receipt of assistance from a local resource contacted voluntarily for such help, defined as help received or help not received.
Level of satisfaction with help received	Expressed level of satisfaction with each resource from which help was received, as measured on a five-point scale, ranging from very dissatisfied to very satisfied.
Continuation/termination of search	Reported occurrence (continuation) or nonoccurrence (termination) of any additional help-seeking activity carried out following receipt of service from a local resource.

*Adapted from Lenz (1984).

in terms of its variable degree of severity, location, and so forth. The indicators for the two different conceptualizations of pain would differ. If pain were defined as an either/or phenomenon, possible indicators might include a patient's positive response to the question, "Are you experiencing any pain?" or whether or not the patient appears to be restricting movement because of discomfort. Defining pain as variable in severity would require indicators of degree, such as on a visual analog or numerical rating scale, or the frequency of requests for pain medication in a 24-hour period.

In Example 1, some dimensions of help seeking were conceptualized as varying in number or degree (e.g., number of activities carried out, level of satisfaction) and others were conceptualized as either/or phenomena (e.g., receipt of help, continuation of search). In Example 2, functional status was conceptualized as a variable phenomenon throughout. In Example 3,

infant development was conceptualized as variable; however, the indicators were stated as behaviors that the infant would or would not perform (either/or). In order to determine an infant's level of development (varying), it would be necessary to sum the number of behaviors that the infant performed or compute a developmental quotient score on the basis of the performed behaviors.

The research and theoretical literature related to a concept is a rich source of possible indicators. A good strategy is to list indicators from the literature, then examine each to determine its degree of fit with the theoretical definition and purpose. For example, assume that one is to operationalize the concept hospital size for the purpose of studying nursing staff turnover. Various indicators that may be found in the literature include number of square feet, number of beds, number of departments or units, total number of employees, number of employees in the nursing department, number of patients served per year, number of bed days per year, and annual budget. Indicators such as number of beds and number of employees would be more relevant for most nursing purposes than those reflecting spatial aspects of hospital size. Because there are several ways in which the number of beds and employees may be counted, one would have to make additional decisions about how to operationalize the concept depending on the purpose of the investigation and the meaning to be conveyed.

The nursing literature often refers to instruments (e.g., questionnaires, checklists, attitude scales, or machines) that have been developed to measure a particular concept. It should not automatically be assumed that these tools will generate appropriate indicators. Considerations to be employed in selecting instruments are included in chapters 11 and 12. These include, among others, congruence with the theoretical definition, the results of evaluations of the instruments or indicators, and, most important, empirical evidence that has accrued over time. In addition to the literature, other sources of potential indicators include one's past experience and the experiences of others, particularly those who are in daily contact with the phenomena being conceptualized and operationalized. Nurses, patients, and family members can suggest indicators and can also help evaluate the relevance and potential observability of indicators derived from the literature in the light of pragmatic experience. It is vital that the selection of indicators not be isolated from reality and common sense.

DEVELOPING APPROACHES TO MEASUREMENT

The fourth step in the process of operationalization is to develop means by which the indicators can be observed and measured. This step constitutes the focus for the remainder of the book. At this point it is sufficient to say that the operations by which a particular indicator can be rendered observable and the rules by which numbers will be assigned to various states or degrees of the indicator must be specified. Having

determined the way in which the concept is to be measured, it is possible to state the operational definition, which expresses the meaning of the concept in terms of the way it will be measured in a particular context.

EVALUATING THEORETICAL AND OPERATIONAL DEFINITIONS

The final step in the process of operationalization is to evaluate the adequacy of the products. Ultimately, judgment of the adequacy with which a concept has been defined and operationalized is made on the basis of accumulated evidence from empirical investigations. Fortunately, the nursing literature is beginning to reflect such cumulativity, and empirical assessments of nursing concepts are becoming more frequent.

Several criteria have been suggested as useful in evaluating the adequacy of an operationalization. They include the following:

1. *Clarity.* The definition, indicators, and operations for the concept are presented in a way that can be easily understood.

2. *Precision.* The observations and operations are explicit and specific. Mathematical formulas are examples of precise operationalizations of concepts, but are rarely used in nursing. Precision should be reflected in verbal operationalizations, such as instructions about how to make a particular observation or carry out an operation.

3. *Reliability.* Observation and operations are repeatable or reproducible.

4. *Consistency.* Terms are used in a consistent manner, and logical reasoning has been used to guide selection of indicators. Linkages among the aspects or dimensions of concept meaning, and between the language meaning of the concept and empirical reality are logically consistent.

5. *Meaning Adequacy.* The meaning designated by a concept and the indicators selected to represent it are congruent, and indicators (as fully as possible) account for the various dimensions of meaning.

6. *Feasibility.* Indicators and operations are capable of being executed. This criterion presents a utilitarian view, which acknowledges the limits imposed by current technology. In determining the feasibility of measures, practical considerations, such as the age, language, culture, cognitive status, and stamina of subjects or patients, are important (see Strickland, 1998).

7. *Utility.* The operationalization is useful within the context of the specific investigation or other activity and, more generally, to the discipline of nursing. Concepts that are operationalized with variable indicators are more useful both theoretically and practically than those operationalized in terms of nonvariable indicators.

8. *Validity.* The observations selected to represent or indicate a concept in fact do so. Assessment of the validity of an operationalization is an ongoing process that requires empirical investigation.

9. *Consensus.* The ultimate test of an operationalization is that it is accepted consensually by the scientific community because of clear and accrued empirical evidence.

SUMMARY

Concepts are abstract verbal symbols that help summarize and categorize ideas, thoughts, and observations. They are basic elements of the complex statements and theories that make up the language of any scientific discipline. They link thought and experience. Nursing concepts designate the subject matter of the discipline but are not necessarily unique to nursing. Because key nursing concepts tend to be complex and relatively abstract, they must be defined and operationalized carefully if they are to be useful in building and applying knowledge.

To operationalize a concept is to delineate what it means and how it will be measured. A multistep procedure is required. The first step is to formulate a theoretical definition that supplies meaning through the use of other concepts. The theoretical definition is developed following a review of the literature, analysis of previous conceptualizations, and identification of examples, which epitomize or are related to

the concept. Through this process essential elements of the concept's meaning are delimited and logically organized. Subsequent steps are to specify variable dimensions of the concept's meaning, identify observable indicators, develop means to measure the indicators, and evaluate the adequacy of the operationalization. The steps are interrelated, in that each logically flows from and builds upon those that precede it. The products of the operationalization process are the theoretical and operational definitions. The latter provides meaning in terms of the observations or operations necessary to measure the concept. Operationalization, including its conceptualization phase, is an ongoing and cumulative process.

Nursing is reflecting increased sophistication in applying a conceptual approach to operationalizing its concepts. Particularly important is the growing body of literature reflecting both careful, theoretically based conceptualizations of key nursing concepts and empirical validation of the adequacy of those conceptualizations and operationalizations. The discipline is moving toward concepts that are defined and operationalized with clarity, precision, reliability, validity, feasibility, and utility.

REFERENCES

Avant, K. C. (2000). The Wilson method of concept analysis. In B. L. Rodgers & K. A. Knafl (Eds.), *Concept development in nursing: Foundations, techniques and applications* (2nd ed., pp. 55–64). Philadelphia: W.B. Saunders.

Beck, C. T., & Gable, R. K. (2001). Ensuring content validity: An illustration of the process. *Journal of Nursing Measurement, 9*(2), 201–215.

Broome, M. E. (2000). Integrative literature reviews for the development of concepts. In B. L. Rodgers & K. A. Knafl (Eds.), *Concept development in nursing: Foundations, techniques and applications* (2nd ed., pp. 231–250). Philadelphia: W.B. Saunders.

Chinn, P., & Jacobs, M. (1983). *Theory and nursing: A systematic approach.* St. Louis: CV Mosby.

Damiano, A. M. (1996). *Sickness impact profile user's manual and interpretation guide.* Baltimore, MD: Johns Hopkins University Press.

Dijkers, M. (1999). Measuring quality of life: Methodological issues. *American Journal of Physical Medicine and Rehabilitation, 78*(3), 286–300.

DiMattio, M. J., & Tulman, L. (2003). A longitudinal study of functional status and correlates following coronary artery bypass graft surgery in women. *Nursing Research, 52*(2), 98–107.

Fawcett, J. (1984). *Analysis and evaluation of conceptual models in nursing.* Philadelphia: F.A. Davis.

Giuliano, K. K., Scott, S. S., Brown, V., & Olson, M. (2003). Backrest angle and cardiac output measurement in critically ill patients. *Nursing Research, 52*(4), 242–248.

Haase, J. E., Leidy, N. K., Coward, D. D., Britt, T., & Penn, P. E. (2000). Simultaneous concept analysis: A strategy for developing multiple concepts. In B. L. Rodgers & K. A. Knafl (Eds.), *Concept development in nursing: Foundations, techniques and applications* (2nd ed., pp. 209–229). Philadelphia: W.B. Saunders.

Hupcey, J. E. (2002). Maintaining validity: The development of the concept of trust. *International Journal of Qualitative Methods, 1*(4), Article 5. Retrieved August 28, 2003, from http://www.ualberta.ca/~ijqm.

Hupcey, J. E., Morse, J. M., Lenz, E. R., & Tason, M. C. (1996). Wilsonian methods of concept analysis: A critique. *Scholarly Inquiry for Nursing Practice: An International Journal, 10*(3), 185–210.

Hupcey, J. E., & Penrod, J. (2003). Concept advancement: Enhancing inductive validity. *Research and Theory for Nursing Practice: An International Journal, 17*(1), 19–30.

Hupcey, J. E., Penrod, J., Morse, J. M., & Mitcham, C. (2001). An exploration and advancement of the concept of trust. *Journal of Advanced Nursing, 36*(2), 282–293.

Kim, H. S. (2000). *The nature of theoretical thinking in nursing* (2nd ed.). New York: Springer.

Leidy, N. K. (1999). Psychometric properties of the functional performance inventory in patients with chronic obstructive pulmonary disease. *Nursing Research, 48*(1), 20–28.

Lenz, E. R., Pugh, L. C., Milligan, R., Gift, A., & Suppe, F. (1997). The middle-range theory of unpleasant symptoms: An update. *Advances in Nursing Science, 19*(3), 14–27.

Lenz, E. R., Suppe, F., Gift, A. G., Pugh, L. C., & Milligan, R. A. (1995). Collaborative development of middle-range nursing theories: Toward a theory of unpleasant symptoms. *Advances in Nursing Science, 17*(3), 1–13.

Maas, J., Johnson, M., & Moorhead, S. (1996). Classifying nursing sensitive patient outcomes. *Image, 28*(4), 295–301.

Meleis, A. I. (1997). *Theoretical nursing: Development and progress* (3rd ed.). Philadelphia: Lippincott.

Miller, J. F., & Powers, M. J. (1988). Development of an instrument to measure hope. *Nursing Research, 37*(1), 6–10.

Morse, J. M. (2000). Exploring pragmatic utility: Concept analysis by critically appraising the literature. In B. L. Rodgers & K. A. Knafl (Eds.), *Concept development in nursing: Foundations, techniques and applications* (2nd ed., pp. 333–352). Philadelphia: W.B. Saunders.

Morse, J. M., Hupcey, J. E., Mitcham, C., & Lenz, E. R. (1996). Concept analysis in nursing research: A critical appraisal. *Scholarly Inquiry for Nursing Practice, 10*(3), 253–277.

Paier, G. S. (1994). *Development and testing of an instrument to assess functional status in the elderly.* Unpublished doctoral dissertation, University of Pennsylvania.

Piper, B. F., Lindsay, A. M., & Dodd, M. L. (1987). Fatigue mechanisms in cancer patients: Developing nursing theory. *Oncology Nursing Forum, 14*(6), 17–23.

Rodgers, B. L. (2000). Concept analysis: An evolutionary view. In B. L. Rodgers & K. A. Knafl (Eds.), *Concept development in nursing: Foundations, techniques and applications* (2nd ed., pp. 77–102). Philadelphia: W.B. Saunders.

Rodgers, B. L., & Knafl, K. A. (Eds.) (2000). *Concept development in nursing: Foundations, techniques and applications* (2nd ed.). Philadelphia: W.B. Saunders.

Sadler, J. J. (2000). A multiphase approach to concept analysis and development. In B. L. Rodgers & K. A. Knafl (Eds.), *Concept development in nursing: Foundations, techniques and applications* (2nd ed., pp. 251–283). Philadelphia: W.B. Saunders.

Scisney-Matlock, M., Algase, D., Boehm, S., Coleman-Burns, P., Oakley, D., Rogers, A. E., et al. (2000). Measuring behavior: Electronic devices in nursing studies. *Applied Nursing Research, 13*(2), 97–102.

Strickland, O. L. (1998). Practical measurement. *Journal of Nursing Measurement, 6*(2), 107–109.

Swartz-Barcott, D., & Kim, H. S. (2000). An expansion and elaboration of the hybrid model of concept development. In B. L. Rodgers & K. A. Knafl (Eds.), *Concept development in nursing: Foundations, techniques and applications* (2nd ed., pp. 129–160). Philadelphia: W.B. Saunders.

Thigpen, L. W., & Drane, J. W. (1967). The Venn diagram: A tool for conceptualization in nursing. *Nursing Research, 16*(3), 252–260.

Walker, L. O., & Avant, K.C. (2005). *Strategies for theory construction in nursing* (4th ed.). Norwalk, CT: Appleton & Lange.

Wilson, J. (1963). *Thinking with concepts.* Cambridge: Cambridge University Press.

3

Measurement Theories and Frameworks

In this chapter we present basic statistical principles and procedures required for understanding the measurement process and measurement theories and frameworks that define the various approaches to measurement.

Measurement problems may range from determining the best method for obtaining the accurate length, weight, and body temperature of a newborn infant, to trying to ascertain the quality of patient care provided on a clinical unit or the level of students' performance in the clinical area. For example, Hymovich (2003) designed a measure to determine how parents of chronically ill children cope with stressors related to their child's illness; Marsh (2003) developed a tool to compare patient satisfaction with health care providers from different disciplines working within the same primary care setting; Wells (2003) constructed a measure for assessing distress during painful medical procedures in adults; and Arnold (1988, 2001) developed an approach to ascertain the diagnostic reasoning process of gerontological nurses. In each of these situations the goal was to describe the kind and/or amount of an attribute possessed by some object.

The focus of measurement is to quantify a characteristic of an object. What is measured is not the object, but a characteristic or attribute of the object. In the examples, the concern is not with measuring the infant, but its length, weight, and body temperature; the clinical supervisor is not concerned with the clinical unit but the quality of patient care administered on the unit; and when a nursing instructor evaluates the level of clinical performance of nursing students, the object is to measure students' ability to perform within the clinical setting, not to measure the students themselves. Similarly, in the published examples the attributes measured were how parents cope; patient satisfaction with the care provided; distress during painful medical procedures; and the diagnostic reasoning process. The attribute to be measured varies in kind and/or amount, and different objects may be assigned to different categories that represent the kind or amount of the attribute possessed. For example, various infants in a nursery have different weights. Similarly, different nursing students in a class will have different levels of ability. Therefore, attributes to be measured are variable and take on different values for different objects. Measurable attributes are often termed variables in scientific language. An attribute must be variable in order to be measured. Measurement provides for meaningful interpretation of the nature of an attribute possessed by an object or event. The results of measurement are usually expressed in the form of numbers.

In nursing and the health professions, there are many attributes of objects that are not easily measured. In such cases, the attribute of concern may be defined in a manner whereby it can be made measurable, that is, the attribute or concept is operationalized. Whenever an attempt is made to measure an attribute it is necessary to define it in qualitative or quantitative terms. A unit of measurement for categorizing the kind and/or amount of the attribute must be established and a measurement rule or procedure must be derived which is congruous with the established unit of measurement. The unit may be a score, a centimeter, a milliliter, a second, a degree Centigrade, or any appropriate unit or category of measurement. The need for the establishment of a suitable unit of measurement, and for precision in measurement, has fostered the development and use of tools such as tests, thermometers, rulers, and balance scales.

Measurement is the process of using a rule to assign numbers to objects or events which represent the kind and/or amount of a specified attribute possessed. The *measurement rule* is the precise procedure used to assign numbers to phenomena, for example, procedures for administering and scoring tests or using a balance scale to measure weight.

SCALES OF MEASUREMENT

Stevens (1946, 1951, 1958, 1960) classified the rules used for assigning numbers to objects to represent the kind and/or amount of a specified attribute possessed by them in a hierarchical manner. From lower to higher levels, the scales of measurement are *nominal, ordinal, interval,* and *ratio.*

In *nominal-scale measurement* objects are placed into categories according to a defined property. Numbers assigned represent an object's membership in one of a set of mutually exclusive, exhaustive, and unorderable categories. Numbers are used for labeling purposes only and have no quantitative significance. Categories used in nominal-level measurement differ in quality rather than quantity; hence, no statement can be made about the amount of the attribute possessed. All members of a category are regarded as similar or equal in some respect. For example, a group of registered nurses may be assigned to categories based on their sex, that is, 1 = male and 2 = female. The basis for classifying is a definition of the class. The basic distinguishing signs for determining inclusion within the class are specified by the definition. Regardless of the number of categories used, two essential conditions should be met. First, a set of categories should be *exhaustive,* that is, every object that is to be classified should belong to at least one category. Second, the designated categories should be *mutually exclusive,* that is, the definition of the categories should be such that no object could be placed in more than one category.

In *ordinal-scale measurement* numbers are assigned to objects according to rank order on a particular attribute. Numbers assigned represent an object's membership in one of a set of mutually exclusive and exhaustive categories that can be ordered according to the amount of the attribute possessed. *Ordinal-scale measurement* may be regarded as the rank ordering of objects into quantitative categories according to relative amounts of the specified attribute. The rankings do not imply that the ranked categories are equally spaced on a scale, nor that the intervals between the scale categories are equal. Ordinal assignment of numbers merely means that the ranking of 1 (for first) has ranked higher than 2 (for second), and since 2 has a higher ranking than 3, then 1 also must rank higher than 3. If, for example, a group of clients are ranked according to their ability to undertake self-care, then a client ranked as 3 would possess less self-care ability than one ranked 2, but would have more ability for self-care than one ranked 4.

An *interval scale* is one for which equal numerical distances on the scale represent equal amounts with respect to the attribute or the object that is the focus of measurement. Numbers assigned in interval-scale measurement represent an object's membership in one of a set of mutually exclusive, exhaustive categories that can be ordered and are equally spaced in terms of the magnitude of the attribute under consideration. However, the absolute amount of the attribute is not known for any particular object, because the zero point in an interval scale is placed in some arbitrary position. In addition to being able to categorize and rank objects, at the interval level one can also order objects according to the size of their numerals and the relative size of the differences between two objects. The Fahrenheit temperature scale is an example of a commonly used interval scale. One can say that two objects having temperatures of 90°F and 100°F are as far apart on the scale as two other objects with temperatures of 50°F and 60°F. One can also say, for example, that a patient's temperature at 6 p.m. is 3 degrees higher than it was at noon, or that the drop in temperature after taking an aspirin was greater than after taking a sponge bath. One cannot say, however, that an object with a temperature of 0°F does not have a temperature at all.

Ratio-level measures give all information that is provided by interval-level measures, but in addition they have absolute zero points, where zero represents an absolute absence of the relevant attribute. The category and rank order of objects with respect to the attribute is known, the intervals on the scale are equal, and the distance or magnitude from the actual zero point is known. Volume, length, and weight are commonly measured by ratio scales and all can be assigned absolute zero values. With a ratio scale one can say that David is two times as heavy as Steven if David weighs 100 lb. and Steven weighs 50 lb.

There is a great deal of controversy about the levels of measurement and the types of statistical operations that can be properly used with the resulting scores. Either the fundamentalist or pragmatist view of measurement rules may be taken. The *fundamentalist view* purports that all measures of attributes can be classified into one of the distinct levels of measurement, and that, once classified, the level of measurement specifies the type of statistical operations that can be properly used. The hierarchical nature of the scales of measurement is considered when statistical operations are applied with scores derived at different levels of measurement. The higher the level of the scale, the broader the range of statistical operations that can be applied with the numbers obtained from measurement. Only nonparametric statistics are considered appropriate with lower level data, that is, nominal or ordinal data; but parametric statistics are permissible with higher level data, that is, interval and ratio data. Frequencies, percentages, and contingency-correlation coefficients are considered permissible at the nominal-scale level of measurement. Ordinal-scale data are believed to allow the same statistical operations permissible with nominal-scale data, but in addition, it is possible to use medians, centiles, and rank-order coefficients of correlation. Practically all of the common statistical procedures are considered permissible with interval and ratio data.

The *pragmatists* point out that most measurement rules are not as clear-cut and easily classified as fundamentalists believe they are, and that it is not practical to waste effort in attempting to classify a variable into a level of measurement. For example, there is some controversy among measurement specialists as to whether scores from psychological tests represent ordinal- or interval-level measurement, because there is no assurance that equal differences between scores represent equal differences in the amount of the attribute of concern, particularly when Likert-type rating scales are used as a basis for scoring. Some contend that test scores simply order subjects according to the amount of the specified attribute possessed, while others purport that test scores represent the magnitude of the attribute possessed. Pragmatists minimize the emphasis on levels of measurement and suggest that the statistical techniques applied to any set of numbers should be determined by the nature of the research question addressed rather than by the level of measurement. We believe that the statistical treatment of any data or set of numbers should be determined by the nature of the scientific inquiry, that is, the research question one is trying to answer, rather than the level of measurement alone. Readers interested in reading further regarding this debate are referred to Nunnally and Bernstein (1994, pp. 20–21).

BASIC STATISTICAL PRINCIPLES AND PROCEDURES

In most instances, measurement results in a number. This number represents the kind and/or amount of some attribute or characteristic of the object or event that is measured. The number that results from measurement may be referred to as either the observed score or the raw score.

In many situations a group of objects is measured on the same attribute, which results in a series or group of observed scores. One might determine, for example, the lung capacity of a group of adult smokers, the arterial pressure of a group of cardiac patients, or the scores on a critical thinking test for a group of nursing students.

Unfortunately, it is difficult to make much sense out of a group of numbers obtained from such situations when they are presented in raw score form. One usually would want to know what the highest and lowest scores are, if the scores are spread out or concentrated at some point along the distribution, and what score occurs most often. Statistical procedures enable one to better understand such groups of numbers and to answer these basic questions about the characteristics of the group of scores. This section presents some basic statistical principles and procedures that are important for understanding measurement and interpreting groups of scores.

Distribution

One step in obtaining information about any group of measures or scores is to arrange them in order from their highest to lowest value and to note how many times a particular score occurs, or whether it occurs at all. This will indicate the *distribution of scores,* which can be represented by a table or graph in which each score is paired with its frequency of occurrence. An illustration of a *frequency distribution* of the hematocrit levels for 50 female patients is shown in Table 3.1. The first column includes scores, that is, the hematocrit values, which are ordered from the highest to the lowest. The sec-

ond column contains the frequencies, that is, the number of patients with each hematocrit value, and clearly displays how many patients had each.

Frequency distributions also can be presented in the form of a histogram. A *histogram* is a bargraph representation of a frequency distribution and makes the shape of the distribution more obvious. Figure 3.1 presents a histogram for the data in Table 3.1. Further discussion of the ways to present frequency distributions is provided in chapter 4.

Distribution Shape

Frequency distributions can occur in various shapes. Because the shape of a distribution provides important information, it is necessary for one to know some of the descriptive terms used to indicate the various shapes. Several common distribution shapes are shown in Figure 3.2. The shape of a frequency distribution can be either symmetrical or asymmetrical. A *symmetrical distribution* is one in which both halves of the distribution are identical in shape. Normal and flat distributions are symmetrical in shape. *Skewed distributions,* that is, distributions in which scores trail off in one direction, are *asymmetrical.*

TABLE 3.1   Frequency Distribution of Hematocrit Values (Scores) for 50 Female Patients

Hematocrit Value or Score	Frequency
48	1
47	1
46	2
45	3
44	6
43	6
42	9
41	7
40	6
39	3
38	2
37	2
36	0
35	2
	$n = 50$

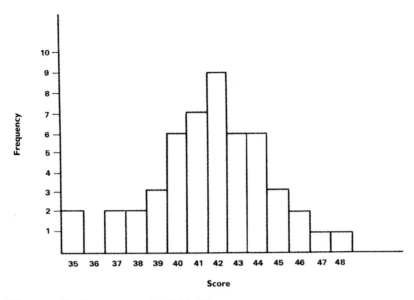

FIGURE 3.1   **Histogram for data presented in Table 3.1.**

A bimodal distribution may be symmetrical or asymmetrical. The extent to which a distribution departs from symmetry is referred to as its degree of *skewness*. The direction of skewness refers to the fact that in some asymmetrical distributions most scores pile up at one end of the scale as far as frequency of occurrence is concerned, while there are fewer scores at the other end. When the frequency of scores is low on the right side of the distribution, it is *positively skewed*. If the frequency of scores is low on the left side of the distribution, then it is *negatively skewed*. Difficult tests or situations in which scores are generally low in a group will result in distributions that are positively skewed. Easy tests or instances in which most scores tend to be high within a group will yield negatively skewed distributions. In instances in which scores occur in the middle range with few scores in the low and high levels, *normal distributions* will result. *Bimodal distributions* will often occur when two distinctly different populations are measured on a selected attribute. For example, if the hematocrit levels of a group of healthy males and females are determined, a bimodal distribution would be likely to result, because males normally have higher hematocrit levels than females. In this case, males and females are actually two different populations, because the variable of interest, that is, hematocrit, is influenced by sex.

In the norm-referenced measurement situation a normal distribution is desirable. A skewed distribution would be expected in a criterion-referenced measurement situation following a specific intervention or treatment. The theoretical basis for the occurrence of these distributions as indicated for each measurement framework is discussed in chapter 4.

The shape of a distribution also may vary in regard to the peakedness of the curve of the distribution as shown in Figure 3.3. *Kurtosis* refers to the peakedness of a distribution's curve.

The curve of a normal distribution, as indicated by curve A in Figure 3.3, is referred to as *mesokurtic* and is used as the standard with which the curves of other distributions are compared to determine their kurtosis. A very peaked slender curve is called *leptokurtic* and is illustrated by curve B. A *platykurtic* curve is flat or broad as shown by curve C. The scores in a leptokurtic curve are closer together, that is, have less variance, than in the normal curve. On the other hand, the scores in a platykurtic curve are more spread out, that is, have more variance, than in the normal curve. If a distribution is bimodal, the kurtosis of each curve is considered separately.

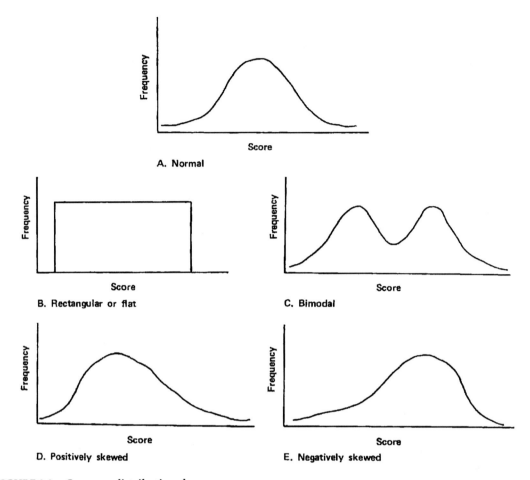

FIGURE 3.2   **Common distribution shapes.**

Measures of Central Tendency

Rarely do all the individual members of a group or population have the same amount of some common attribute. Instead, different objects vary on the attribute of interest. In many instances, one might be interested in the averageness of some specific attribute. For example, one might want to know the average weight and length of a group of newborn infants or the average score on a depression scale for a group of psychiatric clients. The mode, median, and mean are three statistical indices of averageness or central tendency.

The *mode* is the score in a distribution that occurs most frequently. The mode of the scores in Table 3.1 is 9. The mode is determined by inspecting the data to ascertain which score occurs most often. It is the easiest measure of central tendency to calculate.

Occasionally a frequency distribution will have two or more modes rather than one. In some cases more than one score will have occurred at maximum frequency. A distribution in which two scores occur most often is called a bimodal distribution and is illustrated in Figure 3.2. If a distribution has three scores which occur most often, it is referred to as a trimodal distribution.

The *median* is the score value in a distribution above which 50 percent of the scores fall and below which 50 percent of the scores fall. The 50th *percentile* is another label for the median. When a distribution includes an unequal number of scores the median is the middle score. For example, if a distribution included the

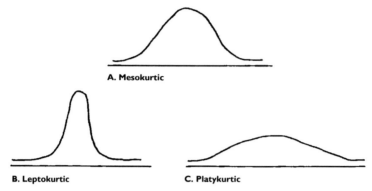

A. Mesokurtic

B. Leptokurtic   **C. Platykurtic**

FIGURE 3.3   Types of kurtosis.

scores 4, 6, 10, 11, 13, 15, and 16, the median would be 11.

Because the median represents the middle score, it may be a value that is not included in the scores in the distribution. This may be the case when the distribution includes an even number of scores. Where there is an even number of scores, the median is calculated in the following manner.

1. The scores in the distribution are arranged from the lowest to the highest value.
2. If no score occurs more than once, the median is the midpoint between the two middle scores. For example, in the case in which the scores are 3, 5, 6, and 8, the median is the midpoint between 5 and 6. Thus:

$$\text{Median} = (5 + 6)/2$$
$$= 5.5$$

3. When tied scores occur, as in Figure 3.4, a frequency tabulation is required.
   a. Determine placement of the median score. In this case the median score is $n/2$ or $40/2$. Hence, the median score will be the 20th score from the bottom of the distribution.
   b. Find the score corresponding to the 20th score.
      (1) The 20th score is located between the score interval from 81 to 85.
      (2) A cumulative frequency of 18 is found in the lower limit of this interval: Thus, $20 - 18 = 2$ points above 18 is required for the 20th score.

(3) The number of frequencies in the interval containing the 20th score is equal to $26 - 18 = 8$ frequencies.
(4) Multiply 2/8 by the width of the interval containing the 20th score, that is, $85 - 81$. Thus $2/8 \times 4 = 1$.
(5) Hence, $81 + 1 = 82$. This is the score equal to the median.

The median has the advantage that its value is not influenced by extreme scores. This makes it a useful measure of central tendency when small samples are used.

The *mean* is the sum of scores in a distribution divided by the number of scores entered into the computation of the sum. A shorthand way to express this definition is presented in Formula 3.1 below.

Formula 3.1: Calculation of mean

$$\bar{X} = \frac{\Sigma X}{n}$$

where $\bar{X}$ = arithmetic mean
Σ = the sum of a series of scores
X = raw score
n = number of scores summed

Example: The mean of 2, 4, 8, 6, 10 is calculated as follows:

$$\bar{X} = \frac{\Sigma X}{n} = \frac{2 + 4 + 8 + 6 + 10}{5}$$

$$= \frac{30}{5}$$

$$= 6$$

SCORE	FREQUENCY	CUMULATIVE FREQUENCY
100	2	40
95	3	38
93	5	35
88	4	30
85	8	26
81	7	18
78	4	12
69	3	7
61	3	4
55	1	1
	$n = 40$	

FIGURE 3.4 **Frequency distribution used for demonstrating computation of median.**

The mean is the balancing point of a distribution. It is the point value where a linear scale would balance as illustrated in Figure 3.5. The more equal the difference between the size of the scores around the mean, the more likely is the mean to be in the center of the scale. However, when extreme scores occur, the mean shifts toward the extreme score away from the middle score on the scale.

The location of the median and mean in a distribution is related to the shape of the distribution. Figure 3.6 illustrates the relationship between the measures of central tendency and the shape of a distribution of scores. The values of the mode, median, and mean are the same in a normal distribution (A). When a distribution is positively skewed (B), the mean is larger than the median and mode, and the mode is the smallest value. In a negatively skewed distribution (C), the opposite occurs; that is, the mean is the smallest value, the median is next, and the mode is the largest.

The mean is usually the preferred measure of central tendency, particularly when large samples are used or when the distribution of scores is nearly symmetrical. The mean also has the greatest stability and can be used for further statistical manipulations. The median is most appropriately used when the distribution shows marked skewness. The mode is best employed in situations in which a rough estimate of central tendency is required quickly or where the typical case is needed. Although these rules are generally appropriate, one should consider each set of data in terms of the specific situation or particular need to determine which measure of central tendency is best to employ.

Dispersion

An important characteristic of any distribution of scores is the amount of spread or scatter among the scores, which is referred to as dispersion. To illustrate this concept further, assume

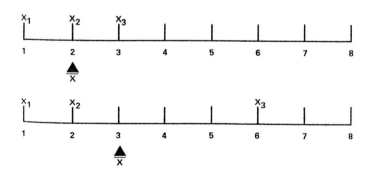

FIGURE 3.5 **Representation of the shift of the mean with extreme scores away from the middle score.**

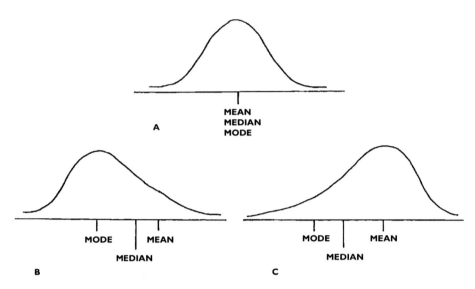

FIGURE 3.6   Relationship between the shape of a distribution and the values of its measures of central tendency.

that fasting blood sugar levels are taken over a 6-month period for two diabetic children. One child has diabetes that is easy to control, and the other has diabetes that is difficult to control. One might obtain distributions of blood glucose levels for the two children similar to the ones shown in Figure 3.7.

Example: Given the infant weights of 6, 10, 8, and 4, with $\overline{X} = 7$ lb.

$$SS_x = (6-7)^2 + (10-7)^2 + (8-7)^2 + (4-7)^2$$
$$= (-1)^2 + (+3)^2 + (+1)^2 + (-3)^2$$
$$= 1 + 9 + 1 + 9$$
$$\sigma_x^2 = \frac{20}{4}$$
$$= 5 \text{ square units}$$

It can be seen from this computational method that the variance is the average of the sum of the squared deviation scores.

Note that the two distributions have means that are equal. However, the spread or dispersion of blood glucose levels for the two children is quite different; that is, the dispersion of the fasting blood glucose levels for the child with diabetes that is difficult to control is more spread out than that of the child with controlled diabetes. The fasting blood glucose levels for the child with easily controlled diabetes are rather consistent and more easily kept within the

normal range with treatment, while the child with difficult-to-control diabetes has fasting blood glucose levels that are sometimes low, sometimes normal, and sometimes high. In other words, the variability of fasting blood glucose levels for the child with difficult-to-control diabetes is greater than those for the child with easily controlled diabetes.

The dispersion of a distribution of scores may be measured by three indices: (1) range, (2) variance, and (3) standard deviation.

The *range* is the distance from the lowest score in a distribution to the highest score. Hence, it is calculated by subtracting the lowest from the highest score. The range is the simplest of the three indices of dispersion and is useful for a quick gross description of a distribution's dispersion. It is limited by the fact that its value is totally dependent upon two extreme scores.

The *variance* and *standard deviation* are based on the deviation of each score in a distribution from the arithmetic mean. A deviation score represents the distance between a subject's raw score and the mean of the distribution. It is calculated by subtracting the mean from the raw score $(X - \overline{X})$. If, for example, infant A weighs 6 lb., infant B, 10 lb., infant C, 8 lb., and infant D, 4 lb., the mean of this distribution of weight is 7 lb. The deviation score, in terms of each infant's weight, is $6 - 7$ or -1 for infant A,

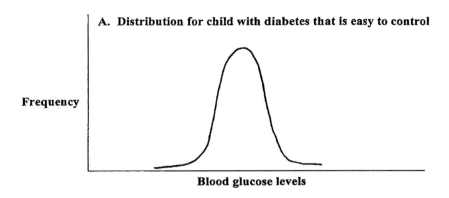

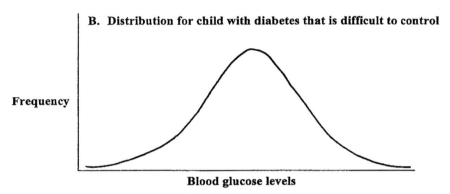

FIGURE 3.7 Hypothetical distributions of fasting blood glucose levels for two children with diabetes.

10 – 7 or +3 for infant B, 8 – 7 or +1 for infant C, and 4 – 7 or –3 for infant D. It should be noted that the sign of the deviation score indicates whether the raw score is above (+) or below (–) the mean. In addition, the sum of the deviation scores in a distribution should always equal zero.

The variance of the distribution of scores may be calculated by using the deviation scores or raw scores. Illustrations of each of these approaches using the example cited above follow.

Formula 3.2: Calculation of variance using deviation scores

$$\sigma_x^2 = \frac{SS_x}{n}$$

where σ_x^2 = variance of the distribution scores

SS_x = the sum of the squared deviation scores

n = the number of scores in the distribution

Formula 3.3: Calculation of variance using raw scores

$$\sigma_x^2 = \frac{\Sigma X^2 - (\Sigma X)^2 / n}{n}$$

where σ_x^2 = the variance of the distribution of scores

ΣX^2 = the sum of the squared raw scores

$(\Sigma X)^2$ = the square of the sum of the raw scores

n = the number of the scores in the distribution

Example

X	X²
6	36
10	100
8	64
4	16
$\Sigma X = 28$	$\Sigma X^2 = 216$

$$(\Sigma X^2) = 28 \times 28 = 784$$

$$\sigma_x^2 = \frac{216 - (784/4)}{4}$$

$$= \frac{216 - 196}{4}$$

$$= \frac{20}{4}$$

$$= 5 \text{ square units}$$

It should be noted that the variance is a square measure rather than linear. To transform a square measure to linear it is necessary to calculate the positive square root.

The *standard deviation* of a distribution of scores is the square root of the variance. Hence, the standard deviation is the linear counterpart of the variance. It is obtained by the following formula.

Formula 3.4: Calculation of standard deviation

$$\sigma_x^2 = \sqrt{\sigma_x^2}$$

where σ_x = standard deviation
$\quad\quad\sigma_x^2$ = variance

Example: The variance of the infant weights of 6 lb., 10 lb., 8 lb., and 4 lb. is 5 square units.

$$\sigma_x = \sqrt{5 \text{ square units}}$$
$$\sigma_x = 2.24$$

The standard deviation is a useful statistic for comparing differences in variability among two or more distributions. For example, if distribution A has a standard deviation of 3, while distribution B has a standard deviation of 5, then one would know that the variability in distribution B is greater than that for A.

The standard deviation also may be thought of as a unit of measurement along the baseline of a frequency distribution. For example, in a normal distribution there are about three standard deviations above the mean and three below. Therefore, the range of the distribution is made up of approximately six standard deviations and all deviations above the mean are positive, and those below the mean are negative. If a distribution has a mean of 20 and a standard deviation of 5, one could divide the baseline into standard units. To do this one would start at the mean and add one standard deviation (5) to the value of the mean (20) to obtain +1 standard deviation, or 25. The raw score 25, then, is exactly one standard deviation above the mean. Likewise, scores that are two and three standard deviations above the mean are 30 and 35, respectively. To determine the value of –1 standard deviation one would subtract one standard deviation (5) from the mean (20) with a result of 15, which is one standard deviation below the mean. The score values for –2 and –3 standard deviations would be 10 and 5, respectively. This is illustrated in Figure 3.8.

The standard deviation is also useful because in normal distributions it is known what percentage of scores lie within specified standard deviations from the mean.

Measures of Correlation

A number of procedures have been developed for assessing the quality of norm-referenced tests and test items that involve the use of the Pearson product-moment correlation coefficient or other measures of linear association. For this reason, Pearson product-moment correlation is discussed to present information necessary for understanding reliability and validity theory and the proper application and interpretation of correlation in measurement contexts.

The linear relationship of two sets of scores can be represented by a *scatterplot* or *scattergram*. Suppose two alternate forms of a 12-item professionalism scale were administered to a group of eight nurses and resulted in scores on the two forms as shown in Table 3.2.

A two-dimensional representation of these scores is presented in the scatterplot shown in Figure 3.9. Although a *scatterplot* provides a good visual illustration of the relationship between two sets of scores, it is often desirable to summarize the extent of this relationship using a numerical index. The statistic most frequently employed to quantitatively summarize scatterplot information is the Pearson product-moment correlation coefficient (r_{xy}). Hence, r_{xy} is a quantitative measure of the linear relationship between two sets of scores. In other words, it measures the extent to which two sets of scores in two-dimensional space follow a straight line trend.

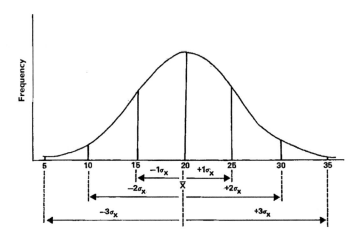

FIGURE 3.8   **Illustration of standard deviation as units along the baseline of normal distribution with a mean of 20 and standard deviation of 5.**

The value of r_{xy} lies between the interval −1.00 to +1.00. If r_{xy} of 1.00 was obtained, it would represent a perfect positive relationship between the two sets of scores and is illustrated by a scatterplot with a line that slopes downward from right to left as shown by scatterplot A in Figure 3.10. If the line slopes downward from left to right, as in scatterplot B, an r_{xy} of −1.00 would result. This represents a perfect negative relationship between the two sets of scores.

If the scores obtained from the same group of subjects on a measure are not perfectly correlated with the scores obtained on a second measure, patterns similar to those shown in scatterplots C and D in Figure 3.10 may occur. Scatterplot C implies that increases in the value of one score (Y) tend to be associated with increases in the value of the other score (X). In scatterplot D, increases in the value of one score (Y) tend to be associated with decreases in the value of the other score (X). In other words, a positive linear relationship indicates that a person who scores high on one measure or test is also likely to score high on the other, and that a person who scores low on one test is also likely to score low on the other. A negative relationship suggests that a person who scores high on one test is likely to score low on the other. When a perfect correlation does not exist it results in a scattering of points away from the straight line which best summarizes the trend. In general, the more widely scattered the points, the closer r_{xy} is to zero.

TABLE 3.2   Hypothetical Scores for Eight Nurses on Alternate Forms of a 12-item Professionalism Scale

Nurse	Score	
	Form A	Form B
A	9	11
B	6	7
C	4	2
D	3	5
E	10	8
F	2	3
G	8	6
H	2	1

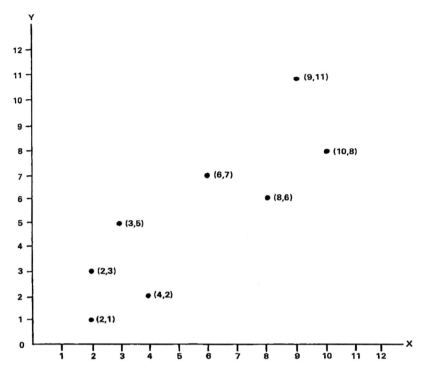

FIGURE 3.9   Scatterplot of scores presented in Table 3.2.

Two types of scatterplot patterns will lead to an r_{xy} of zero (or a value very close to zero): (1) when there is no recognizable pattern in the scatterplots, or (2) when the pattern of the scatterplot is curvilinear, that is, seems to follow a well-defined curve.

An example of the former case is presented in Figure 3.11 in scatterplot A, and an example of the latter case is illustrated by scatterplot B.

When the configuration is an amorphous glob, as in scatterplot A, an r_{xy} value of zero is accurately reflected because there is no useful relationship between the two sets of scores. However, where a curvilinear relationship exists, as illustrated in scatterplot B, an r_{xy} value of zero is very misleading because a useful relationship exists. Statistical indices are available that are appropriate for measuring the degree of curvilinear association between sets of scores, for example, eta (Guilford, 1965).

At this point, attention is given to interpretation of r_{xy}. It is useful to convert r_{xy} to a percentage in order to provide further interpretation. This is done by squaring the r_{xy} value and by changing the result to a percentage. The value that results is the *percentage of explained variance* between two sets of scores. This means that scores obtained from one measure could be used to explain the variance in another measure and vice versa. For example, if the value of r_{xy} is +0.70, then the percentage of explained variance is $r_{xy} = (+0.70)^2 = 0.49$, or 49%. This means that 49% of the variance in the scores from one measure or test would be explained on the basis of the scores from the other measure or test and vice versa.

Potential problems may influence the interpretation of r_{xy}. First, reducing the variability in the distribution of either or both sets of scores (X and/or Y) tends to decrease the value of r_{xy}. This can occur when (1) there is loss of measurement information (e.g., when a nominal level measurement scale is employed rather than a higher level measurement scale), and (2) there is restriction of range in the data, that is, when a homogeneous subset of data points in the scatterplot is used to calculate r_{xy} (Martuza, 1977, p. 76).

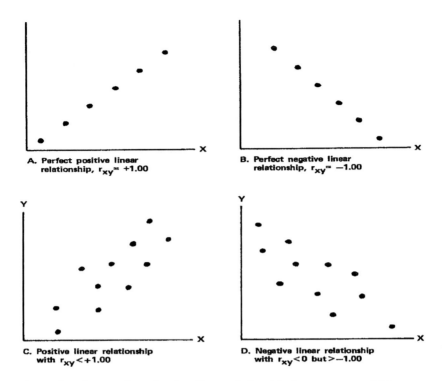

FIGURE 3.10   **Examples of scatterplots of various linear relationships between two variables.**

The effects of restriction of range are illustrated by the scatterplot in Figure 3.12. Suppose the true association between X and Y in a population was as illustrated in Figure 3.12, but r_{xy} was calculated using individuals with scores of 60 or higher on variable X. The value of r_{xy} would be close to zero and, therefore, would misrepresent r_{xy}. This would happen because data points in the included portion of the scatterplot do not exhibit a strong linear trend. In most instances restriction of range will decrease the value of r_{xy}; however, in some instances it may be increased.

The second problem that may be encountered in the interpretation of r_{xy} is that measurement error can affect the value of r_{xy}. Random errors of measurement, that is, factors that can inadvertently increase or decrease the score values obtained from measurement, will distort the value of r_{xy}. When either or both sets of scores have been influenced to a large degree by random error, the true nature of their relationship will be distorted, and so will r_{xy}. The value of r_{xy} may be increased or decreased by random

error of measurement. In most cases, however, a decrease in the value of r_{xy} will result. Random error of measurement is discussed more fully in subsequent sections of this chapter.

The Pearson product-moment correlation coefficient (r_{xy}) can be computed from raw scores in the following manner:

Formula 3.5: Computation of the Pearson product-moment correlation coefficient

$$r_{xy} = \frac{n\Sigma XY - (\Sigma X)(\Sigma Y)}{\sqrt{[n\Sigma X^2 - (\Sigma X)^2][n\Sigma Y^2 - (\Sigma Y)^2]}}$$

where ΣXY = the sum of the products of each person's X and Y scores
(ΣX) = the sum of all X scores
(ΣY) = the sum of all Y scores
n = the number of subjects
ΣX^2 = the sum of all squared X scores
$(\Sigma X)^2$ = the square of the sum of all X scores
ΣY^2 = the sum of all squared Y scores
$(\Sigma Y)^2$ = the square of the sum of all Y scores

Subject	X	Y	XY	X^2	Y^2
A	9	11	99	81	121
B	6	7	42	36	49
C	4	2	8	16	4
D	3	5	15	9	25
E	10	8	80	100	64
F	2	3	6	4	9
G	8	6	48	64	36
H	2	1	2	4	1
	$\Sigma X = 44$	$\Sigma Y = 43$	$\Sigma XY = 300$	$\Sigma X^2 = 314$	$\Sigma Y^2 = 309$

$$(\Sigma X)^a = 1936 \qquad (\Sigma Y)^2 = 1849$$

$$r_{xy} = \frac{n\Sigma XY - (\Sigma X)(\Sigma Y)}{\sqrt{[n\Sigma X^2 - (\Sigma X)^2][n\Sigma Y^2 - (\Sigma Y)^2]}}$$

$$= \frac{8(300) - (44)(43)}{\sqrt{[8(314) - 1936][8(309) - 1849]}}$$

$$= \frac{2400 - 1892}{\sqrt{(2512 - 1936)(2472 - 1849)}}$$

$$= \frac{508}{\sqrt{(576)(623)}}$$

$$= \frac{508}{\sqrt{358848}}$$

$$= \frac{508}{599}$$

$$= 0.85$$

To illustrate the computation of r_{xy}, the scores presented in Table 3.2 will be used. Scores on form A are designated as X, and scores on form B are designated as Y (see above).

If the value 0.85 for r_{xy} is squared, it can then be interpreted to mean that 72% of the variance in X may be explained or predicted on the basis of Y and vice versa. Several variations of r_{yy} can be employed. These coefficients are summarized in Table 3.3. Further information regarding these statistics and their formulas can be found in Kirk (1968), Glass and Stanley (1970), Nunnally (1978), Agresti and Agresti (1979), or Nunnally and Bernstein (1994).

Waltz and Bausell (1981, p. 264) point out that some of the coefficients in Table 3.3, that is phi, r_s, and r_{pb} are equal to r_{xy}, that is, they are simply the product-moment correlation coefficient formula applied to nominal and ordinal data. The remaining coefficients, r_{tet} and r_{bis}, are approximations of r_{xy}.

Now that an introduction to measurement and the basic statistical principles and procedures that undergird measurement has been provided, attention will be given to measurement theory.

MEASUREMENT ERROR AND RELIABILITY AND VALIDITY OF MEASURES

The goal of all measurement is to achieve accurate results. However, this is not completely possible because measurement error, to some extent, is introduced into all measurement procedures. There are two basic types of error that affect the precision of empirical indicators: random error and systematic error.

Random error, also termed *variable* or *chance error,* is caused by chance factors that confound the measurement of any phenomenon. An important characteristic of random error is that it occurs in an unsystematic manner in all measurement. A measurement tool or method affected by random error will yield empirical indicators that will sometimes be higher and sometimes lower than the actual magnitude of the attribute measured. Assume that a nurse takes a patient's oral temperature six times during the course of a day. Also assume that on two measurement occasions the temperature is taken with the patient breathing through the mouth

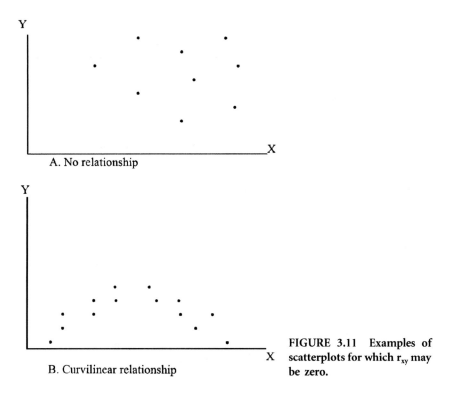

A. No relationship

B. Curvilinear relationship

FIGURE 3.11 Examples of scatterplots for which r_{xy} may be zero.

and on another measurement occasion the temperature is taken immediately after the patient has taken several sips of hot coffee. This is an example of random error because the tempera-

ture readings would sometimes be lower and sometimes higher than the patient's actual body temperature as a result of the introduction of various factors into the measurement

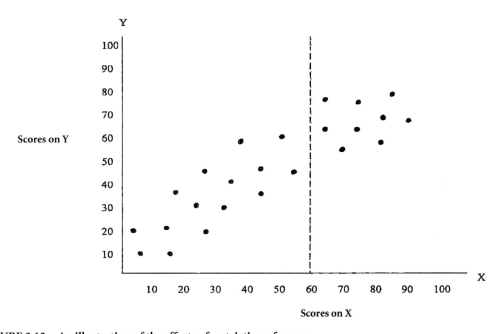

FIGURE 3.12   An illustration of the effects of restriction of range.

TABLE 3.3   Coefficients for Use With Various Types of Data*

		Variable X		
		Nominal	**Ordinal**	**Interval or Ratio**
Variable Y	Nominal	PHI (ø) CONTINGENCY (C) TETRACHORIC (r_{tet})	CURETON'S RANK BISERIAL (r_{rb})	BISERIAL (r_b, r_{bis}) POINT BISERIAL (r_{pb})
	Ordinal	CURETON'S RANK BISERIAL (r_{rb})	SPEARMAN RHO (P, r_s) KENDALL'S TAU (τ)	TAU (τ)
	Interval or Ratio	BISERIAL (r_b, r_{bis}) POINT BISERIAL r_{pb})	TAU (τ)	PEARSON PRODUCT MOMENT (r_{xy})

*From Waltz & Bausell, 1981.

procedure which result in errors of measurement. Even if there were no fluctuations in the patient's true body temperature, the temperature readings obtained from measurement to measurement would not be consistent. Therefore, random error primarily affects the reliability, that is, the consistency of measurements, and consequently validity as well, because reliability is a necessary prerequisite for validity. However, one should recognize that this does not mean that the validity of measures is not affected at all by random error. The introduction of error always affects the validity of specific measures to some degree.

Systematic error, the second type of error that affects empirical measurements, has a systematic biasing influence on measurement procedures. Suppose a patient's thermometer always registers 0.4°F higher than the actual temperature. This is an example of systematic error because repeated temperature readings taken with this thermometer would always be 0.4°F higher than it really should be. A systematic increase of 0.4°F would always be introduced into the results. Hence, the extent to which the thermometer measures what it purports to measure, that is, temperature, is compromised.

Given the above information about the occurrence of random and systematic error, a central question arises about how one can determine the extent to which a given tool or method measures the concept under consideration. Stated in different terms, how well do the results of a measuring procedure represent a given concept? For instance, how can one evaluate the extent to which an instrument designed to measure nursing professionalism accurately represents that concept? Reliability and validity of empirical measurements are two basic aspects of measurement that can be used to examine these questions. The occurrence of random error in measurement procedures is the central threat to the reliability of the measurement. In a similar manner, the validity of a measurement is more threatened by the occurrence of systematic error.

Reliability and Random Error

The reliability of a measurement method is directly influenced by random error. There is an inverse relationship between the amount of random error introduced into measurement and the reliability of the measurement. The higher the reliability of the measurement, the less random error is introduced into the measurement procedure. A large amount of random error decreases the reliability of the measurement.

A measurement tool is reliable for a particular subject population to the extent to which it yields consistent results on repeated measurements of the same attribute. Because reliability refers to the consistency or stability of empirical indicators from measurement to measurement, it naturally follows that empirical indicators obtained from any measurement procedure are reliable to the extent that they are free of random errors. Because sets of measurements of the same attributes for the same objects or events will never exactly duplicate each other, unreliability in measurement is always present to some extent. Thus, the reliability of a measure is a matter of degree. While the amount of random error may be large or small, it is always present. If the random error is large, then the consistency of empirical indicators that result from repeated measurements will be poor and reliability will be compromised. If, however, there is only a small amount of random error, the stability of empirical indicators on repeated measurements will be high and reliability will be high. Stated in different terms, the more consistent and stable the results obtained from repeated measurements, the higher the reliability of the measurement procedure, but the less consistent and more variable the results, the lower the reliability.

The occurrence of random error is a common problem that affects the reliability of any measurement procedure. The following illustrations should clarify how random error is introduced into measurement procedures. First, suppose three nurses are given the task of independently measuring the height of two adult patients to the nearest 1/8 inch on the same day using the same method. It is probable that there will be noticeably different measurements of height obtained by these nurses as long as they are unaware of each other's results. Since height is not likely to change in the same day, obviously discrepancies between findings must be due to measurement errors. You can probably think of a number of chance factors that could influence the results, for example, (1) factors resulting from individual differences in patients, such as height of hair, (2) factors resulting from differences in the nurses' instructions to patients during the procedure, such as instructing patients to stand tall without slumping the back, or (3) differences in the nurses' procedure such as location or placement of the measuring tape on the patients' heads.

Similarly, suppose a nurse takes the same patient's blood pressure twice with the patient lying in a recumbent position in a relaxed manner at a 1-minute interval. It is likely that the two blood pressure readings will vary somewhat without any actual change in the patient's blood pressure. Differences in noise level in the room could affect auditory acuity during the repeated readings. Other factors that could affect the final results are variations in the nurse's eye level in relation to the column of mercury in the sphygmomanometer during readings and differences in the speed at which the blood pressure cuff is deflated on successive measurements.

In both of these examples, certain factors influenced the measurement procedure, which affected the results obtained. In each illustration, if random error had not occurred one could expect error-free results and results would have been the same across measurements. This is not the case in reality. A very important point should be made. Fluctuations in measurement results that occur due to random error do cancel each other out if many independent measurements are made. "They do not directly influence the meaning of the measurement but do directly affect the precision with which the characteristic of interest is being measured" (Martuza, 1977, p. 9). For example, if the heights of 20 adults were measured repeatedly for 3 days in succession, one would not expect each person's height to be precisely duplicated on repeated measurements. However, one would expect that the person who was the tallest on the first day would be among those measured the tallest on the second and third days. Although each person's height would not be exactly the same from measurement to measurement, it would tend to be consistent in relation to the heights of others in the group.

There are numerous sources of random error. Some examples are (1) the manner in which a measure is scored or coded, (2) characteristics or state of the subject or respondent (such as attention span, anxiety, or illness), (3) chance factors affecting the administration or appraisal of measurements obtained (such as fatigue of observers, different emphasis placed on different words by an interviewer, the amount of heat or lighting in the room, or luck in the selection of answers by guessing), and (4) characteristics of the measurement tool or method such as type of items employed in constructing a test or the parameters of a mechanical instrument.

Validity and Systematic Error

In addition to being reliable, it is desirable for a measurement procedure to be valid. Any measurement tool or method is valid to the degree that it measures what it purports to measure. Hence, an empirical indicator of a particular nursing concept is valid to the extent that it successfully measures the intended concept. For example, a rating scale designed to measure maternal behavior would be valid to the extent that it actually measures maternal behavior rather than reflects some other phenomenon.

As noted above, the validity of a specific measurement tool or method is influenced by the degree to which systematic error is introduced into the measurement procedure. There is an inverse relationship between the degree to which systematic error is present during a measurement procedure and the extent to which the empirical indicator is valid. The more systematic error is included in the measure, the less valid the measure will be, and vice versa. Therefore, validity is a matter of degree just as reliability is a matter of degree. The goal of obtaining a perfectly valid empirical indicator that represents only the intended concept is not completely achievable. As previously noted, systematic error causes independent measurements obtained by the same tool or method to be either consistently higher or lower than it ought to be. This clearly presents a problem with validity because there is a common systematic bias in all results obtained by the tool or method, which influences the extent to which the attribute of interest is actually measured.

To illustrate the impact of systematic error on the validity of a measurement, suppose that an oxygen analyzer has an error in calibration so that it consistently registers the percentage of oxygen two points below the actual percentage of oxygen. Even though variations in the concentration of oxygen in a premature infant's isolette would be reflected in repeated measurements, each measurement would be 2 percentage points below the actual level due to systematic error in the measuring device, the oxygen analyzer. The effect is that a constant—2 percentage points—would be subtracted from the value that would be obtained if the oxygen analyzer were properly calibrated. An inference about the absolute concentration of oxygen in the isolette would be invalid.

Similarly, if a measurement procedure that was designed to measure only nausea also measures anxiety, then this would present a problem of validity. The measurement procedure would not be a totally valid measure of nausea because it simultaneously measures anxiety. Thus, systematic bias has been introduced into the results, which do not accurately measure the concept of interest. However, this bias would be included in all measurements obtained with the tool.

There are a number of biasing factors that can contribute to systematic error in measurement. Usually the sources of systematic error are associated with lasting characteristics of the respondent or subject, the measurement tool or method, and/or the measuring process. The sources of systematic error do not fluctuate from one measurement situation to the next as is the case with random error. Examples of systematic sources of error associated with the respondent or subject are chronic illness, test-taking skills, a negative attitude toward completing questionnaires or taking tests, and a poor comprehension of language used in the questionnaire or test items. Characteristics of measurement tools that may systematically bias measurements are the inclusion of items that measure knowledge, skills, or abilities that are irrelevant to the concept being measured, and poor calibration of a measuring device. Another source of systematic error may be the measurement process itself; for example, observer or scorer bias (such as an observer's tendency to rate slim individuals higher than heavy individuals on items related to physical activity).

By now it should be clear that measurement error is central to questions related to reliability and validity. Any tool or method is relatively reliable if it is affected to a minimal extent by random measurement error. Even though high reliability of a measuring instrument is a laudible goal, measures that are reliable are only a portion of the answer to measurement concerns. It is also important that a tool or method be valid for the purposes for which it is used. Systematic error biases the degree to which an indicator measures what it is supposed to measure by reflecting some other phenomenon. Hence, validity is enhanced by the degree to which systematic error is kept to a minimum. While reliability focuses on the consistency of performance of the measure, validity is more of a theoretically oriented issue because it focuses on the crucial relationship between the concept and it's empirical indicator (Carmines & Zellar, 1979).

Two important points should be made about the relationship of reliability and validity. First, a measurement procedure can be highly reliable but have low validity. Consistency of results does not necessarily mean that a tool effectively measures the concept that it is used to measure. Second, a measurement procedure that has low reliability when the measurement situation remains constant cannot have an acceptable degree of validity. As noted by Jennings and Rogers (1989), if a study uses an unreliable outcome measure, the results are not meaningful because it is not possible to know what the independent variables are predicting. The presence of large random error compromises the extent to which an empirical indicator represents the concept it is supposed to measure. Therefore, reliability is a necessary but not sufficient condition for validity.

CLASSICAL MEASUREMENT THEORY

The preceding section examined measurement error and related it to the concepts of reliability and validity. This section presents a discussion of classical measurement theory, which is a model for assessing random measurement error. As noted previously, random error is present in the measurement of any phenomenon. The basic tenet of classical measurement theory evolved from the assumption that random error is an element that must be considered in all measurement. The underlying principle of this theory is that every observed score is composed of a true score and an error score. The true score is the true or precise amount of the attribute possessed by the object or event being measured. The error score reflects the influence that random error has on the observed score. The basic formulation of classical measurement theory is as follows:

Formula 3.6: Classical measurement theory

$$O = T + E$$

where O = observed score
T = true score
E = error score

This equation simply indicates that every *observed score* that results from any measurement procedure is composed of two independent quantities: a *true score*, which represents the precise score that would be obtained if there were no random errors of measurement; and an *error score*, which represents the contribution of random measurement error that happens to be present at the time the measurement is taken.

Consider the following examples as illustrations of true- and error-score components of the observed score. Suppose a nurse attempts to take the pulse of a patient for 1 minute and misreads the second hand on her watch. She counts the patient's pulse rate for 64 seconds rather than the intended 60 seconds, thereby increasing the patient's actual pulse rate of 82 (the true score) to 88 (the observed score). According to Formula 3.6, the error score in this instance is +6 beats, since this is the discrepancy between the patient's true pulse and observed pulse.

$$O = T + E$$
$$88 = 82 + (+6)$$

Suppose that the random error had been in the other direction and the nurse counted the patient's pulse rate for only 58 seconds rather than the intended 60 seconds. Although the patient's actual pulse rate was 82 (the true score), the observed pulse rate was 78 (the observed score). Therefore, the error score in this case is –4.

$$O = T + E$$
$$78 = 82 + (-4)$$

It should be noted that in reality one does not know the true score and the error score values. Only the observed score is known. The above examples are for the purpose of illustration only. Formula 3.6 assumes that the object or event being measured possesses a specific amount of the attribute of interest when the measurement is taken. The precise amount of the attribute is obscured because of the random error, which either increases or decreases the results. The influence of the random error on the observed measurement is called the *error of measurement*. Classical measurement theory assumes that the observed score which is obtained when a measurement is taken is a combination of the true score and the error of measurement. The implication of this assumption is that systematic errors become part of the true score and affect validity but not reliability.

True scores are conceived to be unobservable quantities that cannot be directly measured. When an attribute is measured, the true score is assumed to be fixed. If it were possible for the true score to remain constant while the attribute of interest was measured an infinite number of times, variability in observed scores would result from the impact of random error of measurement that would occur by chance when each measurement was taken. Random disturbances in the observed score due to random error means that some observed scores would be higher than the true score, while other observed scores would be lower than the true score. Classical measurement theory assumes that the mean of error scores is zero and that the correlation between the true score and error score is zero. Therefore, distributions of random error can be expected to be normally distributed; hence, the distribution of observed scores would be normally distributed. The effects of random error can be expected to cancel each other out if many independent measures of the same attribute of an object or event are made and averaged. An average or arithmetic mean of observed scores would be the true score. A hypothetical dispersion of observed scores about the true score is illustrated in Figure 3.13.

The more widely dispersed observed scores are around the true score, the larger is the error

of measurement. If the true score were known and could be subtracted from each observed score, the results would be a set of deviation scores, which would be the errors of measurement. Since the true score is considered fixed and the dispersion of observed scores is due to errors of measurement, subtraction of true scores from observed scores would result in a normal distribution of error scores (errors of measurement) (Figure 3.14). The standard deviation of this distribution of error scores would be an index of the amount of measurement error. This standard deviation of error scores is termed the *standard error of measurement*.

If it were possible to have a measurement procedure that was perfectly reliable, the observed score and the true score would be the same. There would be no error of measurement and, therefore, no error score. In such a case the standard error of measurement would equal zero. The more reliable a measurement procedure is, the smaller will be the standard error of measurement. The less reliable the measurement procedure, the larger the standard error of measurement. The size of the standard error of measurement is an indicator of the amount of error involved in using a particular measurement procedure.

Observed Score Variance

If a large number of persons were measured with respect to the same attribute, the observed scores would not be the same. This is true because there would be real differences in the amount of the attribute possessed by different individuals, and because there would be differences in the effects of random error on each observed score. Since each person's observed score is composed of true-score and error-score components, three different score distributions

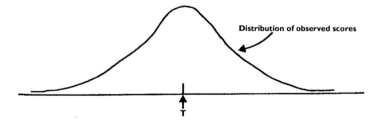

Distribution of observed scores

FIGURE 3.13 The true score and hypothetical distribution of observed scores for a person at a specific point in time.

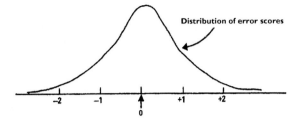

Distribution of error scores

FIGURE 3.14   Hypothetical distribution of errors of measurement.

would result: (1) a distribution of the observed scores, (2) a distribution of true scores, and (3) a distribution of error scores. Figure 3.15 illustrates these distributions of scores. Each person's observed, true, and error scores (e.g., for individuals J and L) are represented in each of the three distributions.

Remember that true scores and error scores are not observable. Only the values of the observed scores are known. Classical measurement theory assumes that the correlation between the true score and error score is zero. If this is the case, the following formula holds.

Formula 3.7: Basic variance formula

$$\text{Var (O)} = \text{Var (T)} + \text{Var (E)}$$

where (O) = variance of the observed-score distribution, also noted as σ_o^2
Var (T) = variance of the true-score distribution, also noted as σ_T^2
Var (E) = variance of the error-score distribution, also noted as σ_E^2

This basic variance formula holds only when true scores and error scores are not correlated; that is, when the true score cannot be used to predict the error score and vice versa.

The Statistical Definition of Reliability

Formula 3.7 can be converted to illustrate the statistical definition of reliability. In order to do this, each term in Formula 3.7 is divided by Var (O). The result is as follows:

$$\text{Var (O)} = \text{Var (T)} + \text{Var (E)}$$

$$\frac{Var(O)}{Var(O)} = \frac{Var(T)}{Var(O)} + \frac{Var(E)}{Var(O)}$$

Formula 3.8: Statistical definition of reliability and unreliability

$$1.00 = \frac{Var(T)}{Var(O)} + \frac{Var(E)}{Var(O)}$$

Note that Var(O)/Var(O) is equal to one. The expression Var(T)/Var(O) is the *statistical definition of reliability*. It is representative of the proportion of variation in the observed score distribution that results because of true-score differences among respondents or subjects. The second ratio in Formula 3.8, Var(E)/Var(O), is the *statistical definition of unreliability*. It is a representation of the proportion of variation in the observed-score distribution that is due to random errors of measurement. A *variance ratio* is equivalent to a squared Pearson r (coefficient of correlation). Therefore, Var(T)/Var(O) may also be written as $r_{(T,O)}^2$, which is the squared correlation of true scores with observed scores. The second ratio, Var(E)/Var(O), may be written as $r_{(E,O)}^2$, which is the squared correlation of error scores with observed scores. Thus, $r_{(T,O)}^2$ is also a statistical representation of reliability and is termed the reliability coefficient. Similarly, $r_{(E,O)}^2$ is a statistical representation of unreliability.

The square root of the reliability coefficient is the correlation between observed scores and true scores for a test or measure. This is usually called the test's *reliability index*. Since a reliability coefficient is conceptually a squared value, the statistic used to estimate it empirically is never squared in practice. Reliability also can be expressed in terms of error variance. Referring to Formula 3.8:

$$1.00 = \frac{Var(T)}{Var(O)} + \frac{Var(E)}{Var(O)}$$

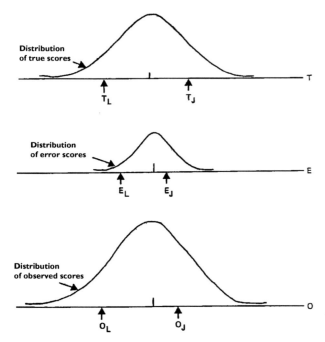

Distribution of true scores

T_L T_J T

Distribution of error scores

E_L E_J E

Distribution of observed scores

O_L O_J O

FIGURE 3.15 Distributions of true scores (T), error scores (E), and observed scores (O) for a population of persons measured for the same attribute.

If Var(T)/Var(O) were transposed to the left side of the equation and 1.00 to the right side, it can be seen that:

Formula 3.9: Reliability of observed score as a measure of score

$$\frac{Var(T)}{Var(O)} = 1.00 - \frac{Var(E)}{Var(O)}$$

Hence, the reliability of the observed score (O) as a measure of the true score (T) is equal to 1.00 minus the error variance. It is obvious then that the reliability of a measure varies between 0 and 1. If the observed score is highly contaminated with random error, then the reliability is decreased and becomes closer to zero. Conversely, if only a small amount of random error occurs in the measurement of a phenomenon, the reliability increases and is closer to 1.00. Reliability coefficients provide an indication of the significance of interindividual differentiation in observed scores. If a reliability coefficient is high, then more credence can be given to interindividual differences in observed scores. A low reliability coefficient reduces the credibility. The variance of error of measurement indicates intraindividual variability in the person's observed score due to the introduction of random error when the measurement was taken (Stanley, 1971, p. 373). When the variance of error of measurement is large, this means that a large amount of random error was introduced into individual scores.

If a nursing instructor used an achievement test with an estimated reliability of 0.85 to test students' knowledge of surgical nursing, this would indicate two things. First, 85 percent of the variance in the distribution of observed scores is due to actual differences in knowledge among the nursing students tested. Second, the remaining 15 percent of variance in the observed score distribution resulted from random errors of measurement, for example, misinterpretation of items or guessing.

The derivation of the statistical definition of reliability for a distribution has been shown. However, it is optimal to compute the reliability coefficient directly with at least two observed scores per subject. When the observed score is a composite of more than one part of a measure, then the consistency among several parts can be examined and a reliability estimate obtained. For example, if a test contained two or more items, one could study how scores on items of the test covary with each other and determine the consistency of the test.

Two conceptual models that have evolved from classical measurement theory are commonly used for the discussion of measurement error: (1) the model of parallel measures, and (2) the domain-sampling model. Both are basic models for the computation of reliability coefficients.

The Model of Parallel Measures

This model purports to determine a measure's reliability by correlating parallel measurements. It is assumed that two measures of the same thing are parallel if (1) they have the same correlation with a set of true scores, (2) variance in each measure that is not due to true scores is strictly the result of random error of measurement, and (3) they have the same standard deviation. For example, if two tools designed to measure depression are parallel, they would yield the same true scores when used in the same measurement situation. The differences in the observed scores on the measures would be due only to random error. Since random errors tend to cancel each other out, the standard deviations reflect true score variance. The model of parallel tests assumes that the correlation between any two tests of a domain is a complete and precise determination of the reliability coefficient rather than only an estimate. A major limitation of this model is that it disregards the fact that reliability cannot be precisely determined by sampling of items in a content domain.

Nunnally (1978, p. 203) points out that the model has limitations because it offers a conceptual dead end for the development of theories of measurement error since true scores are defined by only two tests. He contends that if there are three supposedly parallel tests rather than two, and the three correlations among them are different, what then is the reliability? Since the model explicitly assumes that all parallel tests have the same reliability, one is faced with a dilemma. However, this is not a problem for the domain-sampling model with which this possibility is admitted, and an estimate of the reliability of any one measure is the average of its correlations with other measures.

The Domain-Sampling Model

The domain-sampling model considers any measure to be composed of a random sample of items from a hypothetical content domain which it purports to measure. According to this model, if a 50-item test was designed to measure knowledge of pulmonary physiology, it could be considered to consist of a random sample of 50 items from a domain of all possible items which could test knowledge in this content area. A number of other tests could also be devised by randomly sampling the same domain. Each of the tests that would result from sampling the same domain would have somewhat different means, standard deviations, and correlations because of random error in the sampling of items. Tests or measures composed of items randomly taken from the same content domain are considered randomly parallel tests.

The domain-sampling model indicates that the goal of any measure is to estimate the score a person would obtain if examined on all possible items within the content domain. The score that an individual would obtain if it were possible to be measured with a test composed of all possible items from a domain would be the true score. This is sometimes referred to as the *domain score*. In reality, it is not possible to obtain a domain score. In most instances there are an infinite number of items in a content domain. It also is difficult to randomly sample a domain. Most test items are constructed for each specific measure. However, actual applications of the domain-sampling model do result in accurate predictions.

According to the domain-sampling model, the extent to which any sample of items from the domain is correlated with the true score is an indication of its reliability. If a sample of items has a low correlation with the true score or domain score, then the reliability also would be low. Conversely, a high correlation between a sample of items from the domain and the true score means that the reliability of the sample is high. The domain-sampling model is applicable regardless of the number of items in the sample. Reliability estimates can be obtained if there is only one item in the item sample, or if there are many items.

The only assumption of this model is that the average correlation of each item with all the others in the domain is the same for all items. The degree to which items in the domain measure the same attribute would be indicated by the average correlation of items in the domain. The wider the dispersion of correlations of items about this average, the less likely that the items in the domain measure a common attribute. When the average correlation of items in the domain is zero or close to zero, the items do not have a common element and do not measure one attribute. It is, therefore, desirable for item correlations in the domain to be relatively homogeneous, positive, and greater than zero. When item correlations in the domain are more homogeneous, reliability estimates are more precise. The degree of variance in the correlations among items in the domain is a reflection of random error connected with the average correlation for a particular sampling of items. Errors that would cause variation from item to item, such as guessing, would reduce item correlations and thereby reduce reliability.

Thus far, the discussion of the domain-sampling model has primarily focused on the correlations of single items in the domain. However, these concepts can be extended to whole tests as well. It was noted earlier that this model views tests as consisting of a random sample of items from a content domain. A number of tests generated from the same domain using random selection of items would be considered randomly parallel tests. Each would have means, standard deviations, and correlations with true scores that would differ by chance only. If it were possible to randomly select test items from the domain, the average correlation of a single test with a number of other randomly parallel tests would be an estimate of the average correlation of the test with all other tests in the domain. Conceptually, this would result in the reliability for the tests.

Since the whole test is a summation of its items, the average correlation among whole tests will be larger than the average correlation among items. This will result in higher correlations with true scores for the whole test. The domain-sampling model assumes that the reliability of scores obtained on a sample of items from the domain increases as the number of items sampled from the domain increases (Nunnally & Bernstein, 1994, pp. 230–233). Therefore, longer tests have higher reliability coefficients than shorter tests. However, Nunnally (1978, p. 208) noted that tests with as few as ten items may have rather precise reliability.

On initial examination the model of parallel measures and the domain-sampling model appear quite different. However, Nunnally (1978) notes that the model of parallel measures is a special case of the domain-sampling model. Whereas the basic assumptions of the parallel-measures model result in a specification of a characteristic of measurement error, the domain-sampling model estimates the same characteristic. Any formula obtained from the parallel-measures model can be matched by a formula from the domain-sampling model, which is based on estimation. However, the reverse does not hold. There are many principles and formulas emanating from the domain-sampling model that cannot be provided for by the model of parallel tests.

The model of parallel measures and the domain-sampling model are the best-known conceptual approaches to measurement. Both have evolved from classical measurement theory and have proved to be useful and understandable approaches to the discussion of measurement error. Generalizability theory is another model that deals more fully with the various sources of measurement error and further extends classical measurement theory. The following section presents the central concepts of generalizability theory.

AN INTRODUCTION TO GENERALIZABILITY THEORY

Generalizability theory is an extension of classical measurement theory that is usually employed to analyze the effects of different measurement conditions on the psychometric properties of an instrument or measurement method (Embretson & Hershberger, 1999, p. 3). Generalizability theory (Cronbach, Glesser, Nanda, & Rajaratnam, 1972; Nunnally & Bernstein, 1994), or G theory as it is sometimes called, provides a framework for examining the dependability of behavioral measurements (Shavelson, Webb, & Rowley, 1989). Whereas classical measurement theory partitions score variance into two components (that is, true-score variance and error variance), generalizability theory acknowledges the multiple sources of measurement error by deriving estimates of each source separately. This approach provides a mechanism for optimizing estimates of reliability. The reliability coefficient that is derived is called a "generalizability coefficient."

A fundamental notion of generalizability theory is that a score's usefulness depends on the degree to which it allows one to generalize accurately to some wider set of situations, *the universe of generalization.* One's *universe score* would be the person's mean score over all acceptable observations and would be the best information on which to base decisions about the person's behavior. Instead of focusing on how accurately observed scores reflect their corresponding true scores, generalizability theory is concerned with how well-observed scores permit us to accurately generalize about an individual's behavior in a defined universe of situations (Shavelson, Webb, & Rowley, 1989). "The question of 'reliability' thus resolves into a question of accuracy of generalization, or generalizability" (Cronbach, Glesser, Nanda, & Rajaratnam, 1972, p. 15).

Generalizability theory allows error components in a measurement to be identified and their magnitude estimated. The researcher who is concerned about the quality of measurement

can systematically manipulate certain facets of error, control others, and ignore still others. In a manner similar to the ANOVA (analysis of variance) design, the researcher can isolate sources of error, called "facets," and the levels of the facets, called "conditions." The sources of error depend on the measurement design and procedure. Examples of sources could be raters, forms, items, occasions, and their interactions. Table 3.4 illustrates the decomposition of an observed score in generalizability theory for a design in which raters and items are sources of error.

Analysis of variance procedures can be used to estimate variance components within the design. Only a single source of error, that is, raters or items, can be calculated at a time. However, variance components are calculated for each source of error. For example, if raters are considered the source of error, the score for each person by each rater would be summed over items. Mean squares are provided by the ANOVA for persons and the residual (person x rater interaction confounded with random error). Variance components can be estimated from the mean squares. The degree to which each facet contributes to measurement error is indicated by the magnitude of the variance components. From these estimated variance components specific formulas can be used to calculate a generalizability coefficient that is analogous to a reliability coefficient (Shavelson, Webb, & Rowley, 1989; Nunnally & Bernstein, 1994).

The nature of the decisions to be made with the data is also considered in generalizability

TABLE 3.4   Decomposition of an Observed Score in Generalizability Theory*

Decomposition of Observed Score[†]	Definition
$X_{pri} = u$	Grand mean
$\quad + u_p - u$	Person effect
$\quad + u_r - u$	Rater effect
$\quad + u_i - u$	Item effect
$\quad + u_{pr} - u_p - u_r + u$	Person x rater effect
$\quad + u_{pi} - u_p - u_i + u$	Person x item effect
$\quad + u_{ri} - u_r - u_i + u$	Rater x item effect
$\quad + $ residual	p x r x i, error

*Adapted from Shavelson, Webb, & Rowley, 1989.
[†]Note: p = person; i = item; r = raters; u = constant.

theory. A distinction is made between relative decisions and absolute decisions. In *relative decisions* the focus is on the dependability of the differences among individuals or the relative standing of individuals that results from the measurement procedure. Error components in relative decisions are due to variance associated with the rank ordering of individuals other than the component that is the focus of measurement. *Absolute decisions* are based on the observed score, which reflects the performance of the individual without regard to the performance of others. In this case, error is defined as all variance components associated with a score, except for the component for the object that is the focus of measurement.

In generalizability theory two types of studies are done related to the assessment of measurement error-generalizability studies (G) and decision (D) studies. A G study is primarily concerned with estimating the magnitude of as many potential sources of measurement error as possible and is concerned with the extent to which a sample of measurements generalizes to a universe of measurements. The universe of a G study is usually defined in terms of a set of measurement conditions based on a set of sample measurements obtained. Often this universe is more extensive than the conditions under which the sample was obtained. In G studies all facets that are likely to enter into the generalizations of a diverse group of users are systematically studied. Examples of G studies include studies concerned with the stability of scores over time, the internal consistency or interrelationship of items on a scale or subscales on a scale, and the equivalence of two alternative forms of a measure or tool. Often, the purpose of a G study is to help plan a D study that will have appropriate generalizability (Crocker & Algina, 1986; Nunnally & Bernstein, 1994).

A D study is designed and conducted for the specific purpose of making a decision, such as describing examinees for placement or selection, comparing groups of subjects in an experiment, or investigating the relationship between two or more variables (Crocker & Algina, 1986). "D studies use information from a G study to design a measurement that minimizes error for a particular purpose" (Shavelson, Webb, & Rowley, 1989, p. 923). D studies may have facets that are either fixed or random. If facets are fixed, then the investigator should generalize the results only to those fixed conditions included in the D study. However, when random facets are selected to be included in the study, the investigator can reasonably assume that the conditions in the D study are a sample from a larger number of conditions, and can generalize to all of these latter conditions.

In general, a G study is conducted when a measurement procedure is being developed, while a D study employs the measurement procedure for a specific purpose. Therefore, G studies should be as fully crossed as possible and incorporate all possible facets and variance components. The results from a well-developed and well-designed G study can provide information upon which the generalizability for a wide variety of nested D study designs can be estimated (Shavelson, Webb, & Rowley, 1989). For a full discussion of the specific approaches to the development and implementation of G studies and D studies, see Crocker and Algina (1986), Fyans (1983), and Nunnally and Bernstein (1994).

AN INTRODUCTION TO ITEM RESPONSE THEORY

Item response theory (IRT) is an approach to constructing cognitive and psychological measures that usually serves as the basis for computer adapted testing. In classical measurement theory an attribute is assessed on the basis of responses of a sample of subjects or examinees to the set of items on a measure. Hence, it focuses on test performance. IRT, on the other hand, focuses on item performance and the examinees ability, i.e. predicting how well an examinee or group of examinees might perform when presented with a given item. IRT differs from classical measurement theory with regard to how items are selected for inclusion in a measure and in how scores are interpreted.

IRT is based on two basic premises: (1) an examinee's test performance can be predicted or explained by a set of factors referred to as traits, latent traits, abilities, or proficiencies; and

(2) the relationship between examinees item performance and the set of abilities underlying item performance can be described by a monotonically increasing function called an item characteristic function or *item characteristic curve* (ICC). This curve graphically illustrates that as the level of the ability increases, so does the probability of a correct response to an item (Hambleton, Swaminathan, & Rogers, 1991; Isaac & Michael, 1995). Thus, IRT provides direction for a method of test construction that takes into account item analysis and selection, and a measurement scale for reporting scores.

Isaac and Michael (1995) note that the probability of a person correctly answering a test item is a function of two attributes: (1) the *person attribute* that can be any trait of interest but usually refers to "ability," "achievement," and "aptitude." It is the amount of the trait possessed by the person to correctly answer a certain number of items like the ones on the test, and (2) the *item attribute* that refers to the *difficulty level,* defined as the point on the ability scale where the person has a fifty percent chance of answering the item correctly. The estimate of these two attributes, person ability and item difficulty, is referred to as *calibration* (pp. 119–120). Assumptions underlying IRT include unidimensionality, item independence, equal item discrimination, and no guessing.

Unidimensionality implies that one dominant ability influences test performance or, equivalently, that only one ability is measured by the items that make up the test. It is assumed that items can be arranged in order of difficulty along a single continuum such that the examinees performance on these items can be represented by a single score that is on the same continuum as the items. Thus, different items should be answered correctly by examinees with high ability more often than examinees with low ability.

Item independence, also referred to as *local independence* means that when ability influencing test performance is held constant, examinees' responses to any pair of items are statistically independent. For an examinee of given ability, a response to one item is independent of a response to any other item. Thus, a correct response to one item cannot depend on a correct response to any other item.

Equal item discrimination assumes that items represent equal units when summed to yield a total score.

No guessing assumes that no one correctly guesses an answer. When low ability examinees guess correctly on difficult items, the unidimensionality assumption is not tenable. (Wright & Shaw, 1979; Hambleton, Swaminathan, & Rogers, 1991; Isaac & Michael, 1995).

Many possible item response models exist that vary in the mathematical form of the item attribute function and/or the number of parameters specified in the model. All IRT models contain one or more parameters describing the item and one or more parameters describing the person (examinee). The most popular unidimensional IRT models are the one-, two-, and three-parameter models. These models are appropriate for dichotomous item and response data. The Rasch (1960) *one-parameter logistic model* is the most frequently employed. In this model, items differ only in their difficulty. It is assumed that the only item characteristic that influences examinee performance is item difficulty. Person ability and item difficulty are measured on the same scale, therefore items and persons can be directly related. The ICCs in this case differ only by their location on the ability scale. It is assumed that examinees of very low ability have zero probability of correctly answering the item and no allowance is made for guessing. Figure 3.16 presents a simplified example of an ICC for two items for the one parameter model. The ICC for the three items in Figure 3.16 indicates that item 1 requires a higher level of ability to answer correctly with probability .50 than items 2 and 3.

In the *two-parameter logistic model* developed by Lord (1952) and modified by Birnbaum (1968, 1969), items differ in their difficulty and discrimination. *Item discrimination* is defined by the slope of the ICC. Items with steeper slopes are more useful for separating examinees into different ability levels than are items with less steep slopes. The two-parameter model, like the Rasch model, makes no provision for guessing. Figure 3.17 presents a simplified example of a two-parameter model. In Figure 3.17 the slopes for items 1 and 3 indicate

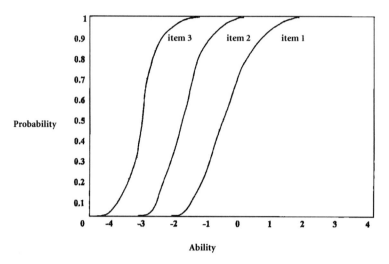

FIGURE 3.16   One-parameter ICC for three items.

they are better able to discriminate among examinees than is item 2. In terms of difficulty, item 2 tends to be the more difficult item (i.e., to answer with probability of .70 requires a higher level of ability as compared with items 1 and 3).

In the *three-parameter logistic model,* items differ in their difficulty, discrimination, and proneness to being answered correctly due to guessing. An ICC, in this case, graphically represents the probability of an examinee getting an item correct

as a function of ability. It reflects the difficulty, discrimination, and proneness to guessing of the item. Figure 3.18 presents a simplified example of an ICC for the three-parameter model. In Figure 3.18, the third parameter, proneness to guessing, is illustrated by item 3, where the probability of respondents with low ability answering the item correctly is .25 as compared with items 1 and 2, where the probability is 0. The three-parameter logistic model also is exemplified in the work of

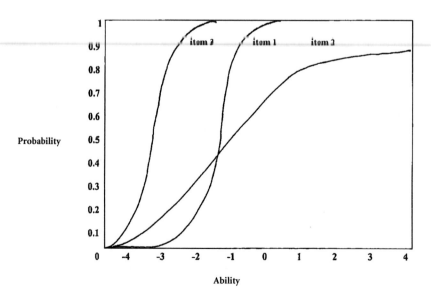

FIGURE 3.17   Two-parameter ICC for three items.

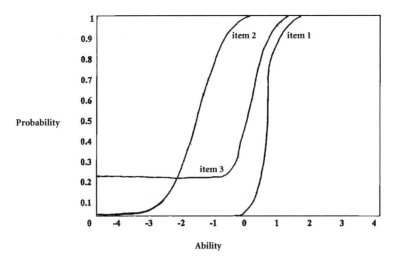

FIGURE 3.18   Three-parameter ICC for three items.

Lord (1968), who performed an analysis of the verbal scholastic aptitude test using Birnbaum's three-parameter logistic model.

The first step in any IRT application is to estimate these parameters. *Item calibration* involves the evaluation of the fit of the item difficulty parameter. *Test calibration* involves the evaluation of the fit of the person abilities to the model and the estimation of the ability parameter corresponding to each test score.

When IRT is employed, the traditional concept of reliability is replaced by the *concept of information*. Examinee interactions with items yield information about their ability. More information means more precise estimates. Information increases as item difficulty approaches examinee ability. For the one- and two-parameter logistic models, maximum information is obtained when item difficulty equals examinee ability. Item information also increases as item discrimination increases. Information increases as the guessing parameter decreases. Item information is additive. Item information functions may be added together to obtain a *test information function* or an *item pool information function*.

An IRT model is usually chosen in one of two ways: (1) by choosing the model with the fewer item parameters that fits the test data adequately, or (2) by choosing the model and then selecting the test items to fit the chosen model.

Checking model data fit usually involves evaluating the assumptions of IRT, unidimensionality, equal discrimination, (Rasch model) and minimal guessing (Rasch and two-parameter models). For example, using data from two samples of examinees an ICC graph can be constructed to compare item difficulty based on Sample 1, with item difficulty based on Sample 2. Expected model features can also be evaluated by comparing invariance of examinee ability parameter estimates and invariance of item parameter estimates. The relative fit of different models can be compared to determine if one model fits significantly better than another model and/or if model predictions of actual data and simulated test results can be compared. Isaac and Michael (1995) noted that while the IRT model continues to gain in use, the two greatest challenges for users are its complex mathematical foundation that makes it extremely difficult to understand and/or explain to nontechnical audiences and emerging problems regarding the underlying assumptions and their empirical validation (p. 121). Readers interested in a more advanced discussion of IRT are referred to Crocker and Algina (1986), Hambleton, Swaminathan, and Rogers (1991), and Embertson and Hershberger (1999). Item response theory is discussed in chapter 23 as it is applied to computer-based testing.

SOURCES OF VARIANCE IN SCORES

There are many sources of variation in scores obtained from measurement. In previous sections of this chapter, a discussion of random and systematic sources of error emphasized how error variance can affect the reliability and validity of measures. The goal of measurement is to obtain measurements in such a manner that variance resulting from error is kept to a minimum. It is desirable that variance reflected in scores be due to actual differences in score values.

Score Variance

For the most part, variance within a set of scores for a group of individuals occurs because different persons manifest different amounts of the attribute of interest. It should be kept in mind that the importance of the reliability coefficient for a measure is that it reflects the proportion of the variance in scores due to true differences within the particular population of individuals on the variable being evaluated. Therefore, it is desirable that measures be constructed and used so that they will be sensitive to real variations in true scores of individuals. The size of variation in true scores between persons is primarily determined by two factors: (1) the frequency of correct or appropriate responses to items, and (2) the correlations between the individual items. A measure will be most sensitive to real differences between persons when variance of the individual items is greatest—that is, when the probability of a correct response is 0.5 for any item chosen at random from the domain. When test items are either too easy or very difficult, score variance between individuals will be small, because such items do not adequately distinguish variations in the attribute of interest. This also is true for measures such as opinion questionnaires and attitude scales that have no correct answers. Each individual can be perceived as having a set probability of either agreeing or disagreeing with each statement. If statements are constructed in such a manner that true differences in opinions or attitudes are not elicited, then variations in scores will be small. True score variance also will be increased when the correlations between items in the domain are large and when the number of items in a measure is large.

It is desirable for measurements to have true score variance, particularly in the norm-referenced case. The magnitude of reliability coefficients depends upon the dispersion of true scores between individuals. Restriction of the range of variability is likely to lower the reliability of a measure in the manner noted earlier in the discussion of measures of correlation.

Error Variance Within a Set of Scores

Error variance within a set of scores obtained on a specific occasion occurs for many reasons. For any measure, error variance due to such factors as general ability to comprehend instructions, test taking skills, and shrewdness in guessing is likely to affect scores. This type of systematic error results from lasting characteristics of each individual and results in stable individual differences in scores. Other such sources of systematic error include familiarity of the subject with test format, the nature of items, and level of comprehension of words, formulas, and generalizations that must be applied to correctly respond to certain items. Temporary characteristics of the individual can result in random error. Fatigue, emotional strain, and condition of the testing environment could result in an inability to concentrate, inadvertent skipping of items, misreading of items, and fluctuations in memory. Differences in standards and approaches to scoring would reduce correlations among items and thereby reduce reliability estimates. Errors in scoring could be assessed within a test if scoring errors tended to reduce correlations among items.

Variations in Scores Between Measurements

In some instances two randomly parallel tests are administered either simultaneously (during one testing period) or at short (e.g., 2-week) intervals. If the attribute of interest is such that there should not be noticeable variations for individuals tested, then the correlation between the two sets of scores should be nearly perfect. This may not be the case, however. Sets of scores on randomly parallel tests, also termed alternative forms, may not be highly correlated for three major reasons.

First, randomly parallel tests may not be truly parallel. There may be actual differences in the content of the two tests. The domain-sampling model envisions that randomly parallel tests are composed of items randomly selected from the same content domain. Since this is not possible in reality, some tests that are developed as parallel measures of an attribute may not be really parallel. Some aspects of the content domain may receive more emphasis in one test than the other, or one test may be constructed in such a manner that the use of certain words or terminology is emphasized more than in the other measure. The correlation between scores on the two tests might be lower because of these differences.

A second reason that variation may occur between measurements is because the conditions under which the tests were administered are markedly different and thereby influence the scores. Different environmental conditions such as a very hot room or noisy distractions may be present at one testing situation and not at the other. Temporary factors that can affect performance have already been discussed. If an entire group of people were tested together on both occasions under markedly different conditions, then the effect could be that a number of people in the group would have quite different observed scores on the two testing occasions. This would decrease the correlation between scores.

A third factor that might lessen correlations of scores between measurements is differences in scoring from one occasion to another. The use of different criteria for scoring either by the same scorer or two or more different scorers might result in somewhat different scores for the same person. This is particularly likely to happen when one scorer or rater is used on one occasion and a different scorer or rater is used on a subsequent occasion. However, even when a single scorer is used, rater drift can occur over time and the scorer can use different rating criteria without realizing that this is the case. For this reason, when raters are used in research studies it is advisable to periodically assess intrarater and/or interrater reliability and retrain raters if indicated.

The Reliability of Change Scores

In some cases, it is desirable to determine the reliability of change scores, such as when one is considering a pretest and a posttest to determine whether there has been a change in the amount of a specific attribute of interest. In such an instance, the change score would be the posttest score of a subject minus the pretest score. To illustrate, suppose a nurse wants to determine if the level of preoperative patient anxiety for a group of patients will decrease after a planned patient-teaching program is given. A state anxiety measure is used to measure patient anxiety prior to the teaching program, and patient anxiety after the patient-teaching program is completed. The raw change score of each patient would be the difference between his posttest and pretest scores. How will the nurse know if any changes that are exhibited are reliable?

One should keep in mind that errors of measurement previously discussed that could increase or decrease both sets of observed scores may have a significant impact on change scores, resulting in an interpretative problem. The obtained difference score equals true-score difference plus error-of-measurement difference. Although the posttest score minus pretest score seems to be the best way to measure change, it is not the best estimator of true change. Errors of measurement that are present in the pretest and posttest measurement procedures can seriously affect the difference score. Two commonly discussed problems associated with the measurement of change are the reliability of the difference score and the systematic relationship between measures of change and initial status.

The reliability of difference scores depends upon the variance and reliability of the pretest, corresponding values for the posttest, and the correlation between the pretest and the posttest scores. When the correlation between the pretest and posttest is high, the difference-score reliability tends to be low. For example, for a pretest and posttest with a common variance and a common reliability of 0.80, the reliability of the difference scores would be 0.60, 0.50, 0.33, and 0.00 when the pretest-posttest correlations were 0.50, 0.60, 0.70, and 0.80, respectively (Linn, 1979, p. 4). Hence, for the measurement of change, the lower the correlation between pretest and posttest scores, the higher the reliability of the measure of change. However, this fact creates a dilemma because the low correlation reduces confidence that one is measuring the same thing on each occasion.

The second problem frequently encountered with difference scores is that they generally are correlated with pretest scores. This is a disadvantage because a goal in the use of difference scores often is to compare the gains of individuals or groups that started with unequal pretest scores by removing initial differences. The problem arises from the fact that the sign of the correlation between the difference and pretest scores depends upon the variances of the pretest and posttest. Where the variances for the pretest and posttest are equal, a negative correlation is to be expected. In this case, persons or groups with low pretest scores will tend to have higher gains than those with high pretest scores, and the initially lower scoring group has a built-in advantage. On the other hand, if the posttest variance is substantially larger than the variance for the pretest, the correlation between the difference score and the pretest will be positive rather than negative. Where the correlation is positive, there is a built-in advantage to the group scoring higher on the pretest when comparisons are made in terms of simple difference scores (Linn, 1979, p. 5). Given the problems associated with using difference scores for the measurement of change, several alternatives have been offered: (1) residualized change scores, (2) estimated true-change scores, and (3) standardized change scores.

Residualized change scores have come into use because of the desire to obtain gain scores that are uncorrelated with initial status or pretest scores. However, they are not true measures of change (Cronbach & Furby, 1970). They are measures of whether a person's posttest score is larger or smaller than the predicted value for that person. Residualized change scores

are based on the assumptions of classical test theory regarding true-score and error-score components of observed scores and involve using the linear regression of the posttest on the pretest in order to determine predicted values (Nunnally & Bernstein, 1994). Major limitations to using residualized change scores are that they can be used only with measures taken at two points in time, and they are not really growth measures or change scores.

Estimated true-change scores are corrected measures of change. Cronbach and Furby (1970), as well as several other authors, have described procedures for estimating true change. They require estimates of reliability for the pretest and posttest for the sample involved. This is viewed as a major drawback of this approach, because good reliability estimates for the sample often are not available (Linn, 1979).

The use of standardized change scores has been suggested as an alternative to raw difference scores by Kenny (1975). Standardized change scores simply are difference scores that have been standardized. This means that difference scores have been converted so that score distributions have means of zero and unit variances. Hence, standardized change scores will have a negative correlation with initial status or pretest scores, because they are based on pretest and posttest scores with variances that have been set equal.

Further information regarding the alternatives to using raw change scores can be found in Burckhardt, Goodwin, and Prescott (1982), Cronbach and Furby (1970), Kenny (1975), and Nunnally and Bernstein (1994). Specific alternatives to the measurement of change have advantages and disadvantages. Selection of an alternative approach should depend upon the nature of the study and the purposes for which change is to be measured. Since change scores are fraught with problems, we discourage their use and encourage the selection of alternative approaches to measurement whenever possible.

SUMMARY

This chapter presented the basic principles of statistics and measurement theory. Measurement is a process that employs rules to assign numbers to phenomena. The rules for assigning numbers to phenomena have been categorized hierarchically as either nominal, ordinal, interval, or ratio. The numbers that result from measurement are referred to as scores. The use of statistical procedures facilitates a better understanding of groups of numbers by providing numerical summaries of scores or data.

A distribution of scores may be described by its shape, measures of central tendency, and dispersion. A distribution's shape may be symmetrical or asymmetrical. The extent to which a distribution departs from symmetry is referred to as its degree of skewness. The peakedness of a distribution is referred to as kurtosis. The mode, median, and mean are three statistical indices of the central tendency of a distribution of scores. The dispersion or amount of spread of a distribution is indicated by its range, variance, and standard deviation. The range is the distance from the lowest to the highest score in a distribution. The variance and standard deviation represent the amount of scatter among the scores within a distribution. The Pearson product-moment correlation coefficient (r_{xy}) is a statistic often used to summarize the relationship between scores within two separate distributions.

Whenever a measurement is obtained, error is introduced into the results to some degree. The two types of error of measurement are random error and systematic error. Random error results from chance factors that affect measurements, and systematic error arises from factors within the measuring tool, measurement process, or subject. Random error primarily influences the reliability of measurements, while systematic error primarily influences the validity of measurements.

Classical measurement theory is a model for assessing random measurement error. It purports that every observed score consists of a true score, which is the precise amount of an attribute possessed by an object, and an error score, which reflects the influence of random error. The model of parallel measures and the domain-sampling model are two approaches to reliability based on classical measurement theory. The model of parallel measures purports to determine reliability by correlating parallel measurements. The domain-sampling model

provides for an estimate of reliability by an average of item correlations within the measure. Generalizability theory is an extension of classical measurement theory that takes into account the multiple sources of measurement error. It provides for the derivation of a generalizability coefficient, which indicates how accurately one can generalize the results of measurement to a specified universe. Item response theory is an approach to constructing cognitive and psychological measures that usually serves as the basis for computer adapted testing. Item response theory focuses on item performance and the examinees ability unlike classical measurement theory that focuses on test performance.

Variation in scores between measurements is due to actual changes in the true score, or to variation in the amount of error introduced into measurements. It is problematic to use posttest minus pretest difference scores to assess change in true scores, because there is a systematic relationship between measures of change and the initial status or pretest, and the reliability of difference scores may be compromised by psychometric properties of the pretest and posttest. Alternative approaches to the measurement of change include residualized change scores, estimated true-change scores, and standardized change scores.

REFERENCES

Agresti, A., & Agresti, B. F. (1979). *Statistical method for the social sciences.* San Francisco: Dellen.

Arnold, J. M. (1988). Diagnostic reasoning protocols for clinical simulations in nursing. In O. L. Strickland & C. F. Waltz (Eds.), *Measurement of nursing outcomes* (Vol. 2, pp. 53–76). New York: Springer Publishing.

Arnold, J. M. (2001). Diagnostic simulations and instruments. In C. F. Waltz & L. S. Jenkins (Eds.), *Measurement of nursing outcomes* (2nd ed.), (Vol. 1, pp. 3–32). New York: Springer Publishing.

Birnbaum, A. (1968). Some latent trait models and their use in inferring an examinee's ability. In F. M. Lord & M. R. Novick (Eds.),

Statistical theories of mental test scores (pp. 397–479). Reading, MA: Addison-Wesley.

Birnbaum, A. (1969). Statistical theory for logistic mental test models with a prior distribution of ability. *Journal of Mathematical Psychology, 6*(2), 258–276.

Burckhardt, C. S., Goodwin, L. D., & Prescott, P. A. (1982). The measurement of change in nursing research: Statistical considerations. *Nursing Research, 31*(1), 53–55.

Carmines, E. G., & Zellar, R. A. (1979). *Reliability and validity assessment.* Beverly Hills, CA: Sage Publications.

Crocker, L., & Algina, J. (1986). *Introduction to classical and modern test theory.* New York: Holt, Rinehart & Winston.

Cronbach, L. J., & Furby, L. (1970). How we should measure "change": Or should we? *Psychological Bulletin, 74,* 68–80.

Cronbach, L. J., Glesser, G. C., Nanda, H., & Rajaratnam, N. (1972). *The dependability of behavioral measurements: Theory of generalizability of scores and profiles.* New York: Wiley.

Embretson, S. E., & Hershberger, S. L. (Eds.) (1999). *The new rules of measurement.* Mahwah, NJ: Lawrence Erlbaum Associates.

Fyans, L. J., Jr. (Ed.) (1983). *Generalizability theory: Inferences and practical applications.* San Francisco: Jossey-Bass.

Glass, G. V., & Stanley, J. C. (1970). *Statistical methods in education and psychology.* Englewood Cliffs, NJ: Prentice-Hall.

Guilford, J. P. (1965). *Fundamental statistics in psychology and education* (4th ed.). New York: McGraw-Hill.

Hambleton, R. K., Swaminathan, H., & Rogers, H. J. (1991). *Fundamentals of item response theory.* Newbury Park, CA: Sage.

Hymovich, D. P. (2003). The coping scale of the chronicity impact and coping instrument. In O. L. Strickland & C. Dilorio (Eds.), *Measurement of nursing outcomes* (2nd ed.) (Vol. 3, pp. 88–100). New York: Springer Publishing.

Isaac, S., & Michael, W. B. (1995). *Handbook in research and evaluation* (3rd ed.). San Diego, CA: EDITS.

Jennings, B. M., & Rogers, S. (1989). Managing measurement error. *Nursing Research, 38*(3), 186–187.

Kenny, D. A. (1975). A quasiexperimental approach in assessing treatment effects in the nonequivalent control design. *Psychological Bulletin, 82,* 345–362.

Kirk, R. E. (1968). *Experimental design: Procedures for the behavioral sciences.* Monterey, CA: Brooks/Cole.

Linn, R. L. (1979). *Measurement of change.* In Educational Evaluation Methodology: The State of the Art. Second Annual Johns Hopkins University National Symposium on Educational Research, Baltimore, Maryland.

Lord, F. M. (1952). *A theory of test scores.* Psychometric Monograph No. 7. Iowa City, IA: Psychometric Society.

Lord, F. M. (1968). An analysis of the verbal scholastic aptitude test using Birnbaum's three-parameter logistic model. *Educational & Psychological Measurement, 28*(4), 989–1020.

Marsh, G. W. (2003). Measuring patient satisfaction outcomes across provider disciplines. In O. L. Strickland & C. Delorio (Eds.), *Measurement of nursing outcomes* (2nd ed.) (Vol. 2, pp. 243–257). New York: Springer Publishing.

Martuza, V. R. (1977). *Applying norm-referenced and criterion-referenced measurement in education.* Boston: Allyn & Bacon.

Nunnally, J. C. (1978). *Psychometric theory* (2nd ed.). New York: McGraw-Hill.

Nunnally, J. C., & Bernstein, I. H. (1994). *Psychometric theory* (3rd ed.). New York: McGraw-Hill.

Rasch, G. (1960). *Probabilistic models for some intelligence and attainment tests.* Chicago: MESA Press.

Shavelson, R. J., Webb, N. M., & Rowley, G. L. (1989). Generalizability theory. *American Psychologist, 44,* 922–932.

Stanley, J. C. (1971). Reliability. In R. L. Thorndike (Ed.), *Educational measurement* (2nd ed.). Washington, DC: American Council on Education.

Stevens, S. S. (1946). On the theory of scales of measurement. *Science, 103,* 677–680.

Stevens, S. S. (1951). Mathematics, measurement, and psychophysics. In S. S. Stevens (Ed.), *Handbook of experimental psychology* (pp. 1–49). New York: Wiley.

Stevens, S. S. (1958). Problems and methods of psychophysics. *Psychological Bulletin, 55*(4), 177–196.

Stevens, S. S. (1960). Ratio scales, partition scales, and confusion scales. In H. Gulliksen & S. Messick (Eds.), *Psychological scaling: Theory and applications.* New York: Wiley.

Waltz, C. F., & Bausell, R. B. (1981). *Nursing research: Design, statistics, and computer analysis.* Philadelphia: F.A. Davis.

Wells, N. (2003). Measuring distress during painful medical procedures: The distress checklist. In O. L. Strickland & C. Delorio (Eds.), *Measurement of nursing outcomes* (2nd ed.) (Vol. 2, pp. 187–195). New York: Springer Publishing.

Wright, B. D., & Shaw, M. H. (1979). *Best test design.* Chicago: MESA Press.

Part II

Understanding Measurement Design

4

Strategies for Designing Measurement Tools and Procedures

As noted in chapter 1, the two major frameworks for measurement are the norm-referenced and criterion-referenced approaches. This chapter focuses on the design and interpretation of each of these types of measures. *Norm-referenced measures* are employed when the interest is in evaluating a subject's performance relative to the performance of other subjects in some well-defined comparison group. How well a subject's performance compares with the performance of other subjects is irrelevant when a criterion-referenced approach is used. *Criterion-referenced measures* are employed when the interest is in determining a subject's performance relative to a predetermined set of target behaviors. For this reason, different strategies are used when designing norm-referenced and criterion-referenced measures.

DESIGNING NORM-REFERENCED MEASURES

Essential steps in the design of a norm-referenced measure are (1) selection of a conceptual model for delineating the nursing or health care aspects of the measurement process; (2) explication of objectives for the measure; (3) development of a blueprint; and (4) construction of the measure, including administration procedures, an item set, and scoring rules and procedures. Since selection of a conceptual model is addressed in chapters 1 and 2, the focus here will be on steps 2 through 4.

Explicating Objectives

The first step in the design of any measure is to clarify the purposes for the measurement. When a conceptual model serves as a basis for the tool's development, this step is more easily undertaken than when it does not. For example, suppose an investigator is interested in assessing a geriatric patient's ability to perform activities of daily living (ADL) upon admission to an assisted living facility. Using self-care theory, activities of daily living are conceptually defined as the patient's capacity to perform various physical (body care) tasks that permit the individual to provide self-care on a daily basis. Further, it is assumed that (1) body care tasks essential in everyday life are related to eating, dressing, bathing, toileting, transfer, walking, and communication; (2) the concept of self-care is not an absolute state but a continuum of ability levels that vary in the frequency with which the help of others is needed; and (3) the geriatric patient's level of ability in performing certain activities of daily living may differ from the same individual's level of ability in performing other activities.

On the basis of this conceptual definition of ADL self care, the investigator is directed to operationalize ADL self-care in the following manner: (1) use a performance-objective type of measure, most appropriately, observation; (2) include in the measure multiple items reflecting salient characteristics or conditions related to each of the identified body care activities essential in every day life; and (3) provide a way for respondents to demonstrate various levels of ability to provide self-care with and without the help of others.

Hence, the objective for the measure is this: Given a series of ADL tasks, the geriatric patient newly admitted to an assisted living facility will demonstrate the frequency with which he/she can perform those tasks, i.e., eating, dressing, bathing, toileting, transfer, walking, and communicating, alone or with the help of others. It should be apparent that this objective derives from, and is consistent with, the conceptual definition of ADL self-care, it defines the relevant domain of content to be assessed by the measure as the geriatric patients' performance of specific and varied ADL activities, and it specifies the type of behavior the subject will exhibit to demonstrate that the purpose of the measure has been met, that is, the frequency with which he/she is able to perform the behavior with and without the help of others. To meet this objective, the investigator looks to the conceptual framework as well as empirical findings from studies defining ADL self-care in a similar manner to identify and list a number of

behaviors salient to the measurement of the geriatric patients' ability to eat, dress, bathe, toilet, transfer, walk, and communicate. This preliminary list is then subjected to scrutiny by experts in ADL for geriatric patients living in assisted living facilities who may add and/or delete behaviors. Each of these behaviors then becomes an item on the measure. Hence, each item included in the measure should be linked to the conceptual definition; that is, items that do not relate directly to the objective for the measure are superfluous and, if included, will tend to decrease validity.

To assess the level of ADL self-care, the investigator employs a five-point rating scale of the frequency with which the geriatric patient requires help from others ranging from never (0) to always (4). A portion of the resulting measure of ADL self-care is illustrated in Figure 4.1. It should be apparent from this hypothetical example that objectives provide the link between theories and concepts and their measurement. Additional examples of this linkage can be found in Waltz and Jenkins (2001) and Strickland and Dilorio (2003a, b). Not only is it

---

Directions: Rate the frequency with which the geriatric patient required help from others in performing ADL during the first week of being admitted to an assisted living facility using the following scale:

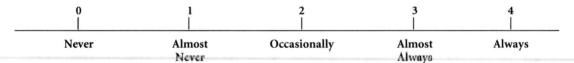

0	1	2	3	4
Never	Almost Never	Occasionally	Almost Always	Always

Place your rating in the blank space next to the item.

Rating	ADL Activity*
_____	Pour liquids
_____	Hold cup or glass
_____	Drink from cup or glass
_____	Open food containers
_____	Hold fork and spoon
_____	Cut food
_____	Raise food to mouth
_____	Place food in mouth, chew, and swallow

*ADL included here are limited and intended only to exemplify a few of the many activities relevant to a geriatric patient in an assisted living facility.

FIGURE 4.1 **A hypothetical sample measure of geriatric patients' performance of ADL in an assisted living facility.**

important to explicate objectives, but it is also paramount that they be stated correctly. A poorly stated objective can be more troublesome than no stated objective. For this reason, attention now turns to approaches for writing objectives that have gained favor with use.

Behavioral objectives are usually stated by using one of two approaches. The first approach is best characterized by the work of Mager (1962). In this view an objective has essentially four components: (1) a description of the respondent; (2) a description of the behavior the respondent will exhibit to demonstrate the accomplishment of the objective; (3) a description of the conditions under which the respondent will demonstrate accomplishment; and (4) a statement of the standard of performance expected to indicate accomplishment. This format for writing objectives is particularly useful when constructing measures of cognition, especially in a criterion-referenced framework, because it forces one to explicate clearly the standard of performance expected prior to the construction of items. It should be noted, however, that its use is not limited to cognitive, criterion-referenced measures and that it has utility as well when constructing measures of affect and performance in a norm-referenced framework. Figure 4.2 illustrates Mager's approach to the formulation of an objective for measuring the performance of a pediatric nurse practitioner student in a pediatric ambulatory care center.

The second approach reflects the views of scholars like Tyler (1950) and Kibler, Barker, and Miles (1970). Although similar to Mager's approach, a behavioral objective in this case is composed of only three components: (1) a description of the respondent; (2) delineation of the kind of behavior the respondent will exhibit to demonstrate accomplishment of the objective; and (3) a statement of the kind of content to which behavior relates. This approach to objective explication is quite useful within a norm-referenced measurement context because it results in an outline of content and a list of behaviors that can then be readily used in blueprinting. Blueprinting is discussed in the next section of this chapter. Figure 4.3 illustrates the same objective written according to the Tyler-Kibler scheme. An example of use of Tyler's (1950) approach to behavioral objectives can be found in Howard (2001).

A *taxonomy* is a useful mechanism for defining the critical behavior to be assessed by an objective in such a manner that all who use the same taxonomy or classifying scheme will assess the same behavior in the same way, thus increasing the reliability and validity of measurement. Numerous taxonomies have been proposed for the cognitive, affective, and psychomotor domains. Attention here will focus briefly on those that have gained favor through empirical use: (1) Bloom's (1956) taxonomy of the cognitive domain; (2) Krathwohl, Bloom, and Masia's (1964) taxonomy for the affective

---

Objective: Given a well child newly admitted to the pediatric ambulatory care center, the PNP student will perform a comprehensive physical assessment as outlined in the center's standards-of-care procedure manual.

Component	Example
1. Description of respondent	PNP student
2. Description of behavior to be exhibited if objective is accomplished	Perform a comprehensive physical assessment
3. Description of conditions under which respondent will demonstrate accomplishment	A newly admitted well child
4. Statement of standard of performance	Perform assessment according to pediatric ambulatory care center standards of care outlined in the procedure manual

FIGURE 4.2   Formulation of an objective to measure performance of a pediatric nurse practitioner (PNP) student using Mager's approach.

Objective: The PNP student performs a comprehensive physical assessment on a newly admitted well child.

Component	Example
1. Description of respondent	PNP student practicing in a pediatric ambulatory care center
2. Description of behavior to be exhibited if objective is accomplished	Perform a comprehensive physical assessment
3. Statement of the kind of content to which behavior relates	An outline of standards of care contained in the center procedure manual was presented to the student in class prior to the PNP's clinical rotation

FIGURE 4.3 Formulation of an objective to measure PNP student performance using the Tyler-Kibler scheme.

domain; and (3) Fitts's (1962, 1964) scheme for the psychomotor domain.

Table 4.1 presents a simplified version of the taxonomy of the cognitive domain. In Bloom's framework, the mental operations are grouped into a small number of simple-to-complex, hierarchically ordered categories: knowledge, comprehension, application, analysis, synthesis, and evaluation. Hence, each subsequent level of mental activity involves the mental operations required at the preceding levels. For example, to be able to analyze, the respondent must first be able to know, comprehend, and apply.

A simplified version of the taxonomy for the affective domain appears in Table 4.2. As with the cognitive taxonomy, levels are hierarchical in nature, and performance at higher levels allows one to assume that the respondent can perform at lower levels as well.

Taxonomies for assessing the psychomotor domain are far less developed than for the other two; however, the approach by Fitts, which is summarized in Table 4.3, shows some promise in this area and is included for this reason. Fitts (1962, 1964) identifies three phases of skill development: cognitive, fixation, and autonomous. Phases overlap to some extent; that is, they are not distinct units—and movement from one phase to another is a continuous process. As a subject proceeds from early to late phases, the performance of the skill becomes progressively more automatic and more accurate, and demands less concerted effort on the part of the subject, allowing attention to be given to other activities concurrently.

From the tables it should be apparent that the use of taxonomies in explicating and measuring objectives provides several advantages. A critical aspect of any behavioral objective is the word selected to indicate expected behavior. A behavioral term by definition is one that is observable and measurable (i.e., behavior refers to any action on the part of an individual that can be seen, felt, or heard by another person). Cognitive and affective objectives, although they are concerned with thinking and feeling, which themselves are not directly observable, are inferred from psychomotor or behavioral acts. In reality, the same behavioral term can be seen, felt, or heard differently by different people. Similarly, since it is impossible to measure every action inherent in a given behavior, different people frequently define the critical behavior to be observed, using a given objective, quite differently. When taxonomies are employed, action verbs and critical behaviors to be observed are specified, hence decreasing the possibility that the behaviors will be interpreted differently and increasing the probability that the resulting measure will be reliable and valid.

A measurement must match the level of respondent performance stated in the behavioral objective; that is, a performance verb at the application level of the cognitive taxonomy must be assessed by a cognitive item requiring the same level of performance. Any discrepancy between the stated objective and the performance required by the instrument or measurement device will result in decreased reliability and validity of the measurement process. For

(text continues on page 93)

TABLE 4.1 A Simplified Version of the Taxonomy of the Cognitive Domain*

Mental Operation Level	Action Verbs	Examples Objective	Examples Measurement	Comments
Knowledge: Measures the subjects' ability to recall or recognize information in essentially the same form as it was presented. The essential learner behavior is remembering.	Action verbs at the knowledge level usually include: Cite Classify Complete Correct Identify Label List Mark Name Read Recall Recite Recognize Show State Tell Write	The newly employed acute care nurse practitioner will cite the hospital standards for performing a comprehensive physical assessment on a newly admitted critically ill adult patient.	*PLC†:* The hospital standards for performing a comprehensive physical assessment are outlined in the procedure manual presented at orientation. *Question:* Cite the hospital standards for performing a comprehensive physical assessment on a newly admitted critically ill adult patient.	This is the lowest level of mental activity. The PLC reflects the information to be acquired by the subjects that is part of the objective stated during the program's development.
Comprehension: Measures understanding at the most rudimentary level, i.e., the subject's ability to use previously acquired information to solve a problem. 1. *Translation:* Ability to paraphrase, present in a different language, or recognize paraphrases or symbolic changes.	Action verbs at the comprehension level usually include: Conclude Convey meaning of Decode Describe in own words Explain Extrapolate Give reasons Illustrate Interpret Reformulate Restate Rewrite	The newly employed acute care nurse practitioner will explain in his or her own words how to perform a comprehensive physical assessment on a newly admitted critically ill adult patient.	*PLC:* During orientation the instructor has explained how a comprehensive physical assessment is performed on a newly admitted critically ill adult patient. *Question:* The orientation instructor assigns subjects to play roles of acute care nurse practitioners and instructor. In a sociodrama the subjects are to act out these roles as explained to them by the instructor.	At this level, the subject must remember the information and use it to solve a novel problem. A key feature at this level is that the item or the context in which it is asked is structured in such a way that the respondent is made aware of the information required to solve the problem. Items are designed to determine whether the learner can solve a novel problem if the information to be used is specified. *(continued)*

TABLE 4.1   A Simplified Version of the Taxonomy of the Cognitive Domain* (Continued)

Mental Operation Level	Action Verbs	Examples			Comments
		Objective	Measurement		
2. *Interpretation:* Measures the subjects' ability to make an inference based on the information in a communication to explain what is meant by the communication or to summarize the information in the communication.	Summarize Tell why Translate	Given a case history of a newly admitted critically ill adult patient and a description of the comprehensive physical assessment performed on that patient, the newly employed acute care nurse practitioner will make conclusions about the patient's status on the basis of the data.	*PLC:* The newly employed acute care nurse practitioner has been taught at orientation to perform a comprehensive physical assessment on a newly admitted critically ill adult patient. The instructor then presents the learner with a case history and a description of a comprehensive physical assessment performed on the patient. *Question:* (True or False) On the basis of the results of the physical assessment, it is evident that the patient has altered mobility.		In Bloom's taxonomy there is a third type of comprehension, which is not dealt with in this simplified version because it is so similar to translation and interpretation. In this simplified version, extrapolation is subsumed under interpretation.
Application: Requires the subjects to use previously acquired information in solving a novel problem. Neither the question nor the context in which it is asked helps the respondents decide what previously acquired information must be used to solve the problem. Questions are aimed at determining whether subjects are able to select the appropriate knowledge	Action verbs at the application level include: Administer Adopt a plan Apply Carry out Compute Demonstrate Employ Make use of Perform Plot Put in action Put to use	The newly employed acute care nurse practitioner will perform a comprehensive physical assessment on a newly admitted critically ill adult patient.	*PLC:* During orientation the instructor has taught the newly employed acute care nurse practitioner to perform a comprehensive physical assessment according to hospital standards. Later in the emergency room, a critically ill patient is admitted and the instructor asks: *Question:* Can you perform a physical assessment on this patient?		Note that if this question were a comprehension item, the instructor would have told the learners to use the procedure for a comprehensive physical assessment outlined in the standards. Application items like comprehension items require the learners to use previously acquired information to solve a novel problem. Unlike the comprehension item, an application item does not

identify for the learners the previously acquired information to be used in solving the problem. Thus, questions at the application level are aimed at determining if the respondents are able to select as well as use knowledge correctly in solving a new problem.

Level description	Action verbs	Instructional objective	PLC example
as well as use it correctly in solving a new problem. *Analysis:* May require the subjects to (1) identify a logical error in a communication (e.g., a contradiction, an error in deduction, an erroneous causal inference) or (2) identify, classify, and/or recognize the relationships among the elements (i.e., facts, assumptions, hypothesis, conclusions, ideas, etc.) in a communication. Items at this level usually assume specific training in a logical process to be used.	Action verbs at the analysis level include: Analyze Arrange in order Combine Compare Contrast Criticize Deduce Designate Detect Determine Distinguish Formulate	After watching a videotape of an experienced acute care nurse practitioner performing a physical assessment on a critically ill adult patient, the newly employed acute care nurse practitioner will list at least five behaviors on the part of the acute care nurse practitioner that may introduce error into the findings and at least five behaviors likely to result in valid conclusions regarding the patient's status.	*PLC:* The newly employed acute care nurse practitioner watches a videotape on strategies and techniques for minimizing errors and maximizing validity of the findings of a physical assessment on a critically ill adult patient. *Question:* List all of the actions taken on the part of the acute care nurse practitioner performing the assessment that are likely to minimize errors and those likely to maximize validity.
Synthesis: Requires the respondent to produce or create: (1) a unique verbal or written communication, or (2) a plan or procedure for accomplishing a particular task.	Action verbs at the synthesis level include: Compose Construct Design Develop Devise Fabricate Form Formulate hypotheses Integrate Propose	The newly employed acute care nurse practitioner will design a procedure for his or her unit to reduce the kind and amount of errors resulting from the nurses' poor performance in conducting physical assessments.	*PLC:* The newly employed acute care nurse practitioner has read extensively regarding the strategies and techniques for maximizing the validity of physical assessments and has participated in staff development programs regarding strategies and techniques for minimizing errors in this regard. *Question:* How can we reduce

(continued)

Understanding Measurement Design

TABLE 4.1 A Simplified Version of the Taxonomy of the Cognitive Domain* (Continued)

		Examples		
Mental Operation Level	Action Verbs	Objective	Measurement	Comments
	Reorganize Restructure		the effect of errors in procedure on the validity of the outcomes of physical assessments performed on this particular critical care unit?	
Evaluation: Requires the subjects to judge the value of ideas, people, products, methods, etc., for a specific purpose and state valid reasons for their judgment (i.e., the learners must state the criteria upon which the judgment is based).	Action verbs at the evaluation level include: Appraise Ascertain value Assay Assess Diagnose Evaluate Fix value of Judge List in order of importance Rank in order of importance	After observing an experienced acute care nurse practitioner perform a physical assessment on a newly admitted critically ill adult patient, the newly employed acute care nurse practitioner will judge the comprehensiveness and accuracy of the results and state the reasons for his or her judgment.	*PLC:* The instructor in staff development demonstrates two contrasting approaches to performing a physical assessment. *Question:* Which do you think is likely to result in the most valid data regarding patient status? State your reasons for choosing the approach that you did.	

*Portions of the material in this table are adapted from Staropoli, C., and Waltz, C. F.: *Developing and Evaluating Educational Programs for Health Care Providers.* FA Davis, Philadelphia, 1978.
†PLC refers to the prior learning condition.

TABLE 4.2 Simplified Version of the Taxonomy of the Affective Domain

Affective Levels	Action Verbs	Examples		Comments
		Objective	Measurement	
Receiving (Attending): Measures the respondent's awareness and/or willingness to receive specified stimuli. Indicates the respondent is capable of directing attention toward specified materials or behavior.	Action verbs at the receiving level include: Accept Attempt Comply Define Identify Limit List Listen Observe Recognize Refrain Reject	The nurse will listen carefully and respectfully to all opinions rendered by the critically ill AIDS patient.	Over time the respondent consistently demonstrates behavior indicating s/he is listening (eye contact, nondirective responses, etc.) respectfully to opinions expressed by the patient with AIDS.	
Responding: Measures the respondent's tendency to respond in a favorable manner to specified stimuli. Response behavior indicates that the respondent has become adequately involved or committed to a specified stimulus. If the respondent consents, seeks, and/or enjoys working with a specified activity, he or she is responding favorably.	Action verbs at the responding level include: Ask Challenge Choose Cite Consult Delay Doubt Hesitate Inquire Offer Query Question Read Repeat Select Try	The nurse will willingly comply with agency suggestions concerning courtesy toward the patient with AIDS.	The respondent seeks out agency suggestions concerning courtesy toward the AIDS patient and performs consistently within agency expectations.	

(continued)

TABLE 4.2 Simplified Version of the Taxonomy of the Affective Domain (*Continued*)

Affective Levels	Action Verbs	Examples		Comments
		Objective	Measurement	
Valuing: Measures reflect that the respondent displays behaviors with acceptable consistency under appropriate circumstances to indicate adoption of a certain value or ideal. In demonstrating the value behavior, the respondent can select from among differing values on specified topics and may demonstrate a high degree of commitment, conviction, or loyalty to the accepted value.	Action verbs at the valuing level include: Consider Display Examine Express Insist Join Participate Persist Practice Pursue Qualify Seek Specify Support Test Undertake Volunteer Weigh	The nurse will voluntarily participate in a hospital-sponsored benefit to raise funds for AIDS research.	The learner volunteers to participate in the benefit and enthusiastically supports the work he or she chooses to undertake.	
Organization: Measures reflect that the learner is able to classify a value concept by (1) determining, comparing, analyzing, comparing its characteristics, and (2) placing all previously	Action verbs at the organization level include: Adapt Analyze Compare Contrast Criticize	The nurse will organize a community-based support group for families of AIDS patients and will incorporate time in his or her weekly schedule to participate in its implementation.	The respondent organizes the group and incorporates time for his or her involvement into a weekly schedule.	

| classified values into a harmonious and ordered relationship, thus building a personal value system. | Deduce
Demonstrate
Designate
Design
Determine
Diagnose
Gather
Identify
Investigate
Order
Organize
Propose | | |
| *Characterization by a Value or Value Complex:* Measures indicate the respondent is able to respond to the complex world and environment about him or her in a consistent, predictable, and comprehensible manner. | Action verbs at the characterization level include:
Construct
Design
Develop
Evaluate
Formulate
Plan
Revise
Synthesize | The nurse will solve problems regarding staff fear or unwillingness to care for the AIDS patient in terms of patient consequences rather than on the basis of rigid principles or emotional feelings. | The respondent consistently solves problems in terms of patient consequences rather than rigid principles or emotional feelings. |

TABLE 4.3 Fitts's Phases of Complex Skill Development

Phase of Development	Objective	Measurement	Comments
		Examples	
1. *Cognitive:* Measures indicate that the subject tends to intellectualize the skill and makes frequent errors in performing it.	The newly employed acute care nurse practitioner performs a physical assessment of a newly admitted critically ill adult patient.	Observation of the acute care nurse practitioner's performance reflects a preoccupation with the examination, and attention to proceeding according to the outline in the procedure manual even when deviation in the sequence of events appears appropriate. Interpersonal interaction with the patient is limited and the nurse makes frequent eye contact with the observer each time an action is taken.	At this phase subjects dwell on the procedure and plans that guide the execution of the skill.
2. *Fixation:* Measures indicate a tendency to practice correct behavior patterns; errors are fewer than during phase 1 and decrease with practice.	The newly employed acute care nurse practitioner performs a physical assessment of a newly admitted critically ill adult patient.	Observation of the newly employed acute care nurse practitioner's performance reflects less preoccupation with the skills and the observer, fewer errors are noted, and a pattern for proceeding with the assessment has emerged.	At this phase practice of the skill is important, and errors decrease with practice.
3. *Autonomous:* Measures indicate increasing speed of performance, errors occur infrequently, individual is able to resist stress and interference from outside activities and is able to perform other activities concurrently.	The newly employed acute care nurse practitioner performs a physical assessment of a newly admitted critically ill adult patient.	Observation of the newly employed acute care nurse practitioner's performance reflects few errors, a pattern of performance that is less rigid than during the preceding stages, interpersonal communication between patient and provider is high, and elements of the health history are considered and elicited in conjunction with the physical assessment.	At this phase, the skill becomes automatic and attention focuses on other aspects of the patient.

example, if the objective for the measurement is to ascertain the ability of practicing nurses to apply gerontological content in their work with aging clients (application level of Bloom's) and if the measure constructed to assess the objective simply requires a statement in their own words of some principles important to the care of the gerontological patient (comprehension level of the taxonomy), the outcomes of the measurement are not valid, in that this tool does not measure what is intended. When taxonomies are employed, this type of discrepancy between the level of objective and level of performance measured is less apt to occur than when taxonomies are not employed.

An example of the use of taxonomies can be found in Sheetz (2001) who employed Bloom's (1956) taxonomy of the cognitive domain, Kratwohl, Bloom, and Masia's (1964) taxonomy of the affective domain, and Harrow's (1972) taxonomy of the psychomotor domain in the development of a rating scale to measure students' clinical competence.

Blueprinting

Given a set of objectives reflecting the process or outcomes to be assessed by the measure and a content outline representative of the domain

of interest, the next step is to develop a blueprint to establish the specific scope and emphasis of the measure. Table 4.4 illustrates a blueprint for a measure to assess a patient's compliance with a discharge plan. The four major content areas to be assessed appear as column headings across the top of the table and critical behaviors to be measured are listed on the left-hand side of the table as row headings. Each intersection or cell thus represents a particular content-objective pairing, and values in each cell reflect the actual number of each type of item to be included in the measure. Hence, from the table it can be seen that three items will be constructed to assess the content-objective pairing patient knowledge of the contents of the discharge plan/general health knowledge.

The scope of the measure is defined by the cells, which are reflective of the domain of items to be measured, and the emphasis of the measure and/or relative importance of each content-behavior pairing is ascertained by examining the numbers in the cells. From the blueprint, one can readily tell the topics about which questions will be asked, the types of critical behaviors subjects will be required to demonstrate, and what is relatively important and unimportant to the constructor. Tables 4.5 and 4.6 present additional examples of blueprints that vary

TABLE 4.4   Blueprint for a Measure to Assess a Patient's Compliance With a Discharge Plan

Objectives	Content				
	General Health Knowledge	**Medications**	**Activities of Daily Living**	**Nutrition**	**Total**
Ascertain patient knowledge of the contents of the discharge plan	3	5	5	5	18
Determine patient attitudes toward the contents of the discharge plan	2	2	2	2	8
Evaluate patient compliance with the contents of the discharge plan	4	10	10	10	34
Total	9	17	17	17	60

TABLE 4.5   Blueprint for the Knowledge Subscale of a Measure of Compliance With the Discharge Plan

Content	Objectives			
	Knowledge	Comprehension	Application	Total
General health knowledge	I	I	I	3
Medications		2	3	5
Activities of daily living		2	3	5
Nutrition		2	3	5
Total	I	7	I0	I8

slightly in format. In Table 4.5, the blueprint for the knowledge subscale of the measure of compliance with the discharge plan is defined by topic area and objective, but in this case, rather than listing the critical behaviors to be assessed, the performance expectations are specified using the levels of Bloom's taxonomy. In Table 4.6, objectives are defined in terms of the steps of the nursing process, content is defined by components of the nursing conceptual model used, and numbers in the cells represent percentages of each type of item to be included rather than the actual number of items.

Given the blueprint, the number (or percentage) of items prescribed in each cell would be constructed. Content validity (discussed in more detail in chapter 6) could then be assessed by presenting content experts with the blueprint and the test and having them judge (1) the adequacy of the measure as reflected in the blueprint—that is, whether or not the domain is adequately represented—to ascertain that the most appropriate elements are being assessed; (2) the fairness of the measure—whether it gives unfair advantage to some subjects over others; and (3) the fit of the method to the blueprint from which it was derived. Additional examples of blueprinting can be found in Toth (2003), Jalowiec (2003), and Jones (2003).

Constructing the Measure

The type of measure to be employed is a function of the conceptual model and subsequent operational definition of key variables to be measured. If, for example, one conceptualizes job satisfaction as a perceptual phenomenon,

the measurement will require use of an affective or typical performance instrument. If, on the other hand, job satisfaction is conceptually defined as a cognitive phenomenon dependent upon one's understanding and comprehension of factors in the work setting, a maximum performance or cognitive measure is appropriate. The essential characteristics of the types of measures are presented in chapter 1, and instrumentation and data collection methods are discussed in detail in chapters 7–23 and will not be given further attention here.

Regardless of type, every measure is composed of three components: (1) directions for administration; (2) a set of items; (3) directions for obtaining and interpreting scores.

Administration

Clemans (1971) presents a comprehensive set of considerations to be made in preparing instructions for the administration of a measure. More specifically, he advocates the inclusion of the following information:

1. A description of who should administer the measure
   - A statement of eligibility
   - A list of essential characteristics
   - A list of duties
2. Directions for those who administer the measure
   - A statement of the purposes for the measure
   - Amount of time needed for administration
   - A statement reflecting the importance of adhering to directions

TABLE 4.6   Blueprint for a Measure of Clinical Performance

Content (King's* Model)	Objectives (Nursing Practices)				
	I Assessment	II Planning	III Implementation	IV Evaluation	Total
(1) Nurse Variables a. perception b. goals c. values d. needs e. expectations	5%	5%	5%	5%	20%
(2) Patient Variables a. perception b. goals c. values d. needs e. expectations f. abilities	10%	10%	30%	10%	60%
(3) Situational Variables a. structure b. goals c. groups d. functions e. physical resources f. economic resources g. climate	10%	5%	2%	3%	20%
Total	25%	20%	37%	18%	100%

*King, I. (1968). A conceptual frame of reference for nursing. *Nursing Research, 17*, 27–31.

- Specifications for the physical environment
- A description of how material will be received and stored
- Specifications for maintaining security
- Provisions for supplementary materials needed
- Recommendations for response to subjects' questions
- Instructions for handling defective materials
- Procedures to follow when distributing the measure
- A schedule for administration
- Directions for collection of completed measures
- Specifications for the preparation of special reports (e.g., irregularity reports)
- Instructions for the delivery and/or preparation of completed measures for scoring
- Directions for the return or disposal of materials

3. Directions for respondents
   - A statement regarding information to be given to subjects prior to the data collection session (e.g., materials to be brought along and procedures for how, when, and where data will be collected)
   - Instructions regarding completion of the measure, including a request for cooperation, directions to be followed in completing each item type, and directions for when and how to record answers
4. Directions for users of results
   - Suggestions for use of results
   - Instructions for dissemination of results (p. 196)

The importance of providing this information as an essential component of any measure cannot be overemphasized. Errors in administration are an important source of measurement error, and their probability of occurrence is greatly increased when directions for administration are not communicated clearly and explicitly in writing. Those readers who desire further specifics on the topic of administration procedures will find Cleman's work extremely useful. Readers interested in examples of directions for administration are referred to Marsh (2003), Delorio and Yeager (2003), Weinert (2003), and Emerson (2001).

Items

Within the context of a given type of measure, there are a variety of specific item formats available, each with its own unique advantages and disadvantages in light of the specific purposes for, and characteristics of the setting in which, measurement is to occur. Most important, an item should be selected because it elicits the intended outcome, that is, the behavior specified by the objective(s). For example, if the objective of a measurement is to assess clinical performance, the item format should elicit performance by respondents in the clinical area. A written multiple-choice test or attitude survey would not be likely to elicit clinical performance on the part of subjects, and hence would not be an appropriate item format for this measurement objective. Similarly, if a cognitive measure derived from behavioral objectives at the synthesis level of Bloom's taxonomy was composed of a set of true-false items, the behavior specified by the objective and the outcome elicited would be incongruent; that is, at the synthesis level respondents are required to construct or create something new, while true-false items only require them to select one of two options on the basis of recall or comprehension.

Conditions surrounding the measurement will also establish parameters for what is an appropriate and useful item format. For example, if a measure is to be administered to diabetics with impaired vision, item formats requiring the reading of lengthy passages would be impractical. Similarly, measures to be administered to patients in acute care settings should be for the most part short and easily administered

and understood so as to avoid fatigue on the part of respondents and/or to avoid conflict with ongoing care activities. The important point is that the personal characteristics of the respondents such as ability to read, ability to perform physical skills, computational skills, and communication skills must be considered, and an item format must be selected that enhances their ability to respond rather than one that hinders some or all of the subjects.

Other factors in the measurement setting are also important in selecting the format. If an instrument is to be administered by individuals without training or experience in measurement, or if it is to be employed by a variety of different people, the format should be selected with an eye to easy administration. For example, an instrument employing only one item format would be likely to require less time and less complex directions with less probability of being misinterpreted than one employing a number of different item formats. If tables or other illustrations are to be used in the tool, resources should be available for preparing them correctly and to scale; that is, incorrectly or inadequately prepared illustrative materials will increase measurement error, reduce reliability and validity, and decrease the subjects' motivation to respond. If space is limited or reproduction of the tool is apt to be problematic, items requiring lengthy explanations or repetitions of rating scales or other content on each page of the tool are impractical. If scoring is to be undertaken by a few individuals without the advantage of computers, an item format that is automatic and requires little or no judgment on the part of the scorer is indicated, for example, multiple-choice or short answers. When computer scoring is employed, attention should be paid to requirements imposed by available computer software programs.

There are as many different sets of conditions to be considered as there are varied measurement settings. For this reason, only a few of the more frequently overlooked have been included here. In all cases, it is essential that careful analysis of the measurement situation be made and an item format be selected that capitalizes on the factors inherent in a given situation. Another example of such accommodations can be found in Jansen and Keller (2003) and in Jalowiec (2003), who measured attitudinal demands in community dwelling elders.

All items can be thought of as on a continuum ranging from objective to subjective. *Objective items*—those allowing little or no latitude in response and hence requiring no judgment in scoring—are often referred to as *selection-type items*. Examples of selection-type formats are true-false, matching, multiple choice, and scaled response. These items are so named because they require the subjects to choose their responses from a set of options presented to them. Table 4.7 illustrates some of the more common varieties of selection-type items. The multiple-choice format is one of the most objective available and for this reason is employed widely, especially for cognitive tools. For this reason, the construction of multiple choice items is discussed in more detail in chapter 17.

Subjective items allow more latitude on the part of respondents in constructing their answer and therefore require more judgment on the part of the scorers. *Supply-type items*—so named because they require the subject to respond by supplying words, statements, numbers, or symbols—best characterize subjective items. The more frequently encountered supply-type item formats are exemplified in Table 4.8 (see p. 108).

When a norm-referenced measure is employed, one designs items that are likely to make fine distinctions between respondents with differing levels of the attribute being measured, so that the distribution of responses to the measure will resemble a normal curve with a few high and low scores and with most scores falling in the middle range. Hence, one wants to avoid items that are too easy or too difficult for most respondents.

The *difficulty* of an item is defined as the percentage of respondents answering that item correctly or appropriately. In other words, if a cognitive test item is answered correctly by 40 of 100 respondents, the item has a difficulty level of 40% or 0.40. Hence, difficulty may vary from 0, in the case where no one responds correctly, to 1.00, in the case where all respondents respond correctly. When affective or performance measures are employed, the term "appropriately" or "as expected" is more meaningful than the term

"correct"; that is, if subjects' responses are to be compared with a well-defined referent group (e.g., first-level baccalaureate nursing students), one might define what is appropriate on a performance measure on the basis of the behavior one would expect to see in the comparison or referent group. Similarly, if one is measuring attitudes toward gerontology patients, one might define as appropriate those responses that reflect behaviors deemed acceptable or desirable by program planners.

Item difficulties for norm-referenced measures as a whole usually range from 0.30 to 0.70 (Martuza, 1977, p. 179). Several factors come into play in determining the optimum difficulty level for a given item, for example, the nature of the trait being measured, the item's correlation with other items on the instrument, and the specific objectives for the measure. Tinkelman (1971) suggested the following guidelines for determining item difficulty level:

1. In a situation in which the measure is designed to differentiate subjects' competence in a field, there is no standard of passing or failing, scores are interpreted as percentile norms or other measures of relative standing in a group, and intercorrelations among items are low. A 0.50 level of average item difficulty and a narrow range of difficulty among items are desirable in order to increase the variance of scores and increase reliability.

2. In situations in which guessing may come into play, the optimum item difficulty level should be such that the proportion of right or appropriate answers by the average subject would be 0.50 after correction for chance; that is, the average item difficulty level before correction for chance would be halfway between the chance probability of success and 1.00 (Lord, 1952). For example, in a 4 option multiple-choice test, the chance probability of success is 0.25. The difficulty level midway between 0.25 and 1.00 would be 0.65.

3. In general, the measure's reliability and the variance of scores increases as the variance of the item difficulties decreases. Thus, it is generally desirable that the items on a measure have a fairly narrow range of difficulty around the average difficulty level.

(text continues on page 109)

TABLE 4.7 Selection-Type Item Formats

Format	Example	Comments
Alternate-Choice		Consists of a statement to be responded to by selecting from one of two options. Format provides for presentation of a large number of items in relatively short periods of time, therefore allowing broader, more representative sampling from the domain. There is a tendency, however, to select materials out of context, resulting in ambiguity and/or measurement of trivia. More in-depth discussion of these items may be found in Wesman (1971), Ebel (1975), Martuza (1977), King (1979), Gronlund (1976).
1. True-False	Moderate excesses of digitalis cause premature heartbeats and vomiting. T or F I usually feel in control of my life. T or F	Consists of a declarative statement that is True (T) or False (F).
2. Right-Wrong	The median is determined using the formula: $$M = \frac{\sum X}{N}$$ R or W The turnover among nurses in this hospital is largely the result of their feeling undervalued by administration. R or W	Consists of a statement, question, equation, or the like that is identified as Right (R) or Wrong (W) by the respondent.
3. Yes-No	It is more appropriate to serve shredded wheat than Wheatena for breakfast to a patient on a 250 mg sodium diet? Y or N It is more desirable for a faculty member in this institution to spend time conducting research than consulting in that person's specialty area? Y or N	Consists of a direct question to be answered by a Yes (Y) or No (N).

4. Cluster

Pulse pressure is:

1. the difference between venous and systolic pressure. T or F
2. the difference between arterial and venous pressure. T or F
3. the difference between diastolic and systolic pressure. T or F
4. pressure and expansion of the artery as blood flows toward the capillaries. T or F
5. all of the above T or F

Consists of an incomplete statement with suggested completions, each of which is to be judged True (T) or False (F).

5. Correction

Lightening usually occurs approximately *4 weeks before* delivery. _____

I am *satisfied* with the policies in this School of Nursing. _____

Combines selection and supply by presenting a statement and directing the respondent to correct false statements by substituting appropriate word(s).

Matching

Consists of a list of words or statements, a list of responses, and directions for matching responses to words or statements. Imperfect and association type are preferred, because they allow assessment of higher level behaviors. Because homogeneity is paramount in writing such items, the desire for homogeneity when heterogeneity is more appropriate may result in a shift in emphasis away from that desired. Additional information regarding this type of item is available in Wesman (1971), King (1979), Gronlund (1976).

1. Perfect matching

On the line before each poison, place the number of the symptoms that usually characterize it.

Poisons	Symptoms
_____ a. acids	1. diarrhea, garlic breath
_____ b. rat poisons	2. restlessness, rapid pulse
_____ c. cocaine	3. drowsiness, flushed cheeks
_____ d. carbon monoxide	4. dyspnea, cyanosis

Each response matches one and only one word or statement.

2. Imperfect matching

Match each term with its definition:

_____ mode   1. score that separates upper 50% of scores in the distribution from the lower 50% of the scores

_____ median

_____ mean   2. score obtained by the largest number of respondents

Some responses do not match any of the words or statements.

(continued)

TABLE 4.7   Selection-Type Item Formats (Continued)

Format	Example	Comments
	3. largest number of respondents selecting a given score 4. sum of scores in a distribution divided by the total number of scores 5. the average	
3. Statement classification	Judge the effects of the nurse's intervention on the patient's physical comfort in each of the numbered situations, using the following: a. Nursing intervention would tend to reduce the patient's physical comfort. b. Nursing intervention would tend to increase the patient's physical comfort. c. Nursing intervention would tend to have little or no effect on the patient's physical comfort. _____ 1. A primigravida in the first stages of labor is encouraged by the nurse to walk around the corridors _____ 2. As labor progresses, the nurse remains with the primigravida, directing her attention to the fact that labor is progressing as expected. _____ 3. As labor progresses, the nurse teaches the patient various breathing and relaxing techniques. _____ 4. The nurse assesses and records the frequency, duration, and intensity of the contractions at regular intervals. _____ 5. The nurse encourages the patient to void at regular intervals.	Requires respondent to use higher level mental operations such as analysis, evaluation.
Multiple Choice		Components of a multiple choice item are: (1) stem—which is an introductory statement or question; and (2) responses or suggested answers. Readers are referred to Ebel (1975), Wesman (1971), Martuza (1977), King (1979), Staropoli and Waltz (1978), and Gronlund (1976), for further reading.

1. Correct answer	The basic service unit in the administration of public health is: a. the federal government b. the state health department c. the local health department d. the public health nurse	Items that require or permit a correct answer are those that eliminate the need for the respondent to make a judgment regarding the correctness of his response, i.e., matters of fact provide a suitable basis for such items.
2. Best answer	The primary responsibility of the instructor in health services is to: a. provide an emotional and social environment that adds a wholesome and healthful tone to the child's school day b. provide emergency or first aid care when a child becomes ill or injured in school c. provide up-to-date material about health as part of the curriculum d. screen for abnormalities and sickness and record the findings	For many of the important questions that need to be asked it is impossible to state an absolutely correct answer within the reasonable limits of a multiple choice item. Even if space limitations were not a factor, two experts would probably not agree on the precise wording of the best answer. The use of this type of item, which has one best answer, permits the item writer to ask more significant questions and frees the writer from the responsibility of stating a correct answer so precisely that all authorities would agree that the particular wording used was the best possible wording.
3. Based on opinion	Advocates of the specialized approach to school nursing point out that: a. the health of the child cannot be separated from that of the family and community as a whole b. specialized nursing care for the child cannot be separated from that for the family and community as a whole c. a specialized program offers greater diversity and challenge to a well-prepared community health nurse d. specialized nursing in the school allows the nurse to function without the disadvantages of a dual channel of administrative responsibility	The responses to this question represent generalizations on the basis of literature written by the advocates of the specialized approach to school nursing. No authoritative sanction for one particular generalization is likely to be available, yet respondents familiar with this literature would probably agree on a best answer to this item.
4. Novel question	The problem of air pollution is most likely to be reduced in the future by which of the following: a. urban population will wear air purifying equipment b. cities will be enclosed to facilitate air purification c. development of processes that will not produce air pollutants d. use of nonpollutant fuels	Requiring the respondent to predict what would happen under certain circumstances is a good way of measuring understanding of the principle involved.

(continued)

TABLE 4.7 Selection-Type Item Formats *(Continued)*

Format	Example	Comments
5. Selective recall	The U.S. Public Health Service was reorganized in 1966 to: a. include the UNICEF program b. include the Agency of International Development c. combine the Voluntary Agency Services with the official ones d. provide leadership or control of disease and environmental hazards and in development of manpower	Unless this item had been made the specific object of instruction, it will function to assess the learner's ability to recall a variety of information about the Public Health Service, to select that which is relevant, and to base a generalization upon it.
6. Descriptive response	The child's socialization may be defined as: a. a behavioral process in which behavior conforms to the social practices of family and extra family groups b. a process of developing an effective set of performances characteristic of self-control c. the genetically determined or hereditary mechanisms that determine the individual's physical traits d. all of the above	Inexperienced item writers tend to seek items having very short responses. This can seriously limit the significance and scope of the achievements measured. In an item measuring the ability to define an important term, it is usually better to place the term to be defined in the item stem and to use definitions or identifications as the responses. The same principle should be applied to other items, i.e., one word responses need not be avoided altogether, but they should seldom be prominent in any measure.
7. Combined response	A school community safety program should be concerned with: a. teaching children how to avoid accidents b. teaching adults and children to eliminate physical hazards that endanger them c. eliminating physical hazards that endanger children and teaching them to avoid accidents d. teaching children and adults to avoid accidents and eliminating physical hazards that endanger them	A difficulty with four-option multiple choice items is that of securing four good alternatives. One solution to this problem is to combine questions with two alternatives each to give the necessary four alternatives.
8. Combined question and explanation	When was the World Health Organization created and why? a. 1954, to prevent the spread of disease from one continent to another b. 1948, to achieve international cooperation for better health throughout the world	This is a variation of the item type in which essentially two or more alternatives each are combined to give four alternatives.

	c. 1945, to structure health privileges of all nations d. 1948, to provide for a liberated population and aid in the relief from suffering	
9. Introductory sentence	When a group is working as a health team, overlapping of activities may occur. What is essential if this is to be prevented? a. auxiliaries will work within a fairly circumscribed field b. the public health nurse will assume responsibility for all phases of the nursing team's activities c. the functions of all personnel will be defined d. maximum skills of each team member will be used	The use of a separate sentence frequently adds to the clarity of the item stem if it is necessary to present background information as well as to ask the question itself. Combining these two elements into a single question-sentence probably would make it too complex.
10. Necessary qualification	Generally speaking, the environmental health program personnel in urban centers are: a. persons with professional training in civil or sanitary engineering b. sanitary inspectors, or nonengineering personnel with indoctrination and orientation by the health department c. public health engineers whose training embraces the public health aspect of both sanitary engineering and sanitary inspection d. all of the above	If this question asked only about environmental health program personnel in general, without qualifying *urban* personnel, it would be difficult for the respondent to give a firm answer to the question, given the existing differences between the environmental health programs in other than urban areas, i.e., county, state, federal.
11. None of above and/or all of above as options	A necessary requirement for receiving funds under the Comprehensive Health Planning Act of 1966 is that: a. state boards of health must have at least 10% lay representation b. the council responsible for developing a comprehensive health plan for the state must have 50% consumer participation c. health and welfare councils, whether or not actively involved in health planning on the state level, must have at least 25% lay representation d. none of the above	Whenever each of the responses can be judged unequivocally as correct or incorrect in response to the question posed in the item stem, it is appropriate to use none of the above as a response. It would be appropriate to use all of the above in a similar situation in which more than one perfectly correct answer is possible.

(continued)

TABLE 4.7 Selection-Type Item Formats *(Continued)*

Format	Example	Comments
12. True statements as distractors	The general purpose of parent education programs is to: a. teach parents information they need to know throughout their children's changing developmental stages b. help parents reinforce their understanding and strengths in regard to themselves and their children c. develop attitudes of healthy family life in parents of young children d. cover a wider range of subject matter, format, and method than is possible on an individual basis	It is not necessary for the incorrect options to a test item to be themselves incorrect statements. They simply need to be incorrect answers to the stem question. Judgments concerning the relevance of knowledge may be as important as judgments concerning its truth. This is particularly useful as a technique for testing achievement which is sometimes thought to be testable only by using essay measures.
13. Stereotypes in distractors	The particular process of interaction between the organism and its environment that results in a specifiable change in both is referred to as: a. homeostasis b. human behavior c. operant behavior d. developmental dynamism	Phrases such as operant behavior and homeostasis, which a respondent may have heard without understanding, provide excellent distractors at an elementary level of discrimination.
14. Heterogeneous responses	The index of economic welfare is: a. square feet of housing space b. per capita national income c. rate of growth of industrialization d. morbidity and mortality rates	The responses to this item vary widely. Because of their wide differences, only an introductory knowledge of indices of economic welfare is required for a successful response.
15. Homogeneous responses (harder item)	Funds for occupational health programs were allocated to state and local health departments as a result of: a. Social Security Act b. Clean Air Act c. Community Health Centers Act d. Occupational Health Act	The homogeneity of the responses in this item requires a considerably high level of knowledge of public health acts and hence makes the item difficult in comparison to an item using heterogeneous options.

16. Multiple clues (easier item)

The amount estimated to eliminate poverty in our country is said to be which of the following:

a. 2% of the gross national product and 1/5 of the cost for national defense

b. 3% of the gross national product and 1/6 of the cost for the national defense

c. 4% of the gross national product and 1/4 of the cost for national defense

d. 5% of the gross national product and 1/3 of the cost for national defense

The use of the values of two variables fitting the specification in the item stem makes it a fairly easy question. That is, the examinee need only know one of the values or know one in each of the three distractors to respond successfully.

Scaled Response

A statement or question is presented and the respondents answer by marking the area on the scale that represents their answer. (See Nunnally, 1967; Nunnally & Bernstein, 1994, pp. 11–27 and 31–81; and chapter 1 for additional discussion of rating scales.)

1. Number anchors

Rate your level of satisfaction with your present job using the following scale:

1	2	3	4	5
not satisfied				very satisfied

The use of numerical anchors facilitates analysis of data by computer as well as serves to remind respondents of the meaning of the scale steps.

2. Percentage anchors

Using the scale: A — None of the time
B — 1–25% of the time
C — 26–50% of the time
D — 51–75% of the time
E — 76–99% of the time
F — all of the time

rate each of the following actions performed by the nurse you observe administering medications on Unit B.

	Rating
1) washes hands prior to administering medications	___
2) selects correct medication to be given at designated time	___
3) checks patient's ID prior to administering medication	___
4) stays with patient until medication is taken	___
5) records administration of medication correctly	___

(continued)

TABLE 4.7   Selection-Type Item Formats *(Continued)*

Format	Example	Comments
3. Degrees of agreement/disagreement	Indicate your degree of agreement with the following statement: Antagonistic behavior on the part of a patient indicates a need on the patient's part for additional attention and time from the nurse. | 1 | 2 | 3 | 4 | 5 | 6 | Completely Completely Agree Disagree	

4. Adjectives	Using the scale: A. No importance
	                 B. Little importance
	                 C. Some importance
	                 D. Importance
	                 E. A great deal of importance
	
	Rate the importance you place on each of the following nursing faculty activities:
	
	_____ Conducting clinical research _____ Teaching graduate students
	_____ Consulting with nursing service staff _____ Practicing clinically
	_____ Teaching undergraduate students _____ Pursuing professional development activities
		See also chapter 1 for the discussion of the semantic differential, a special form of adjective rating scale.

5. Actual behavior	Observe the nurse's intervening with the patients on Unit C and then check the behavior that best describes what you observed. _____ Does not adapt planned intervention to meet changes in patient situation. _____ Adapts implementation with guidance to accommodate changes in patient situation. _____ Adapts implementation independently to accommodate changes in patient situation. _____ Implements independently a preplanned alternate intervention to accommodate changes in patient situation.	

6. Products

Here are four nursing care plans. Indicate the one you believe to be the most reflective of good principles and practices in gerontological nursing.

    A. Care Plan X
    B. Care Plan Y
    C. Care Plan Z
    D. Care Plan O

Context-Dependent

Patients are given a series of pictures portraying behaviors usually observed in children of 2–3 years of age and asked to identify those observed in their own children.

In this case, the item has meaning to the subject only in relation to other material presented, e.g., scenario, picture, graph, table. Readers are referred to Wesman, (1971), for additional discussion. Visual presentation of material, especially pictures, permits the presentation of a problem or situation in a very clear and simple manner, thus eliminating confusion due to reading or inability to adequately describe a phenomenon.

Interpretation

ANOVA Table

Source	df	SS	MS	F
Between groups	9	72	24	1.5
Within groups	84	448	16	
Total	93	520		

1. How many treatments were studied in the above table?
  a. 2
  b. 3
  c. 4
  d. cannot answer from the table
2. How many subjects participated in the study?
  a. 84
  b. 92
  c. 93
  d. 94

Consists of introductory material followed by a series of questions calling for various interpretations, thus provides for measuring ability to interpret and evaluate materials. This type of item allows one to ask meaningful questions on relatively complex topics. Disadvantages stem from the fact that such items are time consuming to administer and difficult to construct. See Wesman (1971) for more information.

TABLE 4.8 Supply-Type Item Formats

Format	Example	Comments
Short Answer		
1. Question	What term is used to designate that portion of the infant's body that lies nearest the internal os? (presentation)	For cognitive tests this format tends to measure only facts. The respondents are presented with a question or incomplete statement written in such a way that it is clear to the respondents what is expected of them, followed by a blank space in which the respondents write what is called for by the directions. Preferably short answer questions should require an answer that is a single word, symbol, or formula. See Wesman (1971).
2. Completion	Normal labor usually is divided into three stages: dilating, expulsive, placental.	
3. Identification/association	After each event indicate the stages of labor during which it usually occurs. a. effacement _____ b. dilatation of the cervix _____ c. fetal descent _____ d. placental separation _____	
Essay		
1. Multiple aspects of a single topic	An adolescent is being discharged from the hospital on insulin and a diabetic diet regimen. When you visit his/her home one week post discharge: (a) what observations will you make; (b) what information will you seek to elicit from the patient and his/her family and how; and (c) what type of evaluation will you expect to make on the basis of the observation and information you are able to obtain.	Essays lend themselves to measuring complex phenomena, especially the ability to organize and communicate information in an area of interest. Problems lie primarily in the area of (1) subjectivity in scoring (but this can be minimized if criteria for scoring are agreed upon prior to administration); (2) time required to respond; and (3) the limited number of questions that can be handled during a given administration, hence reducing the representativeness of the domain sampled. See Coffman (1971).
2. Independent question	Describe your philosophy of nursing and the resulting implications it has for the delivery of nursing practice.	

4. In the case of homogeneous measures (in which high intercorrelations exist between items) or in cases in which heterogeneous groups of subjects respond, a wider spread of difficulty is indicated.

5. In cases in which the purpose of the instrument is to serve a screening function—that is, to select a small percentage of the best—it should be a relatively difficult test for most subjects; if it is designed to screen out the weakest or least appropriate, it should be a relatively easy test for most respondents (pp. 67–69).

It should be noted that the determination of item difficulty levels occurs at the time the measure is designed and constructed, and then the expected is compared with empirical findings via item analysis procedures (which are discussed in chapter 6).

Although the test blueprint specifies the number of items to be included in the measure during the planning stage, it is essential that test length be reconsidered during construction in light of subsequent decisions made regarding administration and item format. Although generally the longer the test, the higher the probability of reliability and validity, there are situations in which length may become a liability. For example, if the setting in which the measure is to be given places time limits on administration, it may be necessary to reduce the number of items proportionally to accommodate the time limits. Equivalently, if the physical condition of the subject precludes lengthy testing periods, the number of items may need to be reduced or subdivided and then administered on more than one occasion. Equivalently, if the most appropriate item format is also one that is time consuming and demanding, length may need to be traded for a format that better elicits the behavior to be assessed. The important point is that the ideal in terms of length may need to be compromised or modified because of conditions surrounding the measurement. When this occurs, it is important that the relative emphasis of the measurement be preserved by reducing the categories of items proportionally, according to the blueprint specifications.

Scoring

Generally, the more simple and direct the procedure used for obtaining raw scores for the norm-referenced measure, the better; that is, although a number of elaborate weighing schemes have been devised for assigning a raw score to a measure, it has been demonstrated empirically that the end result is usually consistent with that obtained by simply summing over items (Nunnally, 1967; Nunnally & Bernstein, 1994, pp. 75–82). For this reason, we recommend the use of summative scoring procedures, whenever it is appropriate, to obtain a total score or set of subscores for a measure.

To obtain a *summative score,* one assigns a score to each individual item according to a conceptual scheme and then sums over the individual item scores to obtain a total score. Usually, the conceptual scheme for assigning item scores derives from the conceptual model. If one designed a measure of faculty influence on nursing students' preferences for practice, using a theory of personal influence, items would be constructed to measure key influence variables, and item responses would be constructed in such a manner that high scores represent more amenability to influence and low scores, less amenability. For example, in his theory of personal influence, Bidwell (1973) suggests a number of conditions under which the teachers' interactions with students are more likely to influence students' attitudes toward the content. One such condition is when the student perceives a direct positive relationship (i.e., a link) between the teachers' attitudes and the content taught. If one presumes that teachers' attitudes toward the content are reflected by their behavior in regard to it, then in operationalizing the theory one might choose to focus on the students' perception of the link between the content taught by the clinical instructors and the instructors' activities. More specifically, for illustrative purposes, suppose the key variable is defined as students' perceptions of their clinical faculty member's application of content to clinical performance. On the basis of the theory that the more students perceive a direct link—that is, the more they perceive that their faculty member applies the content taught to clinical performance—the more likely they are to be influenced.

Students are asked to rate from 1 (not at all) to 6 (very much) the extent to which they think their clinical faculty member is involved in each of the following activities:

1. Publishing materials that relate the content taught to clinical performance
2. Speaking or in some manner presenting the content at professional meetings
3. Consulting in the content area with practicing nurses in the agency where the faculty member has students
4. Using the content in planning and/or developing programs for practicing nurses that deal with nursing and/or patient care
5. Seeking continuing learning experiences that are relevant to the content taught
6. Seeking continuing learning experiences that are relevant to patient care
7. Participating in research regarding patient care and the content area
8. Using the content in providing direct patient care

Thus, the score for each of the eight items is derived in such a manner that the higher the number selected by the respondent, the more amenable to faculty influence the respondent is expected to be, on the basis of the theory underlying the tool's development. Therefore, when individual item scores are summed to obtain a total score, scores can range from a low of 8 to a high of 48, with high scores reflecting students' strong perception of a link between the faculty member's content and clinical performance and, hence, being more amenable to faculty influence; low scores, on the contrary, indicate less of a link and therefore less amenability to influence. Since this is a norm-referenced measure, an individual respondent's score, that is, the respondent's amenability to faculty influence, would be interpreted on the basis of the scores of other respondents in the sample. To accomplish this, one would usually compute the arithmetic mean for the scores of all members of the sample and then use it to give specific meaning to the individual's score—for example, whether an individual is more or less amenable than other members of the sample, or whether a subject's score is above, below, or at the mean

for the comparison group, which in this case is the sample. Published examples of tools whose scoring is conceptually derived as illustrated here may be found in Waltz and Jenkins (2001), and in Strickland and Dilorio (2003a,b).

Hence, in the norm-referenced case, an individual's score takes on meaning when compared with the scores of others in some well-defined referent group. The referent group might be other members of the same sample, or it might be subjects nationwide to whom the same measure was administered. In the latter case, the norm-referenced measure would most likely be a standardized test and the scores of the reference group would have been derived using an appropriate norming procedure for establishing national norms. Since standardized tests and norming procedures are discussed at length in chapter 7, attention here will focus on those instances in which nurses construct norm-referenced measures for their own use rather than select and administer a standardized tool. It should be noted however, that much of what is discussed here holds true in the case of standardized measures as well.

To facilitate the interpretation of norm-referenced scores, the distribution of raw scores is tabulated using a table, graph, or polygon. In each case, each score is paired and its frequency of occurrence in the set of scores is noted. For example, if the same 10-item measure of ability was administered to 30 subjects, the distribution of their scores could be represented as shown in Table 4.9. This table is called an *ungrouped frequency distribution* and is useful because it clearly displays how many subjects obtained each score. When there is a wide range of scores in a distribution or a number of scores are not received by subjects, it is more desirable and economical to group scores according to size in a *grouped frequency distribution*. Table 4.10 illustrates the use of a grouped frequency distribution to tabulate the scores of 30 subjects on a 100-item cognitive measure. Each group in Table 4.10 is called a score class, and the width of each score class interval in this case is 10. Although there are no fixed rules for when a grouped frequency distribution is preferred to an ungrouped one, Glass and Stanley (1970) suggest that the grouped frequency distribution be

TABLE 4.9   Ungrouped Frequency Distribution of Scores on a 10-Item Measure of Anxiety (*n* = 30)

Score	Number of Subjects
10	1
9	4
8	1
7	0
6	4
5	10
4	5
3	1
2	3
1	1

used when there is a large number of scores, 100 or more, and that it is usually best to construct not fewer than 12 nor more than 15 score classes. They state that with fewer than 12 classes one runs the risk of distorting the results, whereas with more than 15 classes the table produced is inconvenient to handle.

In lieu of a frequency distribution, one might opt to present scores using a graph such as that presented in Figure 4.4. The graph in Figure 4.4 is a histogram. It not only displays all the infor-

mation in the frequency distribution, but it has the advantage of making information regarding the shape of the distribution more accessible to the reader (Glass & Stanley, 1970). The *histogram* is a series of columns, each having as its base one score or class, and as its height the frequency or number of subjects in that class. A column is centered on the midpoint of the score/class interval.

A frequency polygon is yet another way that one may choose to represent the scores. A polygon is very similar to a histogram. In the

TABLE 4.10   Grouped Frequency Distribution of Subjects' Scores on a 150-Item Cognitive Measure (*n* = 30)

Score	Number of Subjects
150–141	1
140–131	2
130–121	1
120–111	4
110–101	3
100–91	1
90–81	1
80–71	5
70–61	3
60–51	3
50–41	1
40–31	2
30–21	1
20–11	1
10–0	1

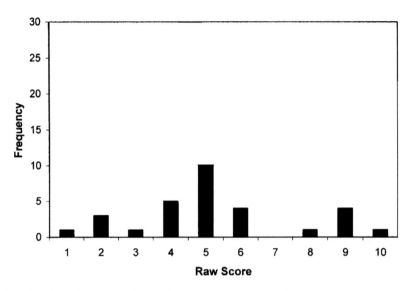

FIGURE 4.4   Distribution of scores on the anxiety measure represented by a histogram ($n = 30$).

histogram, the top of each column is repre-sented by a horizontal line, and the length of one score or class placed at the proper height represents the number of subjects in that class. In the *polygon*, a point is located above the mid-point of each score or class and at the height that represents the frequency at that score. These points are then joined by straight lines. Figure 4.5 illustrates a polygon for the data represented by the histogram in Figure 4.4. The main advan-tage of the polygon over the histogram is that it allows one to superimpose up to three distribu-tions with a minimum of crossing of lines (Glass & Stanley, 1970). Thus, the polygon facilitates comparisons among distributions.

Standards for constructing tables, graphs, and polygons were first published in 1915 by Brinton and have changed little through the years. That report still covers most of the points required for the proper representation of data; thus the following rules are cited from it:

1. The general arrangements of a diagram should proceed from left to right.
2. The horizontal scale should usually read from left to right and the vertical scale from bottom to top.
3. Whenever practical, the vertical scale should be selected so that the zero line appears on the diagram.

4. In diagrams representing a series of observations, whenever possible the sepa-rate observations should be clearly indi-cated on the diagrams.
5. All lettering and figures on a diagram should be placed so they can be read eas-ily from the base as the bottom, or from the right-hand edge of the diagram as the bottom.
6. The title of a diagram should be as clear and complete as possible. (pp. 790–797)

Additional information regarding the tabulat-ing of data can be found in Walker and Durost (1936), Arkin and Colton (1936), Kelley (1947), or Grier and Foreman (1988). Summary statis-tics, described in chapter 3, are then employed to facilitate interpretation of an individual's score and to communicate information about the characteristics of the distribution of scores.

Since in norm-referenced measurement the meaning of an individual's score is dependent upon how it compares with the scores of the other members of the referent group, it is nec-essary to obtain a measure of central tendency for the distribution of scores and then consider an individual's performance in light of it. The mean of the distribution represented in Figure 4.5 is 5.3, the mode is 5, and the median is approximately 5.5. Hence, one knows that an

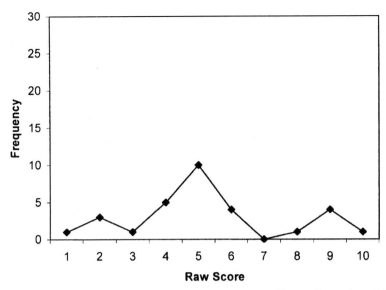

FIGURE 4.5　**Distribution of scores on the anxiety measure represented by a polygon (*n* = 30).**

individual with a score of 3 is below the mean, received an anxiety score lower than most members of the group, and had an anxiety score falling in the lower half of the score distribution. Furthermore, by determining the variance and standard deviation for the distribution, interpretation of the individual's score can be enhanced by referring to how many standard deviations an individual's score lies above or below the mean.

If a norm-referenced measure performs in the intended manner, the resulting distribution of scores ought to display a wide range, large variance, and a shape resembling that of a normal distribution. The *normal distribution* (Figure 4.6) is a symmetric distribution. *Symmetric* means the left half of the distribution is a mirror image of the right half. The normal curve will always be symmetric around its mean; it is bell-shaped, begins and ends near the baseline, but never quite touches it, and therefore is unbounded, meaning there is no beginning and no end. The normal curve is a mathematical construct first used as a model for distributions that closely approximate its characteristics, or would if a very large sample were used. The distributions of scores on the anxiety measure in Figures 4.4 and 4.5 do in fact resemble a normal curve, and their measures of central tendency illustrate another property; that is, in a normal

distribution the mean, median, and mode are equal in value.

Because empirical distributions vary in terms of the extent to which they approximate the theoretical normal curve and because there are a number of normal curves, that is, as many different forms as there are combinations of different means and standard deviations, the use of raw scores for the interpretation of norm-referenced measures can be very problematic. For example, if a tool were administered to two groups of 20 subjects and the distribution resulting from the first administration had a mean of 10 and a standard deviation of 5 and the distribution in the second case had a mean of 20 and a standard deviation of 15, an individual with a score of 15 in the first group would be above average in his or her group, while a subject with a score of 15 in the second would be below average when compared with his or her group. Furthermore, because the standard deviation in the second group is considerably higher than that of the first, more error is present in the first set of scores and, hence, they are less accurate indications of subjects' true amount of the attribute being measured. Therefore, it would be meaningless at best to attempt to compare subjects' scores across groups. For this reason, it is often useful for a norm-referenced measure to transform raw scores to a set of

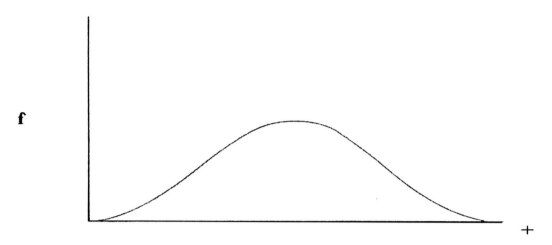

FIGURE 4.6   Shape of the normal curve.

standard scores that allows comparison among different groups of subjects on the same measure as well as facilitates comparison within groups.

Standard scores allow one to describe the position of a score in a set of scores by measuring its deviation from the mean of all scores in standard deviation units. This can be accomplished by converting the raw scores of each subject to a standard score. Any set of n scores with mean and standard deviation $\bar{X}$ can be transformed into a different set of scores with mean 0 and standard deviation 1, so that the transformed score immediately tells one the deviation of the original score from the mean measured in standard deviation units. This is accomplished by subtracting the mean ($\bar{X}$) from the score (X) and dividing the difference by σ_x. The resulting scores are Z scores.

Formula 4.1: Calculation of standard scores (Waltz & Bausell, 1981)

$$Z = \frac{X - \bar{X}}{\sigma_x}$$

where Z = a standard score
X = the subject's raw score
$\bar{X}$ = the mean of the raw-score distribution
σ_x = the standard deviation of the raw-score distribution

Example: The mean and standard deviation of the scores 5, 10, and 18 are 11 and 5.11, respec-

tively. The resulting Z scores are −1.17, −0.19, and +1.36.

$$= \frac{5 - 11}{5.11}$$

$$= \frac{-6}{5.11}$$

$$= -1.17$$

$$= \frac{10 - 11}{5.11}$$

$$= \frac{-1}{5.11}$$

$$= -0.19$$

$$= \frac{18 - 11}{5.11}$$

$$= \frac{7}{5.11}$$

$$= 1.36$$

Aside from being a convenient means for communicating the position of a subject's score, Z scores are a step toward transforming a set of raw scores into an arbitrary scale with a convenient mean and standard deviation. There are many possible scales to which raw scores can be transformed (arbitrary means and standard deviations). For example, intelligence test scores are often transformed to a scale with mean 100 and standard deviation 15 or 16. Similarly, t scores with mean 50 and standard deviation of 10 are used widely.

Formula 4.2: To transform a Z score to any scale of measure:

$$\text{Transformed score} = (\sigma_{sm} \, Z_x) + X_{sm}$$

where σ_{sm} = the desired standard deviation
  Z_x = the Z score that results from $\dfrac{X - \bar{X}}{\sigma_x}$

  X_{sm} = the desired mean

Example: To transform the Z score 1.36 to a t score with mean 50 and standard deviation 10:

$$t = (10)(1.36) + 50$$
$$= 13.60 + 50$$
$$= 63.60$$

A distribution of Z scores is referred to as a *unit normal curve,* which is illustrated in Figure 4.7. It is a unit normal curve because the area under the curve is 1. Its mean and standard deviation are 0 and 1, respectively, and any other normal curve can be moved along the number scale and stretched or compressed by using a simple transformation.

As stated earlier, there is an infinite number of normal curves, a different one for each different pair of values for the mean and standard deviation. The most important property they have in common is the amount of the area under the curve between any two points expressed in standard deviation units. In any normal distribution, approximately:

1. 68% of the area under the curve lies within one standard deviation (σ) of the mean either way (that is $X \pm 1\sigma$).
2. 95% of the area under the curve lies within two σ's of the mean.
3. 97.7% of the area under the curve lies within three σ's of the mean.

It is useful if all references to normal distributions are in terms of deviations from the mean in standard deviation units; that is, when the normal curve is employed, one wants to know how many standard deviations a score lies above or below the mean. The deviation of a score from its mean is $X - \bar{X}$; the number of standard deviations X lies from its mean is $(X - \bar{X})/\sigma_x$ and is called the *unit normal deviate.* The shape of the normal curve does not change when one subtracts the mean and divides by the standard deviation.

Example: What portion of the area lies to the left of a score of 30 in a normal distribution with mean 35 and standard deviation of 10?

It is the proportion of the area that lies to the left of $(30 - 35)/10 = -0.5$ in the unit normal distribution.

Using a table of areas of the unit normal distribution found in most research and statistics books, one can further determine that the area that lies to the left of –0.5 in the unit normal distribution is 0.3085. A table of areas of the unit normal distribution can be found in Waltz and Bausell (1981, Appendix 1, pp. 338–340).

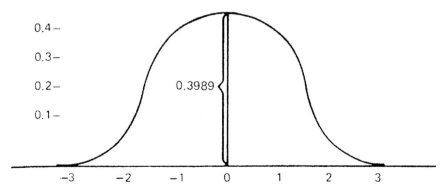

FIGURE 4.7   The unit normal curve (mean = 0; standard deviation = 1).

The Z score is sometimes referred to as a derived score. Two additional derived scores obtained from a raw-score distribution using specific arithmetic operations are percentage scores and percentile ranks. Percentage scores are appropriate for criterion-referenced measures rather than norm-referenced; because they are frequently confused with the percentile rank, which is appropriate for norm-referenced measures, they will be briefly discussed here. A *percentage score* is the percentage of the total number of points available that have been earned by the subject.

The percentage score indicates where the individual's performance is in relation to the minimum and maximum possible values on the raw-score scale. The percentage score is a measure of absolute performance; that is, the percentage score obtained by one subject is completely independent of the percentage scores of all other subjects in the group. Therefore, it is a useful measure of performance in a criterion-referenced context.

In contrast, the *percentile rank* of a particular raw score is the percentage of area in the histogram located to the left of the raw score in question. To determine the percentile rank:

1. Determine how many subjects obtained scores exactly equal to the subject's raw-score value.
2. Divide the number obtained in step 1 by half.
3. Count the number of subjects who obtained scores less than the subject's raw-score value.
4. Add the results obtained in steps 2 and 3.
5. Divide the result of step 4 by the total number of scores in the distribution.
6. Multiply the resulting value by 100.

Example: Find the percentile rank of the raw score 2 in the following distribution:

DISTRIBUTION

Raw Score	Frequency
5	0
4	3
3	2
2	4
1	1

1. Four subjects obtained scores exactly equal to 2.
2. One-half of 4 is 2.
3. Exactly one subject had a raw score less than 2.
4. Adding the results from steps 2 and 3, $2 + 1 = 3$.
5. Because there are 10 scores in the distribution, $3/10 = 0.30$.
6. Multiplying $0.30 \times 100 = 30$, indicating 30 percent of the area of the distribution is located to the left of the raw score 2.

The percentile rank is an indicator of relative performance. The percentile rank of a subject is totally dependent upon the quality of the subject's performance as compared with the performances of the other subjects in the group. Thus, it is an excellent measure in a norm-referenced context, but totally inappropriate for use with criterion-referenced measures.

A *percentile* is simply a point on the raw-score continuum. The Xth percentile is the point or value on the raw-score scale that separates the left most X% of the histogram area from the remainder of the graph. If a subject scored at the Xth percentile, the subject's performance was better than or equal to exactly X% of the performances in the group.

Selected percentiles are sometimes referred to as *quartiles*. That is, the 25th percentile may be called the first quartile, the 50th percentile the second quartile, and the 75th percentile the third quartile. The first, second, and third quartiles are symbolically designated as Q_1, Q_2, and Q_3, respectively. Q_2 is the median of the distribution. Quartiles are useful for summarizing data, because simply reporting that P_{50} is 10 and P_{25} is 15 tells the reader immediately that 50% of the observations are less than 10, and 25% of them lie between 10 and 15. For large groups of data, knowing the quartile values may enable the reader to readily envision the entire collection of observations.

Once the scores resulting from a norm-referenced measure have been transformed to sets of comparable values (e.g., standard scores), a *profile* can be plotted to demonstrate the comparability of two or more scores for the same subject or the comparability of two or more scores for groups of subjects. More specifically, profiles may be used to:

1. Obtain a visual representation of the relative performance of subjects in several different areas.
2. Compare the performance of a single group of subjects on several variables and with a set of norms (e.g., national norms).
3. Provide sample-by-sample comparisons in terms of common variables and with a set of norms (e.g., national norms).
4. Compare a subject's performance in successive years (Angoff, 1971).

Usually a profile is constructed as a chart on which one axis represents the tools and the other axis the scores as standard scores, percentile ranks, or stanines. It must be emphasized that a profile must be based on the scores of subjects from the same or strictly comparable populations to whom the tools were administered at the same time. Because profiles are most often employed with standardized measures, which are a special type of norm-referenced measure, the development of profiles is discussed and illustrated in more depth in chapter 7.

DESIGNING CRITERION-REFERENCED MEASURES

In the preceding sections, the development of norm-referenced measures was discussed. At this point, we turn our discussion to the development of criterion-referenced measures. We will begin by differentiating the nature of criterion-referenced measurement from norm-referenced measures. Next we will discuss the place of criterion-referenced measurement in measuring health and nursing concepts. This will be followed by the specification of the similarities and differences in the approach to designing criterion-referenced measures in comparison with norm-referenced measures. In the past, criterion-referenced and norm-referenced measures were regarded as competing approaches to measurement. However, recently works in the area of instructional diagnostics have recognized that the same test may allow for both

norm- and criterion-referenced interpretation (Glaser, 1994; Hambleton, 1994; Watermann & Klieme, 2002).

The Meaning of Criterion-Referenced Measurement

In criterion-referenced measurement the emphasis is on determining what a person can or cannot do, or knows or does not know, not on how the person compares with others (Bond, 1996). For illustrative purposes, suppose that a nursing instructor wants to know if a student can apply the principles of sterile technique while catheterizing a patient. This is quite a different concern from how well the student can perform this task when compared with classmates. The former concern has a criterion-referenced measurement focus, and the latter is an example of the focus of norm-referenced measurement.

Criterion-referenced measures are used to determine an object's domain status, usually with respect to some predetermined criterion or performance standard. In one sense, criterion refers to the specified knowledge or skills in performing a task that a test or measure was designed to assess. However, in another sense, it means the level of performance that is required to pass a test (Brown & Hudson, 2002). The domain refers to the variable or content area that is the focus of measurement. In criterion-referenced measurement the objective of the test or measure specifies the domain that is being measured, and the emphasis is on the determination of the object's or person's domain status. In the example cited above the criterion or performance standards guide the instructor in determining whether the student can perform the expected set of target behaviors independent of reference to the performance of others. When the criterion-referenced framework is applied to a testing situation, whether an individual passes or fails the test would be defined by a preset standard of performance or cut score. If the student scores above the cut score, the student would pass the test regardless of how many peers scored above or below the cut score. Such tests may be referred to as mastery-referenced tests. Standards-referenced assessment is used to refer to criterion-referenced measurement related to large scale performance assessments (Young & Yoon, 1998). When the content of a criterion-referenced test is based on specific objectives, it may be called an objectives-referenced test. The term "domain-referenced" test or measure refers to those circumstances when a well-established domain has been clearly identified and representative items have been selected from the domain for a test (Brown & Hudson, 2002; Hashway, 1998). The phrase criterion-referenced refers to the general family of measurement strategies used for criterion-referenced interpretation of scores.

Use of criterion-referenced measurement is not limited to testing achievement skills or other similar behaviors, but it is also used to determine an object's status in relation to some specific attribute or property. The criterion-referenced measurement framework is applied when individuals are classified or categorized by sex or social class, or when the nurse specifies fetal position during labor. These are some examples of nominal-level use of criterion-referenced measurement, since the results will serve to simply classify an object in relation to a specified attribute rather than imply quantitative value. In this type of criterion-referenced measurement an object's domain status is determined by distinguishing characteristics or features that have been clearly identified and explicated in terms of the nature of the domain. Such distinguishing characteristics serve as the criterion or standard(s) for measurement.

The primary feature of criterion-referenced measurement is its use of an interpretive frame of reference based on a specified domain rather than on a specified population or group (Popham, 1978). The principle difference between criterion-referenced and norm-referenced measurement lies in the standard used as a reference for interpretation of results (Glaser, 1994). In contrast to norm-referenced measurement, in which results are interpreted in terms of those obtained by others on the same measuring device, interpretation of criterion-referenced measurements is based on a predetermined criterion or standard of performance, that is, on specific tasks or performance behaviors.

Comparison of Criterion-Referenced and Norm-Referenced Measures

Although criterion-referenced and norm-referenced measures are developed so that scores will be interpreted differently, they have characteristics in common as well as having distinct differences. Common characteristics include the following according to Gronlund (1988, p. 4).

1. Both require specification of the achievement domain to be measured.
2. Both require a relevant and representative sample of test items.
3. Both use the same types of test items.
4. Both use the same rules for item writing (except for item difficulty).
5. Both are judged by the same qualities of goodness (validity and reliability), although there are sometimes differences in statistical methods employed.
6. Both are useful in the measurement of health variables and in educational measurement.

Table 4.11 delineates some of the differences between criterion-referenced and norm-referenced measures.

Utility in Health and Nursing Measurement

The use of criterion-referenced measurement in the health fields is a common approach to measurement and has been increasing within the last two decades. The application of criterion-referenced measurement is usually best suited for testing basic skills, such as the ability to do manipulative procedures or to demonstrate simple cognitive skills. However, this should not be taken to de-emphasize the importance and usefulness of criterion-referenced measurement in testing domains that include advanced levels of knowledge. It is the intended use of the results of measurement that should determine whether a criterion-referenced measure should be used rather than the complexity of the content domain.

TABLE 4.11 Differences Between Criterion-Referenced and Norm-Referenced Measures

Characteristic	Criterion-Referenced	Norm-Referenced
1. Type of interpretation	Absolute interpretation. Amount of attribute measured is specified based on known placement in a category or by percent.	Relative interpretation. Amount of attribute measured is compared to others for interpretation.
2. Primary uses	Used to categorize attributes or for mastery testing.	Used primarily to obtain scores for purposes of comparison.
3. Type of measurement	Focuses on a delimited domain or subdomains with a relatively large number of items measuring each task, objective, category, or subscale.	Typically focuses on a large domain, with a few items measuring each task, objective, category, or subscale.
	Interpretation requires a clearly defined and delimited domain.	Interpretation requires a clearly defined group.
4. Purpose of testing	To assess the amount of an attribute or material known by each in isolation of others.	To spread out objects or persons across a continuum on the attribute measured.
	Emphasizes description of objects or individuals on the attribute measured or what a person can or cannot do.	Emphasizes discrimination of objects or individuals on the attribute measured in terms of amount or level of learning.
5. Distribution of scores	Distribution of scores vary, often are not normally distributed.	Normal distribution of scores is expected around the mean.
6. Structure of measure or test	Homogeneous, well-defined item content matched to each domain, subdomain or subscale.	More heterogeneous and relatively longer subtests or subscales.
7. Knowledge of nature of questions if testing	Students know the content to expect test questions to address.	Students have little or no idea of nature of content to expect in questions.

(References: Brown, 1996; Gronlund, 1988, p. 14.)

Health Research

Criterion-referenced measurement is amenable for use in the measurement of variables in health and nursing research, and in many instances it may be the most appropriate measurement framework to use in the operationalization of concepts (Strickland, 1994). Suppose a nurse researcher is conducting a study to determine if adjustment to the parental role by parents who have a child with meningomyelocele is related to their acceptance of the child's condition. In this example both the independent variable (adjustment to the parental role) and the dependent variable (acceptance of the child's condition) can be conceptualized so that the criterion-referenced measurement framework would be the more appropriate framework to use for measurement of the variables. If the conceptualization of the variables indicates that parents either adjust to their role or do not adjust, and the parents either accept their child's condition or do not accept it, the criterion-referenced framework is the better framework to use in the measurement of the variables. This is the case because the variables are conceptualized in a criterion-referenced manner. Crucial in the measurement of the variables would be the specification of critical behaviors that each parent must exhibit in order for the researcher to make the determination that adjustment to the parental role had occurred or not occurred or that acceptance of the child's condition had occurred or not.

Whether a nurse researcher should choose a measuring tool that uses the criterion-referenced measurement framework depends on the conceptualization of the variables under study and the nature of the research questions addressed. However, some researchers have a bias toward using norm-referenced measurement when operationalizing variables, because criterion-referenced measures usually yield nominal and ordinal data. Many variables are best operationalized through the use of criterion-referenced measurement. For example, self-care agency is a concept that is likely to be a focus of study in nursing research. The definition of the concept indicates the need to use a criterion-referenced tool to measure the concept because the focus is on determining capabilities that enable performance of self-care (Orem, 1985). Denyes's Self-Care Agency Instrument (Denyes,1988) was designed so that one could determine strengths and limitations in an individual's abilities to make decisions about and to accomplish self-care. Therefore, the focus of measurement is on specifying the individual's degree of ability related to self-care.

Clinical Practice

In the clinical practice setting criterion-referenced measures are sometimes used to determine client ability to perform specific tasks and skills and to categorize clients in regard to their health status or diagnosis. The criterion-referenced measurement framework is used to classify attributes related to client conditions that may be assessed through direct clinical observation or by laboratory tests. For example, pelvic floor muscle strength has been a clinical variable of interest for nurses who care for women with urinary incontinence as well as those who care for obstetrical patients. The Pelvic Muscle Strength Rating Scale (Sampselle, Brink, & Wells,

1989) and the Circumvaginal Muscles Rating Scale (Worth, Dougherty, & McKey, 1986) are two similar instruments that have been developed to rate or categorize the strength of pelvic floor muscles in women. Also, the results of pregnancy tests are interpreted as either positive or negative; the intensity of a heart murmur may be classified as grade 1, 2, 3, 4, 5, or 6; the measurement of reflexes during a neurological exam may be recorded as 0, 1 +, 2 +, 3 +, or 4 +; a test of the presence of albumin in the urine may be interpreted as either negative, trace, or 1+, 2+, or 3+; and a patient may be categorized as either severely, moderately, or mildly hypertensive based on their blood pressure level. Such criterion-referenced measurements are used on numerous occasions daily in the clinical setting. In most cases, criterion-referenced measures that are used in the clinical milieu provide a means for classifying data for descriptive purposes and to facilitate diagnoses. The criterion standards applied during the classification process have been explicated and incorporated into these procedures so that results will be as accurate as possible. Figure 4.8 illustrates the use of the criterion-referenced framework for the classification of primary skin lesions. Types or classes of lesions have been specified and defined in descriptive terms so that the approach to classification is clear and unambiguous. These criterion standards guide the classification process by the examiner.

Educational Programs

Criterion-referenced measures are particularly useful when the purpose of testing is to ascertain whether an individual has attained minimum requirements, such as for practice or for admission to a specific educational program or course. The NCLEX examination is probably the most commonly used criterion-referenced test in nursing. A cut score is set and each individual must score at that level or above in order to be considered safe to practice and to receive a nursing license. In educational programs, criterion-referenced measurement is best applied when there is a need for tests to examine student progress toward the attainment of a designated skill or knowledge level. Criterion-referenced measurement is better suited for such

Type of Lesion	Criterion or Standard for Classification
Macule	Circumscribed, flat discoloration of the skin that is less than 1 cm in size. Occurs in various shapes and colors.
Patch	Circumscribed, flat discoloration of the skin that is larger than 1 cm in size. Occurs in various shapes and colors.
Papule	Circumscribed, elevated, superficial solid lesion that is less than 1 cm in size. Border and top may assume various forms.
Wheal	Circumscribed, irregular, relatively flat edematous lesion. Color varies from red to pale. Varies in size.
Plaque	Circumscribed, elevated, superficial solid lesion larger than 1 cm in size. Border may assume various forms.
Nodule	Solid, elevated skin lesion that extends below the dermis that is up to 1 cm in size. Borders may assume various shapes.
Tumor	Solid, elevated skin lesion that extends below the dermis that is larger than 1 cm in size. Border may assume various shapes.
Vesicle	Circumscribed elevation of the skin with an accumulation of serous fluid between the upper layers of the skin. Covered by a translucent epithelium, less than 1 cm in size. Occurs in various shapes.
Bulla	Circumscribed elevation of the skin with an accumulation of serous fluid between the upper layers of the skin. Covered by a translucent epithelium, larger than 1 cm in size. Occurs in various shapes.
Pustule	Circumscribed elevation of the skin with an accumulation of purulent fluid between the upper layers of the skin. Covered by a translucent epithelium. Contents appear milky, orange, yellow, or green. Occurs in various shapes and sizes.

FIGURE 4.8   Classification of primary skin lesions.

(Adapted from DeGowin, E. L. and DeGowin, R. I.: *Bedside Diagnostic Examination* (2nd ed.), Macmillan, New York, 1969; and Delp, M. H. and Manning, R. T.: *Major's Physical Diagnosis* (7th ed.), Saunders, Philadelphia, 1968.)

functions than norm-referenced measures. Instruction and evaluation of nursing students in the clinical setting is highly amenable to the use of criterion-referenced measures because of the emphasis placed on the application of knowledge and skills. Clearly the focus of evaluation in the assessment of clinical skills in nursing and other practice disciplines should be on what a person is able to do rather than on how the person compares with others. The application of criterion-referenced measurement for ascertaining clinical skills would require each student to demonstrate critical behaviors before performance would be considered satisfactory.

Mastery testing is used to classify students as masters or nonmasters of a single learning objective. Mastery testing yields an all-or-none score (i.e., pass or fail) that indicates whether a person has attained the predetermined level of skills or knowledge. When basic skills are tested, it is not unusual for nearly complete mastery to be expected. Items on the mastery test should be highly sensitive to instructional goals and should discriminate between those who do and do not master the objective tested. Scores are reported separately in terms of the student's performance in relation to each objective, since students may have adequate skills and knowledge related to some objectives but not others. The methods for setting performance standards or cut scores for mastery are particularly important and involve the identification of critical behaviors related to each objective assessed.

When advanced content is tested, it is virtually impossible to set the cut score or level of mastery completely in terms of critical requisite skills, but this often must be done partly in a normative manner. The mastery level is often determined in a normative manner based on the performance of previous groups or through the judgment of the instructor who is teaching the course.

Developing Criterion-Referenced Measures

Given that the primary goal of criterion-referenced measurement is to accurately determine the status of some object in terms of a well-defined domain, two major assumptions regarding a criterion-referenced measure become apparent. First, the items included in the measure should sample the specified content domain carefully. Second, the preset criteria or standards of performance must estimate the object's domain status. These assumptions encourage one to consider several key points that are crucial for the development of criterion-referenced measures, among which are the need for (1) a clear definition or explication of the content domain tested; (2) the inclusion of a relatively homogeneous collection of items or tasks that accurately assess the content domain as the focus of measurement; and (3) the determination of criteria or performance standards that

define an object's domain status. Figure 4.9 presents the various steps for developing and validating measures. Attention for the remainder of this chapter is concentrated on steps 2 through 6, which focus on the construction of measures. The need to delineate a conceptual model as a basis for tool development is discussed in chapters 1 and 2. Concerns related to establishing reliability and validity will be discussed in detail in chapters 5 and 6.

Specifying the Purpose(s) of the Measure

In order to insure that a test will optimally address the needs for which it is developed the purposes of the measure should be clearly specified. As indicated in chapter 2, the conceptual model that serves as the basis for the development of the measure helps to clarify its purpose and guides the manner in which it is developed. However, when the major purposes are clarified and the priorities among probable uses of the measure are identified, the likelihood increases that the final form of the measure will meet the most important purposes it is intended to serve. When specifying the purposes of the measure, the developer should consider the population with whom it will be used, the circumstances in which it is most likely to be employed, and how the scores that will ultimately result will be

---

1. Specify the conceptual model of the measure.
2. Specify the purpose(s) of the measure.
3. Explicate objective(s) or the domain definition.
4. Prepare test specifications including:
   a. Method of administration
   b. Number or proportion of items that will focus on each objective or subscale
   c. Type of items and how they will be created
   d. Test restrictions and givens
   e. General scoring rules and procedures
5. Construct the measure including:
   a. Develop a pool of items or tasks matched to the objective(s) or subscales
   b. Review items or tasks to determine content validity and their appropriateness
   c. Select items after editing or deleting poorly developed items from the item pool
   d. Assemble the measure (including preparation of directions, scoring keys, answer sheets, etc.)
6. Set standards or cut score for interpreting results.
7. Field-test or administer the measure.
8. Assess reliability and validity of measure (including determining the statistical properties of items, and deleting and revising items further based on empirical data).

FIGURE 4.9   Stages in the development and validation of criterion-referenced measures.

applied. For example, a measure of knowledge of diabetic care might be needed by a nursing instructor who wants to test the knowledge of nursing students or by a clinician who needs to assess the knowledge of patients with diabetes. Although both potential users need to measure the same variable, it would not be appropriate in most circumstances to use the same tool for both. The reason for this is obvious. The nursing instructor would want a test that clearly identifies the knowledge level of nursing students who ultimately will be expected to use that knowledge to make decisions about the care of patients. Most likely, such a test would be administered in a classroom setting to a group of students who are reasonably well educated. Knowledge areas to be addressed by such a measure that would be used with nursing students would be broad and include rather detailed scientific information. In this circumstance, a test with many items that uses high-level terminology would be appropriate. However, in a situation where the focus is on the measurement of patient knowledge of diabetic care, the test developer would have to be sensitive to the broad range of educational levels of patients, many of whom would not understand highly technical and advanced terminology. Also, test length in this situation would be important since it is not likely that circumstances under which patients would be administered such a measure would allow for a long test with many items. Therefore, clarifying the primary purposes for which a measure will be used will influence the characteristics of the items or indicators of the variable in the tool as well as other aspects of the tool, such as its length, reading level, and the manner in which it is to be administered.

Explicating Objectives or Domain Definition

A precise and rigorous domain definition is necessary to maximize the interpretability of the results of measurements. It is the objective of the measure that defines and specifies the domain that is to be assessed. The specific objective(s) for the measure, therefore, must be explicated prior to its construction. Methods for stating behavioral objectives were discussed previously

in this chapter during the discussion of norm-referenced measures, and also apply in the construction of criterion-referenced measures.

Preparation of Test Specifications

It has been noted previously that the objective of a measure defines the content domain that is the focus of measurement. However, the objective, in most instances, is not sufficiently constraining to guide the specifics of the construction of the measure such as method of administration, number or proportion of items testing each objective or subscale, test-item format, test restrictions and givens, or test scoring. That is the purpose of test specifications, which serve a similar function as the test blueprint in the norm-referenced case. When the test constructor has provided a description of all of these components, then the major components of test specifications have been explicated. The approach to developing each of these parts of test specifications are the same as described for norm-referenced measures.

If a measure includes subobjectives that relate to the overall objective, the test developer should make sure that each subobjective is adequately represented on the instrument. This can be done by using a blueprinting approach as described earlier in this chapter.

Popham (1978, 1980) has specified a general format for test specifications and suggests that they generally consist of (1) a general description, (2) a sample item, (3) stimulus attributes (item characteristics), and (4) response attributes and specification supplement.

General Description. The general description specifies what it is that the test measures through a succinct overview of the set of target behaviors. In most criterion-referenced test specifications this is the test objective. Although succinct, the general description provides information about the form of the test and the approach to administration of the measure. The following is illustrative of the general description for a measure of knowledge of fluid and electrolyte balance: "Given a written test of knowledge relevant to the care of clients at risk for fluid and electrolyte imbalance, the student will respond to at least 80% of the items correctly."

Sample Item. A sample item, similar to those offered in the measure, is provided along with complete directions to the examinee or respondent. Usually, it is rather simple to provide a sample item, because most measures consist of relatively short items. Sometimes it becomes difficult to supply a sample item if items are lengthy and complicated. In any case, an illustrative item is provided for two reasons. First, for many measures the general description statement along with the illustrative item can provide enough information about the test to further clarify the purpose, scope, and intended use for the measure. The second reason is that the illustrative item can provide format cues for those who will assist in the generation of items that will constitute the test. It should be noted that criterion-referenced test items may consist of most of the item forms discussed for norm-referenced measures. Below is an example of a sample item that is compatible with the general description provided above.

Example of a Sample Item

Directions: This test presents situations that are followed by sets of related test items. Read each situation carefully and answer the multiple-choice items that follow it, based on the information in the situation. Select only one answer. Write the letter of the answer you select in the designated space on the answer sheet provided.

Situation: Mr. Johnson is a 65-year-old retired farmer who has come to the Rural Health Clinic complaining of weakness, frequent episodes of diarrhea of 5 days duration, and abdominal pains. He says he has not been able to eat and drink fluids well because they "make my stomach hurt." Mr. Johnson has a temperature of 102°F, a thready pulse of 92, and a respiratory rate of 18. His blood pressure is 124/70. Mr. Johnson's skin is dry with poor turgor. There have been no episodes of vomiting.

1. In addition to a deficit of water (fluids), which of the following problems should the nurse be most concerned about in observing Mr. Johnson?
   A. Sodium deficit
   B. Chloride deficit
   C. Potassium deficit
   D. Bicarbonate deficit

Stimulus Attributes. Stimulus attributes (item characteristics) are the factors that constrain or limit the composition of the set of items included in the measure. Generally, the items within a measure are designed to yield a response that is used in the measurement of the phenomenon of interest. Therefore, the attributes of the stimulus materials (i.e., the items) are set forth and described. This means that careful thought must be given to the nature of items in an attempt to identify significant factors associated with the desired item characteristics. Attention must be focused upon content considerations that may influence item characteristics. A decision must be made about how the range of eligible content can be most effectively circumscribed through test items. The following is illustrative of stimulus attributes that might be developed for a nursing test which is to measure knowledge requisite for the care of clients at risk for fluid and electrolyte imbalance and which is to consist of multiple-choice items.

Example of Stimulus Attributes

1. Each multiple-choice item will relate to a nursing situation that describes a client at risk for fluid and electrolyte imbalance. The client's diagnosis, pertinent lab results, physical condition, treatment regimen, and significant history will be presented in each situation.
2. Each item will focus on prevention, assessment, or treatment/care related to clients at risk for fluid and electrolyte imbalance.
3. The item stem will not include irrelevant material. Neither should a negatively stated stem be included, except when significant learning outcomes require it. Item stems will consist of complete sentences.

Response Attributes. Response attributes make up the final component of a set of test specifications and focus on the nature of the examinee's or subject's response to items within the measure. Two types of responses are possible. The subject may either select from a collection of response options presented in the measure (e.g., in multiple-choice or true-false questions), or the respondent may construct a response (e.g., in oral presentations, essay items, short- answer items, or behavioral skills tests). It is within the response-attributes section of the test specifications that rules regarding the two response possibilities are specified.

If the response attribute is the selected response, then specific rules are provided that determine the nature of the correct response and also the nature of the incorrect options. For example, if multiple-choice items are to be used in the measure, guidelines for creating not only the correct response but also the wrong answer options must be carefully explicated. Incorrect responses usually reflect common errors encountered in meeting the objective. Hence, by looking at the wrong answers, diagnostic information may be obtained. Illustrated below are a set of response attributes that are complementary to the set of stimulus attributes.

Example of Response Attributes

1. A set of four short one- or two-word responses or single-sentence response alternatives will follow each item stem. All responses within an item should be approximately the same length and must plausibly relate to the item stem.
2. An item will contain only one correct or clearly best answer. All response alternatives will be grammatically consistent with the stem of the item.
3. The three incorrect response alternatives will lack accuracy or appropriate scope.
4. An incorrect response alternative exemplifies a lack of accuracy when it makes a statement contradicted by information in the textbook or makes a statement incapable of verification.
5. An incorrect response alternative exemplifies the lack of appropriate scope when it does not include all of the important details to fully answer the item stem or when it is too general to account for all of the important details needed to clearly answer the item stem.
6. The correct response alternative must be entirely accurate and have appropriate scope, in that it includes all the important information to answer the stem and is verifiable by agreement of experts in the area.

When the respondent is required to construct a response, the response attributes should explain the criteria that will be used to ascertain a reliable judgment of the adequacy of the constructed responses. These response attributes should be so well formulated that determination of the acceptability of any constructed responses would be a rather simple matter. In reality, depending upon the nature of the measure, this ideal may not be easily approximated.

Specification Supplement. This involves listing supplemental material that is needed to clarify the previous elements of test specifications. This could include a list of vocabulary items, or other information from which the item writer can draw (Brown & Hudson, 2002).

Similar test specifications would need to be developed for a measure of proficiency for performing a skill. Figure 4.10, provides an illustrative set of criterion-referenced test specifications for a measure of skill for inserting a nasogastric tube, which is provided in Figure 4.11. This example presents an illustration of response attributes for the constructed response required in this situation.

Finally, in some cases the nature of the content domain or items may be such that a full description of stimulus attributes or response attributes may be too voluminous to include in a focused presentation of the test specifications. In such cases, key statements could be emphasized within an abbreviated description for these sections, and the detailed specifications would be included in a manual, supplement, or appendix. This approach should be taken when lengthy content citations might distract the reader from focusing on important specification statements.

Clearly, one of the major purposes of test specifications is to facilitate the creation of a measure with items that are homogeneous. Since criterion-referenced measures are supposed to assess one content domain, homogeneity of items within a measure is an important indicator of this desirable characteristic. The more homogeneous the items, the more likely it is that the items within the measure are representative of one domain. On the other hand, the more heterogeneous the items, the greater the likelihood that the measure assesses

General Description

Given a conscious adult, the nurse will insert a nasogastric tube. All necessary actions for safe insertion must be performed.

Sample Item

Directions: You are to insert a nasogastric tube from the nostrils into the stomach of an adult client. You must employ the necessary materials and proceed sequentially through each requisite step of the procedure.

Step 1. Gather necessary equipment. (i.e., Levine type lumen tube, large 30 cc syringe and stethoscope, cup of drinking water)

Stimulus Attributes or Item Characteristics

1. Each item will consist of a necessary step in the procedure and describe the behaviors required of the nurse to complete the step. Each item will be stated in behavioral terms.
2. Each item should be listed sequentially (i.e., will follow the item that should be completed immediately prior to it).
3. Where appropriate, more than one descriptive behavior will be included in an item (step), if either may be correctly employed for the completion of that item.

Response Attributes

1. A correct response to an item occurs if both of the following are observed:
   a. The nurse performs the behaviors as described in the item.
   b. The nurse performs the item in its proper sequence.
2. An incorrect response to an item occurs if any one of the following is observed:
   a. Nurse's behavior is not consistent with behaviors described in the item.
   b. Nurse does not perform the item in its proper sequence.
   c. Nurse omits the item.

FIGURE 4.10 An illustrative set of criterion-referenced test specifications for a measure of skill for inserting a nasogastric tube.

factors outside the domain. Precise and rigorous test specifications help to delimit the domain and thereby facilitate the inclusion of homogeneous items that measure the same domain, even though items may be of various levels of difficulty. However, ambiguous and fuzzy test specifications most often lead to incongruent and heterogeneous test items, which reduce the interpretability and, hence, the validity of results.

Test Restrictions and Givens

The restrictions and givens of the test conditions should be spelled out. Often these are incorporated into the statement of the objective. Restrictions may be placed on resources or aids that can be employed or on the amount of time that may be taken to perform a task or behavior. In some instances time may be an important indicator of the quality of performance, such as in the administering of

medications or certain treatments. For example, the time specification in the objective "The student administers medications within 30 minutes of the scheduled time of administration" is strongly related to quality of performance. However, in most situations, time is not usually an important indicator of the quality of performance. Time restrictions may be placed on some skill or achievement tests. Such restrictions should include a long enough period of time to allow those who normally would have mastered the domain to have a sufficient opportunity to exhibit mastery. In addition to resources that a subject may be prohibited from using, there may be a variety of resources that the subject may use during a testing period. Such resources are referred to as givens. Any givens or restrictions in resources, aids, or time used during the measurement procedure should be clearly communicated.

Case No. _____   Name of Subject _____

Date _____   Name of Rater _____

Behaviors (steps)	Correct	Incorrect
1. Gathers necessary equipment. (i.e., Levine type lumen tube, large 30 cc syringe and stethoscope, cup of drinking water).		
2. Marks distance on tube as measured from the tip of the nose, around the ear, to the xiphoid.		
3. Places client in a sitting position (or as near to sitting as possible).		
4. Maintains position throughout procedure.		
5. Advances tube firmly but gently through the client's nostril to the pharynx.		
6. Has the patient swallow sips of water to carry the tube down the esophagus until tube is in the predetermined distance (see step 2).		
NOTE: Removes tube and begins again if coughing or cyanosis occurs during insertion.		
7. Checks to determine if tube is in the stomach by aspirating gastric juices up the tube. —OR— Putting 20 ml of air into the tube by syringe while listening with a stethoscope over the stomach for a gurgling noise.		
Scoring Key: Pass = Correctly performs all steps (1–7) in procedure. Fail = Incorrectly performs at least one step in the procedure.		

FIGURE 4.11   A measure of skill for inserting a nasogastric tube.

Scoring Rules and Procedures

Once the items have been constructed and matched to objectives, scoring rules should be spelled out. In most instances, the item format dictates the general scoring procedure. If any items must be reverse-scored, those items should be clearly identified in the scoring procedure. The test developer must be careful to specify which items measure which objectives when more than one objective is measured within the context of a single tool. Within the criterion-referenced framework a separate score should be derived for each objective measured by the instrument in order to interpret the result appropriately.

In most instances, the same rules of scoring used for norm-referenced measures will also be relevant for the criterion-referenced case. However, with criterion-referenced measures a cut score that indicates mastery or nonmastery of an objective will often need to be determined. Methods for setting cut scores or standards for interpreting scores derived from criterion-referenced measures are discussed in a later section of this chapter.

In summary, the purpose of test specifications is to communicate the specifics related to the construction of the measure. This includes explication of not only what the items on the measure will assess but also the rules that govern the creation and administration of the measure and scoring procedures. The goals of the developer of test specifications are to be sufficiently specific to communicate the scope and constraints to potential users of the measure; and to be sufficiently targeted and explicit to guide those who might be involved in the construction and development of the measure.

Constructing the Measure

After items are constructed, a preliminary review of all test items (or tasks) should be done once the generation of items has been completed. Items are reviewed by content specialists and those that are not well formulated or congruent with objectives are identified, revised, or discarded in a manner similar to that described for norm-referenced measures. Population representatives should be asked to complete the tool and then specify (1) which items they had difficulty responding to and why, (2) which items they have questions about, (3) revisions they believe should be made, and (4) suggestions for items that should be included. Appropriate revisions should then be made in the measure prior to having it field tested.

In some instances a fairly large number of items may be generated to test one content domain. When a large sample of items is developed to test one objective, a predetermined number may be selected for inclusion in the measure by random sampling. Any sampling method that maintains the domain-referenced status of the test would be appropriate. Once items have been selected, the measure should be assembled including directions for administration, scoring keys, answer sheets, and any other materials necessary for administration and scoring of the tool.

Setting Standards for Interpreting Results

Once the domain of a measure has been defined and items to measure the domain have been generated and selected, the next step in the construction of a criterion-referenced measurement tool often is to establish standards or cut score(s). However, standards or cut scores are not a necessary feature of all criterion-referenced measures (Linn, 1982), for example, those that assess domain status by percentage scores only. A standard or cut score is a point along the scale of test scores that is used to classify a subject to reflect level of proficiency relative to a particular objective. Sometimes several cut scores may be established so that a subject may be assigned to one of several levels of proficiency.

As noted previously in the section on scoring, if a test or measure consists of items that assess more than one objective, different standards will be set in relation to sets of items that measure the different objectives. In other words, items that measure different objectives are separated out and used like individual tests, and cut scores are established to make criterion-referenced interpretations of the results. This is done because one cannot make criterion-referenced interpretations of results when performance on different objectives is reflected in one score. The use of one score to represent performance on a number of different objectives does not communicate what a subject can actually do, because the pooling of results will mask performance relative to each specific objective.

Whenever possible, the domain score is computed for each objective, since it represents knowledge, skills, or attitudes in relation to the specified content domain. A percentage score is a domain score. Whereas the percentile rank is used in norm-referenced measurement as an indicator of relative performance, the percentage score often is used in criterion-referenced measurement as a measure of absolute performance. The percentage score is the proportion of the maximum raw-score points that have been earned by the subject and is calculated by the formula below.

Formula 4.3: Converting a raw score to a percentage score

$$\text{Percentage score} = \frac{\text{subject's raw score on the measure} \times 100}{\text{the maximum possible raw score on the measure}}$$

That is, the percentage score is the subject's raw score on a measure, divided by the maximum possible raw score on the measure, times 100.

Example: A raw score of 10 on a 20-item test is equivalent to a percentage score of:

$$\text{Percentage score} = \frac{10}{20} \times 100$$
$$= 0.50 \times 100$$
$$= 50$$

The percentage score represents the proportion of a content domain that an individual has mastered or responded to appropriately. Hence, it indicates an individual's level of performance in relation to the possible minimum and maximum raw scores on a measure.

How are standards or cut scores determined? The answer to this question will depend on the nature of the measure and the content domain that is the focus of measurement. The key idea in criterion-referenced measurement is to determine critical behaviors that distinguish those objects that possess the attribute in question from those that do not. In some situations it is quite a simple matter to make these distinctions. However, in other situations these distinctions are not clear. It also is apparent that the standard level will vary from measure to measure depending upon the nature of the objective assessed and the critical behaviors or attributes that must be observed in order to make a criterion-referenced interpretation. For instance, it is easier to determine if a child possesses the psychomotor skills to jump double dutch than to determine if the child possesses the psychomotor skills appropriate for his age and stage of development. In the former case, 100 percent mastery of the domain would likely be required in order to make the judgment that the child could indeed jump double dutch. However, making a criterion-referenced judgment in the latter case is not so simple, nor is 100 percent mastery of the items that might be used to measure psychomotor development for a particular age and stage of development a likely expectation.

Because the determination of standards for making criterion-referenced interpretations is often not a simple matter, a number of approaches to standard setting have been suggested. Most standard-setting methods can be categorized as judgmental, empirical, or a combination. *Judgmental* methods subject the individual items on the measure to the inspection of judges who are asked to assess how a person who is minimally competent would perform on each item. When *empirical* methods are used, data are collected and cut scores are based on the results of data analysis. Some blend of both judgmental and empirical methods are used in *combination* methods for setting cut scores.

No matter what standard-setting method is used, judgment is involved, and the standard in that regard is arbitrary. If a standard is set too

high the chances of making false-negative criterion-referenced interpretations and decisions are increased; that is, there will be increased chances of wrongly classifying persons or objects as not meeting the standard when, in actuality, they do meet it. Similarly, false-positive classifications are made when persons or objects are categorized as having met the standard when, in actuality, they have not. When standards are set too low the chances of false-positive results are increased. Figure 4.12 illustrates groups that have been classified as masters and nonmasters of a content domain. The area designated "masters incorrectly classified" represents false-negatives, and the area specified "nonmasters incorrectly classified" indicates false-positive classifications. The optimal outcome in establishing a standard is to set cut scores in a manner whereby the chances of false-positive and false-negative results are at a minimum. However, depending on the use that will be made of the results, standards may electively be set high by the user to reduce the chances of making false-positive interpretations at an increased expense of making more false-negative interpretations, and vice versa.

Several authors have suggested judgmental methods that provide a means for setting a standard or cut score. The judgmental methods offered by Martuza (1977), Nedelsky (1954), and Ebel (1979) will be presented here, because they are rather clear-cut approaches that are recognized and used by measurement specialists.

Martuza (1977, p. 270) suggests a rather simple three-step process to the establishment of cut scores. First, content specialists examine each item and carefully rate its importance relative to the objective on a ten-point scale ranging from "of little importance" to "extremely important". The second step involves averaging each judge's ratings across all items in the test. Finally, the averages are converted into a proportion. The proportion could then be used as a cut score for the test. If more than one judge independently rates the items, the mean of the averages from all judges would be used to calculate the proportion that would be used as a cut score. If the proportion that resulted was 85 percent, then this would be the standard. The cut score might be adjusted upward or downward

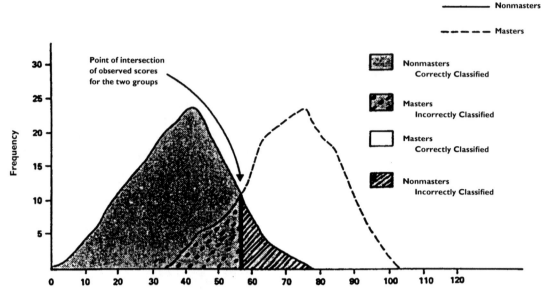

FIGURE 4.12   Frequency polygons of criterion-referenced test scores for masters and nonmasters.

based on the potential for guessing, sampling error, the relative cost of false-negative and false-positive results, or other factors that might influence the results or how they are used.

Ebel (1979) has proposed a judgmental approach to establishing cut scores that requires content specialists to rate each item within a measure along two dimensions: relevance and difficulty. Four levels of relevance (essential, important, acceptable, questionable) are used along with three levels of difficulty (easy, medium, and hard). These results are presented in a 3 × 4 grid with 12 cells. Judges examine each item and locate the items in the proper cell, based upon their level of difficulty and relevance. Once all test items have been located within cells, the judges assign to each cell a percentage that they agree is representative of the percentage of items in the cell to which the minimally qualified subject should be able to respond correctly. The percentage is then multiplied by the number of test items in each cell, and the sum of all the cells is divided by the total number of test items to obtain the standard (cut score). Figure 4.13 presents an example of Ebel's method.

Nedelsky (1954) has offered a method to establish cut scores for tests with multiple-choice items. Judges are asked to review each item and to identify distractors for each item that D-F students or students who are minimally competent should be able to eliminate as incorrect. The reciprocal of the remaining alternatives is the minimum passing level (MPL) on that item for the student who is minimally competent. It is the probability of a correct response as a function of remaining answer choices. For instance, if an item had five options from which the student could select an answer and the judges determined that the minimally competent student could eliminate one distractor as incorrect, this would leave four alternatives from which the student would really have to select. The minimum passing level for that item would be 1/4, or 0.25. If 3, 2, and 1 items remained, the minimum passing level for the items would be 0.33, 0.50, and 1.00, respectively. Once the minimum passing level for each item has been determined by the judges, the minimum passing levels are summed across the test items to obtain a standard. All of the judges' standards are then averaged to obtain a standard or cut score for the test.

Nedelsky recommends a method for adjusting cut scores in order to reduce the chances of false-negative or false-positive interpretations,

		Relevance			
		Essential	Important	Acceptable	Questionable
	Easy	1,20,21 100%	4,15,27,28 100%	3,10 100%	6 100%
Difficulty	Medium	5,14,22,23 100%	2,7,19,16,30 60%	8,13,18 33.3%	17 0%
	Hard	9,26 100%	11,25,29 33.3%	12,24 50%	

$$\text{Standard} = \frac{\Sigma \text{ No. of items in cell } \mathbf{x} \text{ cell percentage}}{\text{Total no. of test items}}$$
(cut score)

$$\text{Standard} = \frac{300 + 400 + 200 + 400 + 300 + 100 + 200 + 100 + 100 + 100}{30}$$
(cut score)

$$\text{Standard} = \frac{2200}{30}$$
(cut score)

$$\text{Standard} = 73.3\%$$
(cut score)

FIGURE 4.13   An example of Ebel's grid for standard-setting.

depending on the user's needs. He assumes that if the standard deviation of the individual judges' standards is computed, a distribution synonymous with the hypothesized distribution of scores of borderline students will result. This standard deviation is then multiplied by a constant K, which is subtracted from or added to the standard. The constant is decided upon by the test user and would regulate the approximate number of borderline students who will pass or fail the test.

Two combination methods for setting standards on classroom tests suggested by Zieky and Livingston (1977) have applicability for other nursing situations as well. They are the borderline-group and the contrasting-group methods. In both methods, experts are used as judges, and standards are based on subjects rather than items. For illustrative purposes, assume that a nursing supervisor is trying to establish a cut score for acceptable performance on a rating scale of staff-nurse team leadership. In the contrasting-group method, the supervisor identifies those staff nurses exhibiting definite acceptable and unacceptable team leadership behavior after

defining minimally acceptable performance. The distributions of scores obtained by the two groups are then plotted. The point of intersection of the two groups is taken as the standard. (Refer to Figure 4.12 for an illustration of the point of intersection.)

In the borderline-group method, the evaluator defines the minimally acceptable performance on the content domain assessed, after which a list is made of a group of subjects who are borderline in performance; that is, their performance is so close to being both acceptable and unacceptable that they cannot be classified into either group. The median of the test scores from this borderline group is taken as the cut score.

As can be noted from the methods presented here, the rigor and applicability of the standard-setting methods vary. Different approaches are required from measure to measure, depending on the purpose, content domain, and intended use of the results. The decision-making context and the resources available to aid in the standard-setting process also need to be taken into consideration. Analysis of the decision-making context consists of viewing the short-term and long-term implications of decisions or conclusions that will be made using the measure. Possible psychological, social, financial, and educational consequences that may result, and the number of people that might be affected, must be given careful thought before making a final decision about the approach to establishing a standard for a measure.

The actual resources that will be needed to implement a standard-setting method also need consideration. The degree to which resources (e.g., personnel, time, effort, money, material, and expertise) are expended would best be determined by the decision context for which the measure will be used and the availability of such resources to carry out the task. The actual number of judges needed for the standard-setting process, when they are used, is usually the decision of the user. However, approximately three or four content specialists should be employed when a high degree of precision is needed in the estimation of the cut score. Hambleton (1980, p. 114) offers several suggestions and insights that are particularly pertinent for the standard-setting process.

Regardless of how technically sound or how content valid the test is, considerable care and attention must be given to the standard-setting process. The best test can be sabotaged by an inappropriate standard. Therefore, the test developer should:

1. Select a standard-setting method that can be efficiently and effectively handled by judges.
2. Ensure that all relevant groups have an opportunity to be involved in standard setting.
3. Train the judges so that they understand their tasks during the standard-setting process.
4. Ensure that the judges understand the purpose of the testing program, know the characteristics of the group of subjects to be tested or assessed, and have the same perspective or definition of a master and a nonmaster of test content.
5. Pilot-test the measure. Decision-validity information should be provided for several standards of test performance. Decision

validity as used in this instance refers to the accuracy with which objects are classified into specific groups based on the set of standard(s) for categorization. Both test results from subjects and independently derived standards from judges can be used to set a revised standard.
6. Review standards occasionally.

Construction of Criterion-Referenced Measures With Descriptive Domains

In nursing many of the criterion-referenced measures that are used assess physical attributes or purely descriptive domains. Specificity and precision in the measurement of descriptive domains are needed in clinical nursing and in nursing research as a means to facilitate precise measurement of client conditions and states. Nominal- and ordinal-level measurements are often employed for descriptive purposes in these situations. A number of examples of such descriptive domains were cited earlier in this chapter—for example, the results of pregnancy tests, which are interpreted as either positive or negative, and the measurement of acetone in the urine, which is given as negative, trace, 1+, 2+, or 3+. Although such measures appear rather simple and easy to construct and use, the reader is reminded that these criterion-referenced measures must adhere to the same measurement principles as are required in the measurement of behavioral domains. In addition, the same principles that undergird the construction of measures to test behavioral domains also apply for descriptive domains, although the approach varies somewhat.

As noted previously, the goal of criterion-referenced measurement is to assess a specified domain and to determine the domain status of some object in regard to the attribute of interest. The outcome or result of criterion-referenced measurement is that the object is classified or categorized according to the attribute that is the focus of measurement. When the attribute is a cognitive or psychomotor skill the person is classified on a pass/fail basis or is categorized in some other relevant manner in terms of the specified content domain. When an object is assessed in regard to a descriptive content domain, the major difference is that a number of items or tasks are not generated in order to determine the domain status of the object. A woman is either pregnant or not. The breath sounds of the lungs are described and categorized by level of intensity, pitch, and duration as vesicular, bronchovesicular, or bronchial, because no clinical measurement equipment exists that can measure this variable as a continuous variable at the interval level of measurement. There is no pool of items or tasks that can be generated to facilitate measurement of these descriptive domains. However, it is desirable that they be assessed in a way that provides an accurate classification of an object's status within the domain.

There are a number of important steps that must be followed in the development of measures with descriptive domains that are similar to those required in the construction of measures that test behavioral domains. When considering the steps, one will notice the marked similarity to those presented in Figure 4.9.

1. Clearly define the conceptual basis of the domain.
2. Formulate the purpose of the measure.
3. Prepare specifications for the formulation of classes or categories.
4. Determine content validity of classes or categories with the assistance of content specialists.
5. Revise classes or categories, if indicated.
6. Administer the measure.
7. Assess the reliability and validity of the measure.

The initial step in the construction of a criterion-referenced measure with a descriptive content domain, as with any other type of measure, is to provide conceptual clarity about what is being measured. Therefore, a clear definition of the central concept or variable that is the focus of the measurement is obtained. The definition must provide conceptual clarity about the scope and limitations in conceptualization of the variable. The purpose of the measure is stated in terms of this definition and thereby further clarifies the content domain of the measure.

The next step is to specify and define the nonoverlapping categories within which phenomena may be classified. The goal is to describe accurately and specifically the distinguishing attributes or dimensions of each category in order to provide a basis for the classification process. Figure 4.8 presents a sample measure for the classification of primary skin lesions. In this example, the descriptions of the categories are based on several dimensions: size, shape, color, and configuration. Descriptions must be precise and unambiguous so that no entity can be classified in more than one category.

The content validity of the classes or categories is judged by content specialists who review each category to determine if there are overlapping categories or one or more categories in which the same object might be classified. The judges also determine if the dimensions used in the categorization scheme are appropriately followed and if there are missing categories. A missing category would be indicated if the categories that had been identified and described did not provide for the categorization of an object or phenomenon that is included in the content domain according to the domain definition. Additional revisions of the classes are made, if indicated, prior to administering the measure. Reliability and validity data can then be investigated.

SUMMARY

The first step in the design of any nursing measure is to clarify the purposes for the measurement. This is facilitated greatly when the measure is derived from a conceptual model. Objectives for the measure should be stated using good form. When taxonomies are employed in writing objectives, action verbs and critical behaviors to be observed are specified, hence decreasing the possibility that the same behavior will be assessed differently by different people.

Specifications regarding the scope, emphasis, and length of the norm-referenced measure are explicated by the process of blueprinting. The blueprint facilitates the construction of items and the assessment of content validity of the resulting measure. When a criterion-referenced measure is employed, test specifications serve the same function as a blueprint and include a general description of the measure, sample item, stimulus attributes, response attributes, and test givens and restrictions that explicate what the items on the measure will assess, as well as the rules that govern the creation and administration of the measure and scoring procedures. The type of measure to be employed is a function of the conceptual model and subsequent operational definitions of key variables to be measured. Regardless of type, every measure has three components: (1) directions for administration, (2) a set of items, and (3) directions for obtaining and interpreting scores. Within the context of a given type of measure, there are a variety of specific item formats available, each with its own unique advantages and disadvantages in light of the specific purposes for and characteristics of the setting in which measurement is to occur. A variety of selection and supply-type formats are presented and exemplified within the chapter.

Summative scoring procedures are advocated whenever it is appropriate to obtain a total score or set of subscores for a measure. A conceptual scheme should be employed for assigning scores and this scheme should derive from the conceptual model for operationalizing key variables. Various procedures for obtaining, tabulating, and summarizing norm-referenced and criterion-referenced scores are presented.

REFERENCES

Designing Norm-Referenced Measures

Angoff, W. H. (1971). Scales, norms, and equivalent scores. In R. L. Thorndike (Ed.), *Educational measurement* (2nd ed., pp. 508–600). Washington, DC: American Council on Education.

Arkin, H., & Colton, R. R. (1936). *Graphs: How to make and use them.* New York: Harper & Brothers.

Bidwell, C. E. (1973). The social psychology of teaching. In R. Travers (Ed.), *Second handbook of research on teaching* (pp. 414–429). Chicago: Rand McNally.

Bloom, B. S. (1956). *Taxonomy of educational objectives, Handbook I, The cognitive domain.* New York: David McKay.

Brinton, W. C. (1915). Preliminary report by the Joint Committee on Standards of Graphic Representation. *Quarterly Publications of the American Statistical Association, 14,* 790–797.

Coffman, W. E. (1971). Essay examinations. In R. L. Thorndike (Ed.), *Educational measurement* (2nd ed., pp. 188–201). Washington, DC: American Council on Education.

Clemans, W. V. (1971). Test administration. In R. L. Thorndike (Ed.), *Educational measurement* (2nd ed., pp. 271–302). Washington, DC: American Council on Education.

Dilorio, C., & Yeager, K. (2003). The epilepsy self-efficacy scale. In O. L. Strickland & C. Dilorio (Eds.), *Measurement of nursing outcomes* (2nd ed.), (Vol. 3, pp. 40–49). New York: Springer Publishing.

Ebel, R. L. (1975). *Essentials of educational measurement.* Englewood Cliffs, NJ: Prentice-Hall.

Emerson, R. J. (2001). Creativity in the application of the nursing process tool. In C. F. Waltz & L. S. Jenkins (Eds.), *Measurement of nursing outcomes* (2nd ed), (Vol. 1, pp. 41–51). New York: Springer Publishing.

Fitts, P. M. (1962). Factors in complex skill learning. In R. Glaser (Ed.), *Training research and education* (pp. 177–198). Pittsburgh: University of Pittsburgh Press.

Fitts, P. M. (1964). Perceptual-motor skill learning. In A. W. Melton (Ed.), *Categories of human learning* (pp. 224–285). New York: Academic Press.

Glass, G. V., & Stanley, J. C. (1970). *Statistical methods in education and psychology* (pp. 28–29, 89, 91). Englewood Cliffs, NJ: Prentice-Hall.

Grier, M. R., & Foreman, M. D. (1988). The presentation of scientific data in nursing research. In I. L. Abraham, D. M. Nadzam, & J. L. Fitzpatrick (Eds.), *Statistics and quantitative methods in nursing issues and strategies for research and education* (pp. 188–197). Philadelphia: W.B. Saunders.

Gronlund, N. E. (1976). *Measurement and evaluation in teaching.* New York: Macmillan.

Harrow, A. (1972). *A taxonomy of the psychomotor domain.* New York: David McKay.

Howard, E. P. (2001). Clinical evaluation tool. In C. F. Waltz & L. S. Jenkins (Eds.), *Measurement of nursing outcomes* (2nd ed.), (Vol. 1, pp. 184–193). New York: Springer Publishing.

Jalowiec, A. (2003). The Jalowiec coping scale. In O. L. Strickland & C. Dilorio (Eds.), *Measurement of nursing outcomes* (2nd ed.), (Vol. 3, pp. 71–87). New York: Springer Publishing.

Jansen, D. A., & Keller, M. L. (2003). Measuring attentional demands in community-dwelling elders. In O. L. Strickland & C. Dilorio (Eds.), *Measurement of nursing outcomes* (2nd ed.), (Vol. 2, pp. 169–184). New York: Springer Publishing.

Jones, L. C. (2003). Measuring guarding as a self-care management process in chronic illness: The SCMP-G. In O. L. Strickland & C. Dilorio (Eds.), *Measurement of nursing outcomes* (2nd ed), (Vol. 3, pp. 150–158). New York: Springer Publishing.

Kelley, T. L. (1947). *Fundamentals of statistics.* Cambridge, MA: Harvard University Press.

Kibler, R. J., Barker, L. L., & Miles, D. T. (1970). *Behavioral objectives and instruction.* Boston: Allyn & Bacon.

King, E. C. (1979). *Classroom evaluation strategies.* St. Louis: CV Mosby.

King, I. (1968). A conceptual frame of reference for nursing. *Nursing Research, 17,* 27–31.

Krathwohl, D. R., Bloom, B. S., & Masia, B. (1964). *Taxonomy of educational objectives, Handbook II, The affective domain.* New York: David McKay.

Lord, F. M. (1952). The relation of the reliability of multiple-choice tests to the distribution of item difficulties. *Psychometrika, 17,* 181–194.

Mager, R. F. (1962). *Preparing instructional objectives.* Belmont, CA: Fearon Publishers.

Marsh, G. W. (2003). Measuring patient satisfaction outcomes across provider disciplines. In O. L. Strickland & C. Dilorio (Eds.), *Measurement of nursing outcomes* (2nd ed.), (Vol. 2, pp. 243–257). New York: Springer Publishing.

Martuza, V. R. (1977). *Applying norm-referenced and criterion-referenced measurement in education.* Boston: Allyn & Bacon.

Nunnally, J. C. (1967). *Psychometric theory.* New York: McGraw-Hill.

Nunnally, J. C., & Bernstein, I. H. (1994). *Psychometric theory* (3rd ed.). New York: McGraw-Hill Inc.

Sheetz, L. J. (2001). Clinical competence rating scale. In C. F. Waltz & L. S. Jenkins (Eds.), *Measurement of nursing outcomes* (2nd ed.), (Vol. 1, pp. 157–161). New York: Springer Publishing.

Staropoli, C., & Waltz, C. F. (1978). *Developing and evaluating educational programs for health care providers.* Philadelphia: F.A. Davis.

Strickland, O. L., & Dilorio, C. (2003a). *Measurement of nursing outcomes* (2nd ed., Vol. 2). New York: Springer Publishing Company.

Strickland, O. L., & Dilorio, C. (2003b). *Measurement of nursing outcomes* (2nd ed., Vol. 3). New York: Springer Publishing.

Tinkelman, S. N. (1971). Planning the objective test. In R. L. Thorndike (Ed.), *Educational measurement* (2nd ed., pp. 46–80). Washington, DC: American Council on Education.

Toth, J. C. (2003). Measuring stress after acute myocardial infarction: The stress of discharge assessment tool, version two (SDAT-2). In O. L. Strickland & C. Dilorio (Eds.), *Measurement of nursing outcomes* (2nd ed.), (Vol. 2, pp. 99–109). New York: Springer Publishing.

Tyler, R. W. (1950). *Basic principles of curriculum and instruction.* Chicago: University of Chicago Press.

Walker, H., & Durost, W. (1936). *Statistical tables: Their structure and use.* New York: Teachers College, Columbia University.

Waltz, C. F., & Bausell, R. B. (1981). *Nursing research: Design, statistics and computer analysis.* Philadelphia: F.A. Davis.

Waltz, C. F., & Jenkins, L. S. (2001). *Measurement of nursing outcomes* (2nd ed., Vol. 1). New York: Springer Publishing.

Weinert, C. (2003). Measuring social support: PRQ2000. In O. L. Strickland & C. Dilorio (Eds.), *Measurement of nursing outcomes* (2nd ed.), (Vol. 3, pp. 161–172). New York: Springer Publishing.

Wesman, A. G. (1971). Writing the test item. In R. L. Thorndike (Ed.), *Educational measurement* (2nd ed., pp. 81–129). Washington, DC: American Council on Education.

Designing Criterion-Referenced Measures

Bond, L. A. (1996). *Norm- and criterion-referenced testing.* ERIC/AE Digest. Washington, DC: ERIC Clearinghouse on Assessment and Evaluation.

Brown, J. D. (1996). *Testing in language programs.* Upper Saddle River, NJ: Prentice-Hall.

Brown, J. D., & Hudson, T. (2002). *Criterion-referenced language testing.* Cambridge, United Kingdom: Cambridge University Press.

DeGowin, E. L., & DeGowin, R. I. (1969). *Bedside diagnostic examination* (2nd ed.). New York: MacMillan.

Delp, M. H., & Manning, R. T. (1968). *Major's physical diagnosis* (7th ed.). Philadelphia: W.B. Saunders.

Denyes, M. J. (1988). Orem's model used for health promotion: Directions for research. *Advances in Nursing Science, 11*(1), 13–21.

Ebel, R. L. (1979). *Essentials of educational measurement.* Englewood Cliffs, NJ: Prentice-Hall.

Glaser, R. (1994). Instructional technology and the measurement of learning outcomes: Some questions. *Educational Measurement: Issues & Practice, 13*(4), 21–26.

Gronlund, N. E. (1988). *How to construct achievement tests* (4th ed.). Englewood Cliffs, NJ: Prentice Hall.

Hambleton, R. K. (1980). Test score validity and standard-setting methods. In R. A. Berk (Ed.), *Criterion-referenced measurement* (pp. 80–123). Baltimore: Johns Hopkins Press.

Hambleton, R. K. (1994). The rise and fall of criterion-referenced measurement? *Educational Measurement: Issues & Practice, 13*(4), 21–26.

Hashway, R. M. (1998). *Assessment and evaluation of developmental learning: Qualitative individual assessment and evaluation models.* Westport, Connecticut: Praeger.

Linn, R. L. (1982, Spring). Two weak spots in the practice of criterion-referenced measurement. *Educational Measurement,* 12–13.

Martuza, J. C. (1977). *Applying norm-referenced and criterion-referenced measurement in education.* Boston: Allyn and Bacon, Inc.

Nedelsky, L. (1954). Absolute grading standards for objective tests. *Educational and Psychological Measurement, 14,* 3–19.

Orem, D. E. (1985). *Nursing: Concepts of practice* (3rd ed.). New York: McGraw-Hill.

Popham, W. J. (1978). *Criterion-referenced measurement.* Englewood Cliffs, NJ: Prentice-Hall.

Popham, W. J. (1980). Domain specification strategies. In R. A. Berk (Ed.), *Criterion-referenced measurement.* Baltimore: Johns Hopkins Press.

Sampselle, C. M., Brink, C. A., & Wells, T. J. (1989). Digital measurement of pelvic muscle strength in childbearing women. *Nursing Research, 38*(3), 134–138.

Strickland, O. L. (1994). The clinical and statistical significance of using norm- versus criterion-referenced measures. *Journal of Nursing Measurement, 2*(2), 105–106.

Watermann, R., & Klieme, E. (2002). Reporting results of large-scale assessment in psychologically and educationally meaningful terms: Construct validation and proficiency scaling in TIMSS. *European Journal of Psychological Assessment, 18,* 190–203.

Worth, A. M., Dougherty. M. C., & McKey, P. L. (1986). Development and testing of the circumvaginal muscles rating scale. *Nursing Research, 35*(3), 166–168.

Young, M. I., & Yoon, B. (1998, April). Estimating the Consistency and Accuracy of Classifications in a Standards-Referenced Assessment. *CSE Technical Report, 475, EDRS.*

Zieky, M. J., & Livingston, S. A. (1977). *Manual for setting standards on the basic skills assessment tests.* Princeton, NJ: Educational Testing Service.

5

Measurement Reliability

A *pretest* is a trial run of a measure that is undertaken to provide information regarding the method's reliability and validity and to reveal problems relating to its content, administration, and scoring. The measure must be pretested on subjects for whom it was designed under conditions that approximate as nearly as possible the conditions expected to exist when it is employed. During the conduct of the pretest, it is important to be attentive to the reactions, comments, and nonverbal communication of respondents that might give clues to problems with the measure. Similarly, observations and concerns during the administration that may suggest needed improvements should be recorded. For example, problems related to maintaining interest, questions raised by respondents, adequacy of the time provided to respond, test length, and the like may come to light during the pretest. It is also most beneficial after the pretest data have been collected to ask respondents to identify difficulties they have encountered in completing the measure, suggestions they may have for improving it, and possible discrepancies between the purpose for which items were constructed and how subjects understood and responded to the items.

In addition, scores should be computed and data compiled and tabulated for interpretation, including the preparation of tables and graphs, so that any difficulties with scoring, interpretation, or preparation of the data for analysis will be evident. Appropriate procedures for estimating the method's reliability and validity should be employed, including item-analysis procedures using the pretest data. On the basis of the information obtained from the pretest, especially the resulting evidence for the measure's reliability and validity, a decision should be made concerning whether the method will be used as is or needs modification before it can be employed. If it is determined that the method needs modifications for improvement, these should be made and the method pretested again prior to its use.

When sufficient evidence for reliability and validity is obtained as a result of the pretest, the measure may then be employed for data collection, but its reliability and validity should still be monitored each time it is employed, using less extensive and more economical procedures than required for the pretest. Should monitoring of the measure suggest that reliability and/or validity are not holding up with use, it is necessary to scrutinize the measure using more rigorous and extensive reliability and validity studies to ascertain needed changes, to make the modifications required, and then to pretest again (Waltz & Bausell, 1981, pp. 84–85). Attention now turns to the determination of the reliability of norm-referenced measures.

Norm-referenced measures are derived from classical measurement theory. In chapter 3, it was noted that in this view, every observed score (O) is composed of a true score (T), which represents the precise amount of the attribute possessed by the subject at measurement time, and an error score (E). If a large number of subjects are measured on the attribute in question and their observed scores plotted, *reliability* would be conceptualized as the proportion of the variance in the observed score distribution that is due to true differences in subjects' possession of the attribute being measured. *Unreliability* would be conceptualized as the proportion of variance in the observed score distribution that is due to error. Hence, in this view every measurement involves some error that, although it can never be eliminated in total, can be reduced.

Measurement error may be random or systematic. If the nurse had only one thermometer and it was accurate, but she misread it while obtaining different measures, the error would be random. *Random errors* limit the degree of precision in estimating the true scores from observed scores and therefore lead to ambiguous measurement and decreased reliability of the measure. In practice, reliability concerns the extent to which measurements are repeatable by the same individual using different measures of the same attribute or by different individuals using the same measure of an attribute. Thus, research and evaluation efforts are limited by the reliability of measuring instruments and/or reliability with which they are employed. More specifically, sources of random error include, but are not limited to, imprecision in the measure itself, temporal factors, individual differences at measurement time, and/or imprecision in the administration or scoring of the measure.

If, in the foregoing example, the nurse employed the thermometer correctly, but the thermometer itself was inaccurate and always registered 0.5 points higher than it should, the error in the nurse's measurement would be systematic. This systematic or constant error would contribute to the mean score of all subjects equally and thus would become part of the true score of each individual. Since validity is defined as the extent to which an instrument measures what it purports to measure, *systematic errors,* because they affect the true scores of all subjects, would decrease the validity of the measure rather than its reliability.

In chapter 3, it was noted that reliability is a necessary but not sufficient condition for validity; that is, a measure that demonstrates evidence for reliability will not necessarily demonstrate evidence for validity as well. The amount of random error places a limit on measurement validity, but even in the complete absence of random errors there is no guarantee of measurement validity; that is, the correlations between a tool and an independent criterion can never be higher than the square root of the product of the reliability of the two and the reliability of the criterion variable (Issac & Michael, 1995, p. 131). Similarly, because random error may occur as a result of circumstances surrounding

the administration of the measure and/or individual differences at measurement time, reliability and validity investigations conducted on one measurement occasion are not sufficient evidence for reliability and validity when measures are employed on other occasions or with different subjects. Thus, evidence for reliability and validity must be determined every time a given measure is employed.

CONCEPTUAL BASIS FOR RELIABILITY

The determination of reliability in the norm-referenced case is conceptualized using *the domain-sampling model.* As noted in chapter 3, this model views any particular measure as composed of a random sample of items from a hypothetical domain of items. For example, an adjective checklist designed to measure anxiety in presurgical patients would be thought of as containing a random sample of adjectives from all possible adjectives reflective of anxiety in that patient group. Obviously, the model does not hold strictly true empirically, because it is usually not practical or feasible to explicate all possible items defining a domain of interest, thus items are actually randomly sampled for a specific measure. The model does however lead to principles and procedures for determining evidence for reliability that have much utility in practice.

On the basis of the domain-sampling model, the purpose for any measure is to estimate the measurement that would be obtained if all the items in the domain were employed. The score that any subject would obtain over the whole domain is his true score. To the extent that any sample of items on a given measure correlates highly with true scores, the sample of items is highly reliable. In other words, specific measures are viewed as randomly parallel tests that are assumed to differ somewhat from true scores in means, standard deviations, and correlations because of random errors in the sampling of items. Thus, in this view, the preferred way to estimate the reliability of a measure is to correlate one measure with a number of other measures from the same domain of content. Since in practice this is often impractical, usually one measure is correlated with only one other measure to obtain an *estimate* of reliability. The domain-sampling model suggests that the reliability of scores obtained on a sample of items from a domain increases with the number of items sampled. Thus, one item would be expected to have a small correlation with true scores, a 10-item measure a higher correlation, and a 100-item measure an even higher correlation.

NORM-REFERENCED RELIABILITY PROCEDURES

In the norm-referenced case, reliability is usually estimated by using a test-retest, parallel form, and/or internal consistency procedure.

The *test-retest* procedure is appropriate for determining the quality of measures and other methods designed to assess characteristics known to be relatively stable over the time period under investigation. For this reason, test-retest procedures are usually employed for investigating the reliability of affective measures. Since cognitive measures assess characteristics that tend to change rapidly, this procedure is not usually appropriate for estimating their reliability.

When a test-retest procedure is employed, the concern is with the consistency of performance one measure elicits from one group of subjects on two separate measurement occasions. To estimate test-retest reliability for a given measure, one would:

1. Administer the instrument or method under standardized conditions to a single group of subjects representative of the group for which the measure was designed.

2. Readminister the same instrument or method under the same conditions to the same group of subjects. Usually the second administration occurs approximately 2 weeks after the first, although the time may vary slightly from setting to setting. It should be noted that it is important to ascertain that no activities have occurred between the first and second administration which may have affected the stability of the characteristic being measured.

3. Determine the extent to which the two sets of scores are correlated. When data are measured at the interval level, the Pearson product-moment correlation coefficient (r_{xy}) is taken as the estimate of reliability. Computation of r_{xy} is discussed in chapter 3. When data are measured at the nominal or ordinal level, a nonparametric measure of association, such as chi square-based procedures or Spearman rho, is used. Discussion of the conditions under which specific correlation coefficients are appropriately used, as well as their computation, may be found in Waltz and Bausell (1981), and in Nunnally and Bernstein (1994, pp. 124–130).

The value of the reliability coefficient resulting from a test-retest procedure reflects the extent to which the measure rank orders the performances of the subjects the same on the two separate measurement occasions. For this reason, it is often referred to as the *coefficient of stability*. The closer the coefficient is to 1.00, the more stable the measuring device is presumed to be.

When it is desirable to employ a more stringent index of test-retest reliability, that is, to determine the absolute agreement between the two sets of scores, the percentage of agreement index is calculated. Engstrom (1988, pp. 383–389) advocates the *percentage of agreement* as an essential index for describing the reliability of physical measures because it reflects both the precision of measurement and frequency of error and has direct and useful clinical meaning. That is, in most clinical situations, some measurement error is acceptable, but there is a limit on the amount of error that can be tolerated without jeopardizing patient safety. This limit, she notes, can be used as an index of agreement. More specific discussion regarding the assessment of the reliability and validity of physical measures is presented in chapter 18.

Whenever two forms of an instrument can be generated, the preferred method for assessing reliability is the *parallel-form* procedure. In parallel-form reliability, the interest is in assessing the consistency of performance that alternate forms of a measure elicit from one group of subjects during one administration. Two measures are considered alternate or parallel if they have (1) been constructed using the same objectives and procedures; (2) approximately equal means; (3) equal correlations with a third variable; and (4) equal standard deviations.

Prior to assessing parallel-form reliability, it is necessary to obtain empirical evidence that the two measures meet these four criteria. To provide empirical evidence for equal means and standard deviations, both measures are administered to the same group of subjects on the same occasion, and a test of the significance of the difference between the means and a homogeneity of variance test are employed. If the resulting means are not statistically significantly different and the variances are homogeneous, evidence that the two measures are parallel is said to exist. Similarly, to obtain empirical evidence that both measures have equal correlations with a third variable, a measure of a third variable believed to be highly correlated with the phenomena being assessed by the parallel measures, which has demonstrated evidence for reliability and validity, is administered to the same group of subjects on the same occasion as the two measures believed to be parallel. Evidence that the two measures are parallel is said to exist if the scores resulting for each of the two measures correlate significantly with the scores resulting from the measurement of the third variable.

Given evidence for parallel forms, to estimate parallel form reliability one would:

1. Administer two alternative forms of a measure to one representative group of subjects on the same occasion or on two separate occasions.
2. Determine the extent to which the two sets of scores are correlated, using an appropriate parametric or nonparametric correlation coefficient as an estimate of reliability.

If both forms of the measure are administered on the same occasion, the value of the resulting reliability coefficient reflects *form equivalence* only. If the measure is administered on two occasions, stability as well as form equivalence is reflected. Values above 0.80 are usually taken as evidence that the forms may be used interchangeably.

Internal consistency reliability is most frequently employed for cognitive measures when the concern is with the consistency of performance of one group of individuals across the items on a single measure. To estimate the internal consistency of a measure, one would administer the measure under standardized conditions to a representative group on one occasion. The alpha coefficient, KR 20, or KR 21 would be calculated as the estimate of reliability.

The *alpha* coefficient is the preferred index of internal consistency reliability because it (1) has a single value for any given set of data, and (2) is equal in value to the mean of the distribution of all possible split-half coefficients associated with a particular set of data. Alpha represents the extent to which performance on any one item on an instrument is a good indicator of performance on any other item in the same instrument. The formula for determining the alpha coefficient is defined below:

Formula 5.1: Determining the alpha coefficient

$$\text{alpha} = \frac{K}{K-1}\left[1 - \left(\frac{\Sigma\sigma^2\ items}{\sigma^2 test}\right)\right]$$

where K = the number of items on the measure
$\Sigma\sigma^2$ item = the sum of the individual item variances
σ^2test = the variance of the distribution of test scores

Example: Five newly diagnosed diabetics are given a 10-item multiple-choice test to assess their knowledge and understanding of diabetic food exchanges and the scores in Table 5.1 are obtained.

The alpha value for this tool is calculated in the following manner:

1. K is equal to 10, since there are 10 items.
2. σ^2test, the variance for the test-score distribution, is calculated in the usual manner using Formula 3.3 in chapter 3.

That is:

$$SS_x = (10 - 7.6)^2 + (8 - 7.6)^2 + (8 - 7.6)^2 + (7 - 7.6)^2 + (5 - 7.6)^2 = 13.20$$

$$\sigma^2\text{test} = \frac{13.20}{5} = 2.64$$

3. σ^2 item, the variance for each item on the test is calculated in the same way using Formula 3.3 in chapter 3.

$$SS_{\text{item 1}} = (1 - 0.4)^2 + (0 - 0.4)^2 + (0 - 0.4)^2 + (1 - 0.4)^2 + (0 - 0.4)^2 = 1.2$$

$$\sigma^2_{\text{item 1}} = \frac{1.2}{5} = 0.24$$

The variance for items 2 through 10 are calculated in the same manner and appear in Table 5.1.

4. Substituting in the formula for alpha:

$$\text{alpha} = \left(\frac{10}{9}\right)\left[1 - \left(\frac{2.04}{2.64}\right)\right] = (1.11)\,(1 - 0.77) = (1.11)\,(0.23) = 0.2553, \text{ rounded to } 0.26$$

The resulting alpha value of 0.26 indicates the test has a very low degree of internal consistency reliability, that is, that the item intercorrelations are low. As a result, performance on any one item is not a good predictor of performance on any other item. A high alpha value is usually taken as evidence that the test as a whole is measuring just one attribute, for example, knowledge of diabetic food exchanges, which in the example is not the case. In the case of tests designed to measure more than one attribute (e.g., those with subscales or components), alpha should be determined for each scale or subset of homogeneous items in addition to the test as a whole.

A number of factors surrounding the measurement situation may affect the alpha value obtained, and for this reason, it is wise to consider the following when alpha is employed:

1. Alpha is a function of test length. The longer the test, that is, the more items included, the higher the resulting alpha value.

2. A spuriously high alpha may be obtained in a situation in which it is not possible for most respondents to complete the test or measure. As a rule of thumb, Martuza (1977) suggests that if less than 85 percent of the subjects respond to all items on the test, alpha should not be used as an estimate of reliability. Equivalently, alpha should not be used when speeded tests are employed.

3. As with all reliability estimates, alpha should be determined each time a test is employed.

TABLE 5.1 Scores Obtained on a Hypothetical Test of Diabetic Food Exchanges

	Item										
Patient	**1**	**2**	**3**	**4**	**5**	**6**	**7**	**8**	**9**	**10**	**Total**
A	1	1	1	1	1	1	1	1	1	1	10
B	0	1	1	1	1	1	1	1	1	0	8
C	0	0	1	1	1	1	1	1	1	1	8
D	1	0	0	0	1	1	1	1	1	1	7
E	0	1	0	0	0	0	1	1	1	1	5
Total	2	3	3	3	4	4	5	5	5	4	38
Mean	0.4	1	1	1	1	1	1	1	1	0.8	7.6
Variance	0.24	0.4	0.4	0.4	0.2	0.2	0	0	0	0.2	2.64

4. From the formula for alpha, it is apparent that alpha is dependent upon the total test variance; that is, the higher the value of the total test variance, the greater the alpha value obtained.

5. Alpha is dependent upon the shape of the resulting distribution of test scores. When a skewed test-score distribution results, variance is usually less than that obtained when the distribution approximates a normal curve, and hence, alpha may be lower in value. Similarly, when alpha is employed with a group of subjects homogeneous in the attribute being measured, alpha will be lower than when a heterogeneous group is measured.

KR 20 and KR 21 are special cases of alpha used when data are dichotomously scored, that is, when each item in a test is scored 1 if correct and 0 if incorrect or missing. The formula for the determination of KR 20 is defined below:

Formula 5.2: Determing KR 20

$$KR\ 20 = \frac{K}{K-1} \left(1 - \frac{\Sigma pq}{\sigma^2 test} \right)$$

where K = the number of items on the measure
     p = the proportion of correct responses to an item
     q = the proportion of incorrect or missing responses
  $\sigma^2 test$ = the variance of the test-score distribution
    pq = the variance for each item
  Σpq = the sum of the item variances

Example: Using the data in Table 5.1, KR 20 is calculated in the following manner:

1. K is equal to 10, since there are 10 items.
2. pq, the variance for item 1, is obtained in the following manner:

    p, the proportion of correct responses to item 1 is 2/5 or 0.4.
    q, the proportion of incorrect responses to item 1 is 3/5 or 0.6.
    pq = p $\times$ q
       = (0.4) (0.6)
       = 0.24

The variances for the remaining nine items are calculated in the same way and are 0.24, 0.24, 0.24, 0.16, 0.16, 0, 0, 0, and 0.16, respectively.

3. The sum of the item variances is 1.44.
4. The variance for the test-score distribution is determined using Formula 3.3 in chapter 3 and is 2.64.
5. Substituting in the formula for KR 20:

$$KR\ 20 = \left(\frac{10}{9}\right) \left[1.00 - \left(\frac{1.44}{2.64}\right) \right]$$
$$= (1.11)\,(1.00 - 0.54)$$
$$= (1.11)\,(0.46)$$
$$= 0.51$$

If one can assume that the difficulty level of all items is the same—that is, p is the same for all items—then KR 21 may be employed. The formula for KR 21 follows below:

Formula 5.3: Determing KR 21

$$KR\ 21 = \frac{K}{K-1} \left(1 - \frac{\overline{X}_{test}\,(1 - \overline{X}_{test}/K)}{\sigma^2 test} \right)$$

where K = the number of items
  $\overline{X}_{test}$ = the mean of the test-score distribution
  σ^2_{test} = the variance of the test-score distribution

Since the p levels for the items in Table 5.1 are not the same, the computation of KR 21 is best exemplified using a different data set.

Example: A 20-item tool is used to assess six students' scores on a nursing research pretest. Items are scored 1 if correct, and 0 if incorrect. The mean of the resulting test-score distribution is 15 and the variance is 25. KR 21 is obtained in the following manner:

1. K is equal to 20, since there are 20 items on the tool.
2. The mean of the test-score distribution is 15.
3. The variance of the test-score distribution is 25.
4. Substituting in the formula for KR 21:

$$KR\ 21\ =\ \frac{20}{19}\left(1-\frac{15(1-15/20)}{25}\right)$$

$$=\ (1.05)\left(1-\frac{15(1-0.75)}{25}\right)$$

$$=\ (1.05)\left(1-\frac{(15)(0.25)}{25}\right)$$

$$=\ (1.05)\left(1-\frac{3.75}{25}\right)$$

$$=\ (1.05)\ (1-0.15)$$

$$=\ (1.05)\ (0.85)$$

$$=\ 0.892,\ \text{rounded to}\ 0.89$$

When a subjectively scored measure is employed, two types of reliability are important, interrater reliability and intrarater reliability.

Interrater reliability refers to the consistency of performance (i.e., the degree of agreement) among different raters or judges in assigning scores to the same objects or responses. Thus, interrater reliability is determined when two or more raters judge the performance of one group of subjects at the same time.

To determine interrater reliability, one would:

1. Employ two or more competent raters to score the responses of one group of subjects to a set of subjective test items at the same time.

2. Use an appropriate correlation coefficient to determine the degree of agreement between the different raters in assigning the scores. If only two raters are used, the Pearson product-moment correlation coefficient (r_{xy}) may be used as an index of agreement among them. When more than two raters are employed, coefficient alpha may be used, with the column headings representing the judges and the row headings representing the subject's performance ratings. Table 5.2 presents an example of alpha employed for the determination of the interrater reliability of six judges of five subjects' performance on a subjective tool.

An interrater reliability coefficient of 0 indicates complete lack of agreement between judges; a coefficient of 1.00 indicates complete agreement. It should be noted that agreement does not mean that the same scores were assigned by all raters, but rather that the relative ordering or ranking of scores assigned by one judge matches the relative order assigned by the

other judges. Interrater reliability is especially important when observational measures are employed as well as when other subjective measures are used, such as free responses requiring categorization, essays and case studies. Raters are often trained to a high degree of agreement in scoring subjective measures using the interrater reliability procedure to determine when the raters are using essentially the same criteria for scoring the responses.

Intrarater reliability refers to the consistency with which one rater assigns scores to a single set of responses on two occasions. To determine intrarater reliability:

1. A large number of subjects are asked to respond to the same subjective tool.
2. Scores are assigned to the responses using some predefined criteria.
3. Answers are not recorded on the respondents' answer sheets and anonymity of respondents is protected as much as possible.
4. Approximately 2 weeks after the first scoring, response sheets are shuffled and rescored a second time by the same rater who scored them on occasion one, using the same predefined criteria.
5. The Pearson correlation coefficient (r_{xy}) between the two sets of scores is determined as a measure of agreement.

A 0 value for the resulting coefficient is interpreted as inconsistency, and a value of 1.00 is interpreted as complete consistency. Intrarater reliability is useful in determining the extent to which an individual applies the same criteria to rating responses on different occasions and should be employed for this purpose by those who use subjective measures. This technique, because of the time lapse between the first and second ratings, also allows one to determine to some extent the degree to which ratings are influenced by temporal factors.

ESTIMATING THE RELIABILITY OF CHANGES IN TEST LENGTH

In many instances, as a result of item analysis that is discussed in chapter 6, it appears that a measure might be improved either by shortening

TABLE 5.2 Example of Alpha Employed for the Determination of Interrater Reliability for Six Judges' Rating of Five Subjects' Performances

Subjects	Judges						Total
	1	2	3	4	5	6	
A	10	5	4	5	10	8	42
B	8	4	4	3	9	7	35
C	10	5	5	4	8	10	42
D	10	4	5	4	10	10	43
E	9	5	5	5	10	8	42
Total	47	23	23	21	47	43	204
Mean	9.4	4.6	4.6	4.2	9.4	8.6	40.8
Variance	0.64	0.24	0.20	0.70	0.64	1.44	8.56

$$\text{alpha} = \frac{6}{5} \quad 1 - \left(\frac{3.86}{8.56}\right)$$
$$= (1.2) \quad (1 - 0.45)$$
$$= (1.2) \quad (0.55)$$
$$= 0.66$$

its length, by eliminating faulty items, or by adding more items. Similarly, when a measure is being developed and tested, the test constructor often will include more items than the number desired for the final form in order to assess by item analysis the performance of individual items with the intent to retain the best items and eliminate faulty items. In these cases it is important to remember that reliability is a function of test length; that is, a longer test tends to demonstrate a higher reliability than a shorter test and vice versa. For this reason, following an item analysis, it is often useful to estimate what the reliability of the measure would be if test length were also varied from the form tested.

The Spearman-Brown formula permits one to estimate the reliability of a shortened or lengthened measure with known reliability. The assumption, when this formula is used, is that while test length is changed, the nature of the test is not.

An original 100-item measure has a known reliability of 0.80 and as a result of item analysis is to be reduced to half its original length or 50 items. The reliability of the shortened version is estimated using formula 5.4.

Formula 5.4: Spearman-Brown formula for estimating the reliability of a shortened test or measure

$$r_{1/2} = \frac{1/2 \, r}{1 + (1/2 - 1) \, r}$$

where r = the original reliability
1/2 = the length of the shortened test
$r_{1/2}$ = the reliability of the shortened test

Example

$$r_{1/2} = \frac{1/2 \, (0.80)}{1 + (1/2 - 1) \, (0.80)}$$

$$= \frac{0.40}{(1/2 - 1) \, (0.80)}$$

$$= \frac{0.40}{1 - (0.40)}$$

$$= \frac{0.40}{0.60}$$

$$= 0.66$$

The reliability of the shortened version is estimated to be 0.66.

Formula 5.5: To estimate the reliability of a lengthened test using the Spearman-Brown formula

$$r_n = \frac{nr}{1 + (n-1)\, r}$$

where r = the original reliability
r_n = the length of the test n times as long

Example: To estimate the reliability of a measure three times as long as the original measure, n in the formula would equal 3. If the original test reliability is known to be 0.20:

$$
\begin{aligned}
r_3 &= \frac{3\,(0.20)}{1 + (3-1)\,(0.20)} \\
&= \frac{0.60}{1 + 0.40} \\
&= \frac{0.60}{1.40} \\
&= 0.42
\end{aligned}
$$

The reliability of the lengthened test is estimated to be 0.42.

It should be noted that whenever a test is to be lengthened, it is important to consider the potential negative effects of increased test length; that is, extreme increases in test length may introduce unwanted factors such as boredom, fatigue, diminished response rate, and other variables that may actually serve to decrease rather than increase reliability.

CRITERION-REFERENCED RELIABILITY PROCEDURES

In criterion-referenced measurement, reliability is concerned with the consistency or dependability with which a measuring device consistently classifies or categorizes phenomena. For this reason, some researchers use the terms dependability or agreement to refer to the reliability of criterion-referenced tests or measures (Brown & Hudson, 2002). In the case of criterion-referenced results, the range of variability is often quite reduced, particularly when scores have been divided into gross categories such as master and nonmaster. In the norm-referenced case, scores are usually highly variable, and reliability is calculated on the basis of parametric correlational analyses. With criterion-referenced measurement the resulting scores are generally less variable than in the norm-referenced case, so reliability is often determined with nonparametric procedures. However, when criterion-referenced scores are reported as percentages, their variability may be similar to those in the norm-referenced case, and most of the procedures used to estimate reliability in the norm-referenced case also are appropriate to assess the reliability of a criterion-referenced measure (Popham, 1978).

In some cases, a criterion-referenced measure may yield scores that are quite variable as far as the actual scores are concerned, but the interpretation of the range of scores would have reduced variability. For example, if a nursing instructor uses a test to determine if a student has mastered the requisite knowledge in a maternity nursing course, the potential score range might be 0 to 100%. However, assume that the cut score for mastery is set at 80%. If the student scores 75% on the test, the student has not mastered the content. Based on the way, in which the scores on the test are interpreted and used, the concern for testing reliability is on the consistency with which the measure classifies the subjects within the specified categories of the content domain. Even if a whole class of 20 students is tested by the measure, with the scores reflecting marked variability, the primary concern would be the consistency with which the measure classifies each student as master or nonmaster in terms of the stated criterion standard, the cut score. This brings to mind another very important point. In the case of criterion-referenced measurement, unless the standard or cut score has high validity, the computation of a reliability index has little significance. A high reliability index in a situation in which the standard has been improperly set may mean only that the measure consistently classifies objects or phenomena incorrectly.

In the criterion-referenced framework, reliability is usually estimated by employing test-retest, parallel forms, and intrarater and interrater agreement procedures.

Criterion-Referenced Test-Retest Procedure

The focus of the test-retest procedure for criterion-referenced measures is on the stability over time of the classification of phenomena by a measure on two separate measurement occasions. In other words, the focus is on the ability of a measure to consistently classify objects or persons into the same categories on two separate occasions. The extent to which a criterion-referenced measure is able to reflect stability of results over time is an indication of the degree to which it is free from random measurement error.

To estimate test-retest reliability for a given criterion-referenced measure, an investigator would follow the same general guidelines in administering the measure as described for the norm-referenced case. However, the calculation of the reliability index would be different because of the difference in the way criterion-referenced test results are interpreted and used.

Two statistics have been identified that may be employed to assess the stability of criterion-referenced test results for the test-retest procedure, regardless of the number of categories established by the measure: P_o is the proportion of observed agreements in classifications on both occasions; K, also referred to as Cohen's K, is the proportion of persons consistently classified in the same category on both occasions beyond that expected by chance. Hence, K is P_o corrected for chance agreements. P_o, also termed percent agreement, is computed by the following formula.

Formula 5.6: Computation of P_o (percent agreement) (Subkoviak, 1980)

$$P_o = \sum_{k=1}^{m} P_{kk}$$

where m = the number of classification categories
P_{kk} = the proportion of objects or persons consistently classified in the kth category

For illustrative purposes, assume that a criterion-referenced measure designed to assess a nurse's attitudes toward elderly clients is administered to 30 nurses at 2-week intervals to determine test-retest reliability. Results are illustrated in Table 5.3. The P_o would be the proportion of student nurses consistently classified with positive/positive and negative/negative attitudes on both testing occasions. Thus, P_o would be the total proportion of the values in cells A and D. Hence:

$$P_o = \frac{15}{30} + \frac{12}{30}$$
$$= 0.50 + 0.40$$
$$= 0.90$$

Therefore, in this example 0.90 or 90% of the classifications made by the measure on both testing occasions were in agreement. However, some small portion of this estimate can be attributed to chance and 0.90 is, therefore, an overestimate of the stability of the test. The proportion of chance agreements (P_c) for data in Table 5.3 can be computed by the product of the corresponding row and column totals as indicated by Formula 5.7.

Formula 5.7: Calculating one proportion of chance agreements (P_c) (Subkoviak, 1980)

$$P_c = \sum_{k=1}^{m} P_k P_k$$

where m = the number of classification categories
$P_k P_k$ = the proportion of objects or persons assigned to category k on each measurement occasion, respectively

In this situation P_c would be computed by the proportions for (A + B) (A + C) + (C + D) (B + D). Thus,

$$P_c = \left(\frac{17}{30}\right)\left(\frac{16}{30}\right) + \left(\frac{13}{30}\right)\left(\frac{14}{30}\right)$$
$$= (0.57 \times 0.53) + (0.43 \times 0.47)$$
$$= 0.30 + 0.20 \ (0.46)$$
$$= 0.50$$

TABLE 5.3   Hypothetical Test Results Matrix for 30 Nurses for Computing P₀ and *K* on a Measure of Nurse Attitudes toward Elderly Clients

		First Administration		
		Positive	**Negative**	**Totals**
Second Administration	Positive	(A) 15	(B) 2	(A + B) 17
	Negative	(C) 1	(D) 12	(C + D) 13
	Totals	(A + C) 16	(B + D) 14	(A + B + C + D) 30

The proportion of nonchance agreements is provided by kappa (*K*) (Cohen, 1960). P₀, observed agreements, and Pc, chance agreements, are used to calculate *K* as follows:

Formula 5.8: Calculating the proportion of nonchance agreements (*K*) (Martuza, 1977; Subkoviak, 1980)

$$K = \frac{P_o - P_c}{1 - P_c}$$

In the present example, *K* is computed by:

$$K = \frac{0.90 - 0.50}{1 - 0.50}$$
$$= \frac{0.40}{0.50}$$
$$= 0.80$$

Several points should be kept in mind regarding the interpretation of P₀ and *K* values. The value of P₀ can range from 0 to 1.00. Total disagreement in observed test classifications is reflected by a P₀ value of 0, while "total agreement" in observed results is reflected by a P₀ value of 1.00. As indicated by the formula for *K*, the value of *K* is always less than or equal to P₀. The size of the difference between P₀ and *K* is always a function of the size of P₀ or chance agreements. The value of *K* always lies within an interval between –1.00 (which represents complete inconsistency of test results) and 1.00

(which reflects total consistency of results) (Hashway, 1998). The upper limit of 1.00 for *K* is fixed; however, the lower-bound value may fluctuate from one situation to another depending upon several influencing factors. Both P₀ and *K* are affected by factors such as test length, number of response alternatives (e.g., when items are multiple choice), the value of the cut score used to classify subjects, and the homogeneity of the group of subjects. At this time, guidelines related to these factors (which would facilitate further interpretation of P₀ and *K* values) have not been explicated. Whenever P₀ and *K* are used to describe the reliability of a criterion-referenced test, these influencing factors should be clearly described because of their impact on the values of P₀ and *K*. However, it should be noted that the size of the difference between P₀ and *K* represents the amount of susceptibility of the decision process to chance factors (Martuza, 1977).

An upper-bound *K* value of 1.00 will result only when the marginal distributions for the two administrations have the same shape or proportions in them, for example, when the proportions in the right upper cell (A + B) and in the bottom left cell (A + C) of the table are the same. One can determine the maximum possible value of *K* for a specific situation by adjusting the values within the cells of the table (cells A, B, C, and D) to reflect the maximum number of possible agreements or consistent test classifications that could be congruent with the observed marginal proportions (marginal proportions are not changed) and by calculating a revised version of K using the adjusted values. When this is done the resulting value is K_{max}, which represents the upper limit value that K could take on with the particular distribution of results. The K_{max} value provides information that can facilitate a better interpretation of a specific K value. When the K/K_{max} ratio is calculated, it provides a value that can be interpreted on a standard scale. The upper limit of this ratio is 1.00. The closer this ratio is to 1.00, the higher the degree of consistency of classifications from administration 1 to administration 2.

The computation of K_{max} for the information provided in Table 5.3 is conducted by first transforming all of the values in Table 5.3 to proportions as shown in Table 5.4. The proportions in the cells of Table 5.4 are then adjusted to reflect the maximum number of agreements in cells A and D that could possibly be congruent with the observed marginal proportions as shown in Table 5.5. At this point K_{max} can be calculated using the formula for K. Hence:

$$K_{max} = \frac{0.53 + 0.43 - [(0.57)(0.53) + (0.43)(0.47)]}{1 - (0.57)(0.53) + (0.43)(0.47)}$$

$$= \frac{0.96 - 0.50}{1 - 0.50}$$

$$= \frac{0.46}{0.50}$$

$$= 0.92$$

The K value for the present example is 0.80 and the K_{max} value is 0.92. Based on these findings it can be assumed that the measure classified the nursing students with a relatively high degree of consistency, since K/K_{max} is 0.87.

Criterion-Referenced Parallel-Forms Procedure

There are some situations when more than one form of a measure is desirable. For instance, in situations in which subjects are measured before and after a nursing intervention, it may be preferable to administer a parallel form on subsequent administrations. The test-retest procedure has a potential pitfall which makes that approach

to the study of the reliability questionable, since significant events may occur during the between testing interval that might interfere with results on the second administration. Also, administration of the test on the first occasion might influence the results on the second testing, particularly if the same measure is used. The use of parallel forms of a measure could help remedy such situations. However, a major concern in instances in which parallel forms of a measure are used is whether the two forms produce a substantial degree of agreement or consistency in the classification of subjects in a specified group.

Two criterion-referenced measures are considered parallel if they assess the same content domain, that is, if they were constructed with the same set of test specifications and if items are relatively homogeneous. Parallel forms of a criterion-referenced measure may be created through random item selection from a pool of items constructed with the same test specifications or the same item-generation rules (Popham, 1978).

The approach to the estimation of the reliability of parallel forms involves administering the two alternate forms of the measure to one specific group on the same measurement occasion. If it is not possible to administer the two forms of the test at the same time, they should be administered under similar circumstances within a short period of time. After the two versions of the measure are administered P_o and K would be calculated in the same manner used in the test-retest case. Data from the two forms would be compiled and placed in a matrix as shown in Table 5.3. However, the label "First Administration" should be changed to "Form 1," and "Second Administration" to "Form 2". If the two forms have high parallel-form reliability, there will be a high consistency in the classification of subjects into categories. In the parallel-forms procedure, high P_o and K values reflect consistency between the alternate forms of a measure.

Criterion-Referenced Interrater and Intrarater Agreement Procedures

As with the test-retest and the parallel-forms procedures, P_o and K can be employed to estimate interrater and intrarater agreement, which

TABLE 5.4   Data from Table 5.3 Expressed as Proportions

		First Administration		
		Positive	**Negative**	**Totals**
Second Administration	Positive	(A) 0.50	(B) 0.07	(A + B) 0.57
	Negative	(C) 0.03	(D) 0.40	(C + D) 0.43
	Totals	(A + C) 0.53	(B + D) 0.47	(A + B + C + D) 1.00

also may be referred to as interjudge and intra-judge agreement (Tindal & Marston, 1990). The focus of interrater agreement in the criterion-referenced case is on the consistency of classifications of two (or more) different raters who classify a specified group of objects or persons using the same measurement tool on the same measurement occasion. For example, if a rating tool designed to measure the environmental safety of nursing units is used, two nurse raters could be employed to independently classify a group of nursing units one at a time as either safe or unsafe. Once results are obtained, P_o and K could be calculated to determine interrater agreement for the classification of the safety of the nursing units. The values of P_o and K are computed in the same manner as indicated previously and used as the index of interrater agreement. Prior to computing P_o and K the data would be set up in a matrix table similar to Table 5.3, but with the appropriate label changes, that is, changing "First Administration" to "Rater 1," "Second Administration" to "Rater 2," "Positive" to "Safe," and "Negative" to "Unsafe".

Intrarater agreement for criterion-referenced measurement situations is the consistency with which a single rater classifies a group of persons or objects, using a specified measuring tool after rating each person or object on two separate occasions. In instances when intrarater agreement is used, there is a danger that the two separate rating situations are not consistent with each other unless the situation has been cap-

tured by a recording device, such as video or audio recordings or written documents from which both ratings can be made. Another danger is that the first rating might affect the second rating. Steps would be taken to minimize this problem by using such techniques as obscuring the identification of the persons or objects being rated, altering the order in which ratings are done, and reordering the pages of the rating tool if appropriate. Data are arrayed in a matrix in the manner discussed previously, with the proper labeling changes. P_o and K are then calculated to provide an index of intrarater agreement (Martuza, 1977).

In cases where criterion-referenced measurement is based on ratings by observers, there are several types of rating errors that can negatively impact the reliability and, thus, the validity of ratings. These include error of standards, halo error, logic error, similarity error, and central tendency error (Shrock & Coscarelli, 1989).

Error of standards result when numerical and descriptive rating scales fail to provide definitions of behaviors specific enough to prevent raters from using their own standards for rating items differently from those intended by the developer of the measure. Hence, different raters would be more likely to rate the same items differently, thereby reducing reliability of ratings between raters.

Halo error occurs when raters allow their opinion of the performer to influence their performance ratings. This may be done subconsciously

TABLE 5.5 Adjustments Required in Table 5.4 for the Calculation of K_{max}

		First Administration		
		Positive	**Negative**	**Totals**
Second Administration	Positive	(A) 0.53	(B) 0.04	(A + B) 0.57
	Negative	(C) 0.00	(D) 0.43	(C + D) 0.43
	Totals	(A + C) 0.53	(B + D) 0.47	(A + B + C + D) 1.00

and may be in a negative or positive direction. Therefore, halo error can affect scores negatively or positively.

Logic error results when a rater rates one characteristic of a performer when another characteristic is supposed to be the focus of the rating. This occurs when the rater is not fully aware of the independence of two performance characteristics. For example, suppose a clinical instructor assumes that a student who takes longer to perform a procedure is less knowledgeable about the procedure. In actuality, speed of conducting the procedure many have nothing to do with the amount of knowledge about the procedure.

Similarity error occurs when a rater has the tendency to rate a performer that they perceived to be similar to them more highly than those whom they perceive to be "different". This error also is referred to as "similarity-to-me error".

Central tendency error is associated with rating scales that allow raters to choose points along a continuum, such as with behaviorally anchored, descriptive, or numerical scales. Raters will often avoid rating performers on the extreme anchors of rating scales and they tend to group ratings more in the middle of the scale. This behavior is so consistent that for most Likert-type scales the extreme positions are often lost; thus, a seven-point scale is responded to as if it were a five-point scale during ratings. For this reason, some psychometricians recommend using only an even number of categories on rating scales (Shrock & Coscarelli, 1989).

Each of the types of reliability procedures are applicable in both norm-referenced and criterion-referenced measurement. The principles for each type of reliability assessment are the same regardless of the measurement framework employed. However, the approach to calculation of the reliability coefficient depends upon the nature of the score that results. As noted previously, since norm-referenced measures result in scores that are at the interval level of measurement, parametric statistical procedures are used. In the criterion-referenced case, nonparametric statistics are employed when categorical scores or classifications result and parametric statistics are permissible when percentage scores result and the distribution of scores are not highly skewed. Table 5.6 summarizes the types of reliability procedures and related statistics that can be applied in the norm- and criterion-referenced cases.

SUMMARY

Every measurement involves some error that cannot be eliminated but can be reduced by using sound approaches to measurement. Random errors of measurement affect reliability. Reliability must be assessed every time a given measure is employed. The domain-sampling model is the conceptual basis of choice for the determination of reliability in the norm-referenced case. Norm-referenced reliability is usually estimated using a test-retest, parallel form,

TABLE 5.6   Types of Norm-Referenced and Criterion-Referenced Reliability Procedures and Related Statistics

Reliability Procedure	Norm-Referenced Statistic(s)	Criterion-Referenced Statistic(s)
Test-Retest: Concerned with consistency of measurements that one instrument or tool elicits from one group of subjects on two separate measurement occasions. (Stability assessment)	Correlation of the two sets of scores using Pearson Product-Moment Correlation.	The percent agreement (P_o) of classification of subjects on the two separate measurement occasions is calculated. Kappa (K), which is P_o adjusted for chance agreements, also can be computed. Pearson's Product-Moment Correlation can be used with percentage scores that are not highly skewed. Nonparametric correlation procedure, i.e., Spearman Rho, can be computed if data are highly skewed.
Parallel Forms Procedure: Concerned with assessing the consistency of measurements that alternate forms of an instrument or tool elicit from the same group of subjects during a single administration. (Equivalence assessment)	Correlation of the two sets of scores obtained from each instrument using Pearson Product-Moment Correlation. Two norm-referenced measures or tools are considered parallel if (1) They were constructed using the same objectives and procedures; (2) Have approximately equal means; (3) Have equal standard deviations; and (4) Have equal correlations with any third variable.	The percent agreement (P_o) in the classification of subjects by the two parallel measures is computed. Kappa (K) also can be computed. Two criterion-referenced measures are considered parallel if: (1) They were constructed with the same set of test specifications; and (2) Items are relatively homogenous in nature. Pearson's Product-Moment Correlation or Spearman's Rho can be used with percentage scores as appropriate.

(continued)

TABLE 5.6 Types of Norm-Referenced and Criterion-Referenced Reliability Procedures and Related Statistics *(Continued)*

Reliability Procedure	Norm-Referenced Statistic(s)	Criterion-Referenced Statistic(s)
Interrater Reliability: Concerned with consistency of performance (i.e., degree of agreement) among different raters or judges in assigning scores to the same objects or behaviors in the same measurement situation using the same tool and/or the same predefined criteria. (Equivalence assessment)	Correlation of the two sets of scores obtained from each rater or judge using Pearson Product-Moment Correlation.	The percent agreement (P_o) of the classification of subjects by the two raters or judges is computed. Kappa (K) also can be computed. Pearson's Product-Moment Correlation or Spearman's Rho can be used with percentage scores as appropriate.
Intrarater Reliability: Refers to the consistency with which one rater assigns scores to a set of behaviors on two occasions (observed under the same conditions) using the same instrument and/or the same predefined criteria. (Stability assessment)	Correlation of the two sets of scores obtained from one rater or judge for the two occasions using Pearson Product-Moment Correlation.	The percent agreement (P_o) of the two sets of classifications obtained from a single rater or judge is computed. Kappa (K) also can be calculated. Pearson's Product-Moment Correlation or Spearman's Rho can be used with percentage scores as appropriate.
Internal Consistency Reliability: Concerned with the consistency of performance of one group of individuals across the items on a single instrument. Alpha is equal in value to the mean of the distribution of all possible split-half coefficients associated with a specific set of test or questionnaire data. (Internal consistency assessment)	The alpha coefficient is calculated. KR 20 and KR 21 are special cases of alpha, which are used when data are dichotomously scored. KR 20 is used when the item difficulty levels *cannot* be assumed to be the same. KR 21 can be used when item difficulty levels *are* assumed to be the same.	KR 20 and KR 21 may be calculated for some criterion-referenced measures *when data are not highly skewed* and are dichotomously scored, e.g., when each item is scored 1 if correct and 0 if incorrect or missing.

Note: The closer the correlation coefficient, alpha, P_o or K are to 1.00 (or 100%) the more reliable the measure or tool is presumed to be.

and/or internal consistency procedure. In addition, when a subjectively scored measure is used, it is important to consider interrater and/or intrarater reliability as well. When variations in the length of a measure result from item analysis, estimations of reliability using the Spearman-Brown formula should be considered prior to actually making such modifications.

When the criterion-referenced measurement framework is used, reliability procedures follow the same general principles as in the norm-referenced case. However, scores are often not as variable since, in many cases, criterion-referenced measures result in classifications or the placement of the objects that are the focus of measurement into categories. In this instance, percent agreement (P_o) and/or Kappa (K) are used as approaches to the calculation of the various types of reliability. When percentage scores are used with criterion-referenced measures, it may be appropriate to use the same statistical approaches as in the norm-referenced case if scores are not highly skewed.

REFERENCES

Brown, J. D., & Hudson, T. (2002). *Criterion-referenced language testing.* Cambridge, United Kingdom: Cambridge University Press.

Cohen, J. (1960). A coefficient of agreement for nominal scales. *Educational and Psychological Measurement, 20*, 37–46.

Engstrom, J. L. (1988). Assessment of the reliability of physical measures. *Research in Nursing and Health, 11*(6), 383–389.

Hashway, R. M. (1998). *Assessment and evaluation of developmental learning: Qualitative individual assessment and evaluation models.* Westport, CT: Praeger.

Issac, S., & Michael, W. B. (1995). *Handbook in research and evaluation* (3rd ed.). San Diego, CA: Edits Publishers.

Martuza, V. R. (1977). *Applying norm-referenced and criterion-referenced measurement in education.* Boston: Allyn & Bacon.

Nunnally, J. C., & Bernstein, I. H. (1994). *Psychometric theory* (3rd ed.). New York: McGraw-Hill.

Popham, W. J. (1978). *Criterion-referenced measurement.* Englewood Cliffs, NJ: Prentice-Hall.

Shrock, S. A., & Coscarelli, W. C. C. (1989). *Criterion-referenced test development: Technical and legal guidelines for corporate training.* New York: Addison-Wesley.

Subkoviak, M. J. (1980). Decision-consistency approaches. In R. A. Berk (Ed.), *Criterion-referenced measurement* (pp. 129–185). Baltimore: Johns Hopkins Press.

Tindal, G. A., & Marston, D. B. (1990). *Classroom-based assessment: Evaluating instructional outcomes.* New York: Maxwell Macmillan International Publishing Group.

Waltz, C. F., & Bausell, R. B. (1981). *Nursing research: Design, statistics and computer analysis.* Philadelphia: F.A. Davis.

6

Validity of Measures

With Karen L. Soeken

Simply defined, validity refers to the extent to which a measure achieves the purpose for which it was intended. In the Standards for Educational and Psychological Testing published by the American Educational Research Association (AERA), the American Psychological Association (APA), and the National Council on Measurement in Education (NCME) (1985, 1999) *validity* is defined as "the degree to which evidence and theory support the interpretation entailed by proposed use of tests" (p. 9). The type of validity information to be obtained depends upon the aims or purposes for the measure rather than upon the type of measure per se. Hence, it is not appropriate to speak of a valid tool or measurement method, but rather of accruing evidence for validity by examining the scores resulting from a measure that is employed for a specific purpose with a specified group of respondents under a certain set of conditions. For any given measure different aspects of validity will be investigated depending upon the measure's purpose(s). That is, "when test scores are used or interpreted in more than one way, each intended interpretation must be validated" (AERA, APA, NCME, 1999). Thus, for any given measure, one or more types of evidence will be of interest. Evidence for the validity of a newly developed measure requires extensive, rigorous investigation using a number of different approaches depending upon the purpose(s), subjects, and the conditions under which it will be used, prior to employing the measure within a research study. In addition, evidence for validity should be obtained within the context of each study in which the measure is used for the collection of data. Therefore, for any given tool or measurement method, validity

will be investigated in multiple ways depending upon the purpose(s) for measurement and evidence for validity will be accrued with repeated use of the measure.

It should be noted that "Validity is a unitary concept. It is the degree to which all of the accumulated evidence supports the intended interpretation of test scores for the intended purpose" (AERA, APA, NCME, 1999, p. 11). Thus, while the content of this chapter is organized in terms of three types of validity—content, construct, and criterion-related—it is important to keep in mind that because validity is a unitary concept, one or more of the three types of validity may be of interest for any given measure depending upon the purpose for measurement. Equivalently, for any given measure, one or more types of evidence for validity may need to be investigated to determine that the intended interpretation of scores for the intended purpose(s) is supported.

When the intent is to determine how an individual performs at present in a universe of situations that the measure is claimed to represent, *content validity* is of import. *Construct validity* is assessed when the purpose is to determine the degree to which the individual possesses some hypothetical trait or quality presumed to be reflected by performance on the measure. When the aim is to forecast an individual's future standing or to estimate present standing on some variable of particular significance that is different from the measure, *criterion-related validity* is investigated (AERA, APA, and NCME, 1985; Nunnally and Bernstein, 1994, pp. 84–101). For a cogent analysis of the revised AERA, APA, and NCME (1999) standards for educational and psychological testing and their components for determining measurement validity, see Goodwin (2002, pp. 100–106).

NORM-REFERENCED VALIDITY PROCEDURES

Content Validity

Content validity is important for all measures and is especially of interest for instruments designed to assess cognition. The focus is on determining whether or not the items sampled for inclusion on the tool adequately represent the domain of content addressed by the instrument and the relevance of the content domain to the proposed interpretation of scores obtained when the measure is employed. For this reason, content validity is largely a function of how an instrument is developed. When a domain is adequately defined, objectives that represent that domain are clearly explicated, an exhaustive set of items to measure each objective is constructed, and then a random sampling procedure is employed to select a subset of items from this larger pool for inclusion on the instrument, the probability that the instrument will have adequate content validity is high. When investigating content validity, the interest is in the extent to which the content of the measure represents the content domain. Procedures employed for this purpose usually involve having experts judge the specific items and/or behaviors included in the measure in terms of their relevance, sufficiency, and clarity in representing the concepts underlying the measure's development. To obtain evidence for content validity, the list of behavioral objectives that guided the construction of the tool, a definition of terms, and a separate list of items designed to specifically test the objectives are given to at least two experts in the area of content to be measured. These experts are then asked to (1) link each objective with its respective item, (2) assess the relevancy of the items to the content addressed by the objectives, and (3) judge if they believe the items on the tool adequately represent the content or behaviors in the domain of interest.

When only two judges are employed, the *content validity index* (CVI) is used to quantify the extent of agreement between the experts. To compute the CVI, two content specialists are given the objectives and items and are asked to independently rate the relevance of each item to the objective(s) using a 4-point rating scale: (1) not relevant, (2) somewhat relevant, (3) quite relevant, and (4) very relevant. The CVI is defined as the proportion of items given a rating of quite/very relevant by both raters involved. For example, suppose the relevance of each of 10 items on an instrument to a particular objective is independently rated by two experts using the 4-point scale, and the results are those displayed in Table 6.1. Using the information from the figure, the CVI equals the proportion of items given a rating of 3 or 4 by both judges or:

$$CVI = 8/10$$
$$= 0.80$$

If all items are given ratings of 3 or 4 by both raters, interrater agreement will be perfect and the value of the CVI will be 1.00. If one-half of the items are jointly classified as 1 or 2, while

TABLE 6.1   Two Judges' Ratings of 10 Items

Judge 2	Judge 1		
	1 or 2 not/somewhat relevant	3 or 4 quite/very relevant	Total
1 or 2 not/somewhat relevant	2	0	2
3 or 4 quite/very relevant	0	8	8
Total	2	8	10

the others are jointly classified as 3 or 4, the CVI will be 0.50, indicating an unacceptable level of content validity (Martuza, 1977).

When more than two experts rate the items on a measure, the *alpha coefficient,* discussed in chapter 5, is employed as the index of content validity. Figure 6.1 provides an example of alpha employed for the determination of content validity for six experts' rating the relevance of each of five items on a measure. In this case, column headings represent each of the six experts ratings (A-F), and the row headings represent each of the five items (1–5) rated. The resulting alpha coefficient quantifies the extent to which there is agreement between the experts' ratings of the items. A coefficient of 0 indicates lack of agreement between the experts and a coefficient of 1.00 indicates complete agreement. It should be noted that agreement does not mean that the same rating was assigned by all experts, but rather that the relative ordering or ranking of scores assigned by one expert matches the relative order assigned by the other experts.

When sufficiency and/or clarity of the specific item and/or behavior included in the measure in representing the concept underlying the measure's development is of interest, the same procedure is employed.

Content validity judgments require subject matter expertise and therefore careful attention must be given to the selection, preparation, and use of experts, and to the optimal number of experts in specific measurement situations. Readers interested in more information in this regard are referred to Berk (1990), Davis (1992), and Grant and Davis (1997).

Content validity judgments are different from the judgments referred to in determining face validity. *Face validity* is not validity in the true sense and refers only to the appearance of the instrument to the layman; that is, if upon cursory inspection an instrument appears to measure what the test constructor claims it measures, it is said to have face validity. If an instrument has face validity, the layman is more apt to be motivated to respond, thus its presence may serve as a factor in increasing response rate. Face validity, when it is present, however, does not provide evidence for validity, that is, evidence that the instrument actually measures what it purports to measure.

Construct Validity

This type of validity is especially important for measures of affect. The primary concern in assessing construct validity is the extent to which relationships among items included in the measure are consistent with the theory and concepts as operationally defined. Activities undertaken to obtain evidence for construct validity include:

- examining item interrelationships
- investigations of the type and extent of the relationship between scores and external variables
- studies of the relationship between scores and other tools or methods intended to measure the same concepts
- examining relationships between scores and other measures of different constructs
- hypothesis testing of effects of specific interventions on scores
- comparison of scores of known groups of respondents
- testing hypotheses about expected differences in scores across specific groups of respondents
- ascertaining similarities and differences in responses given by members of distinct subgroups of respondents

Construct validity is usually determined using (1) the contrasted groups approach, (2) hypothesis testing approach, (3) the multitrait-multimethod approach (Campbell & Fiske, 1959; Martuza, 1977), and/or (4) factor analysis (Rew, Stuppy, & Becker, 1988).

In the *contrasted groups approach,* the investigator identifies two groups of individuals who are known to be extremely high and extremely low in the characteristic being measured by the instrument. The instrument is then administered to both the high and low groups, and the differences in the scores obtained by each are examined. If the instrument is sensitive to individual differences in the trait being measured, the mean performance of these two groups should differ significantly. Whether or not the two groups differ is assessed by use of an appropriate statistical procedure such as the t test or

Subjects	Judges						Total
	A	**B**	**C**	**D**	**E**	**F**	
1	10	5	4	5	10	8	42
2	8	4	4	3	9	7	35
3	10	5	5	4	8	10	42
4	10	4	5	4	10	10	43
5	9	5	5	5	10	8	42
Total	47	23	23	21	47	43	204
Mean	9.4	4.6	4.6	4.2	9.4	8.6	40.8
Variance	0.64	0.24	0.20	0.70	0.64	1.44	8.56

$$\text{alpha} = \left(\frac{6}{5}\right) \left[1 - \left(\frac{3.86}{8.56}\right)\right]$$
$$= (1.2) \quad (1 - 0.45)$$
$$= (1.2) \quad (0.55)$$
$$= 0.66$$

FIGURE 6.1   Example of alpha employed for the determination of content validity for six judges' rating of a five-item measure.

an analysis-of-variance test. For example, to examine the validity of a measure designed to quantify venous access, the nurse might ask a group of clinical specialists on a given unit to identify a group of patients known to have good venous access and a group known to have very poor access. The nurse would employ the measure with both groups, obtain a mean for each group, then compare the differences between the two means using a t test or other appropriate statistic. If a significant difference is found between the mean scores of the two groups, the investigator may claim some evidence for construct validity, that is, that the instrument measures the attribute of interest. Since the two groups may differ in many ways in addition to varying in the characteristic of interest, the mean difference in scores on the instrument may be due to group noncomparability on some other variable that was not measured. Hence, a claim for validity using the constrasted groups approach must be offered in light of this possibility. If no significant difference is found between the means of the high and low groups, three possibilities exist: (1) the test is unreliable; (2) the test is reliable, but not a valid measure of the characteristic; or (3) the constructor's conception of the construct of interest is faulty and needs reformulation.

When the *hypothesis testing approach,* also referred to as the *experimental manipulation approach,* is employed, the investigator uses the theory or conceptual framework underlying the measure's design to state hypotheses regarding the behavior of individuals with varying scores on the measure, gathers data to test the hypotheses, and makes inferences on the basis of the findings regarding whether or not the rationale underlying the instrument's construction is adequate to explain the data collected. If the theory or conceptual framework fails to account for the data, it is necessary to (1) revise the measure, (2) reformulate the rationale, or (3) reject the rationale altogether.

For example, Bidwell (1973) in his theory of personal influence suggests a set of conditions under which a faculty member's interactions with students are more likely to affect or influence students' attitudes toward the content. One such condition is that a faculty member will positively affect students' attitudes toward the content when the student perceives a direct positive relationship or link between the teachers' attitudes and the content taught. This theory, and more specifically the set of conditions, are used as a conceptual framework for identifying variables that may explain variations in students' attitudes toward the content at the completion of a course in clinical nursing. The condition regarding the link is operationalized into a set of questionnaire items that assess students' perceptions of the link between the content taught and faculty activities. For example, students rate from 1 (not at all) to 6 (very much) how much they thought their clinical faculty member or members were involved in the following activities:

- Applying the content they teach to their own clinical performance
- Speaking or in some manner presenting the content at professional meetings
- Consulting with nurses in the agency where they have students, regarding nursing and/or patient care problems in the content area
- Planning and/or developing programs for other nurses that deal with nursing and/or patient care in the content area
- Seeking continuing learning experiences that are relevant to the content they are teaching
- Participating in research in their content area

It is hypothesized that students who respond to the questionnaire items in a manner that indicates they are aware of a positive link (i.e., record higher scores) will demonstrate more positive attitudes toward the clinical content upon completion of the course than will students who respond to the items in a manner that indicates they do not perceive a positive link between faculty activities and the content (i.e., record lower scores). To test this hypothesis a random sample of students is selected from the available population of students and are administered the questionnaire along with a second measure to assess their attitudes toward the clinical content upon completion of the course. The significance of the differences in attitudes between those students who perceive a positive link and those who do not is assessed

using an appropriate statistical technique. If a significant difference is found in the expected direction (i.e., those with high scores on the questionnaire and high scores on the attitude measure, and vice versa), one can say some evidence has been obtained for the construct validity of the measure. It should be noted that this is a simplified example and that in actually designing such a study it would be necessary to control variables such as students' past exposure to faculty in order to test the research hypothesis more precisely.

The *multitrait-multimethod approach* (Campbell & Fiske, 1959) is appropriately employed whenever it is feasible to:

1. Measure two or more different constructs
2. Use two or more different methodologies to measure each construct
3. Administer all instruments to every subject at the same time
4. Assume that performance on each instrument employed is independent, that is, not influenced by, biased by, or a function of performance on any other instrument

Whenever these conditions can be met, the multitrait-multimethod approach to instrument validation is preferred, because it produces more data with more efficiency than other available techniques.

Two basic premises underlying the multitrait-multimethod approach are (1) that different measures of the same construct should correlate highly with each other (the *convergent validity principle*), and (2) that measures of different constructs should have a low correlation with each other (the *discriminant validity principle*). An inherent aspect of the approach, and one that accounts for its popularity over other approaches, is the ability to separate trait from method variance. *Trait variance* is the variability in a set of scores resulting from individual differences in the trait being measured. *Method variance* is variance resulting from individual differences in a subject's ability to respond appropriately to the type of measure used. The size of the correlation between any two measures is a function of both trait and method variance. Validity techniques that focus only on the size of the correlation between two measures are not able to account for the extent to which each of these types of variance are represented in their result. When validity is evident, the correlation between two measures of the same construct will be more a function of trait than method variance. In order to assess whether this is the case, it is necessary to focus not only on the size of the correlation but also on the patterns of the relationships between correlations of measures of the same and different constructs using common and different methods as well.

The multitrait-multimethod approach is best illustrated by example. In the simplest case, suppose a nurse had two instruments designed to measure the construct, maternal-infant bonding, and two instruments designed to measure the mother's incorporation of prenatal learnings into her perinatal care (a second construct). Also, suppose that the format for one measure of each construct consists of a series of behaviors rated on a five-point scale. Each rating indicates the consistency with which a particular behavior is performed. The second measure of each construct is in the form of a performance checklist; that is, all of the behaviors on a standard list that describe the subject's performance are checked.

Each of these four instruments—(1) maternal-infant bonding rating scale, (2) maternal-infant bonding checklist, (3) perinatal care rating scale, and (4) perinatal care checklist—is administered to every member of the validation sample at the same time. The reliability of each instrument is then determined using an index of internal consistency (alpha/KR 20/KR 21), and the correlation (r_{xy}) between each pair of forms is computed. A multitrait-multimethod matrix is constructed and the correlations are entered in the following manner.

The reliability estimate for each form is entered as in Table 6.2 to form what is referred to as the *reliability diagonal*. If these values are sufficiently high, the procedure continues; if not, the procedure terminates because reliability is a prerequisite for validity. The values of the reliability estimates in Table 6.2 range from 0.81 to 0.91, indicating sufficient evidence for reliability and thus the analysis may continue.

Convergent validity is examined by entering in the lower left block of the matrix in Table 6.3 the correlation between the two measures of each construct assessed using different methods to form the *validity diagonal*. The values entered are 0.75 and 0.70, high enough to provide evidence for convergent validity.

The correlation between measures of different constructs employing a rating scale is entered in the upper block of Table 6.3, and the correlation between measures of different constructs using a checklist is entered in the lower right block of the matrix. These coefficients indicate the relationship between measures of different constructs that use the same method of measurement and thus are a function of the relationship existing between the two constructs and the use of a common method. The size of these *heterotrait-monomethod coefficients* will be lower than the values on the validity diagonal if variability is more a function of trait than method variance. Since the values in Table 6.4 follow this pattern, they provide evidence for *construct validity*.

The remaining correlations between measures of different constructs measured by different methods are entered in the lower block in

TABLE 6.2 Reliability Diagonal in Constructing a Multitrait-Multimethod Matrix

		Method 1 (Rating Scale) Bonding	Perinatal Care	Method 2 (Checklist) Bonding	Perinatal Care
Rating Scale	Bonding	0.85			
	Perinatal Care		0.88		
Checklist	Bonding			0.81	
	Perinatal Care				0.91

TABLE 6.3   Validity Diagonal in Constructing a Multitrait-Multimethod Matrix

| | | Method 1 (Rating Scale) | | Method 2 (Checklist) | |
		Bonding	Perinatal Care	Bonding	Perinatal Care
Rating Scale	Bonding	0.85			
	Perinatal Care		0.88		
Checklist	Bonding	0.75		0.81	
	Perinatal Care		0.70		0.91

the left of the matrix as shown in Table 6.5. The values of these *heterotrait-heteromethod coefficients* should be lower than the values in the validity diagonal and the corresponding values of the heterotrait-monomethod coefficients. Since this pattern is apparent in Table 6.5, evidence is present for *discriminant validity.*

In summary, if the information in Table 6.5 resulted from an actual study, it would provide evidence for reliability, convergent validity, construct validity, and discriminant validity— that is, provide more data, more efficiently and economically than what is obtained using other approaches.

Figure 6.2 presents an extension of the example in which a multitrait-multimethod matrix is employed for the analysis of three constructs: bonding, perinatal care, and anxiety. Each construct is measured using two different methods: a rating scale and a checklist. As in the simplest case both the size and patterns of the relationships are examined.

1. The reliability diagonal is examined first and correlations are found to range from 0.81 to 0.91, indicating sufficient reliability for the analysis to proceed.

2. The validity diagonals (in the lower left block of the matrix) indicate that the relationships between measures of the same construct using different methods range from 0.70 to 0.75, high enough to provide evidence for convergent validity.

3. Correlations among measures of different constructs employing a rating scale (upper left block, solid-line triangle) and the correlations among measures of different constructs using a checklist (lower block, solid-line triangle) are examined in light of the values in the validity diagonal. The values of the heterotrait-monomethod triangle are lower than those in the validity diagonal and hence provide evidence for construct validity.

4. The correlations among measures of different constructs measured by different methods

TABLE 6.4   Heterotrait-Monomethod in Correlations in Constructing a Multitrait-Multimethod Matrix

| | | Method 1 (Rating Scale) | | Method 2 (Checklist) | |
		Bonding	Perinatal Care	Bonding	Perinatal Care
Rating Scale	Bonding	0.85			
	Perinatal Care	0.40	0.88		
Checklist	Bonding	0.75		0.81	
	Perinatal Care		0.70	0.35	0.91

TABLE 6.5 **Heterotrait-Heteromethod in Correlations in Constructing a Multitrait-Multimethod Matrix**

| | | Method 1 (Rating Scale) | | Method 2 (Checklist) | |
		Bonding	Perinatal Care	Bonding	Perinatal Care
Rating Scale	Bonding	0.85			
	Perinatal Care	0.40	0.88		
Checklist	Bonding	0.75	0.18	0.81	
	Perinatal Care	0.15	0.70	0.35	0.91

(lower block, broken-line triangles) are examined in regard to the values in the validity diagonal and the heterotrait-monomethod triangles. Since the values in the heterotrait-heteromethod triangles are lower than those in the heterotrait-monomethod triangle, which in turn are lower than those on the validity diagonal, evidence for discriminant validity is present. Hence, from Figure 6.2, it can be seen that extension of the multitrait-multimethod approach from the simplest case to those employing more than two constructs is straightforward.

A word of caution is in order regarding the considerations to be made before employing the multitrait-multimethod approach. One disadvantage of this approach results from the demands it may place on subjects who must respond to multiple instruments at one time. Such a request not only has the potential for decreasing respondents' willingness to participate, hence reducing the response rate, but also introduces the potential for more errors of measurement as a result of respondent fatigue. For this reason, it is important, especially in measuring clinical variables, to carefully consider the appropriateness of using the method in light of the setting as well as the respondents' other needs. A second disadvantage may stem from the cost in time and money necessary to employ the method. One way to reduce the potential cost is to select or design individual measures that are economical and efficient themselves.

Another example of use of the multitrait-multimethod approach to validity assessment can be found in the work of Jones, Cason, and Mancini (2002) who employed the approach to evaluate the validity of a hospital-based nurse competency assessment within the context of a

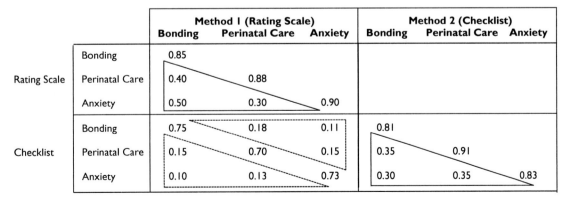

FIGURE 6.2 Example of a multitrait-multimethod matrix employed for analysis of three constructs using two methods.

skills recredentialing program (pp. 22–28). Further discussion of multitrait-multimethod models for investigating validity is available in Eid, Lischetzke, Nussbeck, and Trierweiler (2003, pp. 38–60).

Factor analysis is a useful approach to assessing construct validity when the investigator has designed, on the basis of a conceptual framework, a measure to assess various dimensions or subcomponents of a phenomenon of interest and wishes to empirically justify these dimensions or factors. When factor analysis is employed, the investigator administers the tool to a large representative sample of subjects at one time. An appropriate parametric or nonparametric factor-analysis procedure is then employed. The result of this factoring process is a group of linear combinations of items called factors, each of which is independent of all other identified factors. Once constructed, each factor is then correlated with each item to produce factor loadings. Waltz and Bausell (1981, p. 301) note that it might be helpful to conceptualize these factors as "lumps" of variance taken from items that tend to measure something in common, and the loadings as correlations between these lumps and the items they comprise. Usually, the next step is a process referred to as rotation, in which the factors are repositioned in such a way as to give them more interpretability. Rotated factors are interpreted by examining the items loading upon each, over and above a certain *a priori* set criterion (usually 0.30 is the minimum that will be considered). If evidence for construct validity exists, the number of factors resulting from the analysis should approximate the number of dimensions or subcomponents assessed by the measure and the items with the highest factor loadings defining each factor should correspond with the items designed to measure each of the dimensions of the measure.

All factor analyses do not result in such easily interpretable factors; thus one of the most difficult aspects of this approach is to objectively name or interpret factors without allowing original conceptualization to bias the interpretation, since the interpretation of factors or analyses always involves a certain amount of subjectivity. Some rules of thumb suggested by Waltz and Bausell (1981, p. 304) to avoid such biases include: (1) choosing a minimum loading to interpret, probably no less than 0.30, perhaps as high as 0.50, *before* the analysis is attempted; (2) in naming a factor, consider the relevant items in descending order with respect to the magnitude of their loadings; and (3) never ignorimg an item meeting a predetermined loading criterion simply because it does not "conceptually" fit with the rest of the items loading on a factor. It should also be noted that factors can be notoriously unstable, particularly with small samples, so that the results of factor analysis should be cross-validated. Rew, Stuppy, and Becker (1988) in their article provide a useful discussion of the limitations noted in published studies employing factor analysis for the determination of construct validity (pp. 10–22). Readers are referred to Lauri and Sanna (2002) for another example of the use of factor analysis to obtain evidence for validity for an instrument designed to measure and describe decision making in different nursing fields (pp. 93–100).

CONFIRMATORY FACTOR ANALYSIS
(Karen L. Soeken, PhD)

One of the common methods for assessing the construct validity of an instrument is exploratory factor analysis (EFA), a technique that decomposes the variance of a measure into variance that is shared by the items (common factors) plus variance that is not shared (i.e., uniquenesses). The outcome of this process is the identification of a group of linear combinations of the items that are called *factors*. These underlying factors are defined in mathematical terms so the process is considered data-driven. The ultimate goal is to explain the most variance in the set of variables or items with the fewest number of factors that is determined using a statistical criterion such as eigenvalue greater than 1, or the percent of variance explained. It is possible in EFA for the researcher to move away from a strictly exploratory perspective by specifying *a priori* the number of factors to be extracted. In EFA all items load on or reflect all the extracted factors, with some factor loadings being insignificant. That is, the researcher is not able to specify which items load on which factors, and some items should not load on some factors. In addition, if more than one factor emerges in the analysis, factors are allowed to correlate or not correlate in an all-or-none fashion. Either all factors are permitted to correlate with one another, or all are independent of one another. Finally, EFA does not permit correlated measurement errors. In areas where little is known, EFA can be valuable in suggesting an underlying structure. However, if the structure can be hypothesized, as would be the case for a test developer or a researcher seeking to support the construct validity of a scale, the constraints of EFA are inappropriate.

The test construction process requires an operational definition of the construct so that items reflecting the construct can be written or selected. As a result, one is able to hypothesize not only how many factors there are, but also what the factors are and which specific items belong to or load on each factor. Items need not load on each factor and, in fact, often are considered to reflect only one or maybe two factors. In that case, the item loadings on other factors can be set to 0. The developer might also hypothesize that some factors correlate with one another, while other factors are thought to be independent of one another. Finally, the test developer might speculate that some errors in measurement are correlated, for example, because of a bias in answering negatively worded items or because of the response format. For example, the revised Caregiver Reciprocity Scale II (CRSII) was hypothesized to consist of four factors that correlated with each other: warmth and regard, intrinsic rewards of caregiving, love and affection, and balance within family caregiving (Carruth, Holland, & Larsen, 2003). Each factor consisted of three to seven items, with no item loading on more than one factor. EFA would not permit a direct test of the hypothesis regarding construct validity given that the number of factors was specified along with which item loaded on which factor. However, *confirmatory factor analysis* (CFA) permits each of the above situations, thereby allowing the test developer to use theoretical knowledge in testing the construct validity of the instrument. The intent of CFA is to hypothesize or define the factors

directly and then determine how well the defined measurement model fits the observed data. CFA, then, is *theory-driven* rather than data-driven.

CFA can be thought of as having several steps. In the first step, the hypothesized measurement model is specified and the relationships among variables and constructs are made explicit. Second, the researcher must determine whether the model is identified, that is, whether it is theoretically possible to estimate every parameter in the model. Third, the model is analyzed and parameters are estimated. Finally, the fit of the model is evaluated. Several computer software programs are available for CFA, including the following widely used programs: EQS (Bentler, 1989), AMOS (Arbuckle & Wothke, 1999), and LISREL (Jöreskog & Sörbom, 1996) which stands for LInear Structural RELations.

Specifying the Model

In order to apply CFA, the researcher must explicitly state the hypothesized measurement model using a diagram or a set of equations. In the context of CFA, measured variables or scale items are called *indicators* or manifest (observed) variables. Measured variables are represented in a diagram by squares or rectangles. Constructs or factors are referred to as *latent variables* or unobserved variables, represented by circles in the diagram. Relations among constructs or between constructs and indicators are depicted with arrows ($\rightarrow$) that indicate the direction of the relationship. Curved lines that may have arrows at each end are unanalyzed relationships or associations that have no implied direction.

Consider the measurement model in Figure 6.3 showing one construct with four indicators. Constructs are denoted by ξ (pronounced 'ksi'), and the indicators are represented by X_i. Not all computer programs for CFA require Greek notation, but the notation does provide a useful way of referring to and speaking about the model. Lambda (λ) is a coefficient denoting the effect of ξ on X. These λ are sometimes referred to as the *factor loadings* because they indicate which item "loads" on which factor. A change in the latent variable ξ has an effect on the observed variables X_1, X_2, X_3, and X_4. In fact, lambda is

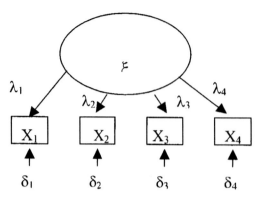

FIGURE 6.3 Measurement model showing one construct with four indicators.

the magnitude of the expected change in the observed variable for one unit of change in the latent variable or factor. In other words, lambda is a measure of the validity of the item as an indicator of the construct. Finally, delta (δ) refers to error in the measurement of X. Each indicator can be expressed in the form of an equation showing its relationship with the construct plus as error term:

$$X_1 = \lambda_1\xi + \delta_1$$
$$X_2 = \lambda_2\xi + \delta_2$$
$$X_3 = \lambda_3\xi + \delta_3$$
$$X_4 = \lambda_4\xi + \delta_4$$

All four equations simultaneously can be expressed using vectors:

$$\mathbf{x} = \Lambda\xi + \delta$$

In this form $\mathbf{x}$ is a vector of the X_i, Λ is a vector that contains the factor loadings, and the vector δ contains the error terms. (CFA is one application of *structural equation modeling* or SEM because of the structural equation system that combines factor analysis and regression-type models.)

The measurement model can be expanded to include multiple factors with a varying number of indicators for each. For example, Figure 6.4 depicts a measurement model with two constructs, each with four indicators or items. In addition, the curved line between δ_1 and δ_2 tells us that the two constructs are correlated with each other.

Identification

Once the model is specified, it is clear which parameters need to be estimated. They are the factor loadings (λ_{ij}), the variances of the measurement errors (δ_1), the variances and, if correlated, the covariances of the factors and, if the model includes correlated measurement errors then the covariances of the errors. In Figure 6.4 there are 19 parameters to be estimated: 8 factor loadings, 8 variances of the measurement errors, 2 variances of the factors, and 1 covariance between the factors. However, each latent variable must have a measurement scale set. This is necessary because the latent variables are not observed and therefore they have no scale. Usually the scaling is accomplished by setting the loading of one indicator for each factor to equal 1.0. This means that a one-point increase in the factor is reflected in a one-point increase on the reference indicator. This process of "setting the scale" reduces the number of parameters that will be estimated; in this example, scaling reduces the number of parameters to 17. An alternative approach to scaling is to fix the variance of each factor to 1.0, in essence standardizing the factor. Using the latter approach the unit of measurement is equal to the population standard deviation.

In CFA parameters can be of three types: free, fixed, and constrained. *Free* parameters have unknown values that must be estimated while *fixed* parameters are set to a constant value by the researcher and are not estimated. For example, the loading of X_1 on ξ_1 is a free parameter that must be estimated; the loading of X_1 on ξ_2 is fixed to 0, i.e., X_1 does not load on ξ_2. *Constrained* parameters are restricted in that they are hypothesized to be equal to one another and must be estimated. For example, a test developer might hypothesize that all the loadings on a factor are equal to one another, a so-called *tau-equivalent* measure. Or, in the case of multiple factors, the developer might hypothesize that the correlations between all pairs of factors are equivalent. Constrained parameters are not completely fixed since they must be estimated, but they are not completely free either since they have some restrictions placed on them.

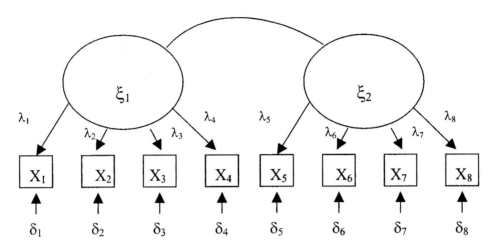

FIGURE 6.4   Measurement model with two constructs, each with four indicators.

The issue of *identification* is critical in CFA. A model is identified if it is theoretically possible to derive a unique estimate for every parameter. You might recall from algebra that one equation with two unknowns such as a + b = 5 does not have a unique solution, but a set of two equations with two unknowns can be solved. The same principle applies in CFA. There must be enough information available to determine unique estimates for the parameters. In CFA the available information comes in the form of the variance-covariance matrix of the observed variables, so there must be enough unique terms in the variance-covariance matrix to be able theoretically to estimate the parameters. (The SEM analysis is sometimes referred to as *analysis of covariance structures* given the dependence on the variance-covariance matrix.) The example includes 8 indicator variables so the variance-covariance matrix will have (8x9)/2 or 36 observations, more than the 17 parameters to be estimated. Note that the use of the term "observation" here refers to an element of the covariance matrix and not to the sample size. As an aside, there is no agreement among researchers as to a desired sample size in CFA. One suggestion offered is a 10:1 subject-to-parameter ratio, or 10 subjects for each parameter estimated (Raykov & Marcoulides, 2000; Kline, 1998).

With "p" indicators, there will be $p(p+1)/2$ unique elements in the variance-covariance matrix, the diagonal consisting of variances and half of the off-diagonal elements that are the covariances. If there are more parameters to be estimated than there are observations, there is insufficient information and the model is *underidentified*. If there is more information than is necessary, the number of observations exceeds the number of parameters, the model is *overidentified* and parameters can be theoretically estimated. Similarly, if there is just enough information for estimating, then the model is *justidentified or saturated*. Saturated models will always fit the data perfectly so the hypothesized model can never really be tested. The model presented in Figure 6.4 is overidentified.

Having enough observations given the number of parameters to be estimated, the so-called "t-rule," is a necessary condition for identification, but by itself this condition is not sufficient to determine whether the model is identified. Several necessary conditions or rules exist to help determine whether a model is identifiable. For example, a single factor model with at least three indictors is identifiable. A two-factor model in which each indicator loads on one factor, measurement errors are uncorrelated, and factors correlate, is identifiable if each factor has at least two indicators. It should be noted, that while it may be theoretically possible to estimate every parameter in a model, there may be other difficulties that keep it from actually happening. (For further discussion of the "rules"or necessary conditions related to identifiability, see, for example, Bollen (1989), Kline (1998), or Raykov & Marcoulides (2000).)

Parameter Estimation

Estimation refers to the process by which the unknown model parameters are estimated. There are four main approaches to estimation: maximum likelihood estimation, unweighted least squares, generalized least squares, and weighted least squares. Each is based on minimizing a fit function. The most widely used approach is *maximum likelihood estimation (ML)*. In ML all parameters in the model are estimated simultaneously so that if they are assumed to be the population values, they maximize the likelihood or probability that the observed data (the covariance matrix) comes from the population. The process is iterative, meaning that an initial solution is derived, and then through subsequent steps the estimates are improved. At each step the parameter estimates are used to compute the relationships among the measured variables. This computed matrix is called the *implied covariance matrix*—implied by the measurement model that has been imposed on the data. The process continues iteratively until the implied covariance matrix comes as close as possible to the sample covariance matrix.

As a rule, with continuous multivariate normally distributed variables, the maximum likelihood procedure has desirable characteristics. Although ML can handle slight to moderate departures from normality, the overall test of the model in the next step is sensitive to violations of the normality assumption. If there are large departures from normality, then other methods for parameter estimation are more appropriate although they require large sample sizes. Another strategy for addressing non-normality is to transform the data to improve the normality. In the case of a Likert-type response scale, which many instruments tend to use, the data can be treated as ordinal and the polyserial correlation (one ordinal and one continuous variable) or polychoric correlation (two ordinal variables) computed and analyzed.

The resulting parameter estimates are unstandardized covariances between factors and unstandardized regression coefficients (i.e., factor loadings) of the direct effect of the factor on the indicator. Using the standard error for each parameter estimate, one can test for the statistical significance of each estimate. Standardized estimates also are presented giving the correlations between factors and the correlation between the factor and the indicator, i.e., the factor loading or *validity coefficient* for the indicator. If an item loads on only one factor, then the standardized estimate can be squared to give the proportion of variance in the indicator explained by the factor, a measure of the *reliability of the indicator*. Another value given is the R^2 for each item, an indication of the proportion of variance in the item explained by all the constructs/factors.

Assessing the Fit of the Model

Evaluation of whether a measurement model fits is not necessarily a simple and straightforward procedure, in part because there is not just one statistical test with a corresponding level of significance. Rather a number of statistical measures of fit have been proposed to evaluate whether the hypothesized measurement model is consistent with the data. Some are measures of overall model fit, while others examine components of the model or the parameter estimates; some can be tested for significance, while others are descriptive; and some are affected by sample size or complexity of the model, while others are not.

The first step in assessing model fit, however, involves looking at the estimates to determine whether they make sense. For example, are the signs (directions) of the estimates what one would expect, and are the sizes (magnitudes) of the estimates reasonable? You might find a correlation between factors that is greater than 1.0 or a variance estimate that is negative—both impossible values. This would be an *improper solution* known as a *Heywood case*, and it might occur, for example, if the sample size were too small or if the model was not correctly specified.

As a test of the overall model fit, we obtain a χ^2 statistic that tests whether the model implied covariance matrix is consistent with the sample covariance matrix. Our goal is to accept the null hypothesis that our model is consistent with the data versus the alternative that it is not consistent. There are some reasons for using caution with the χ^2 test, however. For one, as noted above, multivariate skewness can result in a large χ^2 statistic that would lead to rejection of the null hypothesis. Also, with large samples small differences between the actual and implied covariance matrices can be magnified and lead to a significant χ^2 test statistic. For that reason, the recommendation is to look at the χ^2/df ratio with the goal of having the ratio be less than 3.0. In the example of the Caregiver Reciprocity Scale mentioned above, the $\chi^2 = 193.89$ with 146 df and p < .01 that would suggest the model does not fit, but the χ^2/df ratio = 1.32, well within the acceptable range.

Other fit indices are less sensitive to sample size. One common index is the *Goodness-of-Fit Index* (GFI) that indicates the proportion of observed covariances explained by the model-implied covariances. The *Adjusted Goodness-of-Fit Index* (AGFI) adjusts for the complexity of the model. These indices range from 0–1 with values over .90 recommended, preferably .95 or greater (Hu & Bentler, 1999). Another useful measure is the *Normed Fit Index* (NFI) that is based on the difference of the chi-square value for the proposed model to the chi-square value for the independence model. Although there are no strict guidelines for what supports the model, values greater than .95 are desired (Hu & Bentler, 1999). The *Standardized Root Mean Squared Residual* (SRMR) is based on the average covariance residuals or differences between the observed and model-implied covariances. Values less than .10 are desired (Kline, 1998). There are still other fit indices that focus on different aspects such as adjusting for sample size or for degrees of freedom and indices that are normed versus non-normed. The ones mentioned are probably the most common. At any rate, researchers are advised to report more than one of the fit indices to support the fit of the hypothesized model.

Model Modification

Often an initial model does not fit well, generally because it has not been correctly specified.

Perhaps an indicator has been incorrectly included or linked with the wrong factor. Perhaps an indicator should load on more than one factor. Included in the analysis results are modification indices that are statistical suggestions of how changes to the model would improve the fit. These suggested changes include which items load on which factors as well as whether some error variances or factors should be permitted to correlate. It is important to remember that if the model is modified based on these indices, the analysis has become more exploratory and data-driven. If you decide to modify, then you should use your theoretical expertise along with the empirical guidelines and confirm the modified model using another sample.

OTHER USES OF CFA FOR TESTING MEASUREMENT MODELS

So far the focus has been on what are called first order factors—factors reflected directly by the items or indicators. It is possible that if the factors are correlated, then the factors themselves may reflect a more global or *higher-order factor*. For example, Sousa & Chen (2002) hypothesized that quality of life is explained by a second-order general factor and four first-order factors. A diagram for this model is shown in Figure 6.5.

To assess a second-order factor structure, keep in mind that a second-order structure can never fit better than a first-order structure since it attempts to explain the correlations among the first-order factors with fewer parameters. If the model holds, then quality of life can be conceptualized as being explained by the four first-order factors.

In other situations, the researcher may want to demonstrate that a measurement model or factor structure holds across multiple groups. This is called testing the *invariance of the measurement model* and requires analyzing two variance-covariance matrices simultaneously, one from each sample or group. Parameters are constrained to be equivalent across the samples to determine whether the same model fits both groups. The simplest analysis involves testing

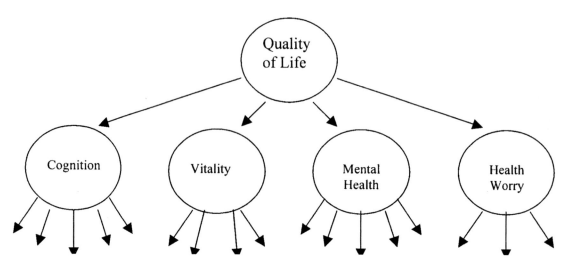

FIGURE 6.5   Hypothesized second-order factor structure (indicators and errors not represented).

the model form or pattern only to determine whether the number of factors is the same in each group with the items loading on the same factors in each group. Knowing that the general model is invariant, one might want to test whether the factor loadings are the same in each group. In this situation the factor loadings for the first group are constrained to be equivalent to the factor loadings for the second group. The correlations among factors or the equivalence of error variances could also be tested. For example, Soeken and Prescott (1991) tested whether the measurement model of the Patient Intensity for Nursing Index was invariant across five different hospitals. Another application might be to test whether a scale has the same factor structure in English-speaking and Spanish-speaking populations. Yet another application is to test the same group at two different times to determine whether the measurement model is invariant across time.

In summary, confirmatory factor analysis is a flexible procedure that directly assesses the link between the theoretical assumptions for a measure with the operational definition of the construct. Because it is theory-driven, CFA can be used to test the hypothesized construct validity of a measure. Individual parameters in a measurement model are tested as well as the overall model.

Criterion-Related Validity

When one wishes to infer from a measure an individual's probable standing on some other variable or criterion, criterion-related validity is of concern. It is important to distinguish between two types of criterion-related validity: predictive validity and concurrent validity. *Predictive validity* indicates the extent to which an individual's future level of performance on a criterion can be predicted from knowledge of performance on a prior measure. *Concurrent validity* refers to the extent to which a measure may be used to estimate an individual's present standing on the criterion. Predictive validity, unlike concurrent validity, involves a time interval during which events may occur; for example, people may gain experience or be subjected to some type of learning experience.

Thus, concurrent and predictive validity differ in the timing of the related criterion measures. For concurrent validity, the measure being tested for validity and the related criterion measure are given within a short period of time and their results compared to make statements regarding present standing in regard to the criterion. With predictive validity the criterion measure is administered much later than the measure being tested for validity, and the results are compared to assess the ability of the measure being tested to predict future standing in regard to the criterion. Activities undertaken to obtain evidence for criterion-related validity include:

- correlation studies of the type and extent of the relationships between scores and external variables
- studies of the extent to which scores predict future behavior, performance, or scores on measures obtained at a later point in time
- studies of the effectiveness of selection, placement, and/or classification decisions on the basis of the scores resulting from the measure
- studies of differential group predictions or relationships
- assessment of validity generalization

In each of the following questions below, the interest is in determining the extent to which performance on a criterion measure can be estimated using information obtained by the measure being tested (the predictor measure).

1. Is performance on a computer-simulated measure of empathy a good predictor of empathetic performance in a patient care situation?
2. Are scores on a confidence index obtained at the completion of an educational experience good predictors of participants' incorporation of skills learned during the program into their future practice?

The criterion against which the predictor measures are to be validated in both questions are higher-order operationalizations of the same construct that the predictor measure is attempting to assess. More specifically, in question 1 the criterion—empathetic performance in a patient care situation—is a higher-order operationalization of empathetic performance on a computer simulation. In question 2, the criterion—confidence to incorporate skills learned during the program into future practice—is a higher-order operationalization of confidence self-reported on a confidence index immediately upon completion of the program. Knapp (1985, pp. 189–192) stresses that in an investigation of the criterion validity of a particular

measure, the criterion against which the obtained scores are to be validated should be a higher-status operationalization of the same construct that the measure is trying to tap, and not an operationalization of some other construct. He cautions that the distinction between criterion-related validity and a substantive research study regarding the relationship between the two variables is a fine one, but one that must be established. The reader is encouraged to read Knapp's article, in which he offers many salient comments regarding the use and misuse of reliability and validity testing citing examples from studies published in the nursing literature.

Similarly in both questions, it is evident that the investigator wants to know the extent to which performance on an important criterion (that is, empathetic nursing practice and confidence in incorporating skills into practice) can be estimated using information from a less costly, more easily obtained measure (that is, computer simulation to measure empathy in patient care and confidence index). If scores on a confidence index administered at the completion of an educational program are found by means of criterion-related validity studies to be a good predictor of participants' future confidence to incorporate learnings into nursing practice, continuing use of the confidence index would be a cost-effective way for those delivering the program to assess incorporation at a time when they might intervene to improve the expected outcome. Similarly, a confidence index is far more economical to administer than a continuing longitudinal study of confidence to incorporate skills into practice using subjects who complete the learning experience. In the case of the measurement of empathetic nursing practice, it is far more convenient and economical to measure empathy using a computer simulation than to conduct an observational study of nursing performance in the clinical setting.

In regard to both questions, criterion-related validity is assessed by measuring the performance of the target population or a representative sample of that population on both the predictor and criterion variables, and then determining the linear correlation, that is, Pearson r or other appropriate correlational and/or regression analyses as a measure or measures of the quality of the predictor for estimating performance on that particular criterion in that target population. The important distinction between the two questions relates to the type of criterion-related validity study indicated by each. Question 1 is a question of concurrent validity; that is, it addresses the extent to which a computer simulation to measure empathy in nursing practice can be used to assess empathy in the delivery of patient care at the present time. Thus, to assess concurrent validity it requires that the predictor measure—the computer simulation—be administered to a representative group of nurses, that a criterion measure of empathetic nursing practice with established reliability and validity be administered to the same group of nurses at the same time or a short time later, and that results on the two measures be compared using the appropriate correlation or regression procedure. The results of this comparison would then be employed to infer the predictor measure's ability to predict present standing on the criterion.

In question 2, the concern is with predictive validity in that the criterion measurement occurs much later than the predictor measurement and the comparison of the two measures' results are employed to predict the ability of the confidence index to predict future confidence to incorporate skills into nursing practice. Predictive validity studies most often employ longitudinal and/or cross-sectional designs and correlation and regression analyses to investigate the relationship between the predictor and criterion measures over time. It should be noted that the utility of most criterion-related validity coefficients is limited by the fact that salient characteristics in most populations are dynamic and changing.

Similarly, the value of the results of criterion-related validity studies is a function of the representativeness of the sample and the choice of a criterion measure. Criterion measures must be valid and, more important, must be reliable and meaningful. Many important nursing and health care variables are difficult to define and measure. Too often a criterion is determined by convenience. For example, when the criterion of interest is not readily available, it is tempting to use a substitute criterion rather than to wait until the desired criterion is available.

The results of criterion-related studies must be carefully evaluated in light of several factors. Factors to be considered in planning and interpreting criterion-related studies relate to (1) the target population, (2) the sample, (3) the criterion, (4) measurement reliability, and (5) the need for a cross validation (Martuza, 1977). More specifically, it should be noted that:

1. Criterion-related validity coefficients obtained at one time must be interpreted in light of other events occurring within the target population at the same time and later, and in most cases will have little or no value later.

An assumption underlying criterion-related validity procedures is that the nature of the target population is relatively static and unchanging. In reality, however, the relationship between any two variables within a particular population is more apt to change than to remain static, rendering the value of most validity coefficients short-lived.

2. Validity coefficients obtained when procedures for sampling the target populations are inadequate will frequently underestimate the true validity of the predictor in question.

The sampling procedure used in criterion-related validity studies must be such that it provides a sample representative of the target population in general and gives each potential subject an equal chance of being selected for inclusion in the sample. Similarly, during the conduct of the study, careful attention must be directed toward assessing the presence of attrition and its potential influence on study results. Selection bias and attrition when present may reduce score variability; that is, they may restrict the range of scores on the predictor and/or criterion variables, thus lowering the value of the resulting correlation coefficient and providing an inaccurate estimate of the true validity of the predictor in question.

3. A given criterion-related validity coefficient is interpretable only in terms of how the criterion is defined in that study.

Important criteria are usually difficult to define and measure in a universally acceptable manner. Occasionally, this fact leads to compromise and results in the selection of a criterion variable that is expedient, convenient, or agreeable to those involved rather than a criterion that is appropriate and of sufficient quality. For example, in nursing, because of the long amount of time often required to collect information (e.g., assessing the incorporation of learning into practice may involve years of costly data collection), it is tempting to use a substitute criterion rather than wait until the desired criterion is available. However, the substitute criterion used may not typically bear the same relevance to the predictors as the desired criterion. In criterion-related validity studies this possibility must be given careful consideration and expediency alone should not rule the conduct of the study.

4. A spurious increase in the validity coefficient may result from criterion contamination.

If criterion contamination is to be avoided, measures of the predictor and criterion variables must be independently obtained and free of bias. Whenever criterion-related studies employ a rating or judging procedure, the probability of criterion-related contamination is present; that is, if raters have knowledge of how members of the sample performed on the predictor, this knowledge may influence their rating on the criterion—high scorers on the predictor tend to be rated high on the criterion and vice versa. The result is an erroneous increase in the correlation between predictor and criterion, providing evidence that the predictor is more effective than it actually is.

5. A reduced validity coefficient may result when the predictor and/or criterion measures have not demonstrated sufficient reliability.

Reliability is a necessary prerequisite for validity. Prior to employing predictor and criterion measures in criterion-related validity studies, each should have been examined for and demonstrate sufficient evidence for reliability. Although there is a formula that exists for estimating the attenuation of a correlation resulting from measurement error (Nunnally, 1967, pp. 217–220), its general use is not recommended. In most practical situations, it is preferable to employ the most reliable predictor and criterion measures one can and then live with the results obtained in that manner, rather than attempt to estimate what might be given an error-free world, that is, to estimate the

correlation that would be obtained if infallible measurement techniques were ever available.

6. Correlation coefficients resulting from criterion-related validity studies tend to overestimate the strength of the predictor-criterion relationship.

In criterion-related validity studies, the validity of a given predictor-criterion relationship in a specific population is simply the linear correlation between the predictor and the criterion in that specific population. As a result, the correlation coefficient tends to overestimate the true predictor-criterion relationship. To obtain a more realistic estimate of the relationship, a cross-validation procedure should be employed whenever possible.

Ideally, two separate and independent samples from the sample population should be employed in a cross-validation procedure. In those instances in which it is not feasible to obtain two samples, it is better to randomly split the existing sample into two subsamples rather than opt not to cross validate at all. Given two samples, cross validation proceeds in the following manner. First, a prediction equation is calculated using data from the first sample. The prediction equation obtained for the first sample is used to estimate the criterion performance for each of the individuals in the second sample (C'). Then, r_{xy} is used to determine the linear correlation among the criterion scores predicted using the second sample (C') and the actual criterion scores (C) obtained for the members of the second sample. This correlation $r_{c'c}$ is then taken as a more precise estimate of the true correlation between the predictor and the criterion in the population of interest.

Validity generalization refers to the extent to which evidence for validity, usually predictive validity, obtained in one setting can be generalized to other settings (Schmidt & Hunter, 1977). Meta-analysis (Glass, McGraw, & Smith, 1981; Hedges & Olkin, 1985; Cooper & Hedges, 1994; Isaac & Michael, 1995) meta-analysis is one approach that can be used to investigate validity generalization if a sufficient database of findings from specific validity studies is available to meet requirements for its use. Meta-analysis is a procedure used to summarize conclusions resulting from a large set of studies investigating a particular variable of interest. Findings from each study are converted to a common statistic, effect size. The mean of effect size is then calculated for all the studies reviewed to provide an estimate of average effect of the variable of interest. Issac and Michael (1995) note that a major disadvantage of the technique is that it does not distinguish between well conducted and poorly conducted studies, but rather treats them equivalently as one body of information (p. 208). Therefore, caution must be exercised in selecting studies for inclusion in the meta-analysis. An example of meta-analysis of studies of nurse faculty job satisfaction can be found in the work of Gormley (2003, pp. 174–178).

NORM-REFERENCED ITEM-ANALYSIS PROCEDURES

Item analysis is a procedure used to further assess the validity of a measure by separately evaluating each item to determine whether or not that item discriminates in the same manner in which the overall measure is intended to discriminate (Issac & Michael, 1995, p. 123). Three item-analysis procedures are of interest in the norm-referenced case: (1) item p level, (2) discrimination index, and (3) item-response chart.

Item p Level

The p level (also referred to as the difficulty level) of an item is the proportion of correct responses to that item. It is determined by counting the number of subjects selecting the correct or desired response to a particular item and then dividing this number by the total number of subjects. For example, a ten-item performance measure is employed to observe the behaviors of 20 nurses working in a pediatric ambulatory center. It is determined that 10 subjects performed correctly in response to item 1; the remaining subjects did not. Thus, the p level for this item is 10/20 or 0.50. p levels may range from 0 to 1.00. The closer the value of p is to 1.00, the easier the item; the closer p is to zero, the more difficult the item. When norm-referenced measures are employed, p levels

between 0.30 and 0.70 are desirable, because extremely easy or extremely difficult items have very little power to discriminate or differentiate among subjects (Martuza, 1975, p. 17–2).

Discrimination Index

The discrimination index (D) assesses an item's ability to discriminate; that is, if performance on a given item is a good predictor of performance on the overall measure, the item is said to be a good discriminator. To determine the D value for a given item:

1. Rank all subjects' performance on the measure by using total scores from high to low.
2. Identify those individuals who ranked in the upper 25%.
3. Identify those individuals who ranked in the lower 25%.
4. Place the remaining scores aside.
5. Determine the proportion of respondents in the top 25% who answered the item correctly (P_u).
6. Determine the proportion of respondents in the lower 25% who answered the item correctly (P_L).
7. Calculate D by subtracting P_L from P_u (i.e., $D = P_u - P_L$).
8. Repeat steps 5 through 7 for each item on the measure.

D values range from -1.00 to $+1.00$. D values greater than $+0.20$ are desirable for a norm-referenced measure (Martuza, 1975, p. 17–2). A positive D value is desirable and indicates that the item is discriminating in the same manner as the total test; that is, those who score high on the test tend to respond correctly to the item, while those who score low do not. A negative D value suggests that the item is not discriminating in the same way as the total test; that is, respondents who obtain low scores on the total measure tend to get the item correct, while those who score high on the measure tend to respond incorrectly to the item. A negative D value usually indicates that an item is faulty and needs improvement. Possible explanations for a negative D value are that the item provides a clue to the lower-scoring subjects that enables them to guess the correct response or that the item is misinterpreted by the high scorers.

Item Response Chart

Like D, the item-response chart assesses an item's ability to discriminate. The respondents ranking in the upper and lower 25% are identified as in steps 1 through 4 for determining D. A fourfold table like the one in Figure 6.6 is then constructed using the two categories, high/low scorers and correct/incorrect for a given item.

Using the information in Figure 6.6, one calculates the chi square value of the resulting proportions.

Formula 6.1: Calculation of chi square (χ^2) values

$$\chi^2 = \frac{N(AD - BC)^2}{(A + B)(C + D)(A + C)(B + D)}$$

$$df = (r - 1)(c - 1)$$

where N = the total number of subjects
A, B, C, D = the values in the cells as labeled in the figure
r = the number of rows
c = the number of columns

Example: Using the information in Figure 6.6:

$$\chi^2 = \frac{20(80 - 1)^2}{(11)(9)(11)(9)}$$

$$= \frac{20(79)^2}{(11)(9)(11)(9)}$$

$$= \frac{124,820}{9801}$$

$$= 12.7$$

$$df = (1)(1)$$
$$= 1$$

Using a table of critical values of the chi square statistic that can be found in most research and statistics books, including Waltz and Bausell (1981, p. 341), and Issac and Michael (1995, p. 250), a value as large as or larger than 1.84 for a chi square with one degree of freedom is significant at the 0.05 level. A significant chi square value of 12.7, as in the example, indicates that a significant difference exists in the proportion of high and low scorers who have correct responses. Items that meet this criterion should be retained, while those that do not should be discarded or modified to improve their ability to discriminate.

Next, one inspects the total response patterns in the item-response chart to identify problems with distractors. Examination of the chart in Table 6.6 suggests that the item does not discriminate well. The incorrect option was selected by only 10% of the subjects. It would therefore be prudent to examine the item to determine if these results are due to some item defect and to revise the item accordingly. Potential problems are that the correct option contains a clue that is used by many of the lower group in responding; or that the incorrect option is grammatically inconsistent with the stem, thus cluing subjects not to select it. If the item appears sound as constructed, it would be useful to analyze the content and procedures to which the item relates for the purpose of determining why the item's discriminating power is marginal.

In addition to its utility in analyzing true/false or multiple-choice measures, the item-response chart is also useful in situations in which affective measures with more than two choices are employed in an attempt to distinguish between the attitudes, values, or preferences of two groups of subjects on a given measure.

For example, one would use an item-response chart like the one in Table 6.7 in the following manner to assess an item's ability to distinguish between practitioners' and educators' preferences for involvement in a particular type of nursing practice.

Example

Item
I prefer working directly with patients to working with students in the clinical area.

Options
A agree (desired response by practitioners)
U undecided
D disagree (desired response by educators)

Response			Totals	
Incorrect		**Correct**		
High	B	A		A+B
1		10	11	
Low	D	C		C+D
8		1	9	
	B+D	A+C		N
Totals	9	11		20

FIGURE 6.6   Item-response chart for a true/false or multiple-choice measure ($n = 20$).

Item-Response Analysis
1. Data are divided into two groups—educators and practitioners

2. A 2 × 3 table is constructed as in Table 6.7.
3. Chi square is determined using Formula 6.2.

Formula 6.2: Determing chi square

$$\chi^2 = \frac{(O - E)^2}{E}$$

$$df = (r - 1)(c - 1)$$

where O = the observed frequencies of responses
E = the expected frequencies of responses, determined by multiplying the column total times the row total for each cell in the table and dividing the resulting product by N
r = the number of rows
c = the number of columns

Group	Disagree	Undecided	Agree	Raw Total
Practitioners	10 (15)	5 (5)	35 (30)	50
Educators	20 (15)	5 (5)	25 (30)	50
Column Total	30	10	60	100

O	E	O – E	$(O - E)^2$	$\dfrac{(O - E)^2}{E}$
10	15	−5	25	1.66
20	15	5	25	1.66
5	5	0	0	0
5	5	0	0	0
35	30	5	25	0.83
25	30	−5	25	0.83

$$\chi^2 = 4.98$$
$$df = 2$$

TABLE 6.6   Example of an Item-Response Chart Indicating an Item Without Discriminatory Power Resulting From a Faulty Distractor

		Response		
		Incorrect	**Correct**	**Totals**
Score	High	5	80	85
	Low	5	10	15
	Totals	10	90	100

A chi square with 2 df is significant at the 0.05 level when the chi square value is 5.99 or larger (Waltz & Bausell, 1981, p. 341; Issac & Michael, 1995, p. 250). In the example, the obtained value of chi square (4.98) does not meet or exceed the critical value and is therefore not significant. Hence, it cannot be concluded that a difference exists in the proportion of practitioners and educators who answered as expected; that is, it was expected that practitioners would agree with the statement "I prefer working directly with patients to working with students in the clinical area" and that educators would disagree. If chi square had been significant, the item would be discriminating as expected and would be retained. The item as it stands, however, needs revision or should be eliminated and replaced by an item with more power to discriminate between practitioners' preferences and educators' preferences for involvement in nursing practice.

Differential Item Function

Differential item function (DIF) refers to "when examinees of the same ability but belonging to different groups have differing probabilities of success on an item" (Hattie, Jaeger, & Bond,

1999, p. 432). When DIF is present it is an indicator of potential item bias, in that an unbiased item, by definition, is one for which the probability of success is the same for equally able respondents regardless of their group membership (e.g., ethnicity or gender). A relatively simple approach to detecting DIF is to compare item discrimination indices (i.e., D, p level, and/or item response charting) across different groups of respondents to determine if responses to the item(s) differ by group membership.

Several additional, more sophisticated, approaches to detecting DIF derived from classical measurement theory include: (1) using hypothesis testing of the differences between two or more groups sampled from the same population who respond to the same measure employing analysis of variance (ANOVA) procedures to examine the interaction of groups' x items, or the chi square statistic to examine the differences between an expected number of respondents in a particular ability category and the actual number observed to respond in that category; in both cases rejection of the null hypothesis of no statistically significant differences is indicative of item bias (Issac and Michael, 1995); (2) performing a distractor response analysis where differences in response patterns of two or

TABLE 6.7   Item-Response Chart for an Affective Measure With More Than Two Responses

	Response			
Group	**Disagree**	**Undecided**	**Agree**	**Total**
Practitioners	10	5	35	50
Educators	20	5	25	50
Total	30	10	60	100

more groups to the incorrect alternative to an item by testing the null hypothesis of no statistically significant differences between group response frequencies in the discrete categories of question distractors; rejection of the null hypothesis suggests item bias is present (Isaac & Michael, 1995); and (3) employing the Mantel-Haenszel procedure (Holland & Thayer, 1988; Silverlake, 1999) where two groups of respondents with similar scores on the same measure are matched, and the performance of each group is compared on each item; items demonstrating differences between groups are presumed to be biased.

Another approach to detecting DIF, based on item response theory, compares item characteristic curves (ICC) for each group of respondents assuming that ICC curves should be similar if items are unbiased (Nunnally & Bernstein, 1994; Embretson & Hershberger, 1999). An example of the use of ICC curves for investigating item score patterns can be found in Meijer (2003, pp. 72–87). Readers interested in a comprehensive discussion of item bias and approaches to detecting DIF are referred to Osterlind (1983).

CRITERION-REFERENCED VALIDITY ASSESSMENT

The validity of a criterion-referenced measure can be analyzed at the item and test levels to ascertain if the measure functions in a manner consistent with its purposes. As Berk (1980b, p. 47) so aptly pointed out, the focus of item validity for criterion-referenced measures is "how well each item measures its respective objective (item-objective congruence)" and helps classify persons or objects into their appropriate category (item discrimination). Test validity focuses on the representativeness of a cluster of items in relation to the specified content domain (content validity), the significance of test results in relation to the initial conceptualization of the measure (construct validity), the decisions that result from the scores on the measure (decision validity), the extent to which future performance on a measure can be predicted from performance on a prior measure (predictive validity), and the extent to which an individual's performance on one measure can be used to estimate an individual's performance on a criterion measure (concurrent validity). Since criterion-referenced measures result in the classification of phenomena in relation to the domain of interest, the validity of standards or cut scores assumes special significance. In essence, validity in terms of criterion-referenced interpretations relates to the extent to which scores result in the accurate classification of objects in regard to their domain status. The measure also must be content valid; that is, its items or tasks must adequately represent the domain that is the focus of measurement. Since validity of the content of the measure is requisite to the validity of the total measure or test, attention is now given to a discussion of content validation of criterion-referenced measures.

Criterion-Referenced Content Validity

Unless the items or tasks in a criterion-referenced measure assess the objective, any use of scores obtained will be questionable. For a measure to provide a clear description of domain status, the content domain must be consistent with its domain specifications or objective. Thus, content validity of a criterion- referenced measure is the first type of validity that should be established and is a prerequisite for all other types of validity.

At the total test level, content validity for criterion-referenced measures relates to the representativeness of the total collection of test items or tasks as a measure of the content domain. In chapter 4, a discussion of test specifications is provided. The major purpose of this approach to the construction of criterion-referenced measures is to facilitate the generation of content-valid test items that are homogeneous. The most frequently used *a posteriori* content validity approach in criterion-referenced measurement uses content specialists to assess the quality and representativeness of the items within the test for measuring the content domain. Content specialists examine the format and content of each item and assess whether it is an appropriate measure of some part of the content domain of interest as determined by test specifications.

Validity Assessment by Content Specialists

Content specialists selected for the evaluation of content in a criterion-referenced measure should be conversant with the domain treated in the measuring tool. The developer of a measure should keep in mind that the ratings of content specialists are only as good as their level of expertise in the area of content measured. One or more poor content specialists can greatly compromise the process of content validation. In most instances, two or more content specialists are employed; however, the number depends on the type of procedure.

In addition to the content validity procedures discussed that primarily place emphasis on the content validity of the test, i.e. group of items within the item-objective congruence measure discussed in a later section of this chapter, focuses on content validity at the item level. Remember that if more than one objective is used for a measure, the items that are measures of each objective usually are treated as separate tests when interpreting the results of validity assessments.

Determination of Interrater Agreement

Rating scales frequently are used to assess the validity of the group of items within a measure. Content specialists are provided with the conceptual definition of the variable(s) to be measured or the domain specifications (or the objectives) for the measure along with the set of items. The content specialists then independently rate the relevance of each item to the specified content domain as described previously in the norm-referenced case. The ratings of two content specialists are used to compute P_0 and K as measures of interrater agreement as described in chapter 5. Suppose the ratings obtained from the judges are as shown in Table 6.8. P_0 then is the proportion of items given a rating of not/somewhat relevant (1 or 2) and quite/very relevant (3 or 4) by both content specialists. Hence, in the case of content validity determination, P_0 is representative of the consistency of judges' ratings of the relevance of the group of items within the test to the specified content domain. As noted previously, K is P_0 corrected for chance agreements.

Once obtained, what do the values of P_0 and K mean? An acceptable level of interrater agreement varies from situation to situation. However, safe guidelines for acceptable levels are P_0 values greater than or equal to 0.80, or K greater than or equal to 0.25. If P_0 and K or either of these values is too low, one or a combination of two problems could be operating. First, this could be an indication that the test items lack homogeneity and that the domain is ambiguous or is not well defined. Second, the problem could be due to the raters who might have interpreted the rating scale labels differently or used the rating scale differently (Martuza, 1977). Refinement of the domain specifications is required if the former is the case. If the latter is the problem, the raters are given more explicit directions and guidelines in the use of the scale to reduce the chance of differential use. The index

TABLE 6.8   Hypothetical Content Specialists Ratings of the Relevance of 30 Items for Assessing Adjustment to Parenthood

		Judge 1		
		not/somewhat relevant (1 or 2)	quite/very relevant (3 or 4)	Totals
Judge 2	not/somewhat relevant (1 or 2)	(A) 3	(B) 2	(A + B) 5
	quite/very relevant (3 or 4)	(C) 1	(D) 24	(C + D) 25
	Totals	(A + C) 4	(B + D) 26	(A + B + C + D) 30

of content validity (CVI), as discussed in the norm-referenced case, can be calculated from the content specialists' ratings and is the proportion of items rated as quite/very relevant (3 or 4) by both judges. In the present case the CVI is 24/30 = 0.80.

As indicated earlier, low values of P_o and K may be due to lack of homogeneity of items because of an inadequate domain definition. A clear and precise domain definition and domain specifications function to communicate what the results of measurements mean to those people who must interpret them, and what types of items and content should be included in the measure to those people who must construct the items. Content specialists' ratings can be used to help check the descriptive clarity of the domain definition of a measure when indicated (Popham, 1978). Suppose that three content specialists are used to judge the congruence of the items in a measure of the specified domain, and that items were developed by ten item writers who contributed three items each. The proportion of homogeneous items, as determined by each rater, will be useful in assessing the adequacy of the domain definition. For each judge the number of items rated as congruent divided by the total number of items in the measure yields the proportion of homogeneous items. For example, if a judge rated 20 of the items in a 30-item measure as congruent, the proportion of homogeneous items would be 20/30 = 0.67. Suppose the proportions of homogeneous items for the three content specialists are 0.67 (20 out of 30), 0.50 (15 out of 30), and 0.60 (18 out of 30). If, upon inspection of the item-by-item ratings of the judges, the majority of the item writers had at least one item that was judged not/somewhat relevant (1 or 2) by the three content specialists, then this would be support for lack of clarity in the domain definition.

Assume that the proportions of homogeneous items for the three content specialists are 0.90 (27 out of 30), 0.93 (28 out of 30), and 0.93 (28 out of 30). After scrutinizing the items, it becomes apparent that each of the items judged to be unlike the rest had been prepared by one item writer. In this case the flaw is not likely to be in the domain definition as specified, but in the interpretations of one item writer.

Average Congruency Percentage

The content validity of a test also can be estimated by an average congruency percentage (Popham, 1978). Suppose four content specialists are identified and asked to read the domain specifications for a measure and then judge the congruence of each item on a 20-item measure with the specifications. The proportion of items rated congruent by each judge is calculated and converted to a percentage. Then the mean percentage for all four judges is calculated to obtain the average congruency percentage. For example, if the percentages of congruent items for the judges are 95, 90, 100, and 100%, the average congruency percentage would be 96.25%. An average congruency percentage of 90 percent or higher can be safely considered acceptable.

When using content specialists' ratings, including a specified number of irrelevant or incongruent items in the item pool can check the accuracy of each content specialist. The number of such aberrant items detected can determine the effectiveness of content specialists. Ratings of any content specialist who does not meet a set minimum level of performance in detecting these bad items are discarded from the analysis.

CRITERION-REFERENCED CONSTRUCT VALIDITY

Measurements obtained through the use of criterion-referenced measures are used to describe and make decisions based on an object's domain status. Even though content validation of a measure is an important initial step in validity assessment, content validity evidence alone does not ensure a measure's construct validity. Hence, evidence of the content representativeness of a measure does not guarantee that the measure is useful for its intended purpose. Although "we may say that a test's results are accurately descriptive of the domain of behaviors it is supposed to measure, it is quite another thing to say that the function to which you wish to put a descriptively valid test is appropriate" (Popham, 1978, p. 159). Thus, the major focus of construct validation for criterion-referenced measures is to establish support for the measure's ability to accurately categorize phenomena in accordance with the purpose for which the measure being used. Approaches used to assess construct validity for criterion-referenced measures are presented below.

Experimental Methods and the Contrasted Groups Approach

Experimental manipulation and the contrasted-groups approach also can be used to generate support for the construct validity of criterion-referenced measures. The basic principles and procedures for these two approaches are the same for criterion-referenced measures as for norm-referenced measures. Since criterion-referenced measures yield nominal or ordinal data, nonparametric statistical procedures are likely to be required when comparative statistical analysis is conducted. Experimental methods or the contrasted-groups approach also may be used to assess the decision validity of a measure, an important type of validity for criterion-referenced instruments.

Decision Validity

The measurements obtained from criterion-referenced measures are often used to make decisions. "Criterion-referenced tests have emerged as instruments that provide data via which mastery decisions can be made, as opposed to providing the decision itself" (Hashway, 1998, p. 112). For example: (1) a student may be allowed to progress to the next unit of instruction if test results indicate that the preceding unit has been mastered; (2) a woman in early labor may be allowed to ambulate if the nurse assesses, on pelvic examination, that the fetal head is engaged (as opposed to unengaged) in the pelvis; or (3) a diabetic patient may be allowed to go home if the necessary skills for self-care have been mastered. These are just a few of the many examples of how criterion-referenced results can be used for decision making. The decision validity of criterion-referenced measures that are used for such decisions takes on special significance, because the consequences of a bad decision can have detrimental effects. The decision validity of a measure is supported when the set standard(s) or criterion classifies subjects or objects with a high level of confidence.

In most instances, two criterion groups are used to test the decision validity of a measure: one group known to be low in the attribute of interest, and the other high. For example, suppose a measure is designed to test mastery of skills for application of aseptic technique. Also, suppose that students in a fundamentals of nursing course, who have no prior exposure to aseptic technique, are randomly assigned to one of two groups: one receiving instruction on aseptic technique and the other receiving no instruction in the area. If the test has decision validity, a much higher percentage of students in the group receiving instruction should be classified as masters after instruction than as nonmasters, and a higher percentage of those receiving no instruction should be classified as nonmasters by the test than as masters. The decision validity of the test would be calculated "by summing the percentage of instructed students who exceed the performance standard and the percentage of uninstructed students who did not" (Hambleton, 1980, p. 98). It is assumed that these are the groups that are correctly classified by the testing procedure. Thus, decision validity can range from 0 to 100%, with high percentages reflecting high decision validity.

Criterion groups for testing the decision validity of a measure also can be created if individuals can be classified prior to testing according to whether they are known by independent means to be low or high on the attribute tested. The congruence between the classifications resulting from the measure and the known classifications are used to calculate the decision validity of the measure. For example, assume that the validity of a nurse's assessments of the position of the fetal presenting part on pelvic examination during labor are considered. Suppose the fetal positions are also determined via sonography. The congruence between the nurse's assessments and the results from sonography is used to determine the decision validity of the nurse's assessments.

Decision validity is influenced not only by the quality of the measure, but also by the appropriateness of the criterion groups, the characteristics of the subjects, and the level of performance or cut-score required. Of course, decision validity is necessary only in instances in which scores or results are used to make decisions (Hambleton, 1980).

Criterion-Related Validity

The functional usefulness of criterion-referenced measures is supported by criterion-related validity evidence. Criterion-related validity, particularly predictive validity evidence, establishes support that a measure functions as it should. Criterion-related validity studies of criterion-referenced measures are conducted in the same manner as for norm-referenced measures. The reader is referred to previous sections on norm-referenced validity for a thorough discussion of criterion-related validity approaches.

CRITERION-REFERENCED ITEM-ANALYSIS PROCEDURES

Some empirical procedures used in the validation of norm-referenced items can be used in criterion-referenced test validation. However, the statistics must be used and interpreted correctly in the context of the criterion-referenced framework. Rovinelli and Hambleton (1977) suggested that empirical methods used for item-discrimination indices have limited usefulness, because they can be used only to identify aberrant items without any intention of eliminating items from the item pool. It is not appropriate to rely on item statistics to select the items for criterion-referenced measures, because theoretically this would alter the content domain and thereby weaken the representativeness of items and, thus, the interpretability of the domain score (Berk, 1980a; Hambleton et al., 1978; Millman, 1974; Popham, 1978). Item-content validity is the extent to which each item is a measure of the content domain. Obtaining content specialists' ratings holds the most merit for assessing item validities for determining which items should be retained or discarded; empirical item-discrimination indices should be used primarily to detect aberrant items in need of revision or correction (Hambleton, 1980).

Item-Objective or Item-Subscale Congruence

The item-objective congruence procedure, which may also be referred to as the item-subscale congruence procedure when used with questionnaires, provides an index of the validity of an item based on the ratings of two or more content specialists (Rovinelli & Hambleton, 1977). In this method content specialists are directed to assign a value of +1, 0, or −1 for each item, depending upon the item's congruence with the measure's objective or subscale. Whenever an item is judged to be a definite measure of the objective or subscale, a value of +1 is assigned. A rating of 0 indicates that the judge is undecided about whether the item is a measure of the objective or subscale. The assignment of a −1 rating reflects a definite judgment that the item is not a measure of the objective or subscale. Hence, the task of the content specialists is to make a judgment about whether or not an item falls within the content domain as specified by the measure's objective or subscale. The data that result from the judges' ratings are then used to compute the index of item-objective congruence or item-subscale congruence.

The index of item-objective congruence provides useful information about the agreement between content specialists' ratings as to whether each item in a test or questionnaire measures the intended objective (or subscale). In this procedure an item is assessed to determine which of several objectives or subscales in a measure it represents. The limits of the index range from −1.00 to +1.00. An index of +1.00 will occur when perfect positive item-objective or subscale congruence exists, that is, when all content specialists assign a +1 to the item for its related objective or subscale and a −1 to the item for all other objectives or subscales that are measured by the tool. An index of −1.00 represents the worst possible value of the index and occurs when all content specialists assign a −1 to the item for what was expected to be its related objective or subscale and a +1 to the item for all other objectives or subscales. An advantage of the index of item-objective congruence (or item-subscale congruence) is that it does not depend on the number of content specialists used or on the number of objectives measured by the test or questionnaire. However, the tool must include more than one objective or subscale in order for this procedure to be used.

The index of item-objective (or item-subscale) congruence is provided by the following formula:

Formula 6.3: Calculating index of item-objective congruence (Martuza, 1977)

$$I_{ik} = \frac{(M - 1)\, S_k - S'_k}{2N\,(M - 1)}$$

where I_{ik} = the index of the item-objective congruence for item i and objective k

M = the number of objectives

N = the number of content specialists

S_k = the sum of the ratings assigned to objective k

S'_k = the sum of the ratings assigned to all objectives, except objective k

Based on the information provided in Table 6.9, the index of item-objective congruence can be calculated in the following manner. It should be noted that in this case:

$$I_{ik} = I_{11}$$
$$M = 4$$
$$N = 3$$
$$S_1 = 2$$

$$S_1 = (-3) + (-2) + (-3) = -8$$

Hence I_{11} = $\dfrac{(4 - 1)\,(+2) - (-8)}{2(3)\,(4 - 1)}$

$$= \frac{6 + 8}{18}$$

$$= \frac{14}{18}$$

$$= 0.78$$

When the index is used to determine which items should be revised or retained during the measure's development process, an index cut-off score to separate valid from nonvalid items within the test should be set. The setting of this index cut-off score is usually derived by the test developer. Hambleton (1980) suggests that this should be done by creating the poorest set of content specialists' ratings that the test developer is willing to accept as evidence that an item is within the content domain of interest. After computing the index for this set of minimally acceptable ratings, the resulting index serves as the index cut-off score for judging the validity of the items. It serves as the criterion against which each item within the measure is judged, based on its index of item-objective congruence, which resulted from content specialists' ratings. If, for instance, the index cut-off score is 0.75, then all items with an index of item-objective congruence below 0.75 are deemed nonvalid, while those with an index of 0.75 or above are considered valid. Those with an index below 0.75 are discarded from the measure or analyzed and revised to improve their validity.

Empirical Item-Analysis Procedures

Criterion-referenced item-analysis procedures determine the effectiveness of a specific test item to discriminate subjects who have acquired the target behavior and those who have not. It is important that the content of the measure be kept as representative of the specified content domain as possible. Therefore, caution should be exercised before items are discarded from a criterion-referenced measure based on empirical item-analysis procedures. The nature of the subjects and the treatment or intervention may result in an item discrimination index that may imply that the item does not function well when it is actually content valid. However, if there is sufficient evidence that an item is not functioning as it should and also is not content valid, it is recommended that it be discarded from the measure or revised.

In criterion-referenced item-analysis procedures, empirical data are obtained from respondents in order to evaluate the effectiveness of the items of the measuring tool. The most commonly used item-analysis procedures employ either pretest-posttest measurements with one group or two independent measurements with two different groups. The selection of the groups

TABLE 6.9   Judges' Ratings of Item-Objective Congruence for a Hypothetical Item I

Content Specialists	Objective			
	1	2	3	4
A	+1	−1	−1	−1
B	+1	−1	−1	−1
C	0	−1	0	−1
S_k	+2	−3	−2	−3

depends upon the purpose of the measure. Groups chosen for item analysis of criterion-referenced measures are often referred to as criterion groups. Two approaches are used for identifying criterion groups: (1) the criterion-groups technique, which also may be referred to as the uninstructed-instructed groups approach, when the focus of measurement is knowledge; and (2) pretreatment/post-treatment measures approach, which in appropriate instances may be called the preinstruction/postinstruction measurements approach.

The criterion-groups technique involves the testing of two separate groups at the same time—one group that is known by independent means to possess more of the specified trait or attribute, and a second group known to possess less. For example, if the purpose of a criterion-referenced measure is to identify parents who have and who have not adjusted to parenthood after the birth of a first child, two groups of parents would be of interest—those who have adjusted to parenthood and those who have not had a previous opportunity to adjust to parenthood. A group of parents who have previously experienced parenthood might then be contrasted with a group of inexperienced parents who have just had their first child. The subjects chosen for each of the groups should be as similar as possible on relevant characteristics, for example, social class, culture, and age. In addition, the proportional distribution of relevant characteristics between groups should be equivalent. The only real difference between the groups should be in terms of exposure to the specified treatment or experience.

The criterion-groups technique has a major advantage in that it is highly practical. Item analysis can be conducted at one time if a group that is known to possess more of the specified trait or attribute is available at the same time as a group that is low or lacking in the trait or attribute of interest. However, one disadvantage is the difficulty of defining criteria for identifying groups. Another is the requirement of equivalence of groups. It is often difficult to randomly assign persons to groups, such as when using instructed and uninstructed groups. Differences in group performance might be attributable to such characteristics as socioeconomic background, age, sex, or levels of ability if groups are not proportionately balanced on relevant characteristics.

The pretreatment/posttreatment measurements approach involves testing one group of subjects twice—once before exposure to some specific treatment (pretreatment), and again after exposure to the treatment (posttreatment). Subjects are usually tested with the same set of items on both occasions, or a parallel or equivalent set of items can be administered on the second testing. In the case in which instruction is the treatment, testing would occur before instruction (preinstruction) and after instruction (postinstruction).

This approach has the advantage of allowing analysis of individual as well as group gains. However, a major limitation is the impracticality of administering the posttest. Item analysis cannot be done until after the treatment or instruction has been completed. A second limitation is the amount of time that may be required between the pretest and posttest. When the period between testing is short, there is a potential problem with testing effect, which could influence performance on the posttest. The use of parallel or equivalent items helps to reduce testing effect. If this is not possible because of practical constraints or the nature of the content domain, the period between administrations might be extended to reduce the carryover effect of memory from the initial testing. The period between the pretest and posttest should not extend beyond 2 months to reduce the chances of a history or maturation effect. Intervening events or simply growing older can influence individual performance or results on the posttest. Improvement in performance due to history or maturation or both can become inextricably mixed with the treatment or effects of instruction. Item analysis is designed to focus only on the change in responses to items because of treatment or instruction (Berk, 1980a).

Item Difficulty

Because of the purpose of criterion-referenced measures, it is appropriate to examine the difficulty level of items and compare them between criterion groups. Separate item p levels should be calculated for each item in the measure for each of the criterion groups. The approaches to calculating item p levels and their interpretation was discussed previously in this chapter in relation to norm-referenced item analysis procedures. The item p levels for each item are compared between groups to help determine if respondents would have performed similarly on an item, regardless of which group they are in. The item p level should be higher for the group that is known to possess more of a specified trait or attribute than for the group known to possess less. Hence, the item p levels should be substantially higher on a measure of parental adjustment for a group of experienced parents, who have had an opportunity to adjust to parenthood previously, than for a group of inexperienced parents. If this were the case, this would be positive evidence of item validity. Likewise, the item p levels of a group should be higher on a posttest after a relevant treatment has been provided than on the pretest.

Item Discrimination

The focus of item discrimination indices for criterion-referenced measures is on the measurement of performance changes (e.g., pretest/posttest) or differences (e.g., experienced parents/inexperienced parents) between the criterion groups. Criterion-referenced item discrimination (generally referred to as D′) is directly related to the property of decision validity, since it is reflected in the accuracy with which persons are classified on the domain of interest. Items with high positive discrimination indices improve the decision validity of a test. Although a vast array of item discrimination indices for criterion-referenced measures has been described in the literature, those discussed here are considered practical in terms of their ease of calculation and meaningfulness for the test development process (Berk, 1980a).

A rather simple item-discrimination index, which can be used with data obtained via the criterion-groups technique, is the criterion groups difference index (CGDI) (also known as the uninstructed/instructed group difference index). The CGDI is the proportion of respondents in the group known to have less of the trait or attribute of interest who answered the item appropriately or correctly subtracted from the proportion of respondents in the group known to possess more of the trait or attribute of interest who answered it correctly.

Formula 6.4: Calculating the criterion groups difference index (CGDI)

$$\text{CGDI} = \begin{matrix}\text{the item p level for} \\ \text{group known to} \\ \text{possess more of} \\ \text{the attribute}\end{matrix} - \begin{matrix}\text{the item p level for} \\ \text{group known to have} \\ \text{less of the attribute}\end{matrix}$$

Three item-discrimination indices that can be employed when the pretreatment/posttreatment measurements approach is used are (1) pretest/posttest difference, (2) individual gain, and (3) net gain. The pretest/posttest difference index (PPDI) is the proportion of respondents who answered the item correctly on the posttest minus the proportion who responded to the item correctly on the pretest.

Formula 6.5: Calculating the pretest/posttest difference index (PPDI)

$$PPDI = \frac{\text{the item p level}}{\text{on the posttest}} - \frac{\text{the item p level}}{\text{on the pretest}}$$

The individual gain index (IGI) is the proportion of respondents who answered the item incorrectly on the pretest and correctly on the posttest. For example, in Table 6.3, which shows the response data on an item by 50 respondents, IGI would be the value in cell C divided by the total number of respondents as given below in Formula 6.6.

Formula 6.6: Calculating the individual gain index (IGI)

$$IGI = \frac{C}{A + B + C + D}$$

$$= \frac{35}{50}$$

$$= 0.70$$

The net gain index (NGI) is the proportion of respondents who answered the item incorrectly on both occasions subtracted from the IGI. Thus, NGI is an extension of IGI that considers the performance of all respondents who answered the item incorrectly on the pretest. Given the information in Table 6.10, the NGI could be calculated in the following manner:

Formula 6.7: Calculating the net gain index (NGI)

$$NGI = \frac{D}{IGI - A + B + C + D}$$

$$= 0.70 - \frac{7}{50}$$

$$= 0.56$$

The selection of an item-discrimination index is determined by the nature of the criterion groups providing the data for analysis. CGDI is the only index discussed for the criterion-groups technique. Of the three indices appropriate for pretreatment/posttreatment groups, NGI

provides the most conservative estimate of item discrimination and uses more information. NGI also provides a greater range of possible values than IGI (Berk, 1980a).

The range of values for each of the indices discussed above is −1.00 to +1.00, except for IGI, which has a range of 0 to +1.00. A high positive index for each of these item discrimination indices is desirable, since this would reflect the item's ability to discriminate between criterion groups.

The nature of the content domain and the measure's objective, along with the method used to compute discrimination, would influence the level at which the item discrimination index should be positive. A summary of criterion-referenced item discrimination indices discussed above is presented in Table 6.11.

A useful adjunct item-discrimination index is provided through the use of P_o or K to measure the effectiveness of an item in relation to the total test in classifying subjects into categories (Martuza, 1977). For example, groups of masters and nonmasters by the test are checked against the proportion of masters and nonmasters on the item. If, for example, the data (expressed as proportions) in Table 6.12 reflect classifications by a specific item and the test for a group of subjects, agreement between these two classifications could be considered an index of item discrimination. Thus, in this case there is 38% agreement between the item and the test as determined by the value of K

$$P_o = 0.70 + 0.10 = 0.80$$

$$P_c = (0.75)(0.85) + (0.25)(0.15) = 0.68$$

$$K = \frac{P_o - P_c}{1 - P_c}$$

$$= \frac{0.80 - 0.68}{1 - 0.68}$$

$$= \frac{0.12}{0.32}$$

$$= 0.38$$

At this point, the value of K_{max} can be calculated to determine the maximum possible agreements consistent with the observed marginal proportions in Table 6.12. The tabular adjustments required are presented in Table 6.13. The

TABLE 6.10   Hypothetical Response Data on an Item by 50 Respondents

		Post-test		
		Correct	**Incorrect**	**Total**
Pretest	**Correct**	(A) 5	(B) 3	(A + B) 8
	Incorrect	(C) 35	(D) 7	(C + D) 42
	Totals	(A + C) 40	(B + D) 10	(A + B + C + D) 50

value of K_{max} in this instance is 0.69. When K is considered in terms of the value of K_{max}, there is evidence that the item discriminates between masters and nonmasters, since K/K_{max} is 0.55.

$$K_{max} = \frac{0.75 + .15 - [(0.75)\,(0.85) + (0.25)\,(.15)]}{1 - [(0.75)\,(0.85) + (0.25)\,(.15)]}$$

$$= \frac{0.90 - 0.68}{1 - 0.68}$$

$$= \frac{0.22}{0.32}$$

$$= 0.69$$

When item p levels and discrimination indices do not support the validity of the item, the problem could be explained in terms of the item itself, the objective, or the nature of the treatment. When an item p level is much higher than expected on the pretest or in a group with less of the specified attribute, it is possible that there has been previous exposure to the content domain. If the p level is much lower than expected on a posttest, the objective may be too difficult or the treatment may have been ineffective. A much lower than expected item discrimination index could be due to one or a combination of problems cited above (Berk, 1980a).

When the item itself is suspected of being faulty, then it must be carefully scrutinized. Usually a negative discrimination index is due to a faulty item. Examination of the structure of the item and each response alternative is in order. Ambiguity, ineffective distractors, and more than one correct answer on a multiple-choice test should be considered. It is a good idea to get item reviews from respondents at the time the tool is administered, when the purpose of the administration is to obtain data for item analysis. Respondents can be asked to identify confusing items, items with no correct answer or more than one correct answer, and other problems encountered while progressing through the test. Such information can be used when identifying and revising poor items.

SUMMARY

Every measurement involves some error that cannot be eliminated but can be reduced by use of sound approaches to measurement. Systematic errors of measurement decrease validity. Validity is a unitary concept. It is the degree to which all of the accumulated evidence supports the intended interpretation of test scores for the intended purpose (AERA, APA, NCME, 1999, p. 11). Validity must be assessed every time a given measure is employed. Three types of measurement validity are: content, construct, and criterion-related. For any given measure, one or more of these types of validity will be of interest. For any given tool or method, validity will be investigated in multiple ways depending upon the purpose for measurement and evidence for validity accrued with repeated use of the measure. Item-response procedures contribute to validity by separately evaluating each item on a measure to determine whether or not that item performs in the same manner as the overall measure is intended to perform. Three item-analysis procedures are used in the norm-referenced

TABLE 6.11 Summary of Selected Criterion-Referenced Item Discrimination Indices

Index	Range of Values	Definition	Comments
Criterion groups difference index (CGDI)	-1.00 to $+1.00$	The proportion of respondents in the group known to possess more of the attribute of interest who answered the item correctly, minus the proportion of respondents in the group known to possess less of the attribute who answered it correctly.	Commonly referred to as the uninstructed/instructed group difference index when used in instructional context. Index is only sensitive to group differences. Does not focus on individual performance differences.
Pretest/Posttest difference index (PPDI)	-1.00 to $+1.00$	The proportion of respondents who answered the item correctly on the posttest, minus the proportion who responded to the item correctly on the pretest.	Index is only sensitive to group changes in performance and not to individual performance gain or loss.
Individual gain index (IGI)	0 to $+1.00$	The proportion of respondents who answered the item incorrectly on the pretest and correctly on the posttest.	Reflects change in performance in group based on performance changes by the individuals within the group who shifted from incorrect to correct response from pretest to posttest.
Net gain index (NGI)	-1.00 to $+1.00$	The proportion of respondents who answered the item incorrectly on both the pretest and posttest subtracted from IGI.	Considers performance of all respondents who answered the item incorrectly on the pretest. Yields values that are more conservative than preceding indices.

Adapted from Berk, R. A.: Item analysis. In Berk, R. A. (Ed.): *Criterion-Referenced Measurement*; Johns Hopkins Press, Baltimore, 1980, pp. 49–79.

TABLE 6.12   Joint Mastery Classifications of Examinees by One Item and the Total Test Score Expressed as Proportions

		Test Classifications		
		Master	**Nonmaster**	**Totals**
Item Classifications	**Master**	**(A)** 0.70	**(B)** 0.05	**(A + B)** 0.75
	Nonmaster	**(C)** 0.15	**(D)** 0.10	**(C + D)** 0.25
	Totals	**(A + C)** 0.85	**(B + D)** 0.15	**(A + B + C + D)** 1.00

case: item p level, the discrimination index, and item-response charts. Differential item function (DIF) is an indicator of item bias. Several approaches are available for detecting DIF based on classical measurement theory and item-response theory.

The concern of criterion-referenced validity is not only with whether a measure assesses what it is purported to measure, but also whether it functions in accordance with the purpose for which it is designed and used. Content validity and the assessment of construct validity and criterion-related and decision validity are important for criterion-referenced measures. As with norm-referenced measures, the validity of crite-

rion-referenced tools may be assessed at the test or item levels. Item validity is a prerequisite to test validity and may be estimated by the determination of item-objective congruence with the use of content specialists or estimated by empirical means. Item validity estimates provide important information that can be used to revise and improve criterion-referenced measures, thereby improving test validity. However, the validity of standards or cut scores takes on special significance and has a direct impact on the validity of the measure, because criterion standards or cut scores are used to classify phenomena in relation to a specified content domain.

TABLE 6.13   Tabular Adjustments Required in Table 6.12 for Computation

		Test Classifications		
		Master	**Nonmaster**	**Totals**
Item Classifications	**Master**	**(A)** 0.75	**(B)** 0.00	**(A + B)** 0.75
	Nonmaster	**(C)** 0.10	**(D)** 0.15	**(C + D)** 0.25
	Totals	**(A + C)** 0.85	**(B + D)** 0.15	**(A + B + C + D)** 1.00

REFERENCES

American Educational Research Association, American Psychological Association, and National Council on Measurement in Education. (1985). *Standards for educational and psychological testing*. Washington, DC: American Psychological Association.

American Educational Research Association, American Psychological Association, and National Council on Measurement in Education. (1999). *Standards for educational and psychological testing*. Washington, DC: American Psychological Association.

Arbuckle, J. L., & Wothke, W. (1999). *AMOS 4.0 user's guide*. Chicago: Smallwaters.

Bentler, P. M. (1989). *EQS program manual*. Encino, CA: Multivariate Software, Inc.

Berk, R. A. (1990). Importance of expert judgment in content-related validity evidence. *Western Journal of Nursing Research, 12*(5), 659–671.

Berk, R. A. (1980a). Item analysis. In R. A. Berk (Ed.), *Criterion-referenced measurement* (pp. 49–79). Baltimore: Johns Hopkins Press.

Berk, R. A. (1980b). Item and test validity. In R. A. Berk (Ed.), *Criterion-referenced measurement* (pp. 47–48). Baltimore: Johns Hopkins Press.

Bidwell, C. D. (1973). The social psychology of teaching. In R. Travers (Ed.), *Second handbook of research on teaching*. Chicago: Rand McNally.

Bollen, K. A. (1989). *Structural equations with latent variables*. New York: John Wiley & Sons.

Campbell, D. T., & Fiske, D. W. (1959). Convergent and discriminant validity by multitrait-multimethod matrix. *Psychology Bulletin, 56*(12), 81–105.

Carruth, A. K., Holland, C., & Larsen, L. (2000). Development and psychometric evaluation of the Caregiver Reciprocity Scale II. *Journal of Nursing Measurement, 8*(2), 179–191.

Cooper, H., & Hedges, L. V. (Eds.). (1994). *The handbook of research synthesis*. New York: Russell Sage Foundation.

Davis, L. L. (1992). Instrument review: Getting the most from a panel of experts. *Applied Nursing Research, 5*, 194–197.

Eid, M., Lischetzke, T., Nussbeck, F. W., & Trierweiler, L. K. (2003). Separating trait effects from trait-specific method effects in multitrait-multimethod models: A multiple-indicator CT-C (M-1) model. *Psychological Methods, 8*(1), 38–60.

Embretson, S. E., & Hershberger, S. (Eds.). (1999). *The new rules of measurement*. Mahwah, NJ: Lawrence Erlbaum Associates, Inc.

Glass, G. V., McGraw, B., & Smith, M. L. (1981). *Meta-analysis in social research*. Beverly Hills, CA: Sage.

Goodwin, L. D. (2002) Changing conceptions of measurement validity: An update on the new standards. *Journal of Nursing Education, 41*(3), 100–106.

Gormley, D. K. (2003). Factors affecting job satisfaction in nurse faculty: A meta-analysis. *Journal of Nursing Education, 42*(4), 174–178.

Grant, J. S., & Davis, L. L. (1997). Selection and use of content experts for instrument development. *Research in Nursing and Health, 20*(3), 269–274.

Hambleton, R. K. (1980). Test score validity and standard-setting methods. In R. A. Berk (Ed.), *Criterion-referenced measurement* (pp. 80–123). Baltimore: Johns Hopkins Press.

Hambleton, R. K., Swaminathan, H., Algina, J., Coulson, D. B. (1978). Criterion-referenced testing and measurement: A review of technical issues and developments. *Review of Educational Research, 48*, 1–47.

Hashway, R. M. (1998). *Assessment and evaluation of developmental learning: Qualitative individual assessment and evaluation models*. Westport, CT: Praeger.

Hattie, J., Jaeger, R. M., & Bond, L. (1999). Persistent methodological questions in educational testing. In A. Iran-Nejad & P. D. Pearson (Eds.), *Review of research in education* (Vol. 24, pp. 393–446). Washington, DC: American Education Research Association.

Hedges, L. B., & Olkin, I. (1985). *Statistical methods for meta-analysis*. Orlando, FL: Academic Press.

Holland, P. W., & Thayer, D. T. (1988). Differential item performance and the Mantel-Haenszel procedure. In H. Wainer & H. I. Braun (Eds.), *Test validity* (pp. 129–145). Hillsdale, NJ: Erlbaum.

Hu, L. T., & Bentler, P. M. (1999). Cutoff criteria for fit indices in covariance structure analysis: Conventional criteria versus new alternatives. *Structural Equation Modeling, 6*(1), 1–55.

Isaac, S., & Michael, W. B. (1995). *Handbook in research and evaluation* (3rd ed.). San Diego, CA: Educational and Industrial Testing Services.

Jones, T., Cason, C. L., & Mancini, M. E. (2002). Evaluating nurse competency: Evidence of validity for a skills recredentialing program. *Journal of Professional Nursing, 18*(1), 22–28.

Jöreskog, K. G., & Sörbom, D. (1996). *LISREL 8: User's reference guide.* Chicago: Scientific Software International.

Kline, R. B. (1998). *Principles and practice of structural equation modeling.* New York: The Guilford Press.

Knapp, T. R. (1985). Validity, reliability, and neither. *Nursing Research, 34*(3), 189–192.

Lauri, G., & Sanna, S. (2002). Developing an instrument to measure and describe clinical decision making in different nursing fields. *Journal of Professional Nursing, 18*(2), 93–100.

Martuza, V. R., et al. (1975). *EDF 660 tests and measurements course manual* (4th rev.). Newark: University of Delaware, College of Education.

Martuza, V. R. (1977). *Applying norm-referenced and criterion-referenced measurement in education.* Boston: Allyn & Bacon.

Meijer, R. R. (2003). Diagnosing item score patterns on a test using item response theory-based person-fit statistics. *Psychological Methods, 8*(1), 72–87.

Millman, J. (1974). Criterion-referenced measurement. In W. F. Popham (Ed.), *Evaluation in education: Current applications* (pp. 311–397). Berkeley, CA: McCutchan.

Nunnally, J. C. (1967). *Psychometric theory.* New York: McGraw-Hill.

Nunnally, J. C., & Bernstein, I. H. (1994). *Psychometric theory* (3rd ed.). New York: McGraw-Hill.

Osterlind, S. J. (1983). *Test item bias.* Thousand Oaks, CA: Sage.

Popham, W. J. (1978) *Criterion-referenced measurement.* Englewood Cliffs, NJ: Prentice-Hall.

Raykov, T., & Marcoulides, G. A. (2000). *A first course in structural equation modeling.* Mahwah, NJ: Lawrence Erlbaum Associates.

Rew, L., Stuppy, D, & Becker, H. (1988). Construct validity in instrument development: A vital link between nursing practice, research, and theory. *Advances in Nursing Science, 10*(8), 10–22.

Rovinelli, R. J., & Hambleton, R. K. (1977). On the use of content specialists in the assessment of criterion-referenced test item validity. *Dutch Journal of Educational Research, 2,* 49–60. Also in Laboratory of Psychometrics and Evaluative Research, Report No 24, 1976. Amherst, MA: The University of Massachusetts.

Schmidt, F. L., & Hunter, J. E. (1977). Development of a general solution to the problem of validity generalization. *Journal of Applied Psychology, 62,* 529–540.

Silverlake, A. C. (1999). *Comprehending test manuals: A guide and workbook.* Los Angeles: Pyrczak Publishing.

Soeken, K. L., & Prescott, P. A. (1991). Patient intensity for nursing index: The measurement model. *Research in Nursing and Health, 14*(4), 297–304.

Sousa, K. H., & Chen, F. F. (2002). A theoretical approach to measuring quality of life. *Journal of Nursing Measurement, 10*(1), 47–58.

Waltz, C. F., & Bausell, R. B. (1981). *Nursing research: Design, statistics and computer analysis.* Philadelphia: F.A. Davis.

7

Standardized Approaches to Measurement

With Theresa L. Dremsa

Standardization, a key process related to measurement, encompasses both uniformity of procedures with administering and scoring tests as well as establishing norms (Anastasi & Urbina, 1997). The standardization process is carried out in a consistent and controlled manner with an extensive variety of situations and subjects (Nunnally & Bernstein, 1994). Standardized approaches to measurement are methodologies that are highly appropriate for answering certain nursing questions and for studying particular relevant phenomena regarding patients, health, and nursing care. They are also relevant in nursing practice, for example, in developing and using consistent approaches with nursing diagnoses and interventions (Avant, 1990; Gordon, 2000; Keenan, Killeen, & Clingerman, 2002; NANDA, 1997; 2001), in evaluating clinical practice (National Quality Forum (NQF), (2003) and educational programs (Baker, 1998, Daniel, 1999; Embretson, 1991; 2001a). Standardized approaches to measurement can also be used in combination with qualitative methods in studies that employ methodological triangulation, described in chapter 9. Standardized measurement techniques have a long history of use in clinical and research laboratory settings to minimize error and assure consistent interpretation of results (Bowling, 2001; Portney & Watkins, 2000). Nursing (Strickland & Dilorio, 2003; Waltz & Jenkins, 2001) and the behavioral sciences (Kerlinger & Lee, 2000) use standardized measures to eliminate bias and reduce error in the research process. In this chapter standardization is defined, and the use and development of standardized measures are detailed.

DEFINITION

Broadly defined, a standardized measure, first proposed by Kelley (1914), is one that is constructed, administered, scored, and interpreted in a prescribed, precise, and consistent manner in order to reduce external influences that compromise reliability (Nunnally & Bernstein, 1994). The defining characteristics of a standardized measure refer to the properties of the measure itself and the way it was developed, rather than to the nature of the entity being measured (Nunnally & Bernstein, 1994). In order to be considered standardized, a measure must be carefully developed, rigorously tested before general use, consistently administered and scored, and interpreted on the basis of established norms. Standardized measures are considered norm-referenced measures, since an individual's score is interpreted by comparing it with scores obtained by other subjects in a well-defined comparison group (Anastasi & Urbina, 1997). Norm-referenced measures are distinguished by the explicit and conscious exercise of control in all aspects of their development, use, and interpretation (Kline, 2000; Nunnally & Bernstein, 1994).

As used in this text, the term "standardized" is applied to measures that have four essential characteristics:

1. A fixed set of items or operations designed to measure a clearly defined concept, attribute, or behavior based on a theoretical framework
2. Explicit rules and procedures for administration and scoring

3. Provision of norms to assist in interpreting scores
4. An ongoing development process that involves careful testing, analysis, and revision in order to assure high technical quality

In light of these criteria a variety of instruments and procedures may be considered standardized measures. Examples include published paper-and-pencil tests designed to measure scholastic aptitude (Scholastic Aptitude Test, 2003); tests designed to measure complex abilities (Embretson & Gorin, 2001) such as verbal and quantitative skill (GRE, 2003) problem-solving (Bowers, Huisingh, Barrett, Orman, & LoGuidice, 1994), abstract reasoning (Embretson, 2001; GRE, 2003), spatial perception (Fasteneau, Denburg, & Hufford, 1999) or manual dexterity; tests to measure personality characteristics (Tellegen, 2003), emotional adjustment (Derogatis, & Rutigliano, 1998; Kamphaus, DiStefano, & Lease, 2003), attitudes (Austin, 2003) and interests (Jastak & Jastak, 2003); tests to assess the developmental level of infants and children (CEED, 2000); observational scales used in client assessment (Bowling, 2001; Stromberg & Olsen, 1997); tests designed to measure anatomical and physiological characteristics (Mancini & Body, 1999; Meek & Lareau, 2003) and measures used in educational program evaluation(AERA, APA, & NCME, 1999) and clinical quality control (National Quality Forum, 2003). Hence, a standardized approach is ideal for measuring a wide range of attributes and behaviors of interest in nursing.

STANDARDIZED VERSUS NONSTANDARDIZED MEASURES

Clearly not all measures used in nursing research are standardized, but may have incorporated one or more of the four essential characteristics required of standardized measures. Such measures will be referred to as *nonstandardized measures*. In this sense, standardization may be considered a matter of degree and one can compare nonstandardized measures with respect to their approximation of the model for standardized measures described below and detailed in Table 7.1.

Comparative Advantages

The comparative differences, advantages and disadvantages of standardized and nonstandardized measures are summarized in Table 7.1. Review of this table suggests that standardized measures are desirable for some purposes but not for others; hence, a standardized measure is not always better by definition than a nonstandardized measure. For example, if a nurse researcher wished to assess the developmental level of an abused child in relation to national norms, a standardized measure of child development would be appropriate. On the other hand, if the purpose were to assess coping strategies of abused children, a standardized measure would be of little value because national norms do not exist.

Because standardized and nonstandardized measures can provide different types of information for use in decision making, evaluating, or understanding a particular phenomenon, the two types of measures are often used simultaneously. For example, schools of nursing often use both nonstandardized teacher-made tests and standardized tests developed by organizations (e.g., National League of Nursing) or proprietary companies (e.g., HESI, ATI) to measure student achievement in a given subfield of nursing. For instance, as a basis for admission decisions, schools may require both standardized aptitude tests (such as Scholastic Aptitude Test [SAT]) and locally developed, nonstandardized aptitude tests related to specific abilities deemed relevant to its particular curriculum. A clinician or researcher wanting to measure preoperative anxiety might combine a standardized laboratory procedure (e.g., measurement of catecholamines in the urine), a standardized measure of anxiety (e.g. the State-Trait Anxiety Inventory (Spielberger, Gorsuch, & Lushene, 1970; Spielberger, 2003), and a nonstandardized measure specific to a particular type of surgical procedure, or verbal self-rating of anxiety on a scale of 1 to 10. Decisions about the use of standardized or nonstandardized measures must be based on the

TABLE 7.1   Comparative Advantages and Disadvantages of Standardized and Nonstandardized Measures

Standardized Measures	Nonstandardized Measures
Construction	
Advantages: Involves input of experts; method of construction is designed to enhance technical quality, reliability, and validity; procedure used in construction and testing is usually described.	Advantages: May be carried out in situations in which time and resources are limited; short span of time is required between planning and use of the measure
Disadvantages: Costly, time-consuming; requires adequate resources	Disadvantages: Construction procedure is variable and does not necessarily assure high quality; procedure generally is not described in detail; amount of expert input is variable and may be unknown
Content	
Advantages: Measures attributes or behaviors that are common to a variety of settings and situations; is applicable to many settings; reflects widespread consensus rather than localized emphasis; is applicable across time and locale; is well-defined and fixed, allowing consistent comparison; parameters are usually specified.	Advantages: Well-adapted to specialized needs and emphasis; flexibility allows adaptation to changes in materials or procedures; allows inclusion of controversial or timely information.
Disadvantages: Inflexible; cannot be adapted to local or specialized situations; may reflect consensus views that are incongruent with specialized needs and purposes; precludes innovative, controversial, or time-bound material	Disadvantages: May reflect unique views or biases that are not deemed relevant by recognized authorities. Time- and situation-specificity precludes widespread use.
Psychometrics	
Advantages: Reliability (internal consistency and test-retest) is high, yielding stable results; procedures to establish reliability and validity are reported, so are known to the user; items and operations have high discriminating power.	Advantages: Technical properties to be optimized are determined based on purposes of the measure (e.g. qualitative studies).
Disadvantages: Stability of scores results in insensitivity to minor fluctuations that may be desirable to measure.	Disadvantages: Technical properties frequently are unknown and may be highly variable, dependent on the construction procedures used.
Administration and Scoring	
Advantages: Established procedures provide consistency, giving comparable results; effects of different testing conditions and environments are minimized; centralized or automated scoring is cost-efficient for large-scale efforts.	Advantages: Procedures can be developed based on specific needs and resources; flexible procedures permit last-minute alterations; local and/or hand scoring is cost efficient for small samples; time lag between administration and scoring is determined by the user
Disadvantages: Inflexibility precludes altering to fit individual circumstances and resources; may be costly and time consuming; scheduling of administration and return of scored results may be controlled externally.	Disadvantages: Consistency between different administrations of the same measure is variable; different rules may be applied in scoring, thus yielding incomparable results.

TABLE 7.1   *(Continued)*

Standardized Measures	Nonstandardized Measures
Interpretation of Scores	
Advantages: Scores can be uniformly compared with norm groups, often at the national level; interpretation is likely to be consistent across applications; explicit instructions may be provided to facilitate interpretation.	Advantages: Comparisons and interpretations can be geared to specific needs and unique circumstances; amenable to situations for which comparison to a defined group is not an appropriate way to assign meaning to a score.
Disadvantages: National norms may be inappropriate for unique purposes; utility for decision-making in specific settings is variable; inappropriate for purposes that do not require comparison with the status quo.	Disadvantages: No established basis for interpretation exists; consistency and accuracy of interpretation is variable, depending on the procedure used and the statistical skill of the interpreter.

purposes for which the information will be used and the types of questions that must be answered.

Construction

Standardized measures are constructed by following a number of sequential steps. Although there is some variation, the following procedure is generally used (Mishel, 1989; Nunnally & Bernstein, 1994):

1. Objectives, specifications, and a blueprint are developed.
2. Items are written and operations identified.
3. The items are pretested and analyzed using item statistics.
4. Acceptable items are assembled into a preliminary form (or preliminary equivalent forms) of the measure.
5. The preliminary form of the measure is experimentally administered to criterion groups of examinees to determine or verify the adequacy of item limits and instructions, difficulty level, discriminating power, reliability, and validity.
6. Revisions are made to eliminate items or operations that are unnecessary, problematic, or do not contribute to the measure's reliability and validity.
7. A final form of the measure is assembled.
8. Uniform mechanisms for administration and explicit instructions for scoring are established.

9. The final form of the measure is administered to carefully selected referent groups in order to develop norms.
10. The final version of the measure, a manual, and supplementary materials are made available for use.

This process is time-consuming and complex, often taking several years. Nonstandardized measures tend to undergo less extensive pretesting and revision, and generally do not have as carefully prescribed instructions for administration and scoring. The most crucial difference between standardized and nonstandardized measures is that the former have established norms that are used to interpret scores. Because of the effort and time involved, standardized measures are usually developed for widespread use. Ideally their development incorporates the collaboration of content and measurement experts throughout. The considerable effort expended is directed toward producing a measurement instrument or device that is of high technical quality and that can be used and interpreted consistently in a variety of settings.

Incidentally, measures that are developed initially as nonstandardized may evolve into standardized measures as they are administered to a variety of subjects over time and information is accrued to establish norms (Portney & Watkins, 2000). Examples of instruments that are well on the way to meeting the criteria for standardization are the Brief Symptom Inventory (BSI) 18 (Derogatis, 1993; 2000) and the

SF-36 (Ware, Kosinski, & Keller, 1994; Ware, 2000; Ware, Kosinski, & Dewey, 2001). These self-report tools are available online at http://www.pearsonassessments.com/tests/; http://www.sf-36.com and are administered to numerous individuals by many investigators in the United States and abroad. The data are being supplied to tool developers, who are continually reevaluating the psychometric properties of the tool and setting up norms. Differences between the two types of measures should become clearer in the following discussion of the development, administration, scoring, and interpretation of standardized measures.

DEVELOPING, ADMINISTERING, AND SCORING STANDARDIZED MEASURES CONTENT

Because they are designed for widespread and consistent use, standardized tests are characterized by content that is (1) sufficiently generic for applicability in a variety of settings, (2) not time-bound or rapidly outmoded, and (3) fixed or predefined (Portney & Watkins, 2000). In contrast, the content of nonstandardized measures is typically specific (geared to use in a given setting) and has the potential to be flexible. Content may be updated frequently and adapted to accommodate minor changes.

Selection of content for any standardized measure is based on a statement of purpose and blueprint that specifies the elements or dimensions of the domain of behavior or cognition that is to be sampled and the relative emphasis that is to be given to each element (Cook & Campbell, 1979; Nunnally & Bernstein, 1994). The purpose of a standardized measure is generally stated in terms that are not situation specific, since they must be acceptable to a variety of potential users. Similarly, the blueprint reflects a definition of the domain that is measured and that is potentially acceptable across settings and defensible on the basis of published research or expert opinion. Such a blueprint would eliminate content that is relevant only in a particular setting or situation or that is specific to a particular theory.

Consider, for example, the difference between the content of a nonstandardized classroom test that is administered in one school of nursing to measure achievement in a critical care nursing course and that of a standardized achievement test designed for administration across the nation to all students studying critical care nursing. The former would reflect a theoretical perspective and content that is defined as important by an individual faculty member or small group or that is included in a required text. It could include reference to a given theory or to specific information taught only in that setting. The standardized test, however, would need to reflect content that is taught in schools nationally in order to be useful. The blueprint for the standardized test would not be based on one person's definition, but on a systematic analysis of a variety of critical care texts and course syllabi, the input of experienced clinicians and educators, and relevant literature in the field. One example of generic content not bound to a particular theoretical perspective and identified for inclusion in a standardized measure is the California Q-Sort (Nunnally & Bernstein, 1994). Careful screening of content using the approaches listed above prevents including conflicting or controversial ideas and new information that has not yet gained widespread acceptance. Neither would be appropriate for a standardized measure.

Since standardized measures are very time-consuming to develop, they are generally used for several years without modification. Hence, content that may become rapidly outdated is generally precluded. Cognitive or affective items that assume or test knowledge of current events or very recent advances in the field are more appropriately included in nonstandardized than in standardized measures.

By definition, the content of a standardized measure is preestablished. "The development of any instrument must be guided by a theory, even if that theory is relatively informal [theory consists of a measurement and a structural component that, respectively deal with the definitions of constructs and their interrelations]" (Nunnally & Bernstein, 1994, p. 107). Items or operations are carefully selected and tested. They cannot be changed or deleted by the user of the measure without modifying its known properties (reliability and validity). To make changes would be to negate the essence of standardization. Nonstandardized measures are not content constrained. Thus, an important difference between the two types of measures is that the content of a standardized test is fixed well in advance of its general use, whereas the content of nonstandardized measures is generally defined by the developer. Consequently, when a nonstandardized measure that has been tested and used previously is modified for subsequent use, it is in effect transformed into a different measure, and *former estimates of reliability and validity no longer apply* (Nunnally & Bernstein, 1994).

Administration

In order to assure consistency, standardized measures are characterized by prescribed administration and scoring procedures. The method for administering the measure is determined in advance by the developer and is then pretested (Nunnally & Bernstein, 1994). In addition, standardized measures are administered to a representative referent group. In actuality, for most standardized measures a series of administrations is required in order to encompass the entire referent sample for establishing norms, which may be geographically dispersed. In each instance the measure is administered according to the same specifications and under conditions identical to those that will be used in subsequent administrations (Portney & Watkins, 2000). For example, if the measure is designed for administration to patients in a home environment and within a specific time limit, these conditions must prevail during each administration in order to assure comparability of results. At the time of the administration, supplementary data about characteristics of the referent sample members are also collected. These data are later used to prepare differentiated norms specific to particular subunits of the referent group. Rigid control over the conditions of administration to assure uniformity is critical to the concept of standardization (Anastasi &Urbina, 1997; Nunnally & Bernstein, 1994). Once it is final, explicit instructions are

provided for users in a test manual. Specific administration procedures include such elements as time limits, directions that are to be given the individual being tested, and for laboratory devices, especially the way in which the instrument is to be used. Detailed instructions for administration and instructions for the subjects must be in final form before the administration of the measure and must be followed precisely.

The requirement for standard administration procedures and conditions places responsibility on the measure's developer to provide explicit instructions that leaves little latitude for error. As noted above, in the case of complex administration procedures, special training and certification may be required to assure consistency. This requirement also places considerable responsibility on the user to become thoroughly familiar with the procedures in advance and to anticipate and try to eliminate potential threats to consistency. Assembling all necessary materials in advance and selecting a quiet location for administering the measure are examples of steps that might be taken to prevent delays and distractions during administration.

Any unanticipated alteration of the prescribed protocol should be noted carefully so that it can be taken into account in interpreting results. Such alterations might include (1) distractions that would affect an entire group of subjects (e.g., fire alarm), (2) systematic errors in executing the procedure itself (e.g., inaccurate time keeping), and (3) influences unique to an individual score (e.g., a subject is called away from the administration momentarily or receives additional instructions). In addition, it may be important to note special circumstances external to the test administration that might alter the performance of an individual or group. For example, if a nurse researcher were measuring staff nurses' job satisfaction, an event such as the recent dismissal of the director of nursing would be likely to influence results and should be noted. Although not all distractions or idiosyncratic circumstances can be eliminated, the user of the standardized measure must (1) try to prevent altering the established procedures to the greatest extent possible, (2) record any unanticipated alterations that do occur, and (3) evaluate the potential impact of any alterations in order to determine whether the results are usable. Many manuals for standardized measures now include instructions about how to handle unexpected problems that may occur during administration.

For some laboratory tests a standard administration may be assured by means of automation (Quest Diagnostics, 2003). Examples of some standardized infant and child development measures that require trained administrators are the Brazelton Neonatal Assessment Scale, (Brazelton, 1973; Brazelton & Sparrow, 2002) Griffiths Scales of Infant Development (Griffiths, 1954; 2003) available online at http://www.aricd.org.uk, and the Nursing Child Assessment Tools (Barnard & Earles, 1979; Shonkoff & Meisels, 2000). Some standardized instruments are now administered electronically, where either the subject or the test administrator responds to the items by keyboard, mouse clicks, or touch-screen methods.

Scoring

As with administration, the procedure for scoring standardized measures is predetermined by the developer. A fixed set of rules is applied so that the same numerical value (score) will be assigned consistently to a given performance on the measure; that is, any number of raters scoring an individual's performance on the measure should arrive at the same result. The primary considerations in scoring are consistency in following the scoring rules and accuracy in computation. Machine scoring by optical scanners and computers is, in general, more accurate and cost efficient than hand scoring. Whether hand- or machine-scoring methods are used, random periodic checks of accuracy are advisable. For machine scoring, this generally entails rescoring a random sample of completed measures by hand or machine and comparing the results with the original computation. For hand scoring, a random sample of measures is selected and rescored by a different individual. The two sets are then compared by computing interrater reliability as described in chapter 5.

Rules for scoring a standardized measure are explicit. For paper-and-pencil tests, scoring keys may be provided if the instrument is to be hand scored. Instruments may be printed on special forms that can be electronically scanned and scored. The data are downloaded into a computer. This method eliminates hand-scoring and transcription errors. In some instances completed instruments, such as health-risk appraisals or aptitude and achievement tests, are mailed to a central scoring facility for computer-assisted scoring (Academy Technologies, 2003; Pearson, 2003; Scantron, 2003). Standardized measures that involve observation include detailed rules for scoring to assure that any given behavior will be assigned the same numerical value by different raters and that identical behaviors will receive the same score (Portney & Watkins, 2000). Machine scoring by optical scanners and computers is, in general, more accurate and cost efficient than hand scoring. Whether hand- or machine-scoring methods are used, random periodic checks of accuracy are advisable. For machine-scoring, this generally entails rescoring a random sample of measure by hand or machine and comparing the results with the original computation. For hand-scoring, a random sample of measures is selected and rescored by a different individual. Computing interrater reliability then compares the two sets.

Technological advances permit highly automated scoring procedures for many physiological laboratory measures; in effect, scoring rules are incorporated in the computer design and are applied automatically in processing the entity to be measured. Computer technology has also simplified scoring procedures in which multiple elements are weighted differently, so it is possible to combine self-report and normed physiological data to determine a single score. The U.S. Army Wellness Check, currently being used routinely to assess the health risk of soldiers stationed throughout the world, is an example of a computer-scored measure that combines self-report data regarding the individual's medical history, family history, and life style with physical measurements (blood pressure, blood glucose levels, ECG, etc.). The computer program for scoring the measure converts raw scores to age- and gender-specific percentile scores, computes a weighted total score, and produces a printout interpreting the results to the individual (Troumbley, 1989; U.S. Army, 2003).

Nonstandardized measures may include uniform procedures for administration and scoring; however, they are usually more flexible and less explicit than procedures for standardized measures. The developer/user generally is free to define the procedures; yet, the same cautions noted above apply in terms of redefining a procedure that was previously established for use as an informal measure. If the administration and scoring procedures differ from one application to another, or from the procedure originally designed by the developer, the results are not truly comparable (Nunnally & Bernstein, 1994).

NORMS

As used in reference to standardized measures, *norms* refer to statistical information that describes the scores earned by members of a defined population or reference group (or generated from a defined set of observations) with which the score earned by a particular individual (or generated from a given observation) can be compared (Nunnally & Bernstein, 1994). Frequently the norm (comparison) group is composed of individuals from widely distributed geographic areas, so that an individual's score is interpreted by comparing it with a national or international distribution. Discussion of norms and standards frequently causes confusion about the correct terminology. A *standard* is an ideal—an object or state defined by an authority or consensus as the basis for comparison. It represents what ought to be, whereas a norm represents what is. For many aspects of physical and chemical measurement (e.g. weight, length, temperature), standards have been established and serve as the basis for scoring a given result. For example, in the measurement of weight, the National Bureau of Standards provides a standard online at http://www.nist.gov/ that serves as the basis for constructing measurement devices (e.g. scales, balances), determining their accuracy, and scoring results.

Norms or distributions of scores describing the body weights of representative samples of objects (including people) also have been generated to depict what is. In addition, values have been generated from actuarial studies to represent ideal weights (standards) for men and women of specific heights (Grinker, 1992; Grogan, 1999). Although they have been criticized as being arbitrary and insufficiently age-specific, such standards are used to answer the question "How does this score compare with the ideal score?" Norms are used to answer the question "How does this score compare with those generated from a representative sample of units measured in the same way with the same instrument?"

Types of Norms

Norms can be classified on the basis of the scope of the population from which they were generated or the units in which they are expressed. National norms are those describing scores earned by a national sample of subjects. They have been established for many of the standardized tests used in nursing and are useful for comparison with individuals from a wide variety of locales and backgrounds (National League of Nursing, 2003). Increasingly, the scope of samples used to establish norms for standardized measures used in nursing education and research is international. Both international and national samples are characterized by their heterogeneity; that is, they contain individuals who vary in sociodemographic characteristics such as age, gender, race, urban-rural residence, social status, and educational background. As a result, national or international norms may be too general to permit specific interpretation and action (Fair Test, 2003). In order to supply information that will be useful, national norms may be provided in terms that display the distribution of the sample as a whole (total group norms) as well as the distributions of subgroups selected according to relevant characteristics (differentiated norms) (International Survey Research [ISR], 2003). Examples of differentiated norms are gender-specific norms, age-specific norms, and occupation-specific norms. National norms may be based on a representative sample of the nation's population or on a nationwide sample of select, but relevant groups of individuals. Norms for the

NLN achievement tests are not based on a sample of the U.S. population but on a sample of students from nursing education programs across the country (National League of Nursing, 2003).

Regional and local norms are those established with more geographically circumscribed samples. Although the developer of a nationally standardized measure may supply norms specific to given multistate regions of the country, local norms generally are established by users themselves: teachers, counselors, administrators, and practitioners. Local norms are established on the basis of samples of subjects in a given school, agency, or district. Because these samples are generally more homogeneous than regional or national samples, local norms are valuable as a basis for decision-making in specific settings. For example, schools of nursing may find local norms for standardized aptitude tests derived from a sample of current students more useful than national norms in admission decisions, because the former constitute a more relevant basis for comparison (American College Test, 1999).

Statistical units for presenting norms may also be used to classify them. Examples are percentile norms and standard-score norms such as T-scores (Nunnally & Bernstein, 1994). The strengths and weaknesses associated with expressing norms in terms of these units were addressed in chapter 4.

Establishing Norms

The process used to establish norms involves several steps carried out after the final version of the instrument has been produced (Nunnally & Bernstein, 1994; Burns & Grove, 1997):

1. A sample group (or groups) of individuals who are representative of those for whom the measure is designed is (are) selected.
2. The final form of the measure is administered to these individuals according to the set procedure or protocol that has been developed and under conditions that are identical to those recommended for administration.

3. Raw scores of the sample individuals are plotted in a frequency distribution and descriptive statistics are computed.
4. A decision is made regarding the statistical units that will be used to express the norms and these statistics are computed (e.g. T-scores, Z-scores).
5. Tables or graphs displaying the norms are prepared.
6. Norms are updated as necessary by reapplying steps 1 through 5.

Since the norming procedures used are critical determinants of the accuracy and usefulness of the norms generated, each of these steps will be addressed in detail.

Selecting the Standardized Sample

The scores of individuals selected for the standardization group or referent group serve as the basis for comparing all subsequent scores on the measures; thus, it is mandatory that these individuals accurately represent the larger population of individuals for whom the measure was designed (Nunnally & Bernstein, 1994). Using the purposes of the measure and the blueprint, the population of intended subjects must be clearly specified (Cook & Campbell, 1979). Because most measures are designed for a specific purpose and are not universally applicable across all ages, cultures, educational levels, and situations, the relevant population is limited to some extent by the test purposes and blueprint (Portney & Watkins, 2000). Many cognitive measures, for example, are designed to be age-specific, that is, they are applicable only to persons from the general population who fall within specific age ranges. Other measures are designed only for persons in specific settings or circumstances or who have had certain experiences. For example, some measures of functional health are disease-specific, designed only for patients with a specific diagnosis, such as rheumatoid arthritis, while others are more generically applicable.

The relevant population is also determined by the scope of the norms to be developed (Nunnally & Bernstein, 1994). Examples of populations appropriate for establishing national norms would be all students enrolled in baccalaureate nursing programs, all adult patients hospitalized in public psychiatric institutions, or all 3-week-old infants with no known birth defects. Populations for local norms might include, for example, all students enrolled in a given school of nursing, all adult patients who have been hospitalized in a given institution, or all persons living in a defined geographic area. The important point is that the relevant population must be specified to include all individuals to whom the measure can appropriately be applied.

In specifying the population for establishing norms for any standardized measure it is important to consider that a variety of personal characteristics of potential subjects may be correlated with scores on that measure. "The term *attribute* in the definition (of an instrument) indicates that measurement always concerns some particular feature of objects . . . one cannot measure objects . . . one measures their attributes" (Nunnally & Bernstein, 1994, p. 4). For example, scores on an aptitude test to measure problem-solving potential may be related to the subjects' educational level, background, age, race, gender, region, or type of residential community. Scores on a measure of job satisfaction may be related to age, stage in career, gender, salary level, type of occupation, and so forth. The specific characteristics that are likely to be correlated with the concept, attribute, or behavior being measured should be identified on the basis of related literature (Nunnally & Bernstein, 1994).

As noted above, some of the correlated characteristics are taken into account in the test purposes and blueprint, and their impact on possible scores controlled or held constant by limiting the relevant population to particular categories of individuals (Nunnally & Bernstein, 1994). Other characteristics that are assumed to be correlated with scores on the measure, but are not held constant by virtue of the population definition could potentially influence scores obtained from the population. Therefore, they must be specified in advance. It is important for the relevant population to include individuals who differ with respect to their status on these correlated characteristics. Let us assume, for example, that it is known that an adult's educational level influences response to paper-and-pencil measures of anxiety. It is necessary to specify that the relevant population for such a measure include adults with a variety of educational levels if, in fact, the measure is to be used across all segments of society. Including those with a range of educational backgrounds would potentially allow a wider range of possible scores. The nature of the population that will ultimately be measured must be specified as clearly as possible and every attempt made to assure diversity of characteristics that may have an impact on scores obtained. Such diversity can be achieved by means of selecting large and heterogeneous subsamples. "Ideally, normative cohorts would be sufficiently large that we would routinely be able to develop distinct norms for different demographic subgroups (e.g. whites, individuals over 40)" (Derogatis, 1987, p. 49).

Selecting the Norming Sample(s)

Once the relevant population for the measure is identified, it is necessary to select a sample that is representative of the population to make up the referent group, that is, the group chosen as the basis for establishing norms (Nunnally & Bernstein, 1994). The selection of a referent group that is truly representative of the individuals for whom the measure is intended is the most important and most difficult task in the standardization process. The norms for the measure are established on the basis of scores from the members of this sample (referent group) and serve as the basis for comparing scores from subsequent administration of the measure. Thus, if a referent sample is atypical of the population that will ultimately be measured, there will not be an accurate basis for interpreting scores. If there is bias in the norms (i.e., if they do not represent the true distribution of the scores in the population), this bias will be transmitted in all subsequent interpretations of a given score.

Certain sampling procedures are more likely than others to yield a referent group that is representative of the test population. Probability sampling refers to a class of sampling procedures in which the process of selecting an individual for the sample is prescribed, such that each individual in the population has a known probability of being selected into the sample (Kerlinger & Lee, 2000). Probability samples are selected at random; that is, the basis for the selection of a given individual is by chance rather than a conscious choice. It is possible to assume that by drawing a random sample any differences between the sample and the population will be randomly (and/or normally) distributed. The primary advantages of using probability sampling for selecting a referent group to establish norms are that bias is minimized and sampling error can be estimated. Several types of probability samples that can be used for selecting referent groups are described in Table 7.2 (Levy & Lemeshow, 1980; 1999).

Those probability sampling procedures that require enumerating each individual in the population (simple random sampling, systematic sampling, or stratified random sampling) are usually impractical for selecting referent groups for most standardized tests because of the large numbers of individuals included (Kerlinger & Lee, 2000). In addition, comprehensive lists of all potential subjects are rarely available. Cluster samples, which involve identifying groups or clusters of individuals as the primary sampling units, are more efficient when the population is large. Such groups or clusters might include political or legal jurisdictions such as cities or census tracts, or organizations such as schools or hospitals, or the classrooms and patient units that comprise them.

Once the clusters in the population are listed, a random sample of clusters is drawn and the individuals within the randomly selected clusters make up the referent group. In establishing national and regional norms that involve a very large population, multistage cluster sampling is usually employed (Levy & Lemeshow, 1999). This is a procedure that involves dividing the initially selected clusters into subunits or secondary sampling units, which are, in turn, randomly selected. The procedure can be continued through several stages involving successively smaller clusters until individuals can be enumerated and randomly sampled. When some characteristics of the population related to the measure are known, it is possible to stratify within each cluster for any stage of the sampling process. This procedure, called multistage stratified cluster sampling, involves dividing the sampling units into homogenous strata or subunits on the basis of one or more characteristics related to the measure (i.e., the score), then sampling at random within strata.

An example of a multistage cluster sampling procedure is included in Figure 7.1. Cluster samples are more convenient and efficient than those that require enumerating the entire population; however, considerably larger sample sizes are required to achieve the same reliability of norms as would be achieved by simple random sampling (Levy & Lemeshow, 1999).

In the example shown in Figure 7.1, let us assume that the size of the hospital in which a nurse works is a variable believed to be related to job satisfaction. In order to introduce more precision into the sampling procedures and to assure that the referent group includes nurses from large and small hospitals, stratification can be employed at stage 2. Once all hospitals are listed, two strata can be formed, provided bed capacity is known. Stratum 1 would consist of all hospitals within the selected state that that have 300 or more beds, and stratum 2 would consist of all hospitals with fewer than 300 beds. Hospitals would be randomly selected from within each stratum. The primary advantage of stratified sampling is that it increases the precision of the norms generated. However, this holds only if the variables selected as the basis for stratification are related to the measure for which norms are being developed. Stratification is frequently impossible because the characteristics of the population are not sufficiently well known to permit subdivision into homogenous groupings.

If the desire is to represent as closely as possible in the sample the proportions of large and small hospitals in the state, it is desirable to use a procedure that involves sampling from each stratum at a rate proportionate to its distribution in the population. Using proportional allocation procedures (PAP) (Kerlinger & Lee, 2000), in the above example we would select into the sample the number of hospitals in each stratum

TABLE 7.2   Probability Samples Used To Select Referent Groups

Type of Sample	Procedure	Comments
1. Simple Random	1. List and number individuals in the population. 2. Randomly select the sample using a random number table or other device.	1. Complete listing is often difficult to construct. 2. The procedure is costly and time consuming.
2. Stratified Random	1. Subdivide the population into two or more groups (strata) that are homogenous with respect to a given characteristic. 2. From each group (stratum) randomly select a sample. 3. Numbers of subjects may be selected in proportion to the size of each stratum in the population (proportionate stratified random sample), or sampling fractions may differ from stratum to stratum (disproportionate stratified random sample).	1. Some characteristics of the population must be known in advance. 2. Can be used to assure representativeness on the selected characteristic(s) used for stratification. 3. Can be used to assure inclusion of sufficient numbers of subjects within selected subgroups. 4. The procedure is costly and time consuming.
3. Systematic	1. List all individuals in the population. 2. Determine the width of the selection interval (K) to be used by dividing the total number of sample cases desired. 3. Select a starting point at random (termed the random start) within the first selection interval using a random number table. 4. After the random start, select every Kth case.	1. Can be applied to stratified or unstratified listings. 2. Generally is more efficient and convenient than simple random sampling. 3. Is subject to bias if there is periodic or rhythmic tendency inherent in the list (e.g., if every Kth element has more or less of a given characteristic than the others). 4. Is subject to bias if there is a linear trend in the list. 5. Effects of periodically and linearity can be minimized by shifting random starts part-way through the list.
4. Cluster	1. List the largest (most inclusive) unit in which population elements are found (termed the primary sampling units). 2. Randomly select a sample of these units. 3. Subdivide the sampled units into smaller units (secondary sampling units). 4. Randomly select a sample of these units. 5. Repeat the procedure in steps 3–4 as many times as necessary until the final stage is reached.	1. In all but the final stage, clusters or groups are sampled rather than individuals. 2. Stratification can be used for any part of the multistage process. 3. Is cost and time efficient, particularly for large, dispersed populations. 4. Sampling errors are greater with cluster samples than with other samples of the same size. 5. Special statistical procedures should be employed for data analysis i.e., hierarchical cluster (analysis [SPSS, 2000]).

Stage	Step	Unit

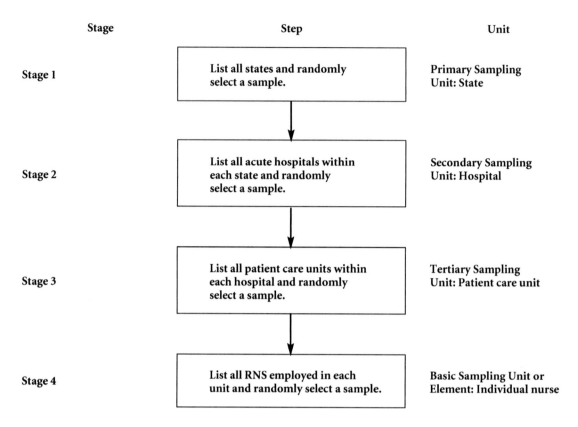

Stage 1 — List all states and randomly select a sample. — **Primary Sampling Unit: State**

Stage 2 — List all acute hospitals within each state and randomly select a sample. — **Secondary Sampling Unit: Hospital**

Stage 3 — List all patient care units within each hospital and randomly select a sample. — **Tertiary Sampling Unit: Patient care unit**

Stage 4 — List all RNS employed in each unit and randomly select a sample. — **Basic Sampling Unit or Element: Individual nurse**

FIGURE 7.1   Steps in selecting a cluster sample.

that corresponds to its percentage of the total number of hospitals in the state. Assuming that small hospitals make up 25% of the 160 hospitals in state A and 50 percent of the 200 hospitals in state B, and that a 10% sample of hospitals is to be drawn, then 4 small and 12 large hospitals would be chosen in state A and 10 small and 10 large hospitals would be selected in state B.

Disproportionate sampling, wherein strata are sampled at rates that are not proportionate to their distribution in the population (e.g., if equal numbers of large and small hospitals had been selected irrespective of their proportions in the population), may be employed to assure sufficient variety in the referent group or to assure inclusion of members of a stratum that may contain only a small number of individuals (or units) who may be theoretically very important (Bowling, 2002; Levy & Lemeshow, 1999). For detailed information about probability sampling procedures the reader is referred to

Cochran (1977), Levy and Lemeshow (1999), Kerlinger and Lee (2000) and Kish (1965, 1995).

Probability sampling is critical to increasing the likelihood that the referent group will be representative of the population for which the measure is intended. However, because it is time-consuming and involves the development of a detailed sampling frame, test developers may employ other sampling methods that are easier but that allow the introduction of bias and will not permit an accurate estimation of error. Examples include:

1. convenience samples, selected on the basis of availability
2. samples in which respondents can volunteer or select themselves
3. purposeful samples, selected because they are thought to be typical
4. samples that experts say represent an appropriate target population

5. samples that are drawn from listings that may incorporate an inherent bias (e.g., telephone directories, voluntary organization rosters, listings of individuals who have contacted a given health agency) (Lyberg, et al., 1997)

Such procedures, although they are in widespread use in nursing research, are likely to result in atypical or nonrepresentative referent groups. Also problematic because of a potential bias are probability samples derived from outdated or incomplete population lists and samples that include a high percentage of nonresponse or nonparticipation (Angoff, 1971).

Sample Size

In addition to the sampling method used to select the referent group, it is necessary to consider the size of the sample to be used (Levy & Lemeshow, 1999). As a general principle, all else being equal, the larger the sample, the more likely it is to be representative of the population. The size of the sample needed is based on a mathematical calculation of sampling error that would result from using a given sample size and a given sampling procedure. In addition, consideration must be given to the degree of precision required in the norms, in light of the purposes for which they will be used and the decisions that will be made. The greater the precision that is required (that is, the smaller the sample error that can be tolerated), the larger the sample size must be (Pedhazer & Schmelkin, 1991). Sample size is, in part, determined by practical considerations such as the time and cost involved.

Norming Administration and Scoring

The term *norming administration* refers to the administration of the measure to the representative referent group in order to generate a frequency distribution that will serve as the basis for comparing and interpreting scores on the measure. Usually a series of norming administrations is required in order to include the entire referent sample, which is generally quite

large and often geographically dispersed. Each norming administration is carried out according to the same procedure as the others, and the scores generated are added to the growing database that will be analyzed in order to generate norms for the measure.

Raw scores earned by the entire referent sample are represented in a frequency distribution, as described in chapter 3. If the measure has several component parts (subscales), a separate frequency distribution is developed for each (Nunnally & Bernstein, 1994). If it is possible that personal characteristics are related to the score on the measure, it is desirable to categorize the referent sample on the basis of one or more of these characteristics and develop separate frequency distributions for each sub-group. Subgroups based on age, occupation, educational level, field of study, and residences are frequently identified, because they are likely to represent distinct subpopulations that differ with respect to the scores earned. There is no set number of variables that should be used to identify subgroups. It is important that data be obtained for as many sub-populations as necessary for comparison purposes, and that the characteristics selected are those that influence the score.

For each frequency distribution, summary statistics are calculated as described in chapter 3. In addition to measures of central tendency (mean, mode, median), statistics that describe the spread of scores (range, variance, standard deviation) and the shape of the distribution (skewness and kurtosis) are computed (Stevens, 1996). The latter statistics allow evaluation of how closely the obtained distribution of scores approximates the theoretical normal curve. The measures of central tendency and dispersion calculated for the referent group (and subgroups) serve as the basis for assigning meaning to any given raw score.

Developers of standardized tests must make decisions about the most meaningful way to communicate to others the nature of the data derived from the standardization administration so that these data can be effectively based on the nature of the measure and its intended use, as well as on statistical considerations. The objective is to describe the data in a manner that is clear and definite and has direct meaning. As noted in chapter 4, raw scores lack meaning and must be converted into some type of derived score in order to be interpreted.

The types of derived scores most commonly used to convey information about referent groups of standardized measures relevant to nursing are percentile scores and standard scores (Nunnally & Bernstein, 1994). These scores describe the standing of a given score in relation to the distribution of scores obtained from the referent group. The computation of percentile and standard scores was described in chapter 4. Percentile scores, which indicate the percentage of scores that fall below the given score, have the advantage of being easily interpretable. However, one limitation is that percentile units are not equal at all points on the scale of raw scores, because a large number of individuals obtain scores near the middle of the distribution. Thus, a percentile difference of 8 points near the middle of the scale (e.g., 48th versus 56th percentile) represents a much smaller difference between raw scores than does a percentage difference of equal magnitude at either end of the distribution (e.g., 5th versus 13th percentile).

Standard scores express the raw score in terms of standard deviation units above or below the mean (Nunnally & Bernstein, 1994). Using standard deviation units has the advantage of providing equal units, such that a given difference between two standard scores represents the same difference between raw scores anywhere along the distribution. This assumption is generally appropriate for referent samples because numbers of subjects are sufficiently large. However, standard scores are not advantageous when a nonnormal distribution of scores in the referent groups reflects the actual peculiarities in the distribution of scores in the referent group measured.

Several types of standard scores can be used as the basis for describing norms. The Z score, described in chapter 4 (using Formula 4.1), ranges between –4.0 (a score 4 standard deviation units below the mean) and +4.0 (a score 4 standard deviation units above the mean). Because of the potential risk of error when minus signs are used, Z scores are frequently transformed to another standard score that uses only positive numbers. Examples of standard scores that use positive numbers are *t scores* and *stanines*. The *t score* is obtained by multiplying the Z score by 10, then adding the product to 50, which is the mean of the *t score* distribution (see Formula 4.2). Stanines present norms on a nine-point scale of equal units, each the width of one half of a standard deviation unit. Stanine scores have a mean of 5 and a standard deviation of 2.

Standard scores have the advantage that, regardless of the value of the mean and standard deviation of a distribution, the interpretation of a given score is consistent (Nunnally & Bernstein, 1994). This feature facilitates comparison across several measures. Standard scores can also be interpreted in terms of percentile rank, assuming a normal distribution. As described in Chapters 3 and 4, each standard deviation unit in a normal distribution contains a fixed percentage of cases. Thus, a raw score one standard deviation above the mean can be expressed as a Z score of +1.0, a *t-score* of 60, a stanine score of 7, or a percentile score of 84.

For some measures of early cognitive and physical development the performance of a referent group may be expressed in terms of age equivalents. These norms are based on the average scores obtained by individuals of different ages. For example, if children in the referent group who are 2 years and 3 months of age have an average score of 30 on the measure, the score 30 is assigned an age equivalent of 2–3. Age equivalents are expressed in terms of two sets of numbers, the first representing the year and the second the month of age. They represent average or typical performance for a given age group. Because patterns of growth vary at different ages, age equivalents do not have uniform meaning across all age groups and are easily misinterpreted. As a result they are being replaced by age-specific norms (i.e., norms differentiated on the basis of age), which are calculated using the frequency distributions for specific age groups and are presented as percentile or standard scores.

Once the decision is made about which types of derived scores will be used to represent the data from the referent group, calculations are usually carried out by computer. For every possible raw score, corresponding derived scores are calculated, thereby assuring that any score earned subsequently will be assigned the same meaning. The exact procedure that was used for transforming raw scores as well as all relevant summary statistics is made available to subsequent users of the measure.

Communicating the Norms

Tables and graphs are prepared to portray the referent group data in a manner that facilitates interpretation by others. The purpose of the tables and graphs that are generated is to communicate the exact nature of the referent group and to facilitate interpreting specific scores. Tables must be accurate and clear, encouraging reliability and validity in score interpretation. Specific instructions for use of the table or graph should be provided, and each table or graph should be labeled clearly enough to stand alone, that is, to be interpreted by the consumer without reference to a complex narrative. Current computer software for calculating statistics has built-in capability to generate graphic and tabular displays for most analyses (e.g., SPSS, 2000).

Updating Norms

Establishing norms for a standardized measure is an ongoing activity, even though it is a time-consuming and costly process. Norms become outmoded due to societal changes (Messick, 1995). Changes in nutrition, sanitation, lifestyle, and health care, for example have made decade-old physiological and weight norms obsolete. Increases in the average level of schooling and changes in educational curricula and media programming tend to affect the scores earned on tests of general mental ability, thus rendering norms established of such measures even 5 years ago inaccurate as a basis for current comparison. Such changes necessitate repeating at periodic intervals the procedure described previously for developing norms. The frequency with which the norming procedure must be repeated and new norms established depends on the likelihood that the attribute or behavior being measured has been influenced by recent changes. In addition to monitoring the occurrence of external or societal events or patterns that might be correlated to the measure, it is desirable to make systematic and ongoing comparisons between distributions of current scores and those of the referent group. Such comparisons are easily made when a measure is centrally scored and all data from subsequent administrations of the measure are available to the test developer and publisher. For example, the Educational Testing Service (ETS) continually updates the norms for its tests. Current research using the measure is another source of comparative information. Some instrument developers give permission for their instruments to be used in research only if the potential user will agree to share the raw data with the developer who continues to cumulate the database of information.

Adequacy of Norms

The process for establishing norms has been described in detail because it provides the basis for judging the adequacy of any set of norms generated. The adequacy of norms is, in turn, a prime consideration when selecting a standardized measure for use and when interpreting results. Criteria for determining the adequacy of norms include the following (Nunnally & Bernstein, 1994; Kline, 2000):

1. The norms were established on the basis of a representative sample from a clearly specified population.
2. The norms were established using a referent group with known (accurately described) characteristics.
3. The norms were established under conditions of uniform administration and scoring.
4. The date of the norming administration is known.
5. The statistical procedures used in deriving the norms were appropriate and accurately described.
6. The norms are clearly presented, with instructions for interpretation provided.
7. Differentiated norms are available to reflect relevant differences among subgroups with specific characteristics.
8. The norms are up-to-date.

Standardized measures vary in the degree to which information is provided to assess the adequacy of the established norms. Ideally information about the method of sampling, the size and characteristics of the norm sample, the conditions of administration, and the date of testing is included with the norm values and table in an accompanying manual, which must be carefully studied. If the publisher, manufacturer, or developer does not automatically supply such information, it is advisable to request it directly and to review published literature related to the measure.

INTERPRETATION OF SCORES

In order to discuss the interpretation of scores on standardized measures, it is necessary to differentiate the meaning of a given piece of information (in this case the score itself) and the use of that information. Ultimately, interpretation takes into account both the generic meaning of the score as it derives from the process of standardization itself and the purposes and context within which the information ultimately will be used. Given the way in which any standardized measure is developed, the meaning of a given score is determined with reference to established norms. The meaning derives from comparison of an individual score with the scores earned by others (the defined referent group) on the same measure. Importantly, the comparison is with performance that is typical of the referent group and should not be construed as comparison with an ideal or standard to be achieved. The generic meaning of any score on a standardized measure, therefore, is always normative, that is defined in terms of interindividual comparison with the typical performance of a referent group (Nunnally & Bernstein, 1994).

The scores on standardized measures are most frequently used to make interindividual or intergroup comparisons. Examples of interindividual comparisons would include ranking a group of applicants prior to selecting the one most qualified for a position or evaluating the anxiety level of a given patient as high or low in comparison with that of the typical adult. An intergroup comparison would be exemplified by the determination that the average satisfaction ratings of students and faculty in doctoral program A are higher than those in program B or are higher than the inter- and intradisciplinary average. In some instances, however, the score on a standardized measure may be used to make intraindividual (also termed ipsative) comparisons, such as comparing scores earned on a number of separate measures or on subscales measuring different dimensions of behavior or cognition (Kerlinger & Lee, 2000).

In some cases a standardized measure score may be used to compare an individual's performance with a standard that has been established on the basis of previously gathered data regarding the relationship between typical performance on the measure and other salient variables. For example, after gathering data about the relationship between the 2003 Scholastic Aptitude Test (SAT) scores of entering students and their grade-point averages throughout an undergraduate nursing curriculum, a school may determine that a particular percentile score on the SAT is necessary for successful completion of the program. Subsequently that score can be used as a standard for comparing the scores of applicants. Similar procedures are used in businesses to select candidates for leadership positions, using data from standardized personality measures. In the realm of clinical practice a given score on a standardized measure could be used to identify individuals who are at high risk relative to a particular condition. In each case, the standard that is used for evaluating performance on the measure is based on normative data and only after systematic study of the ability of the measure to predict outcomes on other variables.

The generic meaning assigned to a score on a standardized measure involves a complex set of considerations related to the procedures used to develop the measure and to establish the norms, the nature of comparison (referent) group, the type of norms established, and the meaning of the statistics used. A score compared with national norms that have been differentiated on the basis of age and converted to percentile ranks would have a different meaning from one that is compared with local norms expressed as age equivalents. Developers and publishers or manufacturers of standardized instruments generally supply aids to help assign meaning to raw scores. These include tables, guidelines, examples, and in some instances even computerized printed explanations that provide the appropriate meaning for a given score (e.g. the MMPI prints out reports). However, it is ultimately the responsibility of the user to make an informed judgment about the meaning of the score. The following guidelines should be kept in mind:

1. The conceptual meaning of whatever derived score is used should be clear to the user.
2. The score has meaning only in relation to the specific measure from which it was derived; thus, the meaning that can be inferred is limited by the purpose, scope, and content of the measure itself.
3. The score has meaning only in relation to the referent group used to establish norms; thus, the characteristics of the referent group must be studied carefully.
4. Measurement error must be taken into account; that is, the subject's true score is recognized to fall not exactly on the point of the obtained score but within a range of scores, the limits of which are one standard error of measurement above and below the obtained score.
5. To the extent that they are provided and address relevant characteristics of the subject(s), differentiated norms should be used as the basis for comparison because they allow for more precise meaning to be inferred.
6. Relevant characteristics of the subject(s), should be taken into account. These include not only demographic characteristics, which help to identify subgroups for whom a given measure or stet of norms may be inappropriate, but also abnormal circumstances which may have influenced performance on the measure.

It was noted above that standardized measures are sometimes used to make intraindividual or ipsative comparisons, that is, comparisons involving two or more scores earned by a single individual (Kerlinger & Lee, 2000). Such comparisons are often used to identify an individual's strengths and weaknesses. In order to assist with interpreting intraindividual comparisons, a profile chart is often developed. This is a graphic representation of the individual's scores on various measures (or subscales of a more inclusive measure), which are plotted on comparable scores scales. The median scores (scores that fall at the 50th percentile) of a group on several measures may also be plotted on a profile. Scores can be displayed either as bands that extend one standard error of measure above and below the obtained score or as specific points on the scale. The former style is preferable, because it allows the interpreter to take into account the inaccuracy of the scores on different measures.

In order to construct a profile based on comparable score scales, it is necessary that the norms be comparable across all measures; that is, they must be converted to the same system of numbers (derived scores) and must have the same shape distribution. Ideally, all measures included in the profile should be normed on the same referent sample and should be independent of one another as well as with those of the referent group (Nunnally & Bernstein, 1994).

An individuals' profile is sometimes compared with the profile of a particular group, with the group profile defined as the medial (50th percentile) score for the group on each measure. While this procedure allows evaluation of whether the individual's scores are different from the central tendency of the group (as defined by the median), it does not permit an accurate assessment of the difference, since the entire array of referent group scores is not represented. Profile charts may be used to depict the comparison of one individual's or group's scores with those of another, or to compare one individual's score at different times. Profile charts are useful because of their flexibility, and because they provide a visual display, which is helpful in interpretation. Caution should be employed to assure that they are used appropriately (Angoff, 1971, pp. 547–548).

The ultimate interpretation of any score on a standardized measure requires taking into account the purposes for which the information will be used. For example, given the generic meaning of a score (say, that a staff nurse scores in the 90th percentile, and hence ranks very high on a standardized measure of quantitative aptitude), that score would be interpreted differently depending upon whether one was selecting applicants for advanced training in budget preparation or conducting research to determine the degree of improvement in medication accuracy resulting from a special training program for nurses with low quantitative ability. The intended use, therefore, provides the context in which a given score is interpreted.

Since the information derived from a standardized measure is often used alone or in conjunction with other measures for decision making, the development of a model defining and setting priorities for the values to be maximized and the information requirements was advocated as a necessary initial step in selecting appropriate measures. It is important to note that such a model also serves as a guide to interpreting scores in the light of the decision to be made. A model developed to set priorities for values and informational needs for admission decisions would provide guidelines, for example, to determine whether subscale scores on a measure should be interpreted individually or whether the total (overall) score should be interpreted. The model would also provide the basis for deciding whether the subscale scores should be given equal weight in the decision or differently weighted in terms of their importance. The model would also specify the ways in which information from multiple standardized measure scores are subject to an indeterminate degree of error because of unmet assumptions and uncontrolled conditions. The best way to avoid making erroneous decisions is to base them on multiple indicators rather than on a single score. Thus, the final interpretation of a given score should be made only after assessing the extent to which it is congruent with other available information.

SELECTING STANDARDIZED MEASURES

In many instances nurses engaged in clinical practice, education, administration, and research do not have sufficient resources (time, money,

expertise) to develop standardized measures themselves, yet seek the technical quality, consistent information, and precise comparative interpretation that a standardized measure can provide. They therefore may select standardized instruments that have been developed by others. In this section of the chapter, procedures and considerations for selecting and using standardized measures are discussed.

Selecting the Measure

Selection of any measure must be based on careful consideration of the nature of the concept, attribute, or behavior about which the information is being sought and the purposes to be achieved by acquiring the information (Nunnally & Bernstein, 1994). The initial step in selecting a measure is to define clearly the kind of information required. This is in itself a time-consuming procedure, which often involves the combined efforts of a variety of people. However, its importance cannot be overemphasized (Cook & Campbell, 1979).

Each standardized measure is unique in its assumptions and specific content and in the aspects of behavior, cognition, affect, or skill that it measures. Similarly, nurses have, within the context of a given situation, unique needs for particular kinds of information. It is critical to remember that only those who require information for particular purposes are in a position to define the exact nature of the information needed and that they must do so before seeking a measure. The defined needs provide the primary criterion for selecting measures to meet them.

Many nursing decisions that are based on information gained from measurement have considerable impact on the decision-makers and others. Examples are educational admissions decisions, promotion decisions in clinical settings, decisions about curricular and program change, and clinical decisions regarding nursing diagnoses and the use of particular nursing interventions. Given the potential impact of such decisions, it is important that the process of defining the need for information be carried out thoughtfully, with attention to goals to be achieved and the consequences of the decisions. During this process it is necessary to identify not only local requirements and conditions, but also the values that underlie the specification of goals. Desired outcomes (goals), of necessity, reflect values whether or not they are recognized and acknowledged. Decision-makers who identify and rank in importance the values that they wish to maximize are able to set priorities for their information needs accordingly. Measures can be selected and their relative importance determined on this basis, heightening the probability that they will yield the information needed for a sound decision (Portney & Watkins, 2000).

Once the information needs are defined and priorities are set, it is necessary to consider which needs are best fulfilled by standardized versus nonstandardized measures. As noted in an earlier section of this chapter, standardized measures are inappropriate for situations in which flexibility, adaptability to specific circumstances, and sensitivity to minor fluctuations are required, and in which interpretation by way of comparison to a defined and relatively heterogeneous reference group is not desired. Given the comprehensive listing of information needs, it is necessary to differentiate those suited for standardized measures from those for which other measures are preferable. Having determined the specific needs to be met by standardized measures, the next step is to identify those measures that have potential to provide the information desired. A number of resources are available to aid in the search and a growing number are available online. Particularly helpful are the well-known publications Tests in Print VI (Murphy, Plake, Impara, & Spies, 2002) and 15th *Mental Measurements Yearbook* (Plake, Impara, Spies, & Pale, 2003). The former includes a description of most standardized tests including title, author, publisher, age levels covered, publication dates, special comments, number and type of scores provided, and references to test reviews and publications using the test. The latter includes evaluative information about the tests as well as additional descriptive information. Other sources of information are compendia of instruments and books that describe standardized instruments, test publishers' and instrument manufacturers' catalogs, and articles in professional journals. Several such publications are described in more detail

in the appendix. One web site that provides links to many of the commonly used standardized measures is: http://www.bridgew.edu/library/testlist.cfm.

Sample sets of those measures deemed potentially useful and accompanying test manuals can be ordered for review and evaluation. These should be examined carefully for evidence of high technical quality and characteristics that are desirable for the particular use intended. Test materials must be reviewed critically and with some skepticism, disregarding evaluative statements unless they are supported by detailed descriptions and statistical evidence.

Table 7.3 includes a set of questions that can be used to guide evaluation of a standardized measure for use in education, practice or research. These questions address the criteria that have been described throughout the chapter. Each measure being considered should be evaluated in the light of these considerations, and its advantages and disadvantages identified. The features deemed most important should be given highest priority in the evaluation. In addition to the general considerations listed above, criteria specific to the particular situation in which the measure is to be used should be identified in order to facilitate the selection process. For example, a faculty group planning an applicant selection process for the graduate program in a school of nursing may determine in advance that it wishes to consider only those standardized aptitude measures that are administered abroad as well as in the United States and that provide norms specific to individuals with an undergraduate major in nursing. A nurse researcher contemplating a health risk assessment of large numbers of adults may decide to consider only measures that are machine-scored by a centralized facility, whereas a group of clinicians choosing a standardized measure to be used during a primary care visit would be more likely to select a measure that that can be hand-scored within a matter of minutes.

SUMMARY

Standardized measures are norm-referenced measures that are constructed, administered,

Table 7.3　Questions to Guide Evaluation of Standardized Measures

Topic	Questions
Purpose	Are the stated purpose and recommended uses congruent with the intended use? Will the measure yield desired information?
Conceptual basis	Is the theoretical model or conceptualization that guided the development of the measure congruent with the conceptualization underpinning the intended use? What are the assumptions and potential biases? What values are inherent in the instrument and are they congruent with the intended use?
Content	Is the content of the measure appropriate without modification for the intended use? Is the content up to date? Is it appropriate for the potential subjects?
Technical quality	Have adequate reliability, validity, specificity, and sensitivity been established? What is the evidence supporting its psychometric properties? Was the measure developed and tested adequately?
Norms	How were norms established? How adequate was the referent group, and how was it selected? Are the norms sufficiently detailed and clear for use as a basis for comparison? Are relevant subgroup norms provided? Are norms updated regularly?
Administration	Are instructions for administration clear and precise? What resources and conditions are required for administration? How easy, costly, and time-consuming is it to administer the measure? Is training required? What about subject burden?
Scoring	Is the measure hand- or machine-scored? How clear are the instructions for scoring? How difficult is the tool to score, and what resources are required? How likely are errors to occur in scoring?
Interpretation	Can scores be interpreted easily, consistently, and accurately? Are materials provided to aid in interpretation and in communicating the meaning of results to the subjects?
Cost	How costly is it to purchase, administer and score the measure? Are costs proportional to the potential value of using the measure and the import of information to be obtained?
Critiques	Have evaluations of the measure been published by experts? What problems, strengths, and weaknesses have been identified? Have viable alternatives been developed and tested?

and scored in a prescribed and consistent manner and that are interpreted with reference to established norms. Because standardized measures are carefully constructed, are of high technical quality, and are designed for widespread use, they have potential utility for measuring many types of nursing phenomena. They are useful for situations in which normative interpretation is required (e.g., when scores are to be interpreted by means of comparison to a defined population) and in which the attributes or behaviors being measured are relatively stable and are common to a variety of situations and settings. They are not designed to be specific to a particular setting or to discern minor fluctuations. Neither the content nor the administration of a standardized measure can be altered to meet local needs.

One of the key advantages of a standardized measure is that norms are provided to aid in interpreting results. Norms are statistics that describe the scores earned by a defined referent group with known characteristics, which is representative of the population of individuals for whom the measure is designed. They are established by administering the measure under controlled conditions. The scores of the referent group serve as the basis for comparing scores earned on all subsequent administrations of the measure and, hence, facilitate consistent interpretation.

The selection of a standardized measure for use in nursing is based on the defined needs for information; the stated purpose, assumptions, and content domain of the measure; its technical quality; the adequacy of the norms; and the costs and procedures required for administration and scoring. Administration and scoring of the selected measures must be carried out with consistent adherence to prescribed procedures. Interpretation of the results occurs within the context of the defined needs. It is guided by the established norms, but also takes into account the characteristics of the referent group and examinee (s) and technical features of the measure. Information gleaned from standardized measures should be interpreted in the light of information gathered from other sources as well.

REFERENCES

Academy Technologies. (2003). *Zip-scan.* Retrieved November 22, 2003, http://www.academytechnologies.com/ZipScan/whatsinitforme.htm

American College Test (ACT). (1999). *Selections from the 1999 National Score Report.* Retrieved November 20, 2003, from http://www.act.org/news/data/99/99data.html

American Educational Research Association (AERA), American Psychological Association (APA), & National Council on Measurement in Education (NCME). (1999). *Standards for educational and psychological testing* Washington, DC: American Educational Research.

Anastasi, A., & Urbina, S. (1997). *Psychological testing* (7th ed.). Upper Saddle River, NJ: Prentice-Hall.

Angoff, W. H. (1971). Scales, norms and equivalent scores. In R. L. Thorndike (Ed.), *Educational measurement.* Washington, DC: American Council on Education.

Austin, J. K. (2003). Child attitude toward illness Scale. In B. K. Redman (Ed.), *Measurement tools in patient education* (2nd ed.). New York: Springer Publishing.

Avant, K. C. (1990). The art and science of nursing diagnosis development. *Nursing Diagnosis, 1*(2), 51–56.

Baker, E. L. (1998). *Understanding educational quality: Where validity meets technology.* ETS William H. Angoff Memorial Lecture Series. Princeton, NJ: Educational Testing Service.

Barnard, K. E. & Earles, S. J. (Eds.). (1979). *Child health assessment, part 2: The first year of life.* Pub. No. (HRA) 79-25. Washington, DC: U.S. Department of Health, Education, and Welfare.

Bowers, L., Huisingh, R., Barrett, M., Orman, J., & LoGiudice, C. (1994). *Test of problem solving—Elementary, Revised (TOPS-E, Revised).* East Moline, IL: LinguiSystems.

Bowling, A. (2001). *Measuring disease* (2nd ed.). Philadelphia: Open University Press.

Bowling, A. (2002). *Research methods in health: Investigating health and health services* (2nd ed.). Philadelphia: Open University Press.

Brazelton, T. B. (1973). *A neonatal behavioral assessment scale.* Philadelphia: J. B. Lippincott.

Brazelton, T. B., & Sparrow, J. D. (2002). *Touchpoints: Both volumes of the nation's most trusted guide to the first six years of life.* United Kingdom: Perseus Press.

Burns, N., & Grove, S. K. (1997). *The practice of nursing research: Conduct, critique, & utilization* (3rd ed.). Philadelphia: W. B. Saunders.

Center for Early Education & Development (CEED). (2000). Measuring growth and development. *Early Report, 27*(2). Retrieved November 16, 2003, http://www.education.umn.edu/CEED/publications/earlyreport/fall00.htm

Cochran, W. G. (1977). *Sampling techniques* (3rd ed.). New York: John Wiley & Sons.

Cook, T. D., & Campbell, D. T. (1979). *Quasi-experimentation: Design & analysis issues for field settings.* Boston: Houghton Mifflin.

Daniel, M. H. (1999). Behind the scenes: Using new measurement methods on DAS and KAIT. In S. E. Embretson & S. L. Hershberger (Eds.), *The new rules of measurement.* Mahwah, NJ: Erlbaum.

Derogatis, L. R. (1987). The Derogatis Stress Profile (DSP): Quantification of psychological stress. *Advances in Psychosomatic Medicine, 17,* 30–54.

Derogatis, L. R. (1993). *BSI: Administration, scoring and procedures manual for the Brief Symptom Inventory* (3rd ed.). Minneapolis, MN: National Computer Systems.

Derogatis, L. R., & Rutigliano, P. J. (1998). Derogatis Affects Balance Scale: DABS. In B. Spilker (Ed.), *Quality of life and pharmacoeconomics in clinical trials* (2nd ed., pp. 169–177). New York: Lippincott-Raven.

Derogatis, L. R. (2000). *Brief Symptom Inventory-18 (BSI-18).* Minneapolis: National Computer Systems.

Embretson, S. E. (1991). A multidimensional latent trait model for measuring learning and change. *Psychometrika, 56,* 495–516.

Embretson, S. E. (2001a). Generating abstract reasoning items with cognitive theory. In S. Irvine & P. Kyllonen (Eds.), *Item generation for test development.* (pp. 219–250). Mahwah, NJ: Erlbaum Publishers.

Embretson, S. E. (2001b). *The second century of ability testing: Some predictions and speculations.* ETS William H. Angoff Memorial Lecture Series. Princeton, NJ: Educational Testing Service.

Embretson, S. E., & Gorin, J. (2001). Improving construct validity with cognitive psychology principles. *Journal of Educational Measurement, 38,* 343–368.

Fair test. (2003). What's wrong with standardized tests? *The National Center for Fair & Open Testing.* Retrieved November 22, 2003, from http://www.fairtest.org/facts/whatwron.htm

Fastenau, P. S., Denburg, N. L., & Hufford, B. J. (1999). Adult norms for the Rey-Oserrieth Complex Figure Test and for supplemental recognition and matching trials from the Extended Complex Figure Test. *The Clinical Neuropsychologists, 13*(1), 30–47.

Gordon, M. (2000). *Nursing diagnosis & classification system development.* Retrieved November 12, 2003, from http://www.aricd.org.uk/index.htm

Graduate Record Exam (GRE). (2003). *Graduate Record Examinations. Educational Testing Service Homepage.* Retrieved December 4, 2003, from http://www.gre.org/splash.html

Griffiths, R. (1954). *The abilities of babies: A study in mental measurement.* England: Amersham, Bucks.

Griffiths, R. (2003). Association for Research in Infant and Child Development. *Online Journal of Issues in Nursing.* Retrieved November 11, 2003, from http://www.nursingworld.org/mods/archive/mod30/cec21.htm

Grinker, J. A. (1992). Body composition measurement: Accuracy, validity, and comparability. In *Institute of Medicine (IOM) body composition and physical performance* (pp. 223–235). Washington, DC: National Academy Press.

Grogan, S. (1999). *Body image: Understanding body dissatisfaction in men, women, and children.* New York: Routledge.

International Survey Research (ISR). (2003). *ISR Benchmarks: National norms.* Retrieved November 20, 2003, from http://www.isrsurveys.com/en/ser_nationalnorms.asp

Jastak, J. F., & Jastak, S. (2003). Wide Range Interest-Opinion Test (WRIOT). *Stoelting Psychological & Educational Tests Homepage.* Retrieved December 4, 2003, from http://www.stoeltingco.com/tests/catalog/WRIOT.htm

Kamphaus, R. W., DiStefano, C., & Lease, A. M. (2003). A self-report typology of behavioral adjustment for young children. *Psychological Assessment, 15*(1), 17–28.

Keenan, G. M., Killeen, M. B., & Clingerman, E. (2002). NANDA, NOC and NIC: Progress toward a nursing information infrastructure. *Nursing Education Perspectives, 23*(4), 162–163.

Kelley, T. L. (1914). Comparable measures. *Journal of Educational Psychology, 5,* 589–595.

Kerlinger, F. N., & Lee, H. B. (2000). *Foundations of behavioral research* (4th ed.). New York: Harcourt.

Kish, L. (1965). *Survey sampling.* New York: John Wiley & Sons.

Kish, L. (1995). *Survey sampling.* New York: John Wiley & Sons.

Kline, P. (2000). *Handbook of psychological testing* (2nd ed.). New York: Routledge.

Levy, P. S., & Lemeshow, S. (1980). *Sampling for health professionals.* Belmont, CA: Lifetime Learning.

Levy, P. S., & Lemeshow, S. (1999). *Sampling of populations: Methods and applications* (3rd ed.). New York: John Wiley & Sons.

Lyberg, L. E., Biemer, P., Collins, M., Leeuw, E., Dippo, C., Schwarz, N., & Trewin, D. (1997). *Survey measurement and process quality.* New York: John Wiley & Sons.

Mancini, I., & Body, J. J. (1999). Assessment of dyspnea in advanced cancer patients. *Support Care Cancer, 7*(4), 229–232.

Meek, P. M., & Lareau, S. C. (2003). Critical

outcomes in pulmonary rehabilitation: Assessment and evaluation of dyspnea and fatigue. *Journal of Rehabilitation Research and Development, 40*(5), 13–24.

Messick, S. (1995). Validity of psychological assessment. *American Psychologist, 50*(9), 741–749.

Mishel, M. H. (1989). Methodological studies: Instrument development. In P. J. Brink & M. J. Wood (Eds.), *Advanced design in nursing research* (pp. 238–284). Newbury Park, CA: Sage.

Murphy, L. L., Plake, B. S., Impara, J. C., & Spies, R. A. (2002). *Tests in print VI: An index to tests, test reviews, and the literature on specific tests (Tests in Print, No. 6).* Lincoln, NB: Buros.

National League of Nursing. (2003). *Shaping the future for nursing education.* Retrieved November 20, 2003, from http://www.nln.org

National Quality Forum (NQF). (2003). Core Measures for Nursing Care Performance. *NQF Brief* (May). Retrieved November 11, 2003, from http://www.qualityforum.org

North American Nursing Diagnosis Association (NANDA). (1997). *Nursing diagnoses: Definition and classification, 1997–1998.* Philadelphia: Author.

North American Nursing Diagnosis Association (NANDA). (2001). *Nursing diagnoses: Definition and classification, 1997–1998.* Philadelphia: Author.

Nunnally, J. C., & Bernstein, I. H. (1994). *Psychometric theory* (3rd ed.). New York: McGraw-Hill.

Pearson (2003). *Applications, services and technologies for education, testing, assessment, business, government.* Retrieved November 22, 2003, from http://www.ncspearson.com/

Pedhazur, E. J., & Schmelkin, L. P. (1991). *Measurement, design and analysis: An integrated approach.* Hillsdale, NJ: Lawrence Erlbaum.

Plake, B. S., Impara, J. C., Spies, R. A., & Pale, B. S. (2003). *Mental measurements yearbook* (15th ed.). Lincoln, NB: Buros.

Portney, L. G., & Watkins, M. P. (2000). *Foundations of clinical research: Applications to practice* (2nd ed.). Upper Saddle River, NJ: Prentice Hall Health.

Quest Diagnostics. (2003). *The nation's leading provider of diagnostic testing, information, and services.* Retrieved November 22, 2003, from http://www.questdiagnostics.com

Scantron. (2003). *Scantron is the leader in data collection systems, testing and assessment and hardware service.* Retrieved November 22, 2003, from http://www.scantron.com/

Scholastic Aptitude Test (SAT). (2003). *About the SAT I: Reasoning and SAT II: Subject tests.* Retrieved November 22, 2003, from http://www.collegeboard.com/student/testing/sat/about.html

Shonkoff, J. P., & Meisels, S. J. (2000). *Handbook of early childhood intervention* (2nd ed.). New York: Cambridge University Press.

Spielberger, C. D. (2003). State-Trait Anxiety Inventory for Adults. *Mind Garden.* Retrieved November 22, 2003, from http://www.mindgarden.com/Assessment/Info/staiinfo.htm

Spielberger, C. D., Gorsuch, R. L., & Lushene, R. (1970). *STAI Manual for the State-Trait Anxiety Inventory.* Palo Alto, CA: Consulting Psychologist Press.

SPSS (2000). *SPSS Base 10.0: Applications guide.* Chicago: SPSS, Inc.

Stevens, J. (1996). *Applied multivariate statistics for the social sciences* (3rd ed.). Hillsdale, NJ: Lawrence Erlbaum.

Strickland, O. L., & Dilorio, C. (2003). *Measurement of nursing outcomes* (2nd ed.) New York: Springer Publishing.

Stromberg, M. F., & Olsen, S. J. (1997). *Instruments for clinical health-care research* (2nd ed). Boston: Jones & Bartlett.

Tellegen, A. (2003). *Building upon a solid foundation: Introducing the new Minnesota Multiphasic Personality Inventory-2™ (MMPI-2™) restructured clinical (RC) scales.* Retrieved December 4, 2003, from http://www.pearsonassessments.com/tests/mmpi2rcscales.htm

Troumbley, P. F. (1989). *A comparison of the health risk and physical fitness of overweight and normal weight soldiers.* Unpublished doctoral dissertation. University of Maryland, Baltimore.

U.S. Army (2003). HOOAH 4 Health. *Program Overview.* Retrieved November 22, 2003, from http://www.hooah4health.com/overview/default.htm

Waltz, C. F., & Jenkins, L. S. (2001). *Measurement of nursing outcomes* (2nd ed.) New York: Springer Publishing.

Ware, J. E. (2000). Health Survey update. *Spine, 25*(3), 3130–3139. Available at: http://www.sf-36.com

Ware, J. E., Kosinski, M. A., & Keller, S. D. (1994). *SF-36 physical and mental health summary scales: A user's manual.* Boston: The Health Institute, New England Medical Center.

Ware, J. E., Kosinski, M. A., & Dewey, J. (2001). *How to score version 2 of the SF-36 health survey.* Lincoln, RI: Quality Metric.

Yates, F. (1981). *Sampling methods for censuses and surveys.* New York: Macmillan.

8

Measurement Issues
in Qualitative Research

Judith E. Hupcey

Qualitative inquiry is an approach to research that focuses on the description and understanding of phenomenon (or concepts) within the social world from the perspective of individuals who are experiencing that world. Qualitative approaches are most appropriate for nursing because they aid in our understanding of phenomena such as the processes associated with health and illness (e.g., grounded theory), how culture influences people's lives and responses to illness (e.g., ethnography), and the essence of a health/illness experience for an individual (e.g., phenomenology). The knowledge and theories developed from this understanding can help advance nursing science with the goal of improving health outcomes by assisting others through similar situations.

There are many issues affecting quantitative inquiry that had been ignored or skirted by qualitative researchers. Over the last 30 years, as qualitative methods have become an accepted means of studying phenomenon of interest to nursing, stricter criteria have been imposed on the qualitative researcher. This has occurred for a number of reasons. The most important reason relates to the advancement of nursing science. Moving nursing science forward requires more than filling our journals with interesting, yet merely descriptive studies. Researchers need to take their work to the next level, which is theory development. This perspective may be pushing qualitative research, as a whole, toward the positivistic end of the qualitative research continuum. However, in order for nursing research to be funded and be useful to nursing science post-funding, issues such as validity, reliability,

and generalizability of qualitative research need to be addressed (Morse, 1999a). Although there are excellent nurse researchers who have opposing paradigmatic views on this (such as autoethnographers, post-modern or feminist researchers), major funding sources (see the NIH [2001] guidelines for qualitative research proposals) require the researcher to address these issues in the same manner as in a quantitative proposal. This chapter will present the more traditional approach to these issues while still describing some of the other terms that may be used by the qualitative researcher (for example, instead of validity, trustworthiness), will discuss threats to validity, reliability, generalizability, and will examine ways to minimize these threats.

OVERVIEW OF QUALITATIVE RESEARCH

Qualitative research is undertaken for a number of reasons. First, when little is known about a concept or phenomenon as a result of limited previous research, or because it is a new area of interest, or is an area that has evolved and prior research and/or theory no longer fit the phenomenon, a qualitative approach would be appropriate. The research could be done simply to explore/describe a phenomenon or could be done with the purpose of theory development or refinement. A second reason for using a qualitative approach is based on the phenomenon/concept under investigation. Many phenomena and concepts are just not suitable for quantitative measurement.

There are numerous characteristics of qualitative research that distinguish it from a traditional quantitative research. The following is a list of some of the hallmarks of a qualitative approach:

- Inductive: the researcher begins with data and builds concept, categories, hypotheses, models, and theory from these data
- Concerned with process and meaning from an emic (participants') view: the purpose is not to show causality or outcomes, but how individuals make sense of their world (thus there are multiple realities)
- Undertaken in the field or naturalistic setting: no controls are placed on extraneous variables or the setting, these variations are intertwined with the phenomenon under investigation, so are important in the understanding of process and meaning
- Uses the researcher as a tool for data collection and analysis: requires that the researcher continually differentiate between his/her own reality and that of the participants and still be close enough to the participants' world to understand and describe it (Creswell, 1998; Morse & Field, 1995; Polit & Beck, 2004)

Although there are numerous qualitative approaches that are used by nurses, several will be used as examples in this chapter and will be briefly described. These include phenomenology, grounded theory, ethnography, focus group, case study, and narrative/storytelling.

Phenomenology

Phenomenology is a qualitative method that is based in philosophy. Its aim is to understand and then describe in detail the essence of the experience as it is lived by the person (Munhall, 1994; Van Manen, 1990). The goal is to accurately describe the phenomenon under study and to transform the lived experience into a textual expression of its essence (this can be done with text, pictures, music, etc.). The phenomenon is described as it is experienced by the person (e.g., the experience of *waiting* by the wife of a critically ill patient), without the use of

theories and to the extent possible, without researcher preconceptions and presuppositions. Data are collected through multiple in-depth conversations with the participant(s), so that the researcher is the primary data collection tool.

Grounded Theory

The methods of grounded theory come from a sociological perspective. They were initially developed by Glaser and Strauss (1967) and subsequently refined by Glaser (1978) and Strauss and Corbin (1998). The primary goal of a grounded theory is to generate explanatory models of human behavior that are grounded in the data. Preexisting theory is not used so the researcher remains open-minded about what concepts will emerge and how they will be organized. A grounded theory documents processes (e.g., the development of trust in health care providers) and change over time in order to link categories and develop models. According to Glaser (1978, 1992), the resultant theory must fit the data, work, have relevance, and be modifiable.

Data are collected using interviews, observations, and field notes. A constant comparative process is used for data collection and analysis. Here data are collected and analyzed simultaneously. Thus the researcher is observing, collecting data, organizing and analyzing the data, and forming theory from the data all at the same time. Hypotheses are compared and tested with incoming data (every piece of information is compared with every other). Within this process the researcher also uses theoretical sampling, where the researcher decides which data to collect next and where to find them, based on the needs of the developing theory.

Ethnography

Ethnography is a branch of anthropology that focuses on the study of cultural groups. The purpose of ethnography is to tell the story of participants' lives from the perspective of the culture of which they are a part (Fetterman, 1989). This investigation involves an in-depth study of the members of the culture through participant observation, interviews, and field notes. The researcher needs to spend time (or possibly live) with the group and become part of the cultural setting in order to collect data and understand the cultural group under investigation.

A focused ethnography is a variation of the traditional ethnography and is an approach that may be more appropriate to nursing. Here the participants are linked by location (e.g., a hospital unit) not a place of residence or culture in the anthropological sense, but share behavioral norms and a common language (Morse & Field, 1995). In a focused ethnography the topic is selected prior to data collection, while in a traditional ethnography it emerges from the data. Data collection, including interviews and observations, are limited to particular events and topics related to the event. The product is an understanding of essential culture schemas.

Focus Groups

A focus group is a technique for data collection that uses group interactions to obtain an understanding of participants' experiences and beliefs. A focus group can be used solely as a technique to collect data (e.g., within an ethnographic study or grounded theory) or as a stand-alone method. Since in-depth data cannot be obtained from each participant, focus groups typically are used for problem identification, program planning, and program evaluation. The group is researcher-controlled in that the topic chosen and questions asked are those of the researcher. However, the discussion and group diversity and consensus come from the group and its discussion (Morgan, 1997).

Case Study

Case studies are an exploration of a "bounded system" or a case (or multiple cases) over time through detailed, in-depth data collection involving multiple sources of information such as interviews, observations, documents, archival records, artifacts, and audiovisual materials (Yin, 1994) that are rich in context (Creswell, 1998). The case can be an individual, an event, program, or organization. The product of a case study is a detailed description of the case,

including chronology, naturalistic generalizations, and lessons learned from the case (Creswell, 1998).

Narrative/Storytelling

A narrative is a method that is used "to give a voice to the silenced" (Frank, 1995) and as a way to study humans' experiences within the social world. Within narrative inquiry, information is gathered for the purpose of storytelling. It is an art of both listening to the narrative and then telling the story (or writing a narrative of the experience) (Riessman, 1993). Data are collected through in-depth interview, field notes, journals, letters, and stories told by the participant. The researcher then writes the narrative of the participant (this may be a collaborative effort between the researcher and participant).

VALIDITY, RELIABILITY, AND GENERALIZABILITY OF QUALITATIVE FINDINGS

As suggested earlier, in order for qualitative inquiry to advance nursing science, methodological and analytic issues such as validity, reliability, and generalizability need to be addressed when a study is designed. Threats to these issues can occur when the study is initially designed (e.g., picking the wrong method for the research question,[1] or not adequately planning the sample), during data collection, and during data analysis. In this section these issues will be defined. This will be followed by a discussion of the threats to validity and reliability during sampling, data collection, and data analysis and how these threats can be minimized.

Validity

In qualitative research, validity can be defined as the "truth value," or trustworthiness of the data and resultant analysis and interpretation,

---

[1]If an inappropriate method is chosen, then the research question cannot be answered; for example, trying to investigate an extremely personal issue in a focus group may result in little or false information being given by the participant.

or the extent to which the findings represent reality (Morse & Field, 1995). Others have broken validity down further. Miles and Huberman (1994) discuss internal and external validity while Maxwell (1992) describes it even further since he believes that internal and external validity reflect positivistic assumptions. He posits five types of understanding and validity: descriptive validity, interpretive validity, theoretical validity, generalizability (this will be discussed separately), and evaluative validity. Each of these types of validity will be discussed below.

Internal Validity

Internal validity asks whether the researchers are measuring or observing what they think they are measuring or observing (LeCompte & Goetz, 1982). In qualitative terms, Miles and Huberman (1994) also refer to internal validity as credibility or authenticity, where the findings need to make sense and be credible to both participants and readers. Internal validity is enhanced during both data collection and analysis when the researcher uses multiple sources of data, links data to the emerging categories and theory, confirms findings with additional data, and looks for negative evidence (tries to find data that may not support the analysis/hypotheses being developed).

External Validity

External validity asks whether the findings and conclusions of the study can be transferred to other contexts, i.e., are they generalizable beyond the present study (applicable across groups) (LeCompte & Goetz, 1982; Miles & Huberman, 1994). Other terms used for external validity are transferability and fittingness (Miles & Huberman, 1994). External validity is enhanced by having an adequate sample, including sample size, sample diversity, and appropriate purposive/theoretical sampling. The findings should be abstract enough to apply to other contexts and contain enough rich description for the reader (or other researchers) to evaluate the findings. For some types of qualitative research (e.g., phenomenology) there are no claims that findings are generalizable beyond the subjects in that particular sample.

Descriptive Validity

Descriptive validity is related to the "truth value," or credibility/authenticity (or valid description) of the data and what was reported from the data (Maxwell, 1992). Here, the researcher needs to carefully collect and corroborate data (this can be done by obtaining feedback about the accuracy of the data and analysis from the original participants or by using secondary participants to confirm the emerging analysis), and present an accurate account of these data.

Interpretive Validity

Interpretive validity relates to meaning or the interpretation of the data (Maxwell, 1992). Does the researcher accurately understand and portray the participant's (emic) view or meaning?

Theoretical Validity

Theoretical validity moves beyond the descriptive and interpretative types of validity to analysis of the validity of a theory (Maxwell, 1992). Thus, does the derived model fit with the data and is it abstract enough to extend theory beyond description?

Evaluative Validity

Evaluative validity applies an evaluative framework to the objects of the study not the study design itself (Maxwell, 1992). Here a judgment is made about the correctness or worth of the meanings or actions. Therefore, how the researcher describes, interprets, or constructs the story or theory is important.

RELIABILITY

Reliability in qualitative research is concerned with consistency over time and across researchers and settings and objectivity and confirmability (Miles & Huberman, 1994). There is a distinction made between internal and external reliability. Internal reliability is defined by LeCompte and Goetz (1982) as "the *degree* to which other *researchers,* given a set of previously generated constructs, would match them with the data in the same way as did the original researcher" (p. 32). Other terms for internal reliability are dependability and auditability. Miles and

Huberman refer to this as "quality control". They ask questions such as: Is the research question clear and does it match the method used? Does the research design specify the role of the researcher? How will data be collected to maximize the phenomenon of interest and to answer the research question (with specific protocols if multiple data collectors are utilized)? When and how will coding checks, data quality checks, and peer reviews take place? Do the findings match across sources of data and the developing theory?

External reliability is defined as "whether independent researchers would discover the same phenomena or generate the same constructs in the same or similar setting" (LeCompte & Goetz, 1982, p. 32). Miles and Huberman (1994) consider this issue as one of "relative neutrality and reasonable freedom from unacknowledged researcher biases" (p. 278). They ask questions that relate to the ability to replicate a study. Are the methods and procedures well described, including the sequence for data collection and analysis and the development of conclusions (is there an audit trial?)? Are researcher biases addressed? Has the researcher linked conclusions to the data and shown potential hypothesis that were refuted and why? Are the data available for others to analyze?

GENERALIZABILITY

Generalizability is often referred to as external validity or transferability. Maxwell (1992) defines generalizability as "the extent to which one can extend the account of a particular situation or population to other persons, times, or settings than those directly studied" (p. 293). Generalizability is applicable with the development of theory from qualitative work and the utility of the theory to other persons in similar situations.

Generalizability has typically been a concern of quantitative researchers, while many qualitative researchers and texts ignore this issue. There are instances when generalizability is not a concern for the qualitative researcher. Some qualitative methods are not intended to produce generalizable findings, but still generate valuable pieces of work (such as with some phe-

nomenologies, individual case studies, and narrative/storytelling). Morse (1999b) points out, however, that for qualitative research to be useable and to advance nursing science, generalizability needs to be addressed. This is particularly true if one of the goals of the qualitative study is to develop a theory. Although the means for how a qualitatively derived theory is developed is different from quantitatively derived theory, the qualitatively derived theory should still meet strict evaluative criteria (Morse, 1997), and thus will be applicable beyond the immediate group studied.

ADEQUACY OF THE SAMPLE

The adequacy of the sample, including both selection and sample size, will influence the credibility (thus validity, reliability, and generalizability) of qualitative results. There is a general misconception that in qualitative research the sample size is small and homogenous and many times not an important issue to address when developing a qualitative research proposal. On the other extreme, some researchers over-compensate and plan a study with a huge number of participants to be comparable to a quantitative study. A sample that is too large and diverse may become cumbersome and will not allow for the in-depth analysis that is one of the hallmarks of qualitative research (Sandelowski, 1995). There is no hidden formula that helps the researcher determine sample size, but Morse (1998) has suggested two principles that need to be considered, First, the more data obtained from each participant, the fewer the number of participants needed, and second, the broader the research topic, the larger the sample will need to be in order to reach saturation or redundancy. Here we will consider those and other factors that should be combined to assist the researcher in determining an adequate sample. The factors that will be addressed are the overall purpose of the study, the research question/topic of interest, the type of purposive sampling to be employed, the sampling unit (e.g., number of participants versus number of interviews or incidents), and the research approach (or method) that undergirds the study.

Purpose of the Research

The purposes of qualitative research studies range from those that aim at pure description (such as in case study, storytelling, narrative, focus group) to the development of theory (such as in phenomenology, grounded theory, ethnography).[2] Thus, sample size would be influenced by the overall purpose of a study. If the purpose of a study is to describe, for example, a person's life or a specific event/phenomenon, few participants may be needed (for a case study even a sample of one may be adequate). In this situation, the quality and quantity of information obtained from each individual needs to be significant, so multiple in-depth interviews need to be collected alone or along with other sources of data such as journal entries. The purpose of focus group research is also descriptive in nature, however the sample size may be larger than with other qualitative methods. This follows Morse's (1998) principle, stated above, that a larger sample is needed when fewer data are obtained from each participant. In focus groups when there are 8–10 participants, limited or superficial information can be obtained from each participant (Morgan, 1998). Thus, the number of participants needed to adequately address a topic is at least 25–30, depending on the topic and homogeneity of the groups.[3] If the purpose of a research project[4] is to develop theory, then the size and diversity of the sample in terms of numbers of participants, number of sampling units (interviews/observations) and data sources needs to be significant.

Research Question/Topic

The research question or topic of interest will also have a major influence on sample selection and the sample size. One of the tenets of qualitative research is to maximize the phenomenon.

The researcher needs to pick the sample that will best answer the research question or best examine the topic of interest. The sample is selected based on the data that can be obtained from the participants. Sampling in this manner is biased in that the researcher is looking for participants who are most knowledgeable, thus have the greatest experience related to the research topic (Morse, 1998). Demographic delimiters such as gender, ethnicity, socioeconomic factors, etc., that are often used in quantitative research *may* hold no analytic value in sample selection strategies for qualitative studies. However, keeping this in mind, within an individual study, some of these demographic factors may actually turn out to influence the participants' experiences. If this occurs, then data for these individual groups need to be collected, and if possible within the constraints of an individual study, sufficient data need to be collected from each group to reach saturation.[5] A second consideration in terms of demographics, particularly age, gender, and ethnicity, is that federal funding guidelines presently mandate the inclusion of adults and children, males and females, and all ethnic groups in research studies. There may be ways to justify the exclusion of certain groups, such as children; however studies may not be funded when ethnic groups are excluded. If the qualitative researcher truly believes that ethnicity is of analytic importance, then the study needs to be designed to address these different groups.

Sample size is also influenced by the research question/topic. A very specific research question would require a smaller sample than a broader topic. For example investigating the experiences of wives of critically ill patients (i.e., only adult patients) would require a smaller sample than a study that explored families' experiences (which would include both adult and pediatric patients). In the wife study, although the researcher may want to include women with a variety of experiences (for example, women of different ages whose husbands were critical as a result of

---

[2]For a comprehensive discussion of levels of qualitatively-derived theory, see Morse (1997).

[3]See Morgan (1998) for greater detail on numbers of groups and sample size.

[4]Notice here I say *project* and not *study,* because although an individual study may begin the process of theory development, numerous studies are needed, to build solid high-level theory (Hupcey & Penrod, 2003).

---

[5]Many small studies do not have the time or resources to collect enough data on each group; in these situations, the researcher must acknowledge this as a limitation of the study and present it as a future avenue for research.

different acute, chronic, or traumatic conditions with varying prognoses), the participant group is still fairly discrete. If the study included all family members, the sample would need to be larger to include some of the same variations as in the wife study, but would also include husbands, children, parents, siblings, etc. Some of these subgroups may not be dissimilar and would not need to be saturated separately, however, until enough data are obtained from these groups, this would not be known.

Type of Sampling

The type of sampling is another factor to consider when designing a study. Purposive sampling is the mainstay of qualitative research and is defined as the selection of data sources to meet the needs of the study. These data sources may be individuals who have knowledge of or experience with the research topic of interest or other types of data that would enhance the researcher's ability to comprehensively understand the topic of interest. According to Sandelowski (1995), there are three variations within purposive sampling: demographic, phenomenal, and theoretical. *Demographic* variation is based on the belief that a demographic factor is analytically important to the study. Participants are selected based on both their experience with the topic of interest and the demographic factor, such as gender. *Phenomenal* variation incorporates dimensions or characteristics associated with the phenomenon of interest. For example, as described above in the study of wives of critically ill patients, some variations would be the prognosis and cause of the critical illness. Participants would be purposely selected to include these variations. Both demographic and phenomenal sampling decisions are made prior to beginning the study. The third variation is *theoretical* sampling. Here, sampling decisions are made based on the analytic needs of the study. The researcher may begin by using some demographic or phenomenal variations, but as the study progresses, subsequent sampling is driven by the developing theory or model. In this case data sources are chosen that have specific characteristics that will expand, validate, or refute the emerging model.

Sampling Units

Sampling unit is a more useful term to consider when designing a qualitative research study. This gives a clearer idea of the sample than simply estimating[6] in a proposal or documenting in the final report the number of study participants. A sampling unit can be an interview, a day of observation or a single unit of observation (when the incident of interest occurs), or some other data source such as an entry in a hospital record or a newspaper clipping. Often reviewers are leery when they read that the sample included "only" 10 participants. What is missing in this type of documentation is the fact that each participant was interviewed three times, wrote daily journals entries, or was observed for eight hours during interactions with multiple family members (so many incidents of interest were observed). When completing a human subjects protection application, an estimate of the number of participants is needed, but for research funding proposals, the addition of the sampling units would strengthen the proposal. So instead of writing, "it is estimated that 15 participants will be needed to reach saturation," the researcher could say, "it is estimated that 30 interviews will be needed" (this could mean 15 participants interviewed twice, 10 participants interviewed three times, or 10 participants interviewed once, and 10 others interviewed twice).[7] These sampling units need to be carefully thought out to ensure that the number of units proposed will be adequate to reach data saturation, yet not so many that the data are "oversaturated" and extensive analysis becomes difficult.

Sample Size Based on Qualitative Approach

There is no set rule that determines sample size in qualitative research; however, there are some

---

[6]Sample size in qualitative research is always estimated, for the researcher does not know a priori the number of sampling units or participants that will be needed to reach analytic saturation. However, the researcher must have a theoretically-based justification for this estimate.
[7]When participants are interviewed a varying number of times, the reason this is anticipated (or occurred) needs to be explained and, at times, justified.

methodological guidelines that may assist the researcher. It must be remembered that sample size alone is not as important as the number of sampling units. For example, in phenomenology, a small sample of less than 10 participants[8] is used; however, multiple interactions (i.e., interviews/conversations, writing samples, journals, or other artistic units such as poetry, art, or music) with the participants are needed. A grounded theory approach would require somewhere between 30 and 50 participants and would include both interviews and observation (Morse, 1994). An ethnographic approach would also require 30 to 50 participants, along with multiple other data sources (Morse, 1994). The number of participants in focus group research depends on the research question and the diversity of the participants. However, the general rule is that five groups of 6–10 participants are needed (Morgan, 1998). Case study research can be undertaken with one participant (i.e., individual, family, or organization), but requires numerous sampling units (i.e., multiple interviews or other data sources). Case studies can also be done with an event or other type of incident (which becomes the case). Here the number of participants and other sources of data will depend on the event chosen and the amount of data needed to fully understand the case (Creswell, 1998). Narrative/storytelling usually uses long detailed descriptions from one or two individuals. These narratives are a result of multiple in-depth interviews or discussions with the participant(s).

DATA COLLECTION

Throughout data collection there are numerous places where threats to validity, reliability, and generalizability can occur. Sources include the research participant, the researcher as the data collector (specifically during interviewing and observations), and the specific techniques used for data collection.

The Research Participant

The quality of the collected data depends on the participant. In order for a participant to provide useful data during an interview, the participant must have had the experience that is being investigated, must have processed and remember the experience, and must be willing and able to articulate that experience. Not all individuals who agree to participate in a research study will fit those criteria. Some people are unable to relay their experiences. There are many possible reasons for this, including:

- They do not want to tell the story
- They have not processed the experience yet, or they are still in the midst of the experience (here observation may be a more appropriate approach)
- They do not remember the event (e.g., due to the trauma of the experience or the severity of an illness)
- The experience was too personal
- Fear that relating the experience will get them or someone else in trouble
- The interview is not being conducted in a private place

Other threats to the validity of the collected data arise when the participants: tell the researcher what they think the researcher wants to hear, listen to clues during an interview and repeat back what they hear (e.g., the researcher uses the word "coping" and participant picks up on it and uses it), and act different than usual, or the way they think they should act, when being observed.

There are a number of ways to minimize these threats to validity and reliability. These include increasing the sample size, performing multiple interviews (this may allow the participant time to process the experience, become comfortable with the interview process and the researcher, and allow time for clarification and/or explanation), doing multiple periods of observation (after a period of time the influence of being watched will decrease), seeking out negative cases (those individuals who do not support the developing hypotheses or model), and performing member checks.[9]

---

[8]According to Morse (1994), approximately six participants are needed to understand the essence of an experience.

The Researcher as Interviewer

The researcher (or person collecting the data) has a major influence on the data collected and the quality and accuracy of that data (in other words, validity and reliability). As in all research, prior to beginning the study everyone involved in data collection needs to understand the study and be trained in the techniques of interviewing and/or observation. During the initial set of interviews and periodically throughout the research study, the interviews are observed or recorded and critiqued for style (e.g., if the interview is unstructured, does it flow as an unstructured interview should), leading questions, advice giving, interruptions, and researcher biases.

Threats to validity and reliability are inherent in the process of interviewing a research participant, as interviews are not neutral tools for data collection.[10] The interview itself is influenced by both the interviewer and interviewee. The interviewer creates the situation under which an interview takes place, that is, questions are asked and answers are given (Fontana & Frey, 2000). Within this situation personal characteristics of the interviewer such as age, race, gender, and profession will influence how well the interviewer and interviewee connect, and thus the data obtained during the interview. How questions are asked and what words[11] are used by the interviewer also will influence the participants' responses.

Using a translator during the interview process may be necessary in some cases but poses problems with data validity (Esposito, 2001). Some of the general threats relate to the interpretation of the question by the translator, including whether the question was understood as it was suppose to be, whether it was translated as it was meant to be, and whether the question was even asked. Other concerns are a result of cultural and language issues (Twinn, 1997). Can the question even be translated or are there words or cultural aspects that do not translate? The same concerns apply to the responses given by the participant. In order to enhance validity, the translator should be trained as an interviewer and should be an active part of the research project. He/she needs to understand the purpose of the study, why certain questions are asked, and what probes are needed to adequately address the research topic. If at all possible, the translator should understand not only the language, but also the culture, so that questions can be preevaluated for their relevance to that particular cultural group. Interview questions also need to be pretested through this translation process to ensure that valid data can be obtained.

Interviewing is an art and researchers need to critique their own interview style. Within this process threats to validity and reliability can be addressed. Some important things to consider are the amount of talking by the interviewer versus the interviewee. A "good" interview will have enormous blocks of interviewee text with minimal talking by interviewer. Other things that are of concern within the interview and which should be avoided are the following:

- Multiple questions being asked at once
- Interrupting the participant before he/she has completed the answer
- Summarizing or verifying what the participant said
- Teaching, preaching, or counseling the participant during a research-related interview (the interviewer is there as a researcher, not as a nurse, and can refer the participant to the appropriate source for information once the interview is finished)
- Changing directions before the participant has told his/her whole story
- Using labels or technical terms
- Asking closed-ended questions (at times, some closed-ended questions are warranted, but for the most part these should be avoided)

---

[9]Member checks are purported to be a way to help enhance the credibility of the analysis by adding evidence that the interpretations of the researchers represent reality. Here, participants are given written or verbal summaries of the findings and asked to validate the emerging themes or models (Polit & Beck, 2004).

[10]For a complete discussion of the types of interviews, see chapter 11.

[11]Spoken words are always ambiguous and may be interpreted differently by the interviewer and participant (Fontana & Frey, 2000).

There also are technical problems that need to be addressed prior to beginning the process of interviewing. All interviewers need to know how to use the tape-recording equipment (e.g., does it have auto-reverse or do you have to flip the tape? Does it make noise when the tape is complete or does it just quietly turn off without you knowing it?), have spare batteries and tapes, and a proper microphone so voice quality will not be compromised if the setting for data collection is less than adequate (always try to do the interview in a quiet setting without distractions). Another problem is loss of data, either the interviewer did not record or it was lost (e.g., erased by accident, lost during transport to the transcriber). Again, knowing how to properly work the equipment should prevent an interview from not being recorded. Making a copy of the interview on a blank tape would provide a backup.

The Researcher as Observer (Participant Observation)

The collection of observational data is more than just a documentation of visual information; it also includes observations using all of the researcher's senses. This technique is used when the information needed to address the research question cannot be obtained by interviews alone and/or when this type of data would augment other types of data (Jorgensen, 1989). Most qualitative observation is done by the researcher (or research assistant) in person, but there are instances when videotaping may be an option (issues related to videotaping will be discussed later). One of the fundamental aspects of participant observation (and one that enhances data validity) is that data collection takes place in the natural context in which it occurs and among those individuals who would naturally be part of that context.

There is a range of participation by the researcher who is collecting observational data, from complete observer to a complete participant. Each level has implications for the quality of the data collected. A complete observer (which is similar to videotaping) does not interact with the individuals or the setting being observed. This has been described as "being a fly on the wall" (Morse & Field, 1995, p. 109). The disadvantage of being a complete observer is that the researcher's ability to interview or clarify why a behavior has occurred is not possible. As the researcher becomes more of a participant (either participant-as-observer where the researcher is part of the setting and acts as a researcher [observer] only part of the time, or observer-as-participant where the researcher is primarily in the setting to observe, but helps out once in a while [Morse & Field, 1995]), other potential threats to validity and reliability can occur. The more a researcher becomes part of a setting, the less objective (or biased) the observations become since the researcher may begin to see events through the eyes of the participants. On the other hand, active participation in a setting may facilitate the acquisition of insider knowledge, so it will help the researcher to determine when the event(s) of interest will occur and potentially what and where to observe.

There are numerous threats to both validity and reliability when using participant observation as a technique for data collection. One threat to validity is behavioral changes on the part of those being observed when the researcher is present. These changes decrease over time, so increasing the length of time in the setting should enhance the "truth value" of what is being observed. It is also important to be allowed to conduct observations at any time that the researcher deems appropriate so that the individuals being observed do not prepare for the visit (Morse & Field, 1995).

Other threats to validity and reliability include not knowing what is important to observe, i.e., observing and documenting the wrong information; missing significant events (because you are observing something else); prematurely determining what is important to observe, and therefore missing the phenomenon of interest; incomplete or incorrect documentation of the phenomenon in terms of field notes.[12]

Participant observation rarely consists of observational data alone. Thus many of the concerns previously raised can be addressed by

---

[12]For a complete description of field notes see Morse and Field (1995), pp. 111–115.

using multiple techniques for data collection such as interviews and documents. Proper documentation of the phenomenon being observed in a field note (so done at regular intervals so information is not forgotten or missed) will also strengthen both the validity and reliability of the data collected. Although the observation itself cannot be critiqued, the field notes from the observatory periods can be evaluated. During this evaluation, questions can be raised as to what has been observed and why, and the comprehensiveness of the field note. This process is extremely important since these field notes are the data that will be used for analysis purposes.

Videotaping has been suggested as a way to address some of the limitations of participant observation. According to Bottorff (1994), three reasons for using videotaping are "when behaviors of interest are of very short duration, the distinctive character of events change moment by moment, or more detailed and precise descriptions of behaviors and/or processes than possible with ordinary participant observation are required" (p. 244). The two advantages of videotape recording are density and permanence (Bottorff, 1994). Density refers to the amount of information that can be simultaneously recorded. Density is significantly higher with videotaping versus participant observation; however, as Bottorff (1994) points out, there are also limitation to this technique. The camera is still only picking up certain events, depending on where it is aimed (so may pick up what's going on in the room, but miss closer facial expressions), microphones may pick up extraneous noises and not the vocalizations of importance, and as with participant observation, behaviors may change because of the camera. Permanence refers to the ability to have the event on tape which allows the researcher to review the event as often as needed and demonstrate the analysis to others. Having a videotape of an event definitely increases data validity and reliability; however, the inability to have data beyond the tape (similar to complete observer) is always present. So as different hypotheses are developed, unless data collection is ongoing, testing will not be possible. Thus, other forms of data collection used along with videotaping are encouraged.

Techniques for Data Collection

One of the most common mistakes made by researchers is not using the appropriate techniques for data collection to adequately investigate the research topic of interest. In order to have valid data that truly reflects reality, multiple sources of data are usually required. Simply interviewing participants may only give a partial picture, since they may not be able to relay the whole story (there are many things that are done unconsciously, so cannot be easily verbalized). Thus, in many instances, participant observation and other sources of data such as medical records are also needed. There are, however, other times when the researcher is interested solely in past experiences, and participant observation is not needed and would provide useless data. Another common error is the use of group interviews or focus groups when in-depth individual interviews are needed to sufficiently explore the topic. And finally, the use of wrong interview structure can pose a serious threat to validity and reliability. Using semistructured or structured interviews too early in a research study when little information is known about the phenomenon of interest can result in the true phenomenon not emerging. Many times the researcher develops a list of structured interview questions that presuppose which concepts are of importance to the participant, thus not allowing them to emerge from the data. On the other hand, if the research is at the point of hypothesis testing and beginning theory development, unstructured interviews will not provide the data needed for this to occur.

DATA ANALYSIS

During the process of data analysis there also are numerous places where threats to validity and reliability can occur. But before data analysis is discussed, data quality needs to be addressed. Of number one importance to data quality is the accuracy of the transcribed interviews and field notes. Accuracy of the data set is the responsibility of the researcher. Each transcribed piece of data needs to be checked for accuracy, since simple things like inaccurate punctuation or a mistyped word can change the entire meaning (Easton, McComish, & Greenberg, 2000). In addition, the researcher needs to fill-in gaps in the transcription (spots where the typist could not understand or hear the tape). The researcher who actually performed the interview is the best person to do this since he/she may be able to reconstruct what was said.

There are areas that researchers should consider when having interviews transcribed. These include which features of the interview are important and need to be part of the transcript and which ones can be ignored (Sandelowski, 1994). For example, how will emotional expression be described? Are pauses important and how will you and the typist determine how to document them? And, does every "uh huh" need to be included? Each of these decisions should be made based on the overall purpose of the research and the method chosen for the study.

The validity and reliability of a study is integrally tied to the process of data analysis. The findings and conclusions of a study need to be cohesively linked to the data. There are key areas that should be addressed during the planning stage of a research project so that validity and reliability will not be compromised once analysis begins. First, the choice of type of analysis needs to match the overall purpose of the study, the methods chosen, and the type of data collected. Thus, a constant comparative analysis will not work for a focus-group study, but is the technique of choice for a grounded theory. Content analysis is appropriate if every participant is asked and responds to the same question. However, if unstructured, open-ended interviews are done, counting the amount of times a word or phrase is used would not work. Second, preplanning how model verification, coding checks, and audit trails are to be conducted will make the process proceed smoothly. Finally, assembling a team to assist with the analysis will help address researcher bias (especially if the team is not all nurses or at least not all nurses from the same specialty area).

Problems that frequently come up during analysis include premature closure of analysis and development of categories/models. Here, either researcher bias comes into play or the researcher observes a pattern of some type early in the analysis process and decides "this is it". When this occurs, data are inaccurately placed into categories (here the researcher begins to work deductively instead of inductively), thus when the real pattern or categories appear they are missed. For a beginning researcher, working with an experienced qualitative researcher and/or a research team should prevent this from occurring. The research team needs to independently code the data and then compare codes and developing categories. Areas of incongruence need to be discussed using specific examples from the data set. If incongruencies continue, further data collection may be needed to examine each area. The experienced researcher should be able to question the research team to ensure that the categories or conclusions are grounded in the data and ask the "what about" questions. The team needs to have rich description from the data to support developing categories to answer questions, such as "You say that this works for situation x, what about in situation y?" (e.g., once trust is established, wives of critically ill patients are able to relinquish care to the nursing staff, does the same hold true for parents?). This back and forth and potential verification with the original participants or secondary informants will help to strengthen the analysis.

SUMMARY

Validity and reliability are important issues to consider when doing a qualitative study. These issues are intertwined and threat to one will result in threats to the other. In order for a qualitative study to be useable and to help advance nursing science, qualitative researchers can no longer avoid these issues. Validity and reliability need to be addressed during the initial project planning, sampling procedures, data collection, and data analysis.

REFERENCES

Bottorff, J. L. (1994). Using videotaped recordings in qualitative research. In J. Morse

(Ed.), *Critical issues in qualitative research* (pp. 224–261). Newbury Park: Sage.

Creswell, J. W. (1998). *Qualitative inquiry and research design: Choosing among five traditions.* Thousand Oaks, CA: Sage.

Easton, K. L., McComish, J. F., & Greenberg, R. (2000). Avoiding common pitfalls in qualitative data collection and transcription. *Qualitative Health Research, 10*(5), 703–706.

Esposito, N. (2001). From meaning to meaning: The influence of translation techniques on non-English focus group research. In J. M. Morse (Ed.), *Qualitative health research: Vol. 11. Meaning and interpretation* (pp. 568–579). Thousand Oaks, CA: Sage.

Fetterman, D. M. (1989). *Ethnography step by step.* Thousand Oaks, CA: Sage.

Fontana, A., & Frey, J. H. (2000). The interview from structured questions to negotiated text. In N. K. Denzin & Y. S. Lincoln (Eds.), *Handbook of qualitative research* (2nd ed.) (pp. 645–672). Thousand Oaks, CA: Sage.

Frank, A. W. (1995). *The wounded storyteller: Body, illness, and ethics.* Chicago: The University of Chicago Press.

Glaser, B. G. (1978). *Advances in the methodology of grounded theory theoretical sensitivity.* Mill Valley, CA. The Sociology Press.

Glaser, B. G. (1992). *Emergence vs. forcing: Basics of grounded theory analysis.* Mill Valley, CA: Sociology Press.

Glaser, B. G., & Strauss, A. L. (1967). *The discovery of grounded theory: Strategies for qualitative research.* Chicago: Aldine Publishing Co.

Hupcey, J. E., & Penrod, J. (2003). Concept advancement: Enhancing inductive validity. *Research and Theory for Nursing Practice: An International Journal, 17*(1), 19–30.

Jorgensen, D. L. (1989). Participant Observation: A methodology for human studies. In L. Bickman & D. J. Rog (Eds.), *Applied social research methods series* (vol. 15). Newbury Park, London: Sage.

LeCompte, M. D., & Goetz, J. P. (1982, Spring). Problems of reliability and validity in ethnographic research. *Review of Educational Research, 52*(1), 31–60.

Maxwell, J. A. (1992). Understanding and validity in qualitative research. *Harvard Educational Review, 62*(Fall), 279–300.

Miles, M. B., & Huberman, A. M. (1994). *An expanded sourcebook: Qualitative data analysis* (2nd ed.). Thousand Oaks, CA: Sage Publications.

Morgan, D. L. (1997). *Focus groups as qualitative research* (2nd ed.). Thousand Oaks, CA: Sage.

Morgan, D. L. (1998). *Planning focus groups.* Thousand Oaks, CA: Sage.

Morse, J. M. (1994). Designing funded qualitative research. In N. K. Denzin, & Y. S. Lincoln (Eds.), *Handbook of qualitative inquiry* (pp. 236–256). Thousand Oaks, CA: Sage.

Morse, J. M. (1997). Considering theory derived from qualitative research. In J. M. Morse (Ed.), *Completing a qualitative project: Details and dialogue* (pp. 163–189). Thousand Oaks, CA: Sage.

Morse, J. M. (1998). What's wrong with random selection? *Qualitative Health Research, 8*(6), 733–735.

Morse, J. M. (1999a). Myth #93: Reliability and validity are not relevant to qualitative inquiry. *Qualitative Health Research, 9*(6), 717–718.

Morse, J. M. (1999b). Qualitative generalizability. *Qualitative Health Research, 9*(1), 5–6.

Morse, J. M., & Field, P. A. (1995). *Qualitative research methods for health professionals* (2nd ed.). Thousand Oaks, CA: Sage.

Munhall, P. L. (1994). *Revisioning phenomenology: Nursing and health science research.* New York: National League for Nursing Press.

National Institute of Mental Health (NIMH). (2001). *Qualitative methods in health research: Opportunities and considerations in applications and review* (NIH Publication No. 02-5046). Available at: http://obssr.od.nih/gov/Publications/Qualitative.PDF

Polit, D. F., & Beck, C. T. (2004). *Nursing research: Principles and methods* (7th ed.). Philadelphia: Lippincott Williams & Wilkens.

Riessman, C. K. (1993). *Narrative analysis.* Thousand Oaks, CA: Sage.

Sandelowski, M. (1994). Focus on qualitative methods: Notes on transcription. *Research in Nursing & Health, 17*(4), 311–314.

Sandelowski, M. (1995). Sample size in qualitative research. *Research in Nursing & Health, 18*(2), 179–183.

Strauss, A., & Corbin, J. (1998). *Basics of qualitative research: Techniques and procedures for developing grounded theory* (2nd Ed.). Thousand Oaks, CA: Sage.

Twinn, S. (1997). An exploratory study examining the influence of translation on the validity and reliability of qualitative data in nursing research. *Journal of Advanced Nursing, 26*(2), 418–423.

Van Manen, M. (1990). *Researching lived experience: Human science for an action sensitive pedagogy.* London: The State University of New York.

Yin, R. K., (1994). *Case study research, design and methods* (2nd ed.). Thousand Oaks, CA: Sage.

Part III

Methods and Instruments for Collecting Data

9

Observational Methods

The events and objects in a person's life are observed daily, and these observations are used to help form opinions, attitudes, and beliefs, and to make decisions. However, in the scientific sense, observation is not a causal matter. Observation is a process whereby data are gathered through the senses in a systematic manner. It involves identifying and recording units of behavior or characteristics occurring in a concrete situation that are consistent with empirical aims of the observer. Behaviors may be observed in naturalistic settings, or observations may be made of experimentally induced behaviors.

In nursing, observations are made of specific events or the behaviors of individuals, and may be used as an alternative to self-reports (Polit & Beck, 2004). Measurement through the use of observations is most prevalent in qualitative research, but is also used in most types of research studies (Burns & Grove, 2001). Observational methods are particularly useful when measurements are taken with noncommunicative subjects, such as with newborns or young children (Lobo, 1992), or with patients who are comatose or whose cognitive functioning may be compromised (Flannery, 2003). Observational measures are also useful in the assessment of physiological phenomena (Dunbar & Farr, 1996) such as the assessment of pressure sores, or other patient behaviors such as in Alzheimer's patients (Sutherland, Reakes, & Bridges, 1999). Most observations are concerned with collecting data about behavior. Behaviors observed include the interactions, communications, activities, and performance of living organisms in various situations. Although behavior is frequently the central focus of observation, environmental surroundings as well as the conditions and characteristics of the individual or event may

be observed. Observational methods may be used in a laboratory or in natural or field settings, and by nurse educators and researchers on a daily basis. Nurses make observations in clinical settings. The nurse may want to observe clients' physical conditions via observations of breath sounds, skin turgor, visual acuity, or other observable signs. Such physiologic characteristics of clients are either directly observed through the senses or aided by equipment such as stethoscopes, x-rays, and other devices. The nurse educator uses observations to ascertain the skill attainment of students in the clinical setting, often aided by rating scales or checklists for recording observations. Observational methods can be employed by the nurse researcher to collect data for the measurement of clinical variables under study, such as behaviors of mothers and infants, communication patterns in clinical settings between practitioners, or mothers' behavioral responses to the attachment behaviors of their infants.

Observations can be conducted either directly by an observer who perceives and records the phenomenon of interest, or indirectly through observing the products of behavior and by collecting reports of behavior with interviews or questionnaires. Direct observation includes rating on-site perceptions and the use of audio and video recording devices, which serve as the basis for making observational rating records. Products of behavior include archive data and physical traces. Examples of archive data sources are records of births, deaths, morbidity, hospital records, and other documents such as newspapers (Tuchman, 1994). Physical traces refer to deposits or erosion of environmental materials that reflect behavior, such as the number of cigarette butts left in a patient's ashtray as a measure of smoking behavior, and the number of pieces of incoming mail as a measure of the extent to which a psychiatric patient had contact with the community. This discussion is concerned only with direct observation as an approach to data collection.

OBSERVER ROLES

There are two observer roles that may be assumed: nonparticipant and participant. The *nonparticipant observer* attempts to adopt a completely passive role while observing phenomena of interest. The goal of the nonparticipant observer is to become an unobtrusive bystander who does not intervene in the phenomenon that is the focus of study while observing and recording information (Polit & Beck, 2004). Hence, the nonparticipant observer simply observes the situation without intentionally influencing the activities and behaviors under study.

Nonparticipant observers may either conceal their role or make no attempt to make observations covertly. Concealment of the observer role may be done to reduce the impact of the observer's presence on the behaviors of interest, because individuals may alter their behavior if they are aware of being monitored. When behavioral distortions occur due to the presence of an observer, this is known as reactivity or reactive measurement effects (Polit & Beck, 2004). A concern associated with concealment of the observer role is the ethics of observing and recording the behavior of individuals without their knowledge.

Participant observers try to become acceptable actors within the activity structure of the group under study. The observer becomes an intimate participant in the experiences of those being studied. An attempt is made to view the world of the subjects from their perspective by taking a flexible and relativistic stance. This demands that the participant observer respect and be sensitive to the subjects' style of dress and modes of gesturing and learn their language.

To immerse themselves in the experiences of their subjects, participant observers use several approaches to reveal all of the relevant aspects of the phenomenon studied. Direct participation in the activities of the subjects is attempted, introspection regarding experiences is used, interviews are conducted, and documents are collected and analyzed when available and direct observation is employed. The participant observer's role may be concealed or revealed to subjects; however, in most cases no attempt is made to conceal the observer's role. Identification of the observer has the advantage of allowing for probing and the elicitation of data that would not be readily available to the concealed observer.

Subject reactivity is perhaps the greatest overall limitation when either the nonparticipant or participant observer approach is used. Responses of subjects have been shown to differ markedly, even in naturalistic situations, when persons are aware that assessments are being made of their behaviors (Atkinson & Hammersley, 1994). The presence of observers may not necessarily influence the behavior of subjects directly but may provide cues to others in the setting who can influence the subjects' behaviors. For example, parents can influence observational data that are obtained on their children.

Some investigators use recording devices such as tape recorders, audiotapes, and still and motion photography to aid observations. Subjects also are reactive to these devices and have been found to respond differently, depending upon whether they knew that recordings were being made or not (Lisovski, 1989).

To reduce subject reactivity, observations should be made as unobtrusively as possible. Several techniques may be employed to reduce reactivity. Whenever possible, continuous direct observation should not be employed. Observations of many phenomena can be made intermittently without negatively affecting the integrity of the data obtained. Observers can be instructed to restrict their observations to a prescribed number of seconds—for example, 10 seconds—and then to look away from the subject. Also, the interval between observations would be specified. Looking at, and then looking away, from the subject reduces reactivity, since the persons observed do not feel that all of their activities are being constantly monitored. This approach will not be useful in situations in which continuous observations are required, such as in the study of some behavioral interactions.

Subjects usually will habituate to an observer's presence after about 10 minutes. Therefore, observers should be in the setting for at least 10 minutes before actual data collection begins. During the preliminary period, observer behaviors should be consistent with those that will be displayed during the observational period. A change in the observer's behavior at any point during the observational period increases the subject's reactivity. Hence, the observer should remain constant in appearance, activity, and smell. Physical movement should be minimized as much as possible, no perfume should be worn, and jewelry should be appropriate for the situation. As much as possible, the observer's clothing and style of dress should be consistent with those worn by subjects in the observational situation. For example, a researcher observing the behaviors of low-income mothers should not wear expensive clothing and jewelry within the observational setting. Whenever the observer is required to leave and reenter an observational setting (e.g., when observations are made over several days or weeks), no major changes in clothing or hairstyle should be made. In most observational situations, clothing should be plain and, whenever possible, the same or a similar style of clothes should be worn during each observational period.

OBSERVING AND RECORDING

The selection of phenomena to be observed depends upon the clinical, educational or research problem that is the focus of investigation. Even after the problem has been specified, there often is a need to further delineate and select the phenomena to be observed. For example, the Clinical Performance Examination for Critical Care Nurses (Mims, 2001) is an observational rating scale developed to measure clinical performance of nurses employed in critical care settings. The tool is composed of five categories of behaviors important in clinical performance of critical care nurses: assessment, clinical/technical skill, communication, documentation, and general employment policies.

Theses categories must be rated by an observer in order to obtain a measure of clinical performance of a nurse in a critical care setting.

When selecting phenomena to be observed, decisions must be made concerning what constitutes a unit. Units of observation range from small and specific behaviors (molecular approach), to large units of behavior (molar approach). The molecular approach might, for example, require recordings of each movement, gesture, phrase, or action, and each of these may be broken down into smaller units. In the molar approach a large unit of behavior, such as seeking help, may consist of a variety of verbal and nonverbal actions that together are construed as signaling the behavior of interest. The molecular approach has the potential disadvantage of causing the investigator to lose sight of a related composite of behaviors that are central to the study at hand. The molar approach has the potential problem of allowing for distortions and errors by the observer because of the likelihood of ambiguity in the definition of units (Polit & Beck, 2004). The approach to selecting units of observation largely depends on the investigator and the purpose for which observations are to be made.

SELECTING SAMPLES

When observational methods are employed, the approach to sampling and data collection will depend upon the problem that is studied, how variables are defined and operationalized, and the setting in which observations are to be made. Decisions about sampling and data collection will directly influence the reliability and validity of results as well as their general application.

Sampling requires the observer to follow specific rules which dictate the nature of the situation to be observed such that the observer is able to record or elicit a set of behaviors which are presumed to have some degree of relevance for addressing a specific concept, hypothesis, proposition, or theory. These rules delineate a procedure that must be followed so that the general application and theoretical relevance of the behaviors to be observed or elicited are increased. The observer may take note of one situation or a series of situations. The investigator draws the sample from a large population of behaviors, social situations, or events, or a small number for intensive observation. Before beginning to sample, the investigator must be able to enumerate the specific units that make up the larger population. This implies that the investigator has a clear definition of the population to which findings are to be generalized. If, for example, one is studying the role and functions of nurses who work in acute care settings, a workable operational definition of acute care settings must be formulated. Depending upon the theoretical intentions of the investigation, an acute care work setting may be operationalized to include all types of units traditionally found in general hospitals, or it may be limited to medical and surgical units. An operational definition of nurse also is required.

After the operational definition of the population under study has been specified, the investigator develops a complete list of all the elements that make up the population. In the example cited previously, this listing would be all of the acute care work settings in the geographical area that is to be sampled. Once the population has been defined and specified, then the investigator *randomly* selects units from that population to be included in the sample for observation. *Random sampling* gives each unit in the population the same chance of inclusion in the final set of observations. Several approaches to random sampling might be employed. Other approaches to sampling may be used, such as cluster sampling and stratified random sampling, described in Polit and Beck (2004).

It should be noted that the sampling process employed in observational approaches most often is multistage. The sampling procedure frequently is constrained by time and place, that is, by a specific time and by a specific geographical locality.

TIME SAMPLING

For some investigations, there may be a need to observe a behavior or activity that occurs continuously over several days, weeks, or months. When this is the case, it is not likely that an observer will be able to monitor the phenomenon of interest continuously. Time sampling can be used to select from the population of times those segments during which observations will be made. The time segments are selected randomly and may be parts of an hour, a day, or a shift, for example. Time segments selected will largely be determined by the focus of the investigation. If mother-infant interactions during feedings are to be studied, it is possible that the times chosen for observation might be for one minute every 5 minutes. If a play-therapy hour for a young child is to be observed, the time segments selected might be the first 10 minutes, the middle 10 minutes, and the last 10 minutes of the hour session.

The observer should consider rhythmicity of phenomena whenever time sampling is used. Certain activities or phenomena may occur on a specific time schedule, or phenomena may be quite different depending upon the time at which observations are made, such as with the administration of medications or treatments. Time of day of the observation may also be important. For example, a nurse researcher studying confusion in the elderly must consider the possibility that late afternoon and evening observations are more likely to reflect higher levels of confusion than observations taken during the morning hours after a restful night of sleep. Depending upon the purpose of the observations, the rhythmicity of phenomena may have a significant impact on the data. For example, data collected about the frequency of nurse-patient interaction on an acute care unit could be quite different from the usual if observations were made only during weekends, when the nurse-to-patient ratio might be lower than usual, or confined to times when medications or treatments were administered and nurse-patient interaction might be higher than usual. With such observations, *random time sampling* becomes particularly important.

EVENT SAMPLING

An alternative approach to time sampling, event sampling may be employed in situations in which events of interest occur relatively infrequently and are at risk of being missed if a strict time sampling procedure is used. In event sampling, integral events or behaviors are specified for observation. The observer must be in a position to take advantage of specific events; therefore, an awareness of the occurrence of the relevant events or behaviors is needed. For example, if an observer is recording the roles and functions of nurses in acute care settings, several events may be selected for observation, for example, change of shift, nursing rounds, care of a dying patient, or nurse-physician interactions. Observation of such events would be likely to provide the observer with data that would not be obtained if a time-sampling procedure were used. Time sampling and event sampling are the most commonly used approaches for selecting observations.

OBSERVATIONAL APPROACHES

There are two basic approaches to the collection of data through observation: structured and unstructured. The structured approach is more amenable to use by the nonparticipant observer, while the participant observer uses the unstructured approach more frequently. Structured *observational* approaches specify behaviors or events for observation in a rather detailed manner, and a protocol for observing and record keeping is delineated in advance. Since structured observations are highly dependent upon the protocol and observational aids developed prior to observations, the kinds of phenomena observed are likely to be restrained. Checklists and rating scales are the most frequently used observational aids employed. Checklists facilitate the classification or categorization of behaviors or characteristics observed. Each categorical system is designed to guide the observer in assigning qualitative phenomena into either a quantitative or qualitative system. Well-developed categorical systems facilitate accurate notation of phenomena within a common frame of reference. In most instances, checklists are devised to prompt the observer to record the absence or presence of a behavior or event; however, the frequency of occurrence may be recorded. The

categorical systems of checklists used in observation should be nonoverlapping, mutually exclusive, and exhaustive.

Rating scales require that the observer classify behaviors or events in terms of points along a descriptive continuum. Observers may use rating scales during direct observations, or the observer may use rating scales to summarize an interaction or event after observation is completed. Rating scales are employed to record quantitative aspects of the phenomenon of interest, such as its intensity or magnitude, and thereby extend category systems beyond those generally found in checklists. For example, Pressler, Hepworth, Applebaum, Sevcik, and Hoffman (1998) used a rating scale format in their adapted scoring of the Neonatal Behavioral Assessment Scale (Brazelton & Nugent, 1995) during their assessment of reflex responses in newborns. Although rating scales are designed to generate more information about the behavior or event observed, immense demands are placed on the observer when the activity level of objects observed is high. In such instances, the use of recording devices can facilitate observation. Recording devices such as video recorders have the advantages of allowing the observer the opportunity to record behaviors frame by frame and review recordings later, particularly for interrater and intrarater reliability assessment of observer ratings.

Unstructured observational approaches involve the collection of large amounts of qualitative information that describe the object, event, or group being observed. There is no specific protocol for observations, nor are specific approaches to observing phenomena delineated. Hence, there are few restrictions on the types of methods used and on the types of data obtained. Interviews, life histories, visits, attendance at social events, and record review may be employed, as well as other appropriate strategies for data collection.

Logs and *field notes* are the most common methods of record keeping; employed with unstructured observations. However, observational aids such as tape recordings, maps, and photographs also may be used. A log is a record of observations of events, objects, or conversations, which is usually kept on a regular basis during the time that the observer is in the observational setting. Field notes are more inclusive than logs and tend to extend observations by analysis and interpretation of relevant occurrences. Use of field notes is a method that combines data collection and data analysis.

Unstructured observation is very useful in exploratory investigations in which the identification and conceptualization of important variables are desired. This approach is flexible and allows the observer to obtain a more complete understanding of the complexities of the situation at hand. Proponents of unstructured observation point out that this approach allows for a better conceptualization of a problem. However, this approach to observation is more highly dependent upon the interpersonal and observational skills of the observer than structured observations. Two major concerns associated with employment of unstructured observation are observer bias and observer influence on the phenomenon that is observed.

RELIABILITY AND VALIDITY OF OBSERVATIONS

When structured observational approaches are used, the reliability and validity of observations depend upon the reliability and validity inherent in the observational aids and in the ability of the observer to identify and record the specified behaviors or events. Thus, the use of well constructed, well-developed observational instruments and well-trained observers takes on special significance. Care should be taken to select reliable and valid observational aids, and observers should be trained prior to the initiation of data collection.

Observer training sessions should be held to familiarize observers with instruments, the nature of behaviors or events observed, the sampling procedure, and the purpose of the project. Trial experience in the use of instruments should be provided until observers have sufficiently mastered the art of observing and recording the phenomenon of interest. If more than one observer is employed, training should continue until there is sufficient interrater reliability. During research studies in which observational

data are collected over several months or years, frequent assessment of interrater and intrarater reliability should be done due to the possibility of observer drift over time. It is not unusual for observers to make subtle unconscious changes in how they rate categories of behavior. When this occurs, the reliability of observation data decreases over time and retraining of observers may be required.

Reliability and validity of unstructured approaches can be facilitated and assessed through the process of triangulation that is discussed in chapter 12. Triangulation involves combining the use of two or more theories, methods, data sources, investigators, or analysis methods in the study of the same phenomenon (Morse, 1991; Sandelowski, 1996). Data triangulation in particular can be particularly useful in this regard. This approach involves the collection of data from multiple sources for the same study or purpose. Such data would need to have the same foci since the various sources of data are intended to obtain diverse views of the phenomenon under study for the purposes of validation. The reliability and validity of findings are evaluated by ascertaining the frequency of an observation by examining data obtained from multiple methods and multiple data sources. The more frequently an observed behavior occurs across time and space, the more likely it will be valid. The lack of multiple instances of observation detracts from the validity of an indicator. Frequency of occurrence of a phenomenon should be observed across subjects over and over again within the same individual. Comparing records from different data sources, for example, interviews, diaries, or other documents, can assess validity of indicators. An indicator that results from an unstructured observation can also be assessed by the observability of behaviors or activities on which it is based. Less credence can be placed on those indicators that result from the observer's imputation of motives, attitudes, or intentions to others.

Lincoln and Guba (1985) suggest the use of member checking to improve the trustworthiness of data and interpretations during naturalistic observation. Member checking involves testing analytic hypotheses, interpretations of data, and conclusions with the subjects from which data were generated. This approach allows subjects to assist the observer in making sense, of the data and subjects are given an opportunity to respond to and assist in the interpretation of the data by getting their feedback regarding the observations made (Connors, 1988; Emerson, 1987).

ADVANTAGES AND DISADVANTAGES OF OBSERVATIONAL METHODS

Several advantages and disadvantages of observation have been addressed during the discussion. This section will serve to highlight some of the major benefits and problems associated with observational approaches. Observation provides a variety, depth, and breadth of information to research that is difficult to obtain with other data-collection methods (Morse & Field, 1995). The approach can be quite flexible and allow an observer to get inside a situation in a manner that can reveal information not readily obtained by other methods. Hence, observational approaches can effectively facilitate and enhance conceptualization and understanding of phenomena. This approach is of particular benefit, because there are many problems that cannot be studied sufficiently by other means. While observational techniques enhance information obtained considerably, observations are often time consuming and costly. Therefore, an investigator needs to carefully weigh the advantages and disadvantages of observation and justify that its advantages outweigh its costs (Morse & Field, 1995).

The major disadvantage of observational approaches is that data obtained through observation are readily amenable to bias and distortion. Perceptual errors by observers and insufficient skill in observing threaten the quality of data. This is less of a problem when the structured approach to observation is used rather than the unstructured. When the observer's presence is known, reactivity to the observer by subjects may distort behavior. However, concealment of the observer's presence or identity presents ethical concerns regarding the subject's consent to be observed. Concealment of observer

identity also can limit the depth and amount of data obtained. The structured approach provides for better control of reliability and validity of measurements than the unstructured approach; however, it limits the kinds of phenomena that will be monitored and recorded. The unstructured approach provides for a large variety of data sources and data collection methods, but reliability and validity of measures are difficult to assess and control.

The problems and difficulties associated with observational methods need not be prohibitive. A clear conceptualization of the problem to be studied, operationalization of key variables, and a logical protocol for observing, recording, and interpreting data can help alleviate or decrease a number of concerns.

ETHICAL ISSUES

Some of the features of observational research make it prone to ethical malpractice. Observations can be done in a rather inconspicuous manner, and observers can easily gather data without the knowledge of the public and without their consent, such as the observation of child behavior in public parks during disguised or covert research. This also applies to misrepresentation by a researcher of his or her identity during the data collection process. Questions have also been raised about areas of life where it may not be ethical to make observations at all. Some scientists question whether observations should be made of suicides, sexual encounters, and other socially sensitive behaviors in private places (Adler & Adler, 1994).

REFERENCES

Adler, P. A., & Aldler, P. (1994). Observational techniques. In N. K. Denzin & Y. S. Lincoln (Eds.), *Handbook of qualitative research* (pp. 377–392). Thousand Oaks, CA: Sage.

Atkinson, P., & Hammersley, M. (1994). Ethnography and participant observation. In N. K. Denzin & Y. S. Lincoln (Eds.), *Handbook of qualitative research* (pp. 248–261). Thousand Oaks, CA: Sage.

Brazelton, T. B., & Nugent, J. K. (1995). *Neonatal behavioral assessment scale* (3rd ed.). London: MacKeith Press.

Burns, N., & Grove, S. K. (2001). *The practice of nursing research: Conduct, critique, & utilization.* Philadelphia: W. B. Saunders Company.

Connors, D. D. (1988). A continuum of researcher-participant relationships: An analysis and critique. *Advances in Nursing Science, 10*(4), 32–42.

Dunbar, S. B., & Farr, L. (1996). Temporal patterns of heart rate and blood pressure in elders. *Nursing Research, 45*(1), 43–49.

Emerson, R. M. (1987). Four ways to improve the craft of fieldwork. *Journal of Contemporary Ethnography, 16*(1), 69–89.

Flannery, J. (2003). The Levels of Cognitive Functioning Assessment Scale. In O. L. Strickland & C. DiIorio (Eds.), *Measurement of nursing outcomes* (2nd ed.), (vol. 2, pp. 34–56). New York: Springer Publishing.

Lincoln, Y. S., & Guba, E. G. (1985). *Naturalistic inquiry.* Beverly Hills, CA: Sage Publications.

Lisovski, M. (1989). In search of the tantrum: The making of the Early Childhood STEP video. *Effective Parenting, 7*(2), 1, 8.

Lobo, M. L. (1992). Observation: A valuable data collection strategy for research with children. *Journal of Pediatric Nursing, 7*(5), 320–328.

Mims, B. C. (2001). Clinical performance examination of critical care nurses. In C. F. Waltz & L. S. Jenkins, *Measurement of nursing outcomes* (2nd ed.), (vol. 1, pp. 120–129). New York: Springer Publishing.

Morse, J. M. (1991). Approaches to qualitative-quantitative methodological triangulation. *Nursing Research, 40*(2), 120–122.

Morse, J. M., & Field, P. A. (1995). *Qualitative research methods for health professionals* (2nd ed.). Thousand Oaks, CA: Sage.

Polit, D., & Beck, C. T. (2004). *Nursing research: Principles and methods* (7th ed.). Philadelphia: JB Lippincott.

Pressler, J. L., Hepworth, J. T., Applebaum, M. I., Sevcik, R. H., & Hoffman, E. L. (1998). A comparison of newborns' NBAS reflex responses using total and individual scores. *Journal of Nursing Measurement, 6*(2), 123–136.

Sandelowski, M. (1996). Using qualitative methods in intervention studies. *Research in Nursing and Health, 19*(4), 359–364.

Sutherland, J. A., Reakes, J., & Bridges, C. (1999). Clinical scholarship abstract. Foot acupuncture and massage for patients with Alzheimer's disease and related dementias. *Image—Journal of Nursing Scholarship, 31*(4), 347–348.

Tuchman, G. (1994). Historical social science: Methodologies, methods, and meanings. In N. K. Denzin & Y. S. Lincoln (Eds.), *Handbook of qualitative research* (pp. 306–323). Thousand Oaks, CA: Sage.

10

Content Analysis

Recorded words and sentences are human artifacts that provide rich data about the personalities, thoughts, and attitudes of their writers (or speakers), as well as extensive information about their interpersonal, social, political, and cultural contexts. Because it provides an approach to accessing the information in a variety of different data sources in a way that is more systematic and objective than intuitive reading or listening, and because of its central position as a data analysis strategy of choice in qualitative research, content analysis is attracting renewed attention as a measurement strategy for nursing research.

Content analysis refers to the set of techniques that are used to identify patterns, categories, and/or themes in recorded language. As used in quantitative research, content analysis involves the systematic and objective reduction or simplification of recorded language to a set of categories that represent the presence, frequency, intensity, or meaning of selected characteristics. It is used for identifying, measuring, describing, and making inferences about specified characteristics within or reflected by written or verbal text. Three key interrelated processes are involved: conceptualizing and identifying characteristics of the content that are to be measured; determining the measures and explicit rules for identifying, coding, and recording the characteristics; and sampling, coding, and tabulating (or otherwise describing) the units (Neuendorf, 2002).

The term content analysis is used to describe both inductive, theory-building techniques (wherein categories for describing data evolve during the analysis), and deductive, theory-testing techniques (wherein theory-based categorical schemes developed before conducting the analysis are used to analyze data from subjects or documents). Inductive approaches to content analysis focus on developing the categories and interpretation as closely as possible to the recorded (printed or verbal) material. As the material is reviewed and analyzed, tentative categories are generated. With the analysis of more material, categories are revised and a final set is determined (Mayring, 2000). Deductive approaches use theoretically derived categories and coding rules. These are applied and revised as necessary. Both inductive and deductive approaches to content analysis can be used in both qualitative and quantitative research.

Content analysis has several distinctive features that make it a useful measurement technique for nursing research, education, and practice. First, it is applied to recorded information, that is, information written as text or recorded in a way that allows exact replay of the original communication. Either preexisting materials that have been written or recorded for another purpose or materials produced for a particular investigation can be used. Examples of materials that can be content analyzed include books, plays, newspaper articles, editorials, films, letters, notes, diaries or other personal documents, speeches, documents such as laws or minutes of meetings, written or tape-recorded responses of subjects to questions, and audiotaped or videotaped recordings of communication. Materials originally produced for a variety of different purposes can be content analyzed to answer questions relevant to nursing and to add richness of meaning to nursing knowledge development.

Second, emphasis is on the content of the written or verbal communication rather than its process or paralingual features (e.g., pitch, volume, rate, accompanying gestures). This is not to negate the importance of process or paralingual elements but to suggest that the procedures of content analysis are best suited to a content focus. Paralingual cues can be adequately analyzed only if they are consistently noted in textual form. Such notations are sometimes present in carefully recorded field notes of qualitative researchers and in some legal proceedings, but are rarely found in documents recorded for other purposes. Process analysis represents a different focus, which is best handled using other tools and techniques designed specifically for that purpose, for example, Bales' Interaction Process Analysis. However, inferences about historical trends and cultural differences can be made by comparing content expressed at different times or by different communicators. The analysis of materials can be directed toward either the manifest (overtly expressed) content of the communication or its latent (unintentionally or unconsciously expressed) content. The analysis of latent content is difficult and somewhat risky, because it requires making inferences about what was intended or meant from that which was actually stated and is analogous to "reading between the lines."

Third, the procedure of content analysis—specifically quantitative content analysis—is designed to achieve relative objectivity by incorporating explicit rules and systematic procedures. The procedure is systematic, in that specified criteria are consistently applied in selecting and processing the content to be analyzed. It is not arbitrary.

Fourth, content analysis involves deliberate simplification or reduction that results in the loss of some of the individuality and richness of meaning in the original material in the interest of discerning regularities, patterns, and themes. The degree to which the material is simplified and the nature of the regularities discerned are determined by the purpose for the analysis and are not inherent in the procedure itself. Finally, content analysis is unobtrusive and can provide insight into complex interactions. It has been used in many disciplines as a research tool.

The earliest applications were in the fields of journalism and political science in studies of the mass media and propaganda, and in anthropological field studies to categorize observational

and interview data. More recent applications have ranged widely from studies of personality and psychological states of individuals to communication patterns within small groups and organizations, comparative cross-cultural studies, and studies of historical trends and social change. Because content analysis can be successfully applied to many types of recorded information, its potential uses in nursing are many. The most frequently cited examples are research oriented and include studies of trends in the profession (e.g., McEwen, 2004), characteristics, opinions, and expressed values of individuals and groups (e.g., Geiger-Brown et al., 2004, Winslow, 2003; Bucknall, 2003); the impact of policy on health care; and current issues and trends (e.g., Kirchoff, Beckstrand, & Anumandla, 2003); and evaluation of the effectiveness of interventions or programs. Content analysis can also be used during the preliminary stages of developing a quantitative measurement instrument, and as a means for validating other measures of the same concept or characteristic.

PROCEDURE

Content analysis involves a multistep procedure that is guided in all of its aspects by the purpose of the investigation, the questions to be answered, and the hypotheses to be tested. For purposes of this discussion it is assumed that the purposes of the investigation have been identified, the data source of relevant recorded information has been located, and the investigator is ready to proceed with the content analysis. The procedure described below focuses primarily on techniques used in quantitative research. A more detailed description of the techniques and strategies used in qualitative research is found in chapter 8.

Step 1: Define the Universe of Content To Be Examined

The universe of content refers to the totality of recorded information about which characteristics will be described or inferences drawn. Examples would include all presidential addresses at American Nurses Association conventions, all nursing ethics texts published in the past decade, all tape-recorded responses to a telephone interview, or all nurses' notes generated by a medical intensive care unit staff during a given month. The universe of content is chosen based on the nature of the information included, its relevance to the purposes of the investigation, its completeness and ease of access, and the conditions under which the materials were produced. In many instances permission must be secured in advance to use the materials for the proposed investigation.

Step 2: Identify the Characteristics or Concepts To Be Measured

These selections are conceptual decisions, so they vary widely from one investigation to another. This step in the analysis consists essentially of answering the question "What do I want to learn about the content of the recorded information?" It is the initial phase of partitioning or subdividing the content into units and categories. There is no limit to the number of characteristics that can be examined; however, the selection should be dictated by the purpose for the investigation.

Step 3: Select the Unit of Analysis To Be Employed

Given the universe of content available and the variables to be measured, a decision must be made about which elements or subunits of the content will be analyzed or categorized. The selection is based on the type of unit that can be used most reliably as evidence for the presence, frequency, or intensity of the characteristics to be studied. Possible units of analysis range in complexity from letters or syllables—used primarily in linguistic research—to entire speeches or texts. The units most potentially useful in nursing are words, items, phrases, and themes. Words are commonly chosen units for analysis, because they are easy to work with and are amenable to computer analysis. They often have multiple meanings and uses, however. A frequently used procedure is to identify words or word combinations that are synonyms for or indicators of a more abstract concept or

characteristic. Themes are sentences or propositions about something. Because they are more complex than words, they are more difficult to use reliably; however, they may impart more meaning than words taken alone. The term "item" refers to an entire production (e.g., story, book, interview, response to an open-ended question) that is analyzed as a whole in terms of one or more given characteristics.

Depending on the number and complexity of the characteristics being measured, more than one unit of analysis can be used to measure a given characteristic. In some instances a given unit may be appropriate for measuring one characteristic of the content but not another, and several units may be used within the investigation, each for a separate subanalysis.

Careful delineation of the unit to be analyzed or categorized is essential if unitizing reliability is to be achieved. *Unitizing reliability* refers to "consistency in the identification of what is to be categorized across time and/or judges" (Garvin, Kennedy, & Cissna, 1988, p. 52). It requires a clear and clearly communicated specification of what is to be coded. The level of unitizing reliability in a content analysis is influenced by the degree of observer inference needed to identify the unit to be coded, the degree of specificity in delineating units, the exhaustiveness of the coding system, and the type of data. In general, the less inference required, the greater the specificity, the more exhaustive the coding system, and the greater the ability of the data to be examined repeatedly (e.g., taped versus untaped live interviews), the easier it is to establish unitizing reliability.

Step 4: Develop a Sampling Plan

Once the unit of analysis has been identified, it is necessary to determine how the universe of content will be sampled. In some instances the entire universe will be examined. This is generally true when content analysis is being applied inductively to interview data. In others, only selected portions will be analyzed. As noted above, unitizing reliability may be easier to achieve if the entire population of units is categorized. A specific plan must be designed with explicit instructions provided as the basis for selecting the content to be analyzed. If sampling is necessary, then random sampling of elements of the universe of content is preferable to non-random procedures. A frequent procedure is to use systematic random sampling. After a randomly determined starting point every nth unit (word, phrase, paragraph, etc.) is sampled. Multistage sampling may be employed. For example, a random sample of textbooks might be selected from those available; then a random sample of three chapters selected from each book; then content of every third paragraph within those chapters analyzed using the themes within each sampled paragraph as the unit of analysis. In the interview example the nurse might select a 5-minute segment from each recorded interview. A decision would have to be made whether to begin the segment at the same point in all interviews (e.g., the first 5 minutes), or randomly select the starting point for the segment (e.g., determine the starting point by a random process such as using a table of random numbers to select a tape-counter reading at which to initiate the analysis).

Step 5: Develop a Scheme for Categorizing the Content and Explicit Coding and Scoring Instructions

In deductive content analysis this step is largely carried out before the data collection begins. Categories are derived from the theory guiding the investigation before the data are analyzed. The coding scheme includes explicit definitions, coding rules, and examples for each coding category. The scheme may be predetermined, but often must be modified partway through the data analysis to accommodate unanticipated nuances in the data. In the case of computer-assisted content analysis, a set of dictionaries must be established, together with the rules for applying them. Either predeveloped dictionaries can be used, or a unique set can be created for the purpose at hand.

In inductive content analysis codes and categories (and ultimately the more encompassing themes) are generated from the data themselves. The process is one of shuffling and sorting data.

Categories "emerge from the data," hence are not preset. The original categories and themes may be subsumed as more data are gathered and compared with the existing scheme. Mayring (2000) recommends revising categories after 10–50% of the data are analyzed. Procedures and strategies for qualitative content analysis are described in detail by Morse and Field (1995), Krippendorff (2004), Graneheim and Lundman (2004), and Neuendorf (2002). Priest, Roberts, and Woods (2002) discuss and compare qualitative content analysis with grounded theory and narrative analysis as three strategies for the interpretation of qualitative data. Inductive and deductive strategies may be combined in a given study. In either case, the categorical scheme links the theoretical or conceptual background of the investigation with the data and provides the basis for making inferences and drawing conclusions.

Having identified the characteristics to be measured (Step 2), the categorical scheme provides the basis for measuring the existence, frequency, intensity, or nature of each characteristic. The categories are constructed so that each unit of the content can be assigned unequivocally to one category; that is, the categories for a given characteristic must be exhaustive and mutually exclusive, and criteria for assigning the content to a category must be clear and explicit. It is generally recommended that the categories in content analysis be as close as possible semantically to the wording in the original text so the meaning is distorted as little as possible.

Several strategies are suggested to aid in constructing a categorical scheme for content analysis:

1. Carefully read or listen to the available material to develop a sense of the language being used and the divisions into which the data might fall, bearing in mind the conceptual orientation underlying the investigation. A myriad of computer programs exist to assist with this process (see Mayring, 2000; Neuendorf, 2002). Examples of programs that assist with qualitative content analysis include ATLAS/ti (www.atlasti.de), winMAX (www.winmax.de), WordStat (www.simstat.com/wordstat.htm),

The Ethnograph, and NUD*IST (handling Nonverbal Unstructured Data by Indexing, Searching and Theorizing; www.qsr-software.com).

2. Examine existing categorical schemes developed by other content analysts. A number of content dictionaries potentially applicable to nursing have already been developed, and some are available as computer programs. These dictionaries group words with similar meanings under a given conceptual heading. The work of Gottschalk (1995) has produced several reliable and valid categorical schemes for measuring psychological traits through the content analysis of verbal behavior.

3. After developing a set of categories, ask experts in the field of the investigation to evaluate the relevance, clarity, and completeness of the scheme.

4. When developing categories from the data themselves in an inductive approach, avoid premature closure by sharing the categories and their basis with a trial audience. Avoid overly delayed closure by keeping the study's purpose and research questions clearly in mind and collaborating with a group of colleagues.

Step 6: Pretest the Categories and Coding Instructions

If the categorical scheme is predetermined, it is pretested by applying it to small portions of the content to be analyzed. Preferably at least two coders should be asked to analyze the same material so that interrater reliability can be assessed and discrepancies clarified. As a result of the pretesting, categories or instructions may have to be redefined, added, or deleted and the entire scheme pretested again before use.

The advantage of a clearly thought out and well-delineated coding scheme is that it enhances the likelihood that interpretive reliability will be achieved. Interpretive reliability refers to the consistency with which units are categorized and meaning assigned to them (Garvin, Kennedy, & Cissna, 1988), and encompasses both intra- and interrater reliability. Interpretive reliability encompasses both global ("the extent to which coders can consistently use the whole coding system across all categories" [p. 54]) and category-specific (the extent to which coders use a given category with consistency) elements. Both global and category-specific reliabilities are improved by clear coding rules, rigid and exhaustive definitions, structuring the coding task as a series of dichotomous decisions, and coder training.

Step 7: Train Coders and Establish an Acceptable Level of Reliability

Careful coder selection and training is an essential step if persons other than the investigator are to be used to perform the analysis. Neuendorf (2002) recommends that during an initial training session coders' ability to agree on coding of variables be assessed, then they should be asked to code independently in order to assess interrater reliability. They should be asked to discuss any coding decision with which they encountered difficulty or ambiguity. Subjective perception, which is influenced by culture and experience, plays a rule in much content analysis; therefore, it is crucial that explicit instructions be provided and several trial runs be carried out before the actual analysis begins. Interpretive (both inter- and intrarater) reliability must be assessed throughout the training period and acceptable levels established before training ends. In some instances it may be necessary to limit the number of categories and/or coders to maintain acceptable interpretive reliability.

Step 8: Perform the Analysis

The data are coded according to prescribed procedures or subjected to computer-assisted analysis. Each element of the content universe being analyzed (i.e., each document, book, verbal response) is coded using the same procedure. If many content characteristics are being examined, the same content may be processed several times to extract all of the information needed. Because fatigue, boredom, and concurrent experience may influence coding, periodic checks of interrater and intrarater reliability must be performed throughout the coding. It is suggested that at least 10% of the material be coded by more than one individual to allow assessment of interrater reliability. Refresher training may be needed. Because intrarater reliability tends to decline over time, the investigator working alone should periodically reassess it.

In more quantitative applications of content analysis, tabulation of data often involves, as a first step, a frequency count of the recorded or observed occurrences of each category or quality. The nature of subsequent analyses is determined by the purpose of the investigation. Such frequency counts may also be used in analyses that are primarily qualitative.

Computers are increasingly being used in both qualitative and quantitative content analysis. Computer software is extensive and is useful for coding and analyzing data, automatic indexing, text-oriented data retrieval and database management, concordance generation, and idea processing. Automatic data analysis can also be executed through use of software programs that count frequencies of word use, observations, or content categories. Although several published content-category dictionaries exist, it is generally recommended that the researcher create a context-specific dictionary for the particular study. Published dictionaries, however, are efficient and provide standardized classification instruments that can facilitate comparison across studies.

RELIABILITY AND VALIDITY

In content analysis both unitizing reliability (consistency in identifying the unit[s] to be categorized) and interpretive reliability (consistency in assigning units to categories) are important. The former is a precondition for the latter (Garvin, Kennedy, & Cissna, 1988). Both unitizing and interpretive reliability come into play in determining the level of more traditional types of reliability in content analytic schemes and procedures. Stability reliability (assessed by intrarater and test/retest techniques) and reproducibility reliability (assessed by interrater techniques) are both relevant for the content analysis, and require clear delineation of the unit(s) to be categorized and the rules for assigning them to categories. Split-half reliability assessment techniques are not appropriate for content analysis (Krippendorff, 2004).

As applied to content analyses, validity refers to the correspondence of variation inside the process of analysis to variations outside that process, correspondence of findings and conclusions to the data, and generalizability of results. Validity is heavily context dependent. Types of validity include: (1) data-related validity—how well the data analysis method represents the information inherent in the available data; (2) semantic validity—how sensitive the method is to relevant symbolic meanings; (3) sampling validity—degree to which the data are an unbiased sample for a universe of interest; (4) pragmatic validity—how well the method works under various circumstances; (5) predictive validity—agreement of predictions with observed facts; and (6) construct validity (Krippendorff, 2004). Computer-assisted techniques for content analysis enhance reliability but require attention to building in context specificity if validity is to be achieved. For a more thorough discussion of reliability and validity of qualitative content analysis, see chapter 8.

ADVANTAGES AND DISADVANTAGES

Major advantages of content analysis as a data collection and analysis technique include the following:

1. The technique allows use of existing information that is available and easily accessible at relatively low cost. Available information can be used for multiple purposes.
2. Characteristics of individuals and groups can be studied unobtrusively, that is, without requiring subjects to do anything out of the ordinary or even making them aware that they are being studied.
3. Information produced for nonscientific purposes can be made usable for scientific inference.
4. Available data sources cover long time frames, thereby allowing study of trends not otherwise amenable to analysis.
5. Computerized approaches are available that greatly simplify difficult categorization and coding procedures.

6. Categorical schemes are generally developed or modified after data are collected and thus do not constrain or bias the data.

Major disadvantages are as follows:

1. The procedure is very time consuming and labor intensive; however, computer applications are markedly reducing the time and effort involved.
2. Many materials have been prescreened or edited by others and, hence, are subject to incompleteness or bias.
3. Data in the original sources may not have been compiled systematically. When doubt exists about the accuracy or completeness of a data source, it is recommended that either multiple sources be content analyzed or content analysis be combined with other techniques.
4. Judgment is required in order to reduce the data and interpret the meaning of another's communication. There is a risk of losing or modifying the meaning of the communication, due to incomplete information and/or subjectivity on the part of the coder or analyst. Accuracy of interpreting the meaning of another's communication can be hampered when subcultural differences exist.
5. Legal or ethical problems may be encountered regarding the use of information gathered for another purpose.
6. Analyses may disregard the context that generated the text, and hence may compromise the validity of the interpretation.
7. Methods of analysis, particularly those used in inductive qualitative analyses, have tended to be individualistic, relying heavily on the interpretive skill of the researcher. Computer software has helped reduce idiosyncratic interpretations, but the process does not lend itself easily to standardization.

REFERENCES

Bucknall, T. (2003). The clinical landscape of critical care: Nurses' decision-making. *Journal of Advanced Nursing, 43*(3), 310–319.

Garvin, B. J., Kennedy, C. W., & Cissna, K. N. 1988). Reliability in category coding systems. *Nursing Research, 37*(1), 52–55.

Geiger-Brown, J., Trinkoff, A. M., Neilson, K., Lirtmunlikaporn, S., Brady, B., & Vasquez, E. T. (2004). Nurses' perception of their work environment, health and well being: A qualitative perspective. *AAOHN Journal, 52*(1), 16–22.

Gottschalk, L. A. (1995) *Content analysis of verbal behavior: New findings and clinical applications.* Hillside, NJ: Lawrence Erlbaum Associates.

Graneheim, U. H., & Lundman, B. (2004). Qualitative content analysis in nursing research: Concepts, procedures and measures to achieve trustworthiness. *Nursing Education Today, 24*(2), 105–112.

Kirchoff, K. T., Beckstrand, R. L., & Anumandla, P. R. (2003). Analysis of end-of-life content in critical care nursing textbooks. *Journal of Professional Nursing, 19*(6), 372–381.

Krippendorff, K. (2004). *Content analysis: An introduction to its methodology* (2nd ed.). Thousand Oaks, CA: Sage.

Mayring, P. (2000, June). Qualitative content analysis: Forum Qualitative Sozialforschung/ Forum: *Qualitative Social Research.* Retrieved from http://www.qualitative-research.net/ fqs-texte/2-00/2-00mayring-e.htm

McEwen, M. (2004). Analysis of spirituality content in nursing textbooks. *Journal of Nursing Education, 42*(1), 20–30.

Morse, J. M., & Field, P. A. (1995). *Qualitative research methods for health professionals* (2nd ed.). Thousand Oaks, CA: Sage.

Neuendorf, K. A. (2002). *The content analysis guidebook.* Thousand Oaks, CA: Sage.

Priest, H., Roberts, P., & Woods, L. (2002). An overview of three different approaches to the interpretation of qualitative data: Part I: Theoretical issues. *Nurse Researcher, 10*(1), 30–42.

Winslow, B. W. (2003). Family caregivers' experiences with community services: A qualitative analysis. *Public Health Nursing, 20*(5), 341–348.

11

Interviews

The interview is the method most often used by nurses in their practice to obtain information. It is a face-to-face[1] verbal interchange in which one individual, the interviewer, attempts to elicit information from another, the respondent, usually through direct questioning. Because interviewing is such a commonplace occurrence, it is easy to forget the care and precision that must be used when interviewing in the context of research. In this book the interview is considered to be a measurement instrument designed to yield data to accomplish specified purposes, so it is subject to the same considerations of reliability and validity as other measurement tools.

The interview is used for a variety of purposes in nursing: to obtain factual (as perceived by the respondent) information, or to learn the respondent's definition of a given situation or perception of events. Because it is flexible, the interview is particularly useful for gathering information from respondents who may have difficulty recalling specific events or may be explaining or reconstructing complex processes or situations. The interview also allows topics to be pursued with considerable depth and detail.

Interviews may be used to elicit an individual's attitudes, opinions, level of knowledge, and standards. Although similar kinds of information and characteristics can be gathered and assessed using questionnaires, the interview is often the method of choice, because misinterpretation or inconsistency can often be identified "on the spot" and communication clarified. The interview is uniquely useful for several populations of interest to nursing research and practice. For example, interviews are very useful for gathering information from persons who cannot read or write, or have difficulty concentrating or understanding or expressing complex ideas (e.g., young children, the very ill, the elderly, the blind, the illiterate, patients with dementia) (see Paterson & Scott-Findlay, 2002; Acton, Mayhew, Hopkins, & Yank, 1999; Docherty & Sandelowski, 1998).

The interview has some limitations as well. For example, because the interview usually involves face-to-face interaction, the respondent is always aware that information is being sought and responses noted; therefore, it is difficult for the researcher to be unobtrusive about information gathering. Also because the interview is an interpersonal interaction, the respondent is always influenced to some degree by the verbal and nonverbal behaviors of the interviewer, the nature of the questions asked, and the setting in which the interview occurs (Yong, 2001). All of these issues may make the interview problematic when anonymity is desirable, for example, when conducting research on sensitive, embarrassing, or stigmatizing topics, such as sexual practices, illegal behaviors, or emotionally painful events. Although many strategies have been recommended to help increase willing and accurate responses in such situations (see chapter 20 and Lee [1993] about collecting sensitive information), the interview may be less useful than more impersonal approaches in situations where willingness to respond and truthfulness of response would be compromised by a personal method of measurement. In some cases, because the respondent is aware of being studied, the very act of being interviewed may alter usual behavior, hence the natural course of events. If that would be problematic, a less obtrusive approach to data collection would be preferable.

---

[1]In some cases interviews are conducted by telephone or computer, and therefore do not involve face-to-face interaction in the strict sense of the word.

The interview is one of the key instruments used in various types of qualitative research, including ethnographic, phenomenological, grounded theory, and historical studies. Therefore, it is important to consider its strengths, limitations, construction, testing, and properties. The following discussion relates to the use of the interview in both quantitative and qualitative studies; however, its use in qualitative research is covered in greater detail in chapter 8.

TYPES OF INTERVIEWS

Interviews are typically classified according to the degree of standardization involved. As discussed in chapter 7, standardization varies in degree; it refers to the control that is exercised regarding the development, content, administration, scoring, and interpretation of a measure. Interviews vary greatly in the degree to which the content and the procedures for administering, recording, and scoring responses are prescribed. There is a continuum ranging from highly standardized (structured) to unstandardized (unstructured) interviews. The two polar extremes are described below, along with their uses, advantages, and disadvantages. Also see Bernard (2000), Gubrium and Holstein (2002), Denzin and Lincoln (2003), and Fielding (2003).

Structured (Standardized) Interview

Structured interviews are those in which the investigator exercises a maximum of control by predetermining a fixed wording and sequence for all questions, and usually by preestablishing the array of possible response alternatives that can be recorded. The interview is presented in the same form to all respondents. The U.S. Census is an example of a structured interview, in which the interviewer is not at liberty to change the wording or order of the questions, and many of the response possibilities are preestablished. In the structured interview the interviewer asks the question exactly as it is designed. If a respondent does not understand the question, the interviewer is not free to elaborate, but generally can only repeat the question or

substitute a predefined alternative. Probes (questions, phrases, or words added to the original question in order to encourage additional or more complete responses) may be included in a standardized interview; however, they are specified in advance and are generally not left to the discretion of the interviewer.

The standardized interview embodies several assumptions. For example, it is assumed that a given verbal stimulus, such as an item or word, will elicit the same range of meanings for each respondent, and that a given wording will be equally meaningful to all respondents. If the meaning of each item is to be identical for every respondent, then the sequence must be identical. Because respondents can differ markedly in their cultural and experiential backgrounds, these assumptions are often erroneous and can be met only when respondents are homogeneous and share characteristics and experiences, allowing them to interpret the meaning of questions from the same frame of reference. To the extent that the assumptions are not met when a standardized interview is used, response error is a problem. Response error occurs when respondents' answers to the items on the interview do not measure what the instrument developer or researcher intends to measure.

A major reason for standardizing an interview is to allow comparability across respondents. If the interview is standardized and differences are discerned among respondents, then it is possible, at least theoretically, to draw the conclusion that any differences found are attributable to actual differences in response, rather than in the instrument or the way it was administered. In fact, the structured interview generally has higher reliability than less structured forms. Since all questions are prescribed, there is less likelihood that differences in the way the interview is conducted will be a source of unreliability. Additionally, there is less likelihood of interviewer bias, which refers to systematic differences that occur from interviewer to interviewer in the way questions are asked and responses are elicited and recorded. Interviewer effects are not eliminated by structuring an interview, although they may be lessened. Another advantage of the highly structured interview is that interviewer training can be less extensive than for less structured forms, because so little is left to the discretion of the interviewer.

Structured interviews vary in the extent to which the arrays of possible responses, as well as the questions themselves, are standardized. The range is from completely structured response alternatives, in which the respondent must choose a prespecified response, to a completely open-ended response situation, in which the respondent answers as he or she wishes, and the response is recorded as delivered. Between the two extremes are items in which the respondent's answer is coded by the interviewer into one of a defined set of response alternatives. Since the interviewer is responsible for recording the response, the more structured the response alternatives, the more reliable the interview tends to be. However, structured response alternatives may force the respondent to answer in a way that does not reflect the "true" response, and validity may be compromised.

The primary disadvantage of the structured interview is its inflexibility. If the interviewer realizes that a respondent is misinterpreting a question or senses that the wording of an item may be offensive, the interviewer does not have the latitude to make changes unless the contingency has been anticipated and an explanation or alternative wording has been provided in advance. It can be frustrating to both interviewer and subject if the interviewer is unable to explain a question or to fit the respondent's answer to the available response alternatives, or the respondent cannot select the "true" answer (rather than simply the best of those provided). The interviewer should note concerns about respondents' misinterpretation or lack of understanding when they occur, because the validity of the interview and the comparability of responses may be seriously compromised.

The structured interview is used most appropriately when identical information is needed from all respondents, when comparisons are to be made across respondents who are relatively homogeneous in background and experience, and when large or geographically dispersed samples are used. The structured interview is often used in hypothesis-testing research and when rigorous quantification of information is required. For detailed information regarding the structured interview see Gubrium and Holstein (2002), and Foddy (1993).

Unstructured (Nonstandardized) Interview

The unstructured interview is one in which the wording and sequence of the questions are not prescribed, but are left to the discretion of the interviewer. There are varying degrees of structure, even in an unstructured interview. The partially structured interview (sometimes called a focused interview) generally begins with a list of topics to be covered. The list serves as an interview guide; however, the interviewer may move freely from one topic area to another and allow the respondent's cues to help determine the flow of the interview. Although the interviewer may work from a list, the way in which questions are phrased and the order in which they are asked are left to the discretion of the interviewer and may be changed to fit the characteristics of each respondent. The interviewer has freedom to pursue various topics to different degrees with each respondent, and to try various approaches to encourage the respondent to elaborate. However, the expectation is that all topics or questions will be covered to some degree. Partially structured interviews are often used in clinical history-taking, applicant selection, and in some types of marketing and qualitative research.

Completely unstructured interviews are those in which respondents are encouraged to talk about whatever they wish regarding the general topic being pursued by the researcher. A list of possible questions may be used, but it is not necessary that all be covered with each respondent. The unstructured interview is designed to elicit subjects' perceptions with minimal imposition of the investigator's input or perspective. The completely unstructured interview allows a conversational or story-telling approach, which is compatible with several philosophical perspectives that underlie qualitative research (see chapter 8; Denzin & Lincoln, 2003; Crotty, 1998). It is a particularly useful adjunct to participant observation in ethnographic or field research.

The assumptions that underlie the unstructured interview are essentially the opposite of those underlying the structured interview. For example, in the unstructured interview standardization of meaning stems not from administering uniform wording to every respondent, but from the latitude to change words to fit respondents' comprehension, language and culture. It is assumed that no single sequence of questions is satisfactory for all respondents. Instead, the best sequence is determined by the interviewer, based on the respondent's readiness to discuss a particular topic. Finally, if all respondents are exposed to essentially the same topics, it is assumed that they are exposed to the same stimuli, regardless of the specific order or wording used. This assumption may or may not be important, depending on the type of research being conducted. For example, it would be irrelevant in phenomenological research.

The primary advantage of the unstructured interview is its flexibility. It allows the interviewer to change questions to fit the respondent's comprehension, probe the meaning of given responses in depth, and respond to individual differences and changes in the situation. The other major advantage is that it allows the respondent to express his or her perceptions and priorities freely; thus, it is ideal for studies that are focused on subjective meaning and the individual's definition of the situation. Disadvantages of the unstructured interview include inability to make systematic comparisons across respondents, particularly quantitative comparisons; difficulty in establishing reliability; likelihood of interviewer bias; requirement for skilled interviewers; difficulty in analyzing data; time required to elicit systematic information; and the time and expense required to train interviewers. The unstructured interview is desirable when respondents differ sufficiently in background to preclude consistent interpretation of meaning, when extensive and in-depth information is needed from each respondent, and when the respondent's meanings and definitions of the situations are important data. The unstructured interview is often used in descriptive and exploratory studies to increase understanding of phenomena that are not well understood. It is also used in preliminary stages of tool development to help generate the items and response alternatives that will later be used in more structured instruments.

Another type of interview that deserves special mention is the telephone interview. Long used as the primary vehicle for consumer marketing research, it is being used increasingly in other types of nursing research, including health services research (e.g., outcome studies). Telephone interviewing has the advantage of being less expensive and time consuming than face-to-face interviews. It also allows respondents in a wider geographic area to be surveyed. An important advantage is the ability to elicit responses regarding sensitive topics with minimal response bias. Telephone interviews have been found to be as effective in eliciting sensitive information as more expensive, in-home audio computer-assisted self-interviews (Ellen et al., 2002). Both tend to elicit more frequent reporting of stigmatized behaviors than face-to-face interviews (Newman et al., 2002). On the other hand, some characteristics, such as level of physical disability, may be underreported in phone interviews, compared with face-to-face interviews. In the latter, the respondents' functional level can be directly observed and their responses validated (Korner-Bitensky, Wood-Dauphinee, Shapiro, & Backer, 1994). Other comparisons have revealed that telephone and face-to-face interviews yield equivalent findings, including information that can be validated with direct observation (Rintala & Willems, 1991).

A disadvantage of the telephone interview is that potential respondents are limited to those with phones. Segments of the population (e.g., the poor, the transient, the homeless) may be excluded. The extent to which this omission is a problem depends on the purpose of the study. For example, community-based epidemiological research surveys may be badly biased by the omission of these subpopulations, and the results may therefore present an inaccurate representation (Donovan, Holman, Corti, & Janneh, 1997). For detailed discussion of the telephone interview the reader is referred to Dillman (1978, 2000).

Recent advances in computer technology have expanded the repertoire of modes available for conducting interviews, particularly structured interviews. The ease of providing audio delivery of computerized information, and innovations in touch screen technology to facilitate interaction between respondent and computer, have greatly expanded the use of computer-assisted self-interviews (CASI) in hospital, ambulatory, and home settings. Although the technology is relatively expensive because of equipment and software design costs, it is ultimately cheaper than one-on-one interviews, particularly if respondents are numerous, geographically distant, or dispersed. The availability of audio computer output means that a respondent need not be literate to use computer-assisted interviewing, and could conceivably have sight limitations. It also means that the interview can be conducted in another language without a bilingual interviewer being present. Lack of respondent computer experience does not seem to pose a serious limitation for computer-assisted interviewing, even for economically or socially disadvantaged populations (Thornberry et al., 2002). A disadvantage of computer-assisted self-administered interviews is that computers must be available, secured, and located in places (e.g., kiosks or booths with earphones supplied) that will allow privacy during data collection. The evolution of handheld devices (e.g., personal digital assistants or PDAs) has increased the feasibility of conducting computer-assisted interviews cost-effectively and in areas with limited space. Many participants have been found to prefer handheld computer-assisted self interviews (H-CASI) over paper-and-pencil questionnaires (Bernhardt et al., 2001).

TYPES OF QUESTIONS OR ITEMS

The basic element of the interview is the question or item. There are two major types of questions included in interviews: the fixed-alternative or closed-ended (structured response alternatives) question, and the open-ended (no response alternatives) question. A semistructured question contains elements of the other two types: that is, some response alternatives are provided, but the respondent is not constrained to choose one of the given answers. There is usually an open-response category included, usually designated "other." The closed-ended question is one that supplies the respondent with two or more specified alternative responses from which to choose. Dichotomous, multiple-choice, and scale items are included in this category. The open-ended question has no specified alternative responses, so the respondent is free to word the answer. Sometimes the question is worded to sound as though it is open-ended, even though there are fixed-response alternatives into which the interviewer must place the respondent's answer. In this case it is the interviewer, not the respondent, who determines the fit of the answer to the response alternatives, thus permitting potential for interviewer bias. The structured interview includes either closed-ended or open-ended items, or a combination of the two types. The unstructured interview generally includes open-ended questions but may include both types. Examples of open-ended questions are as follows:

- What sensations did you experience during your endoscopy? Please give me some words that describe the sensations you felt as the scope was inserted.
- How would you describe your relationship with your nurse manager?
- What are the things you do to reduce stress now that you have stopped smoking?

From a measurement perspective the two types of questions have strengths and weaknesses. The closed-ended question provides uniformity, therefore increased reliability. It is easier to code responses to closed-ended questions; however, the questions themselves may be more difficult to construct, because an appropriate set of response alternatives must be developed. This may take considerable time and effort, often involving preliminary qualitative research. The activity may also be highly subject to cultural bias. It is possible that some responses may be overlooked, and some superfluous responses may be included. These problems can often be minimized by subjecting the questions to experts for review, and by including one open-ended category among the response alternatives. It should be noted that the experts who are most helpful in reviewing response alternatives are often those experiencing the phenomenon being studied. Advisory groups of patients with a given diagnosis or from a given ethnic group may provide very helpful input regarding the relevance, completeness, comprehensibility, clarity of meaning, and appropriateness of both questions and response alternatives.

Closed-ended questions are used most appropriately when the range of possible alternative responses is known, limited, and clear-cut. Since the question writer determines the possible responses available to the respondent, the closed-ended question helps establish the respondent's frame of reference, thereby avoiding responses that are irrelevant or incomparable. On the other hand, since responses are predetermined, they may not be valid indicators of a particular respondent's view. Validity may also be compromised when a subject is forced to choose a response, recognizing that it does not reflect the "true" answer that would be given under other conditions. Validity is also compromised when the respondent is enabled (or forced), by virtue of the response alternatives provided, to address a subject on the basis of little or no knowledge. The inclusion of filter questions may help eliminate this problem. A filter question is used to determine an individual's level of information about, or experience with, a given topic before proceeding to other questions about it. For example, a question such as "Have you ever had surgery?" might be used as a filter to limit portions of the interview to those with prior surgery experience.

Generally closed-ended questions are more efficient to administer and score than open-ended questions. More can be asked and answered in a given period of time. Closed-ended questions are particularly useful for addressing sensitive or stressful topics about which respondents may be reluctant to talk at length. Income is an example of a topic that may best be measured using preestablished categories, rather than an open-ended question. On the other hand, use of closed-ended questions may result in information loss. A respondent who is not constrained by a closed-ended question might provide additional, valuable information.

The open-ended question is easier to construct; however, responses are more difficult to record and analyze reliably. Responses to open-ended questions are often long and complex, therefore cannot be recorded accurately without an audio recorder. The procedures of content analysis are generally employed in order to code and score responses, which can be communicated quantitatively or qualitatively (see chapter 10). In qualitative research, elaborate strategies and special software may be employed to help identify themes in the data, and to validate the meaning of the information with the respondent (see chapter 8). Considerations of interrater reliability are crucial in recording, coding, and interpreting responses to open-ended questions.

The open-ended question "sets the stage" for the respondent's answer, but provides only the frame of reference or context to which the respondent replies. Therefore, the respondent may interpret the question differently from the question writer's intent or may go off on a tangent in answering it. If these problems occur in an unstructured interview, the question can be reinterpreted or the respondent redirected by the interviewer. In the structured interview, however, such tactics are not possible. Therefore, structure must be built into the questions by developing orienting sentences or funnel questions to help orient the thinking of the respondent. A funnel is a list of questions concerning a given topic that are arranged in order of decreasing generality. The inclusion of broad questions allows the respondent to express views without being influenced by subsequent questions.

An advantage of the open-ended question is that it provides a framework within which respondents can use their own words to express their ideas. Open-ended questions yield the rich qualitative descriptions that are enhancing understanding of nursing phenomena. Because of their flexibility, open-ended questions are most appropriate for examining complex issues or processes, when relevant dimensions of responses are unknown, and when the paradigmatic and theoretical underpinnings of a study make it necessary to probe respondent perceptions.

PROCEDURE FOR DEVELOPING THE INTERVIEW SCHEDULE

The suggested procedure for developing an interview schedule is described below. A brief overview of each step is provided. More detailed information about designing and conducting interviews can be obtained from one of many excellent resources, for example, Gubrium and Holstein (2002), Bernard (2000), and Denzin and Lincoln (2003).

Step 1: Determine the Information To Be Sought

The first step in designing an interview is to determine what information is needed from respondents. The decision is based on the objectives for the investigation, the question it is designed to answer, or the variables and hypotheses that have been identified to be measured. As described in chapter 2, it is helpful to construct a blueprint, table of specifications or, at the very least, a content outline listing all of the types or categories of information needed.

Step 2: Develop the Questions or Items

After the needed content has been specified, the next step is to draft the actual questions to be asked and the potential responses, if any are to be provided. This is not an easy task. It involves both translating the purposes into questions that will yield the needed information and designing "lead-ins," or explanatory statements, that will motivate the respondent to provide the information requested. The wording of each question is crucial, since the meaning must be clear to the respondent and sufficiently precise to convey what is expected without biasing the content of the response. Several guidelines are suggested below:

1. Be sure that the wording accurately conveys the meaning intended. If meaning is potentially problematic, ask others the question and have them interpret what they think it means.

2. Keep sentences, phrases, and questions short, because some people have difficulty understanding and remembering complex ideas.

3. Use simple terms that can be understood by the least educated respondent. If technical terms are necessary, clearly define each one before asking the question in which it is included, and list possible synonyms if necessary.

4. Limit each question to only one idea; avoid questions with multiple parts.

5. Avoid words with multiple or ambiguous meanings.

6. To the greatest extent possible avoid terms that are derogatory, emotionally laden, or that might trigger biased responses.

7. Do not ask questions in ways that suggest an answer.

8. Avoid personal or delicate content that the respondent may be reluctant to answer. If such content must be addressed, word the questions as delicately as possible.

9. If a closed-ended format is used, clearly define the entire set of responses. This may be done verbally as part of the question. However, if the list of possible responses is long or complex, they should be written on a card or booklet and shown to the respondent.

10. Try to minimize the effect of social desirability by avoiding questions that lead respondents to express sentiments that imply approval of things generally considered good or behaviors that are expected by society. (See chapter 25 for a more thorough discussion of social desirability.)

11. Use filter questions to be sure that respondents are not being asked to provide answers about topics with which they are unfamiliar.

12. Identify probes that can be used to elicit additional information or clarification (see Price, 2002).

Lead-in or introductory information is provided at the beginning of the interview and additional, reorienting information is sometimes periodically included throughout the interview to set the stage for the questions that are to come and help provide a context in which the respondent is to interpret the question. Such information is helpful when the interview shifts from one topic to another. In a structured interview the script is provided for the interviewer to read identically to each respondent. In unstructured interviews, the interviewer may be permitted to design lead-in or transitional statements that are individualized for each respondent.

As an example, during an interview to assess a new mother's social support network, a statement such as the following might be used to help reorient the mother's thinking:

> For the past few minutes you have been telling me about the help and support you think you might be able to receive from your family, friends, and coworkers if you needed it. Now I would like you to think about the help you have actually received during the past month, specifically from one important person—your spouse/partner.

This statement alerts the respondent to two changes in orientation: (1) from hypothetically available support to that which has actually been received, and (2) from the support network as a whole to a focus on one support provider.

Step 3: Determine the Sequence of the Questions

Once the questions have been designed, an appropriate sequence is determined. The main criterion for determining the sequence is that questions or items be arranged in a logical and realistic fashion so that they make sense to the respondent. For example, if the interview is designed to elicit information about a sequence of events that the respondent carried out, the questions should be arranged so that events occurring earliest in the sequence are asked about before those coming later. The order that is generally suggested is to begin with questions that are likely to capture the interest of the respondent and increase motivation to cooperate. Less interesting questions and those that

may be difficult to answer should come later in the interview. Sensitive or personal questions are generally asked near the end of the interview, since a respondent who is offended or disturbed by them may terminate the interview. Traditionally, sociodemographic information is requested near the end of the interview.

In order to make the interview more logical and less confusing, it is desirable to cluster questions concerning a particular topic. Within clusters, open-ended questions should precede closed-ended questions, and general questions should precede more specific ones. The reason for this ordering is to avoid earlier questions suggesting responses to those that follow, thus minimizing bias in the response. There are exceptions to the general-to-specific ordering. For example, some scales require questions to be randomly ordered, and specific questions may help trigger a respondent's recollection of past events.

Step 4: Draft the Interview Schedule

The interview schedule contains both the questions to be asked and any introductory statement, explicit instructions for the interviewer and respondent, and a closing statement. Introductory information is directed toward providing the basis for informed consent. It is usually presented in writing, but may also be covered verbally. It should address the purpose of the interview, what will be done with the information obtained and who will have access to it, risks and benefits to the respondent and others (if any), an explicit statement that participation is voluntary and that the respondent can refuse to answer any question or terminate the interview at any time, an estimate of the time involved, and an orientation to the interviewing and recording procedure. (See chapter 24 for more detailed information about informed consent and ethical considerations in measurement). It is appropriate to end the interview by expressing appreciation for the respondent's time, help, and cooperation. In some cases, the investigator offers to share the findings with the respondent when the study is complete.

Instructions to the respondent should be explicit. New instructions are required whenever there is a change in format or topic. Instructions to the interviewer must also be detailed and precise. These should include such matters as whether questions may be repeated or reworded, lists of probes, and instructions about how to record or code the response. A particularly important aspect of interview instructions in nursing, especially in research interviews, is whether or not the interviewer is permitted to provide any assistance or health-related information or advice to the respondent either during or after the interview. Nurse interviewers often find it difficult to not intervene with respondents who have obvious problems.

Step 5: Pilot-Test the Interview

Pilot testing an interview actually involves several activities. First it is advisable to subject the questions on the interview schedule to review by measurement experts and experts in the content area. Measurement experts can often spot ambiguous or unclear wording or questions that are unlikely to yield the desired response. Content experts, who may include nurse clinicians and researchers, scholars in other disciplines, and advisory groups of patients, are able to evaluate the clarity of wording, appropriateness of the question to the content area, and completeness and appropriateness of the response alternatives. It also may be helpful to have individuals who are not familiar with the content of the interview review the questions for clarity of meaning and use of readily understandable terms. Such individuals may also suggest additional responses to consider.

A second pilot-testing activity is to try out the interview with individuals with characteristics and experiences like those for whom the interview is designed. The pilot test provides the opportunity to detect problems with the wording of the instructions or questions, determine the time involved, and assess the reliability and validity of the instrument. An opportunity should be provided to "debrief" the pilot-test subjects in order to elicit their opinions of the interview. Since the nature of the setting in which the interview is conducted influences the kind and amount of information that the respondent reveals, it is advisable to conduct the pilot study in a setting which is similar to that in which the interview ultimately will be carried out, in order to assess barriers and facilitators in the setting.

Step 6: Train Interviewers

Subjects' reluctance to answer questions and variations among interviewers in how they conduct the interview are two additional sources of response error. According to Collins, Given, Given, and King (1988), adequate training and supervision of interviewers can be a major factor in reducing these two sources of error and cannot be overemphasized. Selection of interviewers is also important.

The interview is an interpersonal action. Particularly in unstructured interviews the interviewer represents one aspect of the instrument. Therefore, it is essential that interviewers be carefully selected and thoroughly trained before contacting respondents and administering the interview. Selection of appropriate interviewers must take into account the nature of the anticipated respondents and the complexity of the interview situation. Research has shown that the gender, age, race, social class, intelligence, experiential background, appearance, level of expertise or authority (i.e., lay versus professional health care provider), and voice of the interviewer influence respondents' willingness to participate in the interview and the nature of the information received from them; however, the results are mixed, depending on the particular population being studied (Korner-Bitensky, Wood-Dauphinee, Shapiro, & Becker, 1994; Denzin & Lincoln, 2003; Clark, Scott, Boydell, & Goering, 1999; Bray, Powell, Lovelock, & Philip, 1995; Instone, 2002). In general, the more congruent the characteristics and experiences of interviewer and respondent, the more likely is the respondent to cooperate, and the more valid are the responses obtained.

Interviewers must be carefully trained. The training period may vary in length from a few hours to several weeks, depending on the complexity and degree of structure of the interview and the prior experience of the interviewer.

Highly structured interviews may require training periods lasting from one hour to a full day. For unstructured interviews longer periods of training are usually necessary, particularly if the interviewer must code or interpret the data. Training includes not only instruction and practice in administering the questions and recording and coding the responses, but also consideration of verbal and nonverbal communication skills, appropriate appearance and dress, control of distracting environmental elements, and techniques for securing cooperation and for motivating respondents. Although some general guidelines pertaining to virtually all interview situations should be included in interviewer training (see Fielding, 2003) a large portion of the training is specific to the requirements of the particular study and interview.

When research interviewers are clinicians, it is also advisable to include a discussion of the differences between clinical and research interviews. When sensitive questions are to be addressed or the population is vulnerable, special consideration of ethics, human rights, and ways to handle difficult situations should be included in the training. For research interviews, it is advisable to familiarize the interviewers with the research project; however, one should be careful not to share information that might bias the interviewers or compromise their objectivity in reporting and scoring the information. Acceptable levels of interrater and intrarater reliability must be established before training can be considered complete.

Adequate training is imperative from a measurement perspective, because the interviewer controls much of the information obtained. Interviewer bias can be a substantial threat to reliability, as can factors in the interviewer-respondent interaction that might inadvertently discourage the respondent from answering completely and truthfully. Problems may occur because of inter- or intrainterviewer differences in the way questions are asked, responses are elicited and recorded, respondents perceive interviewers and questions, interviewers perceive respondents, and in the interview settings. Conversely, an interviewer's ability to listen effectively, maintain an objective stance, and establish a sense of trust, can be instrumental in eliciting valid responses.

With a highly structured interview schedule in which considerable control is built into the instrument itself, the interviewer must ensure that the schedule is administered and responses recorded consistently across all respondents in order to achieve reliable and valid results. Even with structured interviews, reliability and validity are dependent not just on the instrument, but also on the human beings involved in the interview interaction. With unstructured interviews the interviewer holds considerable discretionary power. Therefore, thorough understanding of the purposes of the interview and considerable communication skill are essential. Regardless of the degree of structuring, personal characteristics and behaviors of the interviewer (e.g., gestures, posture, facial expression, verbal intonation, and voice quality) can influence responses.

If the study is to take place over a period of weeks, it is not sufficient to train interviewers before the study begins. Periodic updates of the training are needed, particularly if and when interrater reliability begins to decline. Periodic assessment of inter- and intrarater reliability and periodic retraining and updating sessions are essential ingredients in a comprehensive interviewer training program. Reliability may be checked by having one other person accompany the interviewer and record and code responses or by recording the interview for another individual to code. In telephone interviews, interrater reliability is checked by having another individual listen to the interview and code the information simultaneously. Reliability coefficients are then computed using the two sets of scores.

Step 7: Administer and Code the Interview

The final step in the interview process is to administer the interview and record, code, and score responses. In addition to the interpersonal factors noted above, several elements in the interview situation itself may influence the reliability and validity of responses. For example, the timing, duration, and scheduling of the interview in relation to other demands and events may influence the information obtained.

A respondent who feels rushed to complete the interview quickly because of time pressures, or one who is preoccupied by personal problems, may be unwilling or unable to supply accurate and complete information. Interviews that are too long may create respondent burden, particularly for respondents who are ill or emotionally distraught, therefore compromising the validity of their responses. Interviewing children requires special, age-dependent, techniques (see Kortesluoma, Hentinen, & Nikkonen, 2003; Instone, 2002). Particularly when the interview addresses sensitive information, intense emotional experiences, or a traumatic event, its timing relative to the event in question affects the respondent's willingness and ability to share information or express feelings (Cowles, 1988). During the initial phases of such experiences, respondents may be unable to discuss their thoughts and feelings.

The setting for the interview is also important. Considerations are convenience for the respondents, degree of privacy available, possible distractions or interruptions, and the potential influence of the setting on the content of the response (e.g., Yong, 2001). For example, a respondent might reply differently to questions about sexual behavior with and without the spouse present. Respondents would be likely to answer differently about their hospital experience if interviewed in the hospital rather than at home, in part because of the cuing effect of the environment. Some environments, such as busy clinics that provide little privacy, have been found to obstruct the free flow of information in patient–health provider interaction, so one can assume that they would similarly impede the flow of information for all types of interviews.

The means used to record responses also influence reliability and validity. Reliability is generally higher for closed-ended than open-ended questions, because responses are recorded on a precoded format. Open-ended questions require that the interviewer take notes or use a voice recorder. In general, the more complex the information, the more rapid the information flow, and the greater the likelihood of unanticipated responses, then the more preferable is the use of a recording device, despite the increased time and cost involved in transcription. Subjects may find the use of a voice recorder to be distracting, particularly in the early stages of the interview, or may prefer that their responses not be taped. The interviewer must secure permission for taping in advance, being sure to communicate to the respondent what will be done with the recording. In order to increase reliability and validity, open-ended interview data should be transcribed and coded as soon as possible after the interview. The transcript should be checked and, if necessary, clarified or corrected by the interviewer. Coding can be done either by the interviewer or another individual.

RELIABILITY AND VALIDITY

As with all measurement instruments, reliability and validity are crucial considerations in the interview. Reliability assessment includes consideration of inter- and intrarater reliability (determined at the time of pilot testing the interview schedule, during interviewer training, and periodically throughout use of the interview with respondents), and reliability of the instrument itself. The latter assessment generally is carried out for structured interviews using the procedures of test/retest reliability, wherein the same respondent is interviewed more than once using the same schedule and results are compared. This is a time-consuming procedure that makes considerable demands on the respondent; therefore it is generally carried out only during the pilot phase of instrument development. It is advisable to compute test/retest reliability periodically on a small sample of interviews during the administration phase as well. Parallel forms reliability assessment may also be employed for structured interviews; however, split-half reliability is generally not appropriate. Given the intent of the unstructured interview to focus with few imposed constraints on the perceptions and priorities of the respondent and given inconsistency in the questions asked, traditional reliability assessment is virtually precluded.

Validity of interview information is a complex issue that entails consideration of the interview itself as well as the issue of self-reported information. Sources of invalidity in the interview include (1) lack of commonly comprehended meanings, (2) differences in situations and settings, (3) reactive effects of the interview itself (respondents modify their responses simply because they are being interviewed), and (4) respondents' modifying their responses to fit their perceptions of social requirements or the interviewer's preferences. Careful instrument design, with attention to the wording of questions and the input of experts, can minimize some of these sources of invalidity (Hutchinson & Wilson, 1992).

Interviews most often elicit self-reported data, that is, information reported by the respondent about himself or herself. Self-reports are subject to error due to the tendency to respond in a socially approved manner, the tendency to acquiesce or agree with a statement without careful consideration, and varying ability to engage in self-focused attention and accurate self-appraisal. It is not necessarily easy to assess the validity of factual information reported by respondents. In most instances it must simply be assumed that the respondent is telling the truth; however, this assumption may be problematic when recall is difficult, sensitive issues are involved, or the response may cast an unfavorable light on the respondent.

There are several ways in which the validity of self-report information can be assessed. For example, within the context of the interview itself, the interviewer can observe whether the respondent is disturbed by certain questions or hesitates to answer. Such observations should be noted, so they can be taken into account in interpreting the information. Inconsistencies in response can also be noted, carefully called to the respondent's attention, and clarified in order to increase validity. Likewise, in many cases inconsistencies between self-reports and behavior can also be noted by the interviewer. For example, an elderly respondent may verbally report no difficulty in moving around the house, yet can be observed holding onto furniture for balance. A diabetic patient may claim to self-administer insulin daily, yet be unable to locate the medication or a syringe when asked. Validity can also be assessed by gathering information external to the interview situation to check the accuracy of responses. Family members can be asked to validate respondents' self-reports, recognizing that the family members themselves may have inaccurate or incomplete information. Hospital records can be consulted to validate reports of factual information about the hospital visit. Other measures of the same behavior or characteristic can be employed in conjunction with the interview as a means for assessing concurrent validity (see discussion of triangulation in chapter 25 and Scisney-Matlock et al's [2000] discussion of the use of electronic devices to measure behavior).

Qualitative researchers point out that the procedures used to assess the reliability, validity, and rigor of quantitative data collection instruments are not adequate for evaluating qualitative approaches. Different concepts and criteria must be applied (e.g., Davies & Dodd, 2002). In many different types of qualitative research, the key data are the respondent's perceptions and definitions of the situation; therefore, only the respondent is truly able to validate the data and the way they have been analyzed and interpreted. Approaches to assessing the reliability and validity of interviews and interview data in qualitative studies are discussed in greater detail in chapter 8.

REFERENCES

Acton, G. J., Mayhew, P. A., Hopkins, B. A., & Yauk, S. (1999). Communicating with individuals with dementia: The impaired person's perspective. *Journal of Gerontological Nursing, 25*(2), 6–13.

Bernard, H. R. (2000). Interviewing: Unstructured and semi-structured interviews. In H. R. Bernard (Ed.), *Social research methods: Qualitative and quantitative approaches* (pp. 189–225) Thousand Oaks, CA: Sage.

Bernhardt, J. M., Strecher, V. J., Bishop K. R., Potts, P., Madison, E. M., & Thorp, J. (2001). Handheld computer-assisted self-interviews: User comfort level and preferences. *American Journal of Health Behavior, 25*(6), 557–563.

Bray, J., Powell, J., Lovelock, R., & Philip, I. (1995). Using a softer approach: Techniques for interviewing older people. *Professional Nurse, 10*(6), 350–353.

Clark, C. C., Scott, E. A., Boydell, K. M., & Goering, P. (1999). Effects of client interviewers on client-reported satisfaction with mental health services. *Psychiatric Services, 50*(7), 961–963.

Collins, C., Given, B., Given, C. W., & King, S. (1988). Interviewer training and supervision. *Nursing Research, 37*(2), 122–124.

Crotty, M. (1998). *The foundations of social research: Meaning and perspective in the research process.* Thousand Oaks, CA: Sage.

Cowles, K. V. (1988). Issues in qualitative research on sensitive topics. *Western Journal of Nursing Research, 10*(2), 163–179.

Davies, D., & Dodd, J. (2002). Pearls, pith, and provocation: Qualitative research and the question of rigor. *Qualitative Health Research, 12*(2), 279–289.

Denzin, N. K., & Lincoln, Y. S. (Eds.). (2003). *Collecting and interpreting qualitative materials* (2nd ed.). Thousand Oaks, CA: Sage.

Dillman, D. A. (1978). *Mail and telephone surveys: The total design method.* New York: Wiley.

Dillman, D. A. (2000). *Mail and Internet surveys: The tailored design method.* New York: Wiley.

Docherty, S., & Sandelowski, M. (1998). Focus on qualitative methods: Interviewing children. *Research in Nursing and Health, 22*(2), 177–185.

Donovan, R. J., Holman, C. D. A., Corti, B., & Jalleh, G. (1997). Face-to-face household interviews versus telephone interviews for health surveys. *Australian and New Zealand Journal of Public Health, 21*(2), 134–140.

Ellen, J. M., Gurvey, J. E., Pasch, L., Tischman, J., Nanda, J. P., & Catania, J. (2002). A randomized comparison of A-CASI and phone interviews to assess STD/HIV-related risk behaviors in teens. *Journal of Adolescent Health, 31*(1), 26–30.

Fielding, N. (Ed.). (2003). *Interviewing.* Thousand Oaks, CA: Sage.

Foddy, W. (1993). *Constructing questions for interviews and questionnaires: Theory and practice in social research.* Cambridge, UK: Cambridge University Press.

Gubrium, J. F., & Holstein, J. A. (2002). *Handbook of interview research: Content and method.* Thousand Oaks, CA: Sage.

Hutchinson, S., & Wilson, H. S. (1992). Validity threats in scheduled semistructured research interviews. *Nursing Research, 41*(2), 117–119.

Instone, S. L. (2002). Growth and development: Developmental strategies for interviewing children. *Journal of Pediatric Health Care, 16*(6), 304–305.

Korner-Bitensky, N., Wood-Dauphinee, S., Shapiro, S., & Becker, R., (1994). Eliciting health status information by telephone after discharge from hospital health professionals versus trained lay persons. *Canadian Journal of Rehabilitation, 8,* 23–34.

Kortesluoma, R., Hentinen, M., & Nikkonen, M. (2003). Conducting a qualitative child interview: Methodological considerations. *Journal of Advanced Nursing, 42*(5), 434–441.

Lee, R. (1993). *Doing research on sensitive topics.* London: Sage.

Newman, J. C., DesJarlais, D. C., Turner, C. F., Gribble, J., Cooley, P., & Paone, D. (2002). The differential effects of face-to-face and computer interview modes. *American Journal of Public Health, 92*(2), 294–297.

Paterson, B., & Scott-Findlay, S. (2002). Pearls, pith, and provocation: Critical issues in interviewing people with traumatic brain injury. *Qualitative Health Research, 12*(3), 399–409.

Price, B. (2002). Laddered questions and qualitative data research interviews. *Journal of Advanced Nursing, 37*(3), 273–281.

Rintala, D. H., & Willems, E. P. (1991). Telephone versus face-to-face mode for collecting self-reports of sequences of behavior. *Archives of Physical Medicine and Rehabilitation, 72*(7), 477–481.

Scisney-Matlock, M., Algase, D., Boehm, S., Coleman-Burns, P., Oakley, D., Rogers, A. E., et al. (2000). Measuring behavior: Electronic devices in nursing studies. *Applied Nursing Research, 13*(2), 97–102.

Thornberry, J., Bhaskar, B., Krulewitch, C. J., Wesley, B., Hubbard, M. L., Das, A., et al. (2002). Audio computerized self-report interview use in prenatal clinics: Audio computer-assisted self-interview with touch screen to detect alcohol consumption in pregnant women: Application of a new technology to an old problem. *Computers, Informatics, Nursing, 20*(2), 46–52.

Yong, V. T. F. (2001). Interviewing men on sensitive issues. *Contemporary Nurse, 11*(1), 18–27.

12

Questionnaires

The questionnaire is a form or document containing questions or other types of items to which the subject supplies a written response. The questionnaire, unlike the interview, is self-administered by the respondent. Since it does not entail verbal interchange, a questionnaire can be mailed, administered by computer, or simply handed to a respondent. It is therefore more impersonal than an interview, and anonymity can be assured. Questionnaires are always structured, in that the questions or items and their order are predetermined and fixed. Although they are structured, questionnaires can be quite versatile. Either closed-ended or open-ended questions can be included, as can a variety of types of scales including checklists, semantic differentials, Likert and Guttman scales, and sociometric measures.

Like the interview, the questionnaire is a relatively direct method of obtaining information. It is used to elicit factual information, attitudes, beliefs, opinions, intentions, and standards, and to assess level of knowledge. It is commonly used to gather self-report data. Because no personal interaction is required for its use, the questionnaire is often the method of choice for large-scale surveys and for eliciting information and opinions about sensitive or controversial topics. On the other hand, because there is often no interpersonal contact, the questionnaire may not be appropriate for eliciting information about complex processes or events that the respondent may have difficulty remembering. It is, of course, useless for individuals who are unable to read or write.

Because it is structured, the questionnaire is useful in situations in which a high degree of consistency is required for description or comparison. The printed format of the questionnaire makes it ideal for scales such as the visual analog scale that are visual representations, or

for those that require the respondent to rank or compare numerous items or to select responses from a long or complex array of response alternatives. Examples of uses of questionnaires in nursing include research studies of the knowledge, attitudes, and behaviors of patients, families, and nurses; patient opinion surveys; health-history and health risk appraisals; student and peer evaluation of courses and programs in schools of nursing; and surveys to assess the health problems and resource needs of groups and communities. The fact that it can be mailed makes the questionnaire efficient for large surveys that are either community-based or target a geographically dispersed population, e.g., a survey of all certified nurse practitioners.

PROCEDURE FOR DEVELOPING THE QUESTIONNAIRE

The procedure for developing the questionnaire is very similar to that for developing the interview (see chapter 11), and many of the considerations for each step are identical. Consequently, the only elements of the procedure that will be detailed here are those that are specific to the questionnaire. For detailed information about constructing questionnaires and the various types of items that can be included in them, the reader is referred to Babbie (1990), Dillman, (2000), Foddy (1993), Hague (1993), Meehan (1994), Oppenheim (1992), Newell (1993), and Salant and Dillman (1994).

Step 1: Determine the Information To Be Sought

This step is identical to the interview, in that objectives are to be specified and a blueprint or table of specifications developed. A determination is made of the importance of each content area, the number of questions needed, and the level of specificity desired.

Step 2: Develop the Questions or Items

In developing questions or items to be included in a questionnaire it is important to consider clarity of meaning, the language used, the ability of the respondent to comprehend and answer the questions, the potential for biasing responses, and the best ways to elicit sensitive or personal information. The guidelines suggested for writing interview questions apply equally to questionnaire items, and are even more important because there is no individual present to help the respondent understand what is being asked or to clarify misperceptions. It is even more crucial in questionnaires than in interviews to word each item clearly, avoid ambiguous and technical terms, define terms with which the respondent may be unfamiliar, avoid double-barreled questions (those that ask for a single answer to more than one question), keep sentences short, avoid negative wording, and provide explicit instructions about how the responses are to be recorded. The questions must be scrutinized to assure that they are relevant to the potential respondents, are not biased or misleading, and that they do not include potentially objectionable wording. Because of one's own cultural and disciplinary biases, it is may be very difficult to identify questions that are problematic or culturally insensitive, and it may be helpful to use the assistance of others, preferably persons with experiential backgrounds and characteristics similar to the potential respondents, to identify such problems at a very early stage of questionnaire development. Special considerations for developing questions to collect sensitive information are addressed in chapter 25.

For closed-ended questions it is necessary to indicate clearly the set of response alternatives. As in the interview that uses closed-ended questions, the array of potential responses should be represented as completely as possible, responses should be constructed so as to be mutually exclusive, and there should be a rationale for the order in which responses are listed. Although responses can be longer with a questionnaire than with an interview, brevity is desirable. In the instructions or in the body of a question, it is necessary to specify the number of responses that may be chosen (e.g., choose one answer, check all that apply) and the way in which the respondent is to indicate the chosen responses (e.g., circle the response, check the response, fill in the space on the response sheet, or in the case of computer-administered questionnaires, click on the desired response or touch the screen next to the desired response).

For open-ended questions it may be helpful to include a list of suggested topics, examples, or subquestions in order to cue the respondent about the kind of information expected or the aspects of the question to consider in formulating a response. Although there are some exceptions, open-ended questions that demand a complicated, detailed, or long response are less frequently included on questionnaires than in interviews, primarily because subjects find it difficult or cumbersome to respond in great detail. If such detailed information is to be elicited via questionnaire, a successful approach is to break down the more general question into a series of more specific questions, each of which has a narrower scope and is easier to answer in a sentence or two. Unless the topic is highly salient and the respondent highly motivated, it is difficult to elicit richly descriptive data from a questionnaire.

With a questionnaire one cannot draw on the interpersonal skills of an interviewer to motivate or encourage response. Therefore, the questions themselves must be clear and compelling, and worded to facilitate a correct interpretation and willing response. A number of techniques can be used to personalize questionnaire items; for example, using conversational sentence structure, using first- and second-person pronouns, and italicizing or underlining words for emphasis. Because it is not possible to correct a respondent's answers, introductory phrases or sentences help provide the context for the question.

Since the questionnaire is printed or typed, the format for questions and sets of possible responses is an important consideration. Clarity, ease of reading, and ease of following instructions are key criteria. Response alternatives are typically separated from the question and are usually aligned vertically. Filter questions assess the respondent's level of familiarity or experience with a phenomenon before proceeding to other questions about it. (For example: Have you been hospitalized within the past year?) They also direct the respondent to different portions of the questionnaire based on the response selected. (For example: If yes, go to question #10; if no, skip to question #18.) Filters are often difficult for respondents to handle without confusion unless the instructions about how to proceed are very clear.

The format, appearance, or sequence of responses may inadvertently confuse, bias or unintentionally cue the respondent. For example, the space provided for the response to an open-ended question indicates the approximate length of the response expected. According to Topf (1986), respondents make a number of common errors when they answer questionnaires, and these errors can be reduced considerably through careful questionnaire construction. A major source of response bias is carelessness due to fatigue or lack of motivation. Suggestions to reduce carelessness include keeping the number of questions to a minimum, keeping the questionnaire interesting by putting less interesting items at the end and alternating different types of scales and questions. Another source of problem is social desirability, or the tendency for respondents to give the most socially acceptable answer. A possible solution is to include on the questionnaire some items to measure social desirability, then correlate the responses to these items with other variables. Significant correlations suggest that respondents have a tendency to base their responses on social desirability. Another alternative is to make it clear throughout that there are no right or wrong answers and provide anonymity. A third problem is acquiescence, or the tendency to agree with positively worded items. To prevent this problem, positively and negatively worded items can be combined on the questionnaire.

Step 3: Determine the Sequence of the Questions or Items

Guidelines for sequencing questionnaire items are somewhat different from those for the interview. In a self-administered questionnaire, it is best to begin with the most interesting topic and questions in order to capture the attention of the respondent (Babbie, 1990). Remember that the sequence in which questions are asked can influence the responses.

Step 4: Subject the Questionnaire to Review

As with the interview, the opinions of measurement and lay and professional content experts, as well as persons unfamiliar with the content, should be sought in order to assess the clarity and completeness of questions and response alternatives. It is generally desirable to compile a preliminary draft of the questionnaire for review, so that it can be examined as a whole and the format evaluated. Revisions are made on the basis of input received.

Step 5: Draft the Questionnaire and Cover Letter

The questionnaire is compiled in the form that will be used for respondents. Ideally it should be spread out and include plenty of "white space." Explicit instructions about how it is to be self-administered and how responses are to be recorded should be included on the questionnaire. This means that prior decisions must be made about how the data are to be gathered and handled. For example, use of optical scanning sheets may be preferable to having the responses to closed-ended questions recorded on the questionnaire itself if the instrument is to be used with a large sample. The format for the questionnaire should be clear, legible, and uncrowded to avoid respondent frustration. Once assembled it is advisable to submit the questionnaire to an editor for review.

If the questionnaire is to be mailed, a cover letter must be drafted. The cover letter is designed to introduce to the respondent the purpose of the questionnaire and its intended uses. Information is also included about such human subject protection issues as the risks and benefits to the respondent and others, provisions for confidentiality and anonymity, and the right to refuse to participate or to answer some questions (see discussion of research ethics in chapter 24). The letter should also provide an estimate of the time required for completion, and explicit instructions about what the respondent is to do with the questionnaire when it has been completed. Since the cover letter replaces the personal contact, it must be worded carefully and in a manner that is likely to motivate the respondent to reply. If the questionnaire is to be handed to the respondent rather than mailed, a script is prepared for an introductory verbal statement containing the same kind of information as a cover letter.

The decision about whether to mail a questionnaire or distribute it via personal contact is based primarily on the nature of the population or sample of respondents who are to receive it. If the respondents can be easily reached by personal contact, it is generally preferable to mail distribution, because response rates are likely to be higher. Personal distribution by the investigator or other cooperating individuals is feasible for many nursing applications of the questionnaire, for example, those that involve patients or staff in local hospitals or health agencies or intact community or student groups. For large or geographically dispersed samples, mail distribution may be the only practical approach, despite the problems involved. The primary problems are low response rates and the cost of postage. Strategies for increasing response rates for mailed questionnaires are addressed below. Mailing costs must be weighed against the costs incurred in personal distribution, that is, expenditures of time and possibly money for travel. When sensitive topics are being addressed and anonymity is desirable, either mail distribution or a combined approach using personal distribution with a mailed return is generally preferable, because anonymity can be guaranteed. On the other hand, for some sensitive or personal topics, personal distribution may be preferable, because it permits rapport to be established with the respondent before or as the questionnaire is distributed and also allows a debriefing

session after data collection is complete. Comprehensive discussions of mailed surveys and techniques for maximizing their reliability, validity, and response rates can be found in Dillman and Sangster (1991), Dillman (1991), and Salant and Dillman (1994).

Step 6: Pretest the Questionnaire

The questionnaire is pretested with a small sample of individuals who are similar to those for whom the instrument is designed, in order to assess clarity, adequacy for the research to be conducted, and freedom from problems and bias. The pretest may be conducted by mail; however, it is generally preferable to distribute the questionnaire to the pretest sample in person, then to follow the administration with an interview in which the respondents are asked to indicate their reactions to the questions and format, identify any portions of the questionnaire with which they had difficulty, and suggest improvements. The personal approach to pretesting also allows validation of the estimated time needed to complete the questionnaire. Item analysis, and reliability and validity assessments, are computed following the pretest and necessary revisions are made. If the revisions are extensive, it is desirable to conduct a second pretest.

Step 7: Administer and Score the Questionnaire

Once a final version of the questionnaire has been prepared, decisions must be made about the administration procedure. One of the key characteristics of the questionnaire is its standardization, which allows one to make the assumption that all respondents are presented with identical stimuli. If the information from the questionnaire is to be used for comparison across respondents, it is essential that the conditions of administration be as standard as possible. In the case of a personally distributed questionnaire it would be important to maintain as much consistency as possible in the individuals distributing the questionnaire, the types of settings in which it is distributed and completed, and the way in which the questionnaire is introduced and cooperation secured. For example, if nursing administrators in each of several hospitals were to distribute a questionnaire to staff nurses, it would be important to select administrators who were in identical positions and to instruct each one to read the predefined introductory statement in the same way to all potential respondents in similar types of settings. If one group was told to complete the questionnaires on site during a staff meeting and another was asked to complete them at home, the different conditions of administration could potentially influence the results and render the two sets of data incomparable.

Mailed questionnaires should be packaged identically and sent to similar settings (e.g., either work address or home address, but not a combination of the two) in order to standardize administration conditions as much as possible. It should be noted that with a mailed questionnaire the investigator has no control over the specific conditions under which the respondent chooses to self-administer the instrument. Considerable variation can occur in the degree of input or help that is sought from others, the order in which the questions are answered, the setting in which the instrument is answered, and the amount of distraction in the environment. Thus, complete standardization is impossible to achieve. The same may be true for computer-administered questionnaires, particularly those that are sent via the Internet to respondents' homes or workplaces. Mail and Internet surveys are discussed in detail by Dillman (2000) and Salant and Dillman (1994).

A problem that continues to plague researchers who use questionnaires is nonresponse. Three types of nonresponse have been identified: Noncoverage, a sampling problem in which some sampling units (e.g., individuals) are omitted from the sampling frame; unit nonresponse, in which some sampling units yield no data because of noncontact or refusal to participate; and item nonresponse, when the sampling unit participates but fails to answer some of the questions or answers them in a way that makes the data unusable (Elliot, 1991). Barribal and White (1999) have developed an explanatory model of data loss in surveys to display the relationships among these three types of nonresponse and factors that influence their occurrence.

Unfortunately, and particularly when questionnaires are mailed, unit nonresponse is common. It is not unusual to encounter response rates as low as 30%. The result is not only a diminished sample size, but also a set of responses that may be atypical of the sample as a whole, since nonresponse is not a random process. Several techniques can improve response rates with mailed questionnaires. These include (1) supplying a self-addressed and stamped return envelope, (2) following up the original administration with one or two mailed or telephone reminders (including another copy of the questionnaire), and (3) offering incentives or rewards (e.g., small amounts of money or inexpensive gifts) either in advance or upon receipt of the completed questionnaire. Strategies already mentioned, such as carefully wording the cover letter to establish rapport and providing a clear and attractive questionnaire, also enhance response rates. A number of experiments have been conducted to determine the effects on response rates of specific variables such as paper color, type of envelope and stamp, type of letterhead, typed versus written address, incentives, and timing and type of follow-up on response rates. The findings are inconclusive. However, some common sense principles are advisable; for example, response is encouraged by a questionnaire that is appealing in appearance, interesting in content, easy to understand, and not overly demanding in time or difficulty. Dillman (2000) and Groves (2002) suggest strategies to enhance response in surveys.

Response rates are predictably problematic with mailed questionnaires. It is helpful to make provision at the time of administration for estimating the nonresponse bias that may exist because of systematic differences between those who respond and those who do not. For example, a record should be kept of the date when each questionnaire is returned, because late respondents have tended to be similar to nonrespondents. Early and late responses can be compared to detect bias. If data are available about some characteristics of the entire sample to whom questionnaires were sent, then the characteristics of those who returned questionnaires can be compared with those of nonrespondents to determine differences, and with the sample as a whole to determine representativeness. Once the degree of potential bias is assessed, it can be taken into account in interpreting the information obtained. A detailed discussion of survey nonresponse and its impact, factors that contribute to it, and strategies to minimize it can be found in Groves (2002).

The coding and scoring procedures for questionnaires with closed-ended questions are straightforward but do require prior decisions about how to handle such common complicating occurrences as item nonresponse, responses that are unclear or unreadable, or obvious misinterpretation of instructions (e.g., checking multiple responses instead of one for each question). The important point is that all questionnaires should be treated identically, with guidelines identified in advance. Knapp (1998) and Groves (2002) provide detailed information about item nonresponse, approaches to dealing with missing data in analysis, and various models for imputing data. Coding and scoring open-ended questions is more complex and time consuming, requiring application of content-analysis techniques to the responses (see content analysis discussion in chapter 10).

Once the data have been obtained from the questionnaire, reliability and validity are assessed using the approaches detailed in chapters 5 and 6. Some of the cross-checking procedures described for the interview can also be employed to assess the validity of factual information provided on the questionnaire. Examples include checking responses against external sources of information such as hospital or clinic records and including consistency checks within the questionnaire itself, whereby the same information is requested in more than one way.

ADVANTAGES AND DISADVANTAGES

The questionnaire has several advantages as a measurement instrument. Major advantages are its cost efficiency and convenience, particularly when the sample is large and/or geographically dispersed, and time and funds are limited. The questionnaire is more time efficient and convenient than the interview, not only for the investigator, but also for the respondent, who is often able to plan the self-administration time, pace, and setting independently. Certainly the time and cost savings for the investigator is considerable when the questionnaire comprises exclusively closed-ended questions that can be scored by a scanning device or administered via computer, including touch screens. Computer administration permits immediate scoring and tabulation of results (see Thornberry et al., 2002). Another advantage is that its impersonal and standardized format assures that all respondents are exposed to uniform stimuli. Such a feature increases reliability, facilitates comparison across respondents, and removes the threat to validity that results from interviewer bias. The questionnaire also allows complete anonymity to be preserved, a feature that is believed to increase the validity of response, especially to sensitive issues and personal questions.

The disadvantages of the questionnaire include low response rates, high rates of missing data, inability to rectify respondents' misunderstandings, inability to adapt questions and their wording to respondents' individual needs and styles, inability to probe complex issues in depth, and, for mailed questionnaires, inability to control the conditions of administration. Problems related to clarity of meaning may not be identified until after data are collected; however, this disadvantage can be largely eliminated through careful pretesting. The questionnaire can be used only by literate respondents, a factor that limits its use for many populations of interest in nursing practice and research.

REFERENCES

Babbie, E. (1990). *Survey research methods* (2nd ed.). Belmont, CA: Wadsworth.

Barribal, K. L., & White, A. E. (1999). Nonresponse in survey research: A methodological discussion and development of an explanatory model. *Journal of Advanced Nursing, 30*(3), 677–686.

Dillman, D. A. (1991). The design and administration of mail surveys. *Annual Review of Sociology, 17*, 225–249.

Dillman, D. A. (2000). *Mail and Internet surveys: The tailored design method* (2nd ed.). New York: Wiley.

Dillman, D. A., & Sangster, R. L. (1991). *Mail surveys: A comprehensive bibliography, 1994–1989.* Chicago: Council of Planning Librarians.

Elliot, D. (1991). *Weighting for non-response.* London: Office for Population Census and Surveys.

Foddy, W. (1993). *Constructing questions for interviews and questionnaires: Theory and practice in social research.* Cambridge: Cambridge University Press.

Groves, R. M. (Ed.). (2002). *Survey nonresponse.* New York: Wiley.

Hague, P. (1993). *Questionnaire design.* London: Kogan Page.

Knapp, T. R. (1998). *Quantitative nursing research.* Thousand Oaks, CA: Sage.

Meehan, T. (1994). Questionnaire construction and design for surveys in mental health. *Australian and New Zealand Journal of Mental Health Nursing, 3*(2), 59–62.

Newell, R. (1993). Questionnaires. In N. Gilbert (Ed.), *Researching social life* (pp. 94–115). London: Sage.

Oppenheim, A. N. (1992). *Questionnaire design, interviewing and attitude measurement* (2nd ed.). London: Pinter.

Salant, P., & Dillman, D. A. (1994). *How to conduct your own survey.* New York: Wiley.

Thornberry, J., Bhaskar, B., Krulewitch, C. J., Wesley, B., Hubbard, M. L., Das, A., et al. (2002). Audio computerized self-report interview use in prenatal clinics: Audio computer-assisted self-interview with touch screen to detect alcohol consumption in pregnant women: Application of a new technology to an old problem. *Computers, Informatics, Nursing, 20*(2), 46–52.

Topf, M. (1986). Response sets in questionnaire research. *Nursing Research, 35*(2), 119–121.

13

The Delphi Technique

The *Delphi technique* is a survey method designed to structure group opinion and discussion (Goodman, 1987), generate group consensus (Isaac & Michael, 1995), and quantify the judgments of experts, assess priorities, or make long-range forecasts (Linstone & Turoff, 1975). In addition, Linstone and Turoff (1975) suggest the following variety of applications for the Delphi technique:

1. Gathering current and historical data not accurately known or available
2. Examining the significance of historical events
3. Evaluating possible budget allocations
4. Exploring planning options
5. Planning program and/or curriculum development
6. Collating the structure of a model
7. Delineating the pros and cons associated with potential policy options
8. Developing causal relationships in complex economic or social phenomena
9. Distinguishing and clarifying real and perceived human motivations
10. Exposing priorities of personal values and/or social goals (p. 4)

In its conventional form, the Delphi technique, also referred to as the *Delphi exercise,* is used in the following way:

1. A panel of experts on the topic of interest is identified. Selection of this panel of experts proceeds with care and concern that a variety of personalities, interests, perceptions, demographics, and the like are represented by those chosen to participate in order to avoid biases as a result of panel membership.

2. Each expert who agrees to participate is then asked to complete a questionnaire designed to elicit opinions, estimates, or predictions regarding the topic. In no instances do participants meet or discuss issues face to face, and in most instances they are geographically remote from one another. The format usually, but not always, is a structured, formal questionnaire, constructed by the investigator, participants, or both, that may be administered by mail, in a personal interview, or at an interactive on-line computer console. The questionnaire is accompanied by a set of instructions, guidelines, and ground rules, and contains a series of items using quantitative or qualitative scales concerned with study objectives. Some questionnaires may include open-ended requests for information as well. The questionnaire is constructed using measurement principles and practices outlined in chapter 12.

3. Responses when received are tabulated, summarized, and returned to the experts. Statistical feedback usually includes a measure of central tendency, a measure of dispersion, and in some instances, the complete frequency distribution of responses for each item. The reliability and validity of the questionnaire is also assessed using the appropriate procedures discussed in chapters 5 and 6. The anonymity of individuals' responses to items is preserved, but the investigator may list respondents' names and office locations as part of the study. In some cases those providing extreme responses (i.e., outliers) may be asked by the investigator to provide written justification for their responses.

4. Using the combined information of all members of the panel, as reflected in the primary round, each expert again predicts, comments, and responds to the new information in

another questionnaire, which is returned to the investigator for analysis.

5. This process is repeated until the resulting data reflect a consensus of opinions, predictions, or beliefs among all the experts on the panel. It should be noted that when an interactive computer is employed, the procedure is often referred to as a *Delphi conference*. By programming a computer to administer and compile panel results it is often possible to eliminate the delay and, hence, reduce the cost accrued in summarizing each round of the Delphi.

Thus, the Delphi technique has four characteristics that distinguish it from other group decision-making processes: anonymity, interaction with feedback, statistical group responses, and expert input (Goodman, 1987).

Linstone and Turoff (1975), suggest the following as circumstances in which the Delphi is most appropriately employed:

- the problem to be addressed does not lend itself to precise analytical techniques but can benefit from subjective judgment on a collective basis
- the individuals needed to contribute to the examination of a broad or complex problem have no history of adequate communication and may represent diverse backgrounds with respect to experience or expertise
- input is needed from more individuals than can effectively interact in a face-to-face exchange
- time and cost make frequent group meeting infeasible
- disagreements among individuals are so severe or politically unpalatable that the communication process must be refereed and/or anonymity assured
- the heterogeneity of the participants must be preserved to assure validity of the results, i.e., avoidance of domination by quantity or by strength of personality ("bandwagon effect") (p. 4)

The Delphi technique is appealing because of its adaptability to a variety of data collection settings. Experts are usually those individuals who are most involved in a variety of undertak-

ings, are busy, and are located in varied and scattered geographical locations. Hence, this approach affords an opportunity to gain input from experts without the difficulties inherent in gaining personal access to such a population. Similarly, experts need not adjust their busy schedules to attend a meeting, be subject to influence by other experts, or relinquish their anonymity—all factors tending to further minimize biases in the resulting data. Anonymity is viewed as advantageous by some who believe that it encourages opinions that are not influenced by peer pressure or other extrinsic factors (Goodman, 1987); others, including Sackman (1975), believe that anonymity leads to a lack of accountability. He notes that in the majority of Delphi studies, where individuals are recruited because of their expertise, less accountable responses may be minimized. Another advantage of the method stems from the fact that it provides for condensing the opinions of many and varied experts on a topic into a few precise and clearly defined statements. Critics of the Delphi method assert that results represent the opinions of experts and may or may not be consistent with reality. Similarly, Linstone (1975) notes that there are uses of the Delphi technique for which it is obvious that experts do not exist, such as quality of life studies where, he states, one would want to ensure representation of all relevant social and cultural groups. Attention to variance in the selection of the panel members as well as precision and care to avoid overgeneralization in reporting of findings can do much to minimize these concerns. Opinions regarding use of the Delphi technique have been varied. Some (Delbecq, 1975; Janis, 1978; Chaney, 1987) characterize the Delphi as fast, inexpensive, understandable, and versatile, while others believe a major disadvantage of the technique relates to the need for multiple data collections, analyses, and processing that is to a large extent dependent upon a speedy response by busy experts. Prior to using the Delphi technique it is wise to ascertain if the benefits to be gained from the effort outweigh the actual cost.

Several authors have noted potential pitfalls to be avoided when using the Delphi technique. These include but are not limited to:

1. Overstructuring the Delphi by the investigator, thus disallowing the respondents an opportunity to contribute other perspectives related to the problem
2. Excessive vagueness of the Delphi, reducing the information produced by respondents
3. Using inadequate techniques for summarizing and presenting group responses
4. Ignoring and not exploring disagreements so that discouraged dissenters drop out and an artificial consensus results
5. Underestimating the demands on respondents to participate and failing to properly compensate them for their time if the Delphi is not an integral aspect of their job function
6. Overgeneralizing results
7. Taking inadequate care to obtain a large, representative sample of experts (Linstone & Turoff, 1975, p. 6; Linstone, 1975, pp. 573–586; Sackman, 1975, pp. 5–27)

In some cases, modifications of the Delphi technique, if undertaken with an eye to preserving the basic integrity of the method, may be more desirable than the specific steps of the conventional procedure outlined. For example, Turoff (1975) points out that the Delphi as originally designed was intended to deal with technical topics and to obtain consensus among homogeneous groups of experts. When employed for delineating the pros and cons associated with potential policy options, the Delphi instead seeks to generate the strongest possible opposing views on the potential resolutions of a major policy issue. He asserts that a policy issue is one for which there are no experts, only informed advocates and referees. Hence, in this case the expert is redefined as an advocate for concerned interest groups within the society or organization involved with the issue. Furthermore, the policy Delphi rests on the premise that the decision maker is not interested in having a group generate his decision, but rather, in having an informed group present all the options and supporting evidence for his consideration; that is, the policy Delphi is a tool for the analysis of policy issues and not a tool for making a decision, it is a decision-analysis tool versus a decision-

making tool. Hence, generating consensus is not the prime objective, and in some cases the design of the Delphi may be altered to inhibit consensus information (pp. 84–101). Those interested in an example of how the Delphi technique has been employed in the area of health policy formulation will find an article by Moscovice (1978) useful.

The Delphi technique has been employed in nursing for more than three decades. In an early effort to determine the direction of future nursing research, primary clinical areas in need of research were identified using a Delphi survey conducted by the Western Interstate Commission for Higher Education (WICHE) (1974). The resulting priorities proved instrumental in guiding the design of clinical nursing research (Brockopp & Hastings-Tolsma, 2003). Lindeman (1975) reported in *Nursing Research* the results of a Delphi survey of priorities in clinical nursing research obtained from a panel of 433 nurses and nonnurse experts. Potential panel members were sought through correspondence to nursing organizations, military officials, allied health organizations, funding agencies and foundations, personal contact, and review of published rosters and membership lists. Expert was operationally defined as a person knowledgeable about clinical practice as well as one who had an appreciation for research. The Delphi procedure in this study consisted of four survey rounds:

Round I: Identification of burning questions about the practice of nursing

Round II: Response to a 150-item questionnaire answering the following questions:

  a. Is this an area in which nursing should assume primary research responsibility?
  b. How important is research on this topic for the profession of nursing?
  c. What is the likelihood of change in patient welfare because of research on the topic?

Round III: Response to the same questionnaire with statistical summary of Round II responses

Round IV: Response to the same questionnaire with statistical summary of Round III response and minority report (p. 436)

The scale underlying responses to the 150-item questionnaire ranged from 1 to 7 with the higher number referring to the greater value or impact of the question. Statistical summaries provided during rounds III and IV included for all three questions and for each item: the individual panel member's response; the median for the total panel; the response range; and the interquartile range. In round III respondents were asked to comment on statements for which they answered outside the interquartile range and then round IV included a 79-page minority report of all the comments of respondents who were outside the interquartile range in round III of the study. The first round of the study began in March 1974, and the final input was completed by September 1974. The report of this study provides numerous examples of questionnaire items and procedures that would be worthwhile reading for those interested in employing the Delphi method.

Another example of the use of the Delphi technique in nursing appeared in a 1981 issue of the *Journal of Nursing Administration*. In this instance, Ventura and Walegora-Serafin reported on the results of a Delphi survey of 347 nursing administrators, clinical nursing staff, and nursing researchers in Veterans Administration (VA) hospitals nationwide in order to identify priorities for nursing research specifically related to the care of the veteran. Potential participants in this study were identified by letters sent to the chiefs of nursing service in 170 VA medical centers and independent clinics. The Delphi procedure included three rounds. During round I each nurse willing to participate submitted three questions related to the nursing care of the veteran believed to warrant study. A group of three nurses then classified the questions into general topic areas and developed 73 statements related to the care of the veteran patient. In rounds II and III nurse participants reviewed and rated each of the 73 statements using a scale of 1 to 7 in terms of the question "What would be the magnitude of the impact on the care of the veteran patient if increased knowledge was available in this area?" A rating of 1 indicated the least impact and 7 the greatest impact. In addition, during round III, respondents reviewed feedback consisting of their own individual rating and the group median for each of the 73 statements from round III (p. 31).

Larson (1984, 1986) used a Delphi survey of practicing nurses on caring behaviors and a study of patients' perceptions of nurse caring behaviors as a preliminary step in identifying nurse caring behaviors that served as the basis for the subsequent development of the Caring Assessment Report Evaluation Q Sort that is still widely employed in nursing research and practice (Watson, 2003). Melnyk (1990), interested in the reasons why people do or do not seek health care, employed a Delphi technique to operationalize the concept of barriers, and recently Kim, Oh, Kim, and Yoo (2002) employed a Delphi procedure to determine priorities for nursing research in Korea.

REFERENCES

Brockopp, D. Y., & Hastings-Tolsma, M. T. (2003). *Fundamentals of nursing research* (3rd ed). Sudbury, MA: Jones and Bartlett Publishers.

Chaney, H. L. (1987). Needs assessment: A Delphi approach. *Journal of Nursing Staff Development, 3*(2), 48–53.

Delbecq, A. (1975). *Group techniques for program planning.* Glenview, IL: Lecht Foresman & Co.

Delphi survey of clinical nursing research priorities. (1974). Boulder, CO: Western Interstate Commission for Higher Education (WICHE).

Goodman, C. M. (1987). The Delphi technique: A critique. *Journal of Advanced Nursing, 12*(6), 729–734.

Isaac, S., & Michael, W. B. (1975). *Handbook in research and evaluation* (3rd ed). San Diego, CA: Educational and Industrial Testing Services.

Janis, I. (1978). *Victims of group think: A psychological study of foreign policy decision and process.* Boston: Houghton Mifflin.

Kim, M. J., Oh, E., Kim, C., & Yoo, J. K. I. (2002). Priorities for nursing research in Korea. *Journal of Nursing Scholarship, 34*(4), 307–312.

Larson, P. (1984). Important nurse caring behaviors perceived by patients with cancer. *Oncology Nursing Forum, 11*(6), 46–50.

Larson, P. (1986). Cancer nurses' perceptions of caring. *Cancer Nursing, 9*(2), 86–91.

Lindeman, C. (1975). Delphi survey of priorities in clinical nursing research. *Nursing Research, 24*(6), 434–441.

Linstone, H. (1975). Eight basic pitfalls: A checklist. In H. Linstone & M. Turoff (Eds.), *The Delphi method techniques and applications* (pp. 573–586). Wellesley, MA: Addison-Wesley.

Linstone, H., & Turoff, M. (Eds.) (1975). *The Delphi method techniques and applications.* Wellesley, MA: Addison-Wesley.

Melnyk, K. A. M. (1990). Barriers to care: Operationalizing the variable. *Nursing Research, 39*(2), 108–112.

Moscovice, I. (1978). Health services research for decision-makers: The use of the Delphi technique to determine health priorities. *Journal of Health Politics, Policy and Law, 2*(3), 388–409.

Sackman, H. (1975). *Delphi critique: Expert opinion, forecasting, and group process.* Lexington, MA: Lexington Books.

Turoff, M. (1975). The policy Delphi. In H. Linstone & M. Turoff (Eds.), *The Delphi method techniques and applications* (pp. 84–101). Wellesley, MA: Addison-Wesley.

Ventura, M., & Walegora-Serafin, B. (1981). Setting priorities for nursing research. *The Journal of Nursing Administration,* June, 30–34.

Watson, J. (2003). *Assessing and measuring caring in nursing and health science.* New York: Springer Publishing.

14

Q Methodology

In recent years, Q methodology has gained interest for use in studying significant phenomenon in a variety of nursing and health care situations (Popovich & Popovich, 1996), in health care informatics (Valenta & Wigger, 1997), as a tool for strategic planning (Popovich & Popovich, 1996), in organizational development (Felkins, Chakiris, & Chakiris, 1993), and in planning public policy (Gargan & Brown, 1993). For example, Larson (1984) developed the Caring Assessment Report Evaluation Q Sort (CARE-Q) to measure, by ranked importance, the differences and similarities in perceptions that nurses and patients have of identified nurse caring behaviors. Watson (2000, pp. 25–47) notes that this tool was the first quantitative caring tool cited in the nursing literature, the one most frequently used, and the one that has generated additional empirical research in different settings, with different patients, and across cultures. Specifically, CARE-Q has been employed in the study of caring from the perspective of nurses (Larson, 1984, 1986; Komorita, Doehring, & Hirchert, 1991); coronary care patients (Rosenthal, 1992); oncology patients (Widmark-Patersson, von Essen, & Sjoden, 1998); in the U.S. and in other countries including Sweden (von Essen & Sjoden, 1991); China (Holroyd, Yue-Kuen, Sau-wai, Fungshan, & Wai-wan, 1998); and Botswana (Hulela, Akinsola, & Sekoni, 2000).

Q methodology is based on the premise that subjectivity can be studied in an objective, orderly, and scientific manner (Stephenson, 1953; Dennis, 1985; Broom & Dozier, 1990; Mickey, 1995). Dennis (1985) notes that "Q methodology encompasses a great deal more than the Q-sort form of instrumentation that is used to gather data" and that "Q methodology is a totally different research tradition than quantitative or qualitative methodologies as they are widely known" (p. 7). When Q methodology is employed, the domain is subjectivity, the emphasis is on the individual, and the methods are unique. Q methodology enables the investigator to develop and understand the dimensions of subjective phenomena from the individual's intrinsic perspective, to determine what is statistically different about those dimensions, to identify characteristics of individuals who share common points of view (Dennis, 1985), and to explore alternative perspectives as well as potential differences or disagreements before consensus is sought (Nutt, 1989). For example, Valenta and Wigger (1997) employed Q methodology to identify and categorize the opinions of primary care physicians and medical students to better understand their reasons for acceptance and/or resistance to adapting information technologies in the health care workplace.

Q methodology differs from other methodologies in the following ways. Quantitative (R) methodology is based on classical measurement theory, conceived from the perspective of the investigator, characterized by descriptive, correlational, and experimental studies, and involves the study of individual differences usually employing norm-referenced measurement to ascertain how respondents differ from each other by quantitative degree. This methodology does not generally value the uniqueness of the individual and treats such variance as part of the within-groups error term which is minimized by the investigator in order to better detect the significance of the differences in the phenomenon of interest. Q methodology, in contrast, focuses on the unique perspective of the individual, highlighting during statistical analysis rather than incorporating into the error term the unexpected and individual meanings subjects may attach to the phenomenon of interest (Brown, 1980; Dennis, 1985).

Q methodology, like qualitative methodology, identifies dimensions of subjective phenomenon from the viewpoints and experiences of individuals and during the data analysis categorizes findings as they emerge from the data inductively through insights into tones and feeling states. Unlike qualitative methodology, however, when Q methods are employed, subjects respond to specific items given by the investigator, resultant categories are derived statistically, and the categories have statistically significant differences among them (Dennis, 1985; Mickey, 1995).

When Q methodology is employed, a universe of statements is derived and a sample of these is placed along a continuum by the respondent using a Q sort. Q sorts obtained from several individuals and/or the same individual are factor analyzed to identify factors reflective of both dimensions of the phenomenon as well as clusters of individuals who sorted the items in a similar manner. Explanation of the factors is made on the basis of commonly shared viewpoints (Brown, 1980; Dennis, 1985).

The Q sort is often employed in order to (1) assess the degree of similarity between different subjects' or groups of subjects' attitudes, expectations, or perceptions at a given time, or (2) determine the change in subjects' or groups of subjects' attitudes or perceptions over time. For example, with regard to the first purpose, one might be concerned with the question of how nurse A's attitudes toward the SARS patient compared with those of nurse B. Do they agree? Disagree? To what extent are their attitudes the same? On what basis do they disagree? Similarly, comparisons might be made between responses by any two relevant subjects' or groups of subjects' Q sort. For example, nurse A might be compared with physician A, or staff nurses as a group might be compared with SARS patients' families as a group. Examples of questions addressed by the second purpose are: (1) How does nurse A agree with his or her own responses to the Q-sort when it is administered a second time after his or her attendance at an infection

control program on SARS? And (2) Do attitudes of families who are having difficulty coping with a member who has SARS change as a result of counseling? In this case the Q-sort is generally used as a measure of the effectiveness of various methods or interventions designed to change attitudes.

The Q-sort technique usually proceeds in the following manner:

1. A subject is presented with 25 to 75 3 x 5-inch index cards, each of which contains a descriptive statement. The statements or items may be derived in a variety of different ways, for example, from personality inventories, case histories of patients with similar health problems, statements recurring in the course of nurse-client interactions, or statements emanating from a particular theoretical or conceptual framework.

2. The subject is asked to sort a specified number of cards into a predetermined number of different categories or piles, usually 9 to 11, according to the study purpose.

3. Summary statistics (e.g., mode, median, and mean ranks, and interquartile range) are determined for each item. The similarity of responses is examined using factor analysis.

Although this procedure, on the surface, appears relatively straightforward and simple to employ, several factors need careful consideration when it is used. More specifically, attention needs to be given to (1) how items are selected, (2) the type of response required, (3) the arrangement of piles, (4) scoring, analysis, and interpretations that can be made on the basis of the measure, and (5) reliability and validity.

ITEM SELECTION

The Q-sort is an ordinal scaling technique conceptually based on small sampling theory. The study population consists of traits, characteristics, and attitudes for a small number of subjects. An advantage of Q methodology according to McKeown and Thomas (1990) is that it does not require a large population to produce meaningful results and that a Q sample of

30–50 individuals can accurately depict a range of perspectives of a topic. The unit of analysis or "n" for the Q study is the number of items referred to as the Q set rather than the number of persons. It is generally assumed that the universe or domain to be sampled is known and finite. To facilitate comparison of the items with each other, the Q-sort is particularly useful when the universe is greater than 25 items but less than or equal to 75 (Fox, 1976, p. 235). The identification of the items to be rated is an especially important consideration; hence, the development of the cards is an extensive and very critical undertaking. The most important concern in the selection of items for the Q-sort is that those selected be truly representative of the universe to be measured, thus providing a reliable and valid measure of the variable of interest. Sources for item selection usually include the literature, extant measures, and/or preliminary interviews with significant others. In developing the CARE-Q, Larson (1984) identified items using a Delphi survey of practicing nurses' caring behaviors and a study of patients' perceptions of nurse caring behaviors that resulted in the identification of 69 nurse caring behaviors which later were reduced to 50 behavioral items. These items were then ordered in six subscales of caring that included: accessible (6 items); comforts (9 items); anticipates (5 items); trusting relationship (16 items); monitors and follows through (8 items) (Watson, 2000, p. 26). Content validity was investigated by an expert panel of nurses who were graduate students and faculty, and a panel of nurses and patients on an oncology unit and test/retest reliability was obtained from a random sample of nurses in a national oncology organization (Kyle, 1995; Andrews, Daniels, & Hall, 1996; Beck, 1999). Limitations of the Q methodology resulted from the forced choice format that led to difficulties in selecting one item over another as the most important (Kyle, 1995) as well as length of time to complete and problems related to the fact that some participants did not sort according to directions (Beck, 1999).

The results obtained by the use of the Q-sort will vary widely with the nature of the universe of statements from which items are selected.

Mowrer (1953, pp. 358–359) exemplifies a potential problem in this area likely to result if one selects items from the domain of what he refers to as "universally applicable" and "universally inapplicable" statements. Such statements for a population of normal subjects might be: "I usually walk in an upright position," "I eat regularly," "I frequently hold my breath for as much as 10 minutes." By selecting such items for a Q-sort and using a dichotomous distribution, one could ensure the finding that different persons correlate highly, that is, are quite homogeneous. On the other hand, he points out, if one selects "idiosyncratic" characteristics such as "place and date of birth," "address of present residence," and "full name of spouse" as items, one could ensure the finding that the correlation between persons would be very low; that is, that persons are very heterogeneous. Similarly, by selecting characteristics that fall in the middle range of universality, one could ensure results that would group individuals into societies or into special roles such as professions or political parties.

Mowrer suggests as one solution to this dilemma the selection of items that refer to state characteristics, that is, those with respect to which the subjects are likely to change, rather than trait characteristics that are stable over time and not amenable to change. After the item universe is thus defined, the items selected should be pretested to ascertain that they are understandable, representative, and workable.

Stephenson (1953) proposed that items for inclusion in the Q sort be selected in the following manner. First, all statements that by some operational criterion fall within the chosen domain are collected and listed. Then from this exhaustive list, sample items are selected at random to serve as statements for inclusion in the Q-sort. In his own research of Jungian types, Stephenson aggregated approximately 2,000 statements used by Jung in discussing introverts and extroverts and then selected, strictly at random, samples of items which then served as the Q sets in subsequent research.

In nursing, Freihofer and Felton (1976) used a similar selection approach in their study of nursing behaviors in bereavement. More specifically the nursing behaviors of the Q-sort were obtained from nurse experts and an exhaustive review of the professional and lay literature on loss, grief, and crisis intervention. In this manner they compiled a list of 125 descriptive statements appropriate for use as helpful nursing behaviors toward the bereaved. From these areas a three-tiered classification system was derived to order client-oriented nursing behaviors: (1) promoting patient comfort and hygiene; (2) indicating understanding of patient emotional needs; and (3) indicating understanding of grief, grieving, and loss of the bereaved. From the total 125 items generated, 88 were selected for the Q-sort and assigned to one of the three specified categories. Items were pretested prior to their use in the study.

The advantages of this type of selection method stem from the fact that the procedure is clearly specified, consequently replicable, and the Q sets derived are truly representative of the delimited universe (i.e., successive sampling from the universe results in comparable Q sets). A primary disadvantage results from the cost involved in delimiting all items in the universe. Another disadvantage cited by Block (1961) is that the method fails to consider the nature of the universe it samples. He contends that when a universe is operationalized to render it measurable, there is no guarantee that the resulting aggregate will properly express the underlying abstractly defined universe. The consequences of this purely empirical approach to item selection may be redundancies in the coverage of certain portions of the domain and inadequate coverage of others, resulting in a Q-sort that does not adequately represent the true universe. This, of course, is a danger whenever a measure is solely empirically derived and highlights the importance of a conceptual framework to guide the operationalization of a phenomenon.

Yet another approach to the problem of selecting a representative set of items for inclusion in the Q-sort was employed by Block (1961) and his associates in developing the California Q-sort. The California Q-sort (CQ) is a standardized measure designed to provide a description of individual personality in terms of the relative salience of personality dimensions. Initially, in an attempt to comprehensively delimit the personality domain as measured by

contemporary clinicians, 90 personality variables were expressed in item form. A number of these items were adapted from an established Q-sort derived earlier for use by assessors in a study of Air Force officers (MacKinnon, 1958). Block notes, in discussing this process, that this initial item collection represented and was somewhat biased by the personal theoretical preferences of the item writers.

For this reason, the 90 items were then subjected to scrutiny by two psychologists and a psychoanalyst who attended to each item's clarity and psychological importance and its implications for the sufficiency of the total item set. This step of the process according to Block took approximately 60 hours of meetings. Next, the item choices of the three-person group of experts were submitted to a larger group of practicing clinical psychologists who again scrutinized the items from their own perspectives in the same manner as the group of experts. The 108-item Q set resulting from these efforts was then empirically tested in a research study over a 14-month period of time. Revisions were then made on the basis of the findings from the pilot research resulting in another revised CQ set consisting of 115 items. The 115-item CQ set was then used in research and clinical practice over a period of three years before it was revised by incorporating suggestions accumulated during that time. In addition, the measurement properties of all of the CQ sets were empirically investigated at the same time, and the present form containing 100 Q items resulted.

Popovich and Popovich (1996) employed yet another approach to selecting items for their Q sort when employing Q methodology within a hospital strategic planning process to address issues of health care reform and the potential impact it would have on the organization. Q methodology in this case was employed to identify consensus areas among their stakeholders as well as any alternative perspectives that might arise. Sixty-eight participants (7 board members, 25 physicians, and 36 hospital managers) attended an evening retreat for dinner and discussion. Members of each stakeholder group were seated at table in a way that enabled them to co-mingle at each table. The response question, which asked what the hospital needed to do to survive and prosper under the constraints proposed in various health care reform proposals, was placed on each table along with tablets for recording responses. A facilitator was assigned to each table to record statements and seek clarification if required. Respondents were asked to frame their responses to the question in terms of routine versus complex activities, and short-term versus long-term implications.

As a result of this process, 149 statements were generated by participants and subsequently edited into 77 statements. Because of constraints in the time allotted for the retreat, another meeting of administrative staff was held the next week, where sorts were distributed and completed. Q-sort response sheets and the sorts were then mailed to the medical staff and board participants for completion, and each participant was asked to rank the 77 statements on an 11-point, most agree (+5)/most disagree (−5) scale. The completed sorts were returned by 56 (82%) of those present at the retreat.

Other approaches to Q-sort item selection are suggested by the work of Whiting (1955), and Dunlap and Hadley (1965). Dunlap and Hadley, using Q-sort methodology in self-evaluation of conference leadership skill, derived their items from two major sources: (1) program objectives, and (2) responses to preself and postself conception instruments used in the first year of their three-year program. Whiting, using the Q-sort to determine the way in which nurses' duties, functions, and interpersonal relationships are perceived by nurses themselves and by others outside of nursing, derived items for his Q-sort on the basis of available empirical findings in this area of concern.

In summary, there are a number of varied approaches to identifying appropriate items for the Q-sort. The utility of a given approach is largely a function of the probability that it will lead one to comprehensively identify and include the Q-sort items that are truly representative of the domain or universe to be measured.

The rubric Q-sort is applied to a number of different types of sorts that require subjects to respond in different ways. In fact, the literature on Q-sort is abundant with arguments regarding what can legitimately be referred to as a Q-sort and what cannot. For this reason, it is important when applying the technique to be aware of the various types of sorts referred to in the literature, to be clear regarding the purpose for the measure in the context of a particular situation, and to ensure that what the subject is asked to do in the way of sorting is consistent with the measurement purpose.

The *S-sort*, also referred to as the *S procedure* and *self-sort*, requires the subject to arrange the items in terms of how he or she views them at a given time. The *ideal sort* asks the subject to sort the cards according to his or her ideal of the best possible in regard to the attitude being measured. The subject usually is asked to sort the cards in terms of their applicability to other persons or social stereotypes. When a variation of this type of sort, called a *self-ideal sort*, is used, the respondent is directed to answer in terms of how he or she would like to be. Self-sorts and ideal sorts are often obtained from the same individual or group and correlated to determine agreement. The *prediction sort* asks the subject to sort the cards according to the manner in which he or she predicts another subject will make the sort. The prediction sort is often compared with the self-sort of the other subject, for example, having the nurse complete a prediction sort and then comparing the results with the self-sort of a patient may be used as an index of how well the nurse understands the patient's expectations and is sensitive to the patient's views. The term *before and after treatment sorts* is used to refer to those instances in which a sort is obtained prior to the implementation of a particular treatment geared to changing attitudes and then is compared with one obtained posttreatment. Self-sorts are often employed as before and after sorts.

Subjects are deliberately selected with the expectation that they will hold different points of view in regard to the phenomenon of interest. As indicated earlier, small sampling theory is the basis of subject selection when Q is employed. The subjects are referred to as the P set. The number of subjects to be included in the P set derives from the need for enough persons to define the factors that emerge from factor analysis of the Q-sorts. Because items are the unit of analysis when the Q-sort is employed, concern for the subjects-to-factors ratio replaces the subjects-to-variables ratio at issue in R methodology (Dennis, 1985). Brown (1980) suggests as a rule of thumb that there be at least four or five persons defining each factor and that, beyond that, additional subjects add very little (p. 260). Since no more than seven factors, and usually fewer, emerge from the data in most Q studies, relatively small numbers of subjects are required. Dennis (1985) notes that since items are the unit of analysis, Q methodology is valuable for single subject studies (i.e., $n = 1$) in which one subject performs multiple Q-sorts according to different frames of reference. Nunnally and Bernstein (1994), on the other hand, caution that when using Q methodology it is more difficult and more costly to obtain large amounts of time from small numbers of subjects than with more conventional approaches that require smaller amounts of time from larger numbers of subjects, especially in subject pools (p. 529).

THE ARRANGEMENT OF PILES

The Q-sort differs from the more frequently encountered rating scale in that it requires the subject to order or rank a set of items in clusters rather than singly as in the case of the rating scale. In most instances, the sorting into clusters or piles is prespecified in such a way that the resulting distribution is normal in shape. For example, suppose a Q-sort is developed to determine what subjects believe to be the most important to the least important characteristics of a nurse practitioner. One hundred statements each describing one characteristic from the universe of nurse practitioner attributes are typed on cards and presented to the subject. The subject is then asked to sort the 100 items into nine piles according to the following scheme:

In pile 1, on the extreme left, place the one item you feel is the least important characteristic of a nurse practitioner.

In pile 9, on the extreme right, place the one item you feel is the most important characteristic of a nurse practitioner.

Next, in pile 2, place the four next least important items and in pile 8, place the four next most important items.

Then in piles 3 and 7, place the 11 next least and most important items, respectively.

In piles 4 and 6, place 21 items each in terms of their being less or more important.

In pile 5, place the remaining 26 items that you believe are of medium importance.

Hence, in this manner, the subject is forced to arrange the statements into an approximately normal curve, beginning with consideration of the extremes and moving toward the middle. This example illustrates only one of many possible item-pile arrangements that will lead to an approximately normal distribution of results.

It is obvious from this example that the phrasing of directions to the subject is both a difficult and important task. Reliability and validity of Q-sort data are endangered if directions are not clearly specified in a manner that is readily understood and followed by the subject. For this reason, users of the Q-sort have tried a variety of approaches to simplify this task. For example, Freihofer and Felton (1976) combined written instructions with a video cassette demonstration tape of how to do the Q-sort, making both available to subjects for reference during the entire sorting period.

Critics of the Q-sort technique note that the greatest precision in the sorting occurs at the extremes while discriminations between middle piles are generally less precise. This, they contend, permits only the study of extremes (for example, most and least important) and provides little or no information regarding the items in between. Whiting (1959) attempted to introduce more precision into his sorting, and hence minimize this disadvantage, by changing instructions concerning sorting from one step of sorting nine piles of varying numbers of items to four steps of sorting items into three different piles; that is, first the subject was asked to sort 100 cards into three piles of high, medium, and low, the high and low containing 16 cards each, and the medium pile 68. Then subjects were asked to sort the 16 cards in the high pile into three piles containing 1, 4, and 11 items each, with the highest item going into the first pile, and the remaining 11 into the third pile. The same procedure was carried out for the cards in the low pile. Then the medium pile of 68 cards was separated into 3 piles of 21, 26, and 21 cards. The first pile containing 21 items was considered slightly greater than medium, the second 26 items neither high nor low, and the third 21 items slightly less than medium (p. 72).

An important consideration in sorting relates to the optimal number of piles or categories. Although studies indicate that subjects can reliably discriminate up to 20 points on a rating scale, most users of the Q-sort have found 9 to 11 to be the optimal number. Another factor often overlooked is that although the desired distribution shape is usually a normal curve, depending upon the purpose of the measure, other distributions may be prescribed as well. In addition to the normal distribution, other symmetric distributions of interest might include:

1. A unimodal distribution in which there is piling of items in the middle categories
2. A rectangular distribution in which there are an equal number of items in each of the categories
3. A U-shaped distribution in which the bulk of the items is placed in the extreme categories with few in the middle

A debate in the literature on Q-sorts that should be noted here relates to whether sorting should be forced, as in the preceding discussion, or unforced, as when the number of piles or items to be placed in piles is left to the subjects' discretion. Block (1961) empirically investigated the alternative consequences of the forced and unforced sorting procedures and found that:

1. Forced sorting permits a clearer assessment of the degree of similarity between sorts than does unforced.
2. Unforced sorting tends to provide fewer discriminations than the forced sort and, consequently, is more susceptible to the Barnum effect (Meehl, 1956), that is, the tendency to say very general and very generally true things about an individual.
3. Unforced sorting, contrary to its advocates' claims, is not likely to be more reliable than forced.
4. Unforced sorting does not, as some argue, provide more information or information that is as easily accessed as with the forced sort.
5. Unforced sorting provides data that are often unwieldy and at times impossible to work with, while forced sorting provides data in a convenient and readily processed form (p. 78).

SCORING, ANALYSIS, AND INTERPRETATION

After the sorting, each item is usually assigned a score corresponding to the pile into which it was placed; that is, if a particular item was placed in pile 4, it would be assigned a score of 4, while one placed in pile 9 would be scored 9. Each subject's sort for each item is thus computed. Summary statistics including measures of central tendency, variance, and standard deviation are determined to examine each item's placement across all subjects. For example, a mean of each statement might be calculated and the statements ranked according to their mean. The standard deviation for each item is examined to assess those items where scores were more diversified (higher standard deviation) and those where there was less variance in how individual subjects viewed them. To determine similarity between subjects' rankings of statements, factor analysis procedures are employed. When factor analysis is employed for Q methodological investigations, the factors are the observable or operant form of the thoughts, feelings, or other kinds of subjectivity, and factor loadings are persons rather than items. That is, when subjects load together significantly on the same factor, it is because their Q-sorts are similar and highly correlated. Conceptually, this indicates that they share a common perspective and define the categories that emerge as dimensions of the phenomenon (Dennis, 1985). Stephenson (1953) and Brown (1980) advocate the use of centroid factor analysis with hand rotation, while Dennis (1985) suggests that principle factoring with varimax rotation be employed since by definition the dimensions or factors in Q are orthogonal. She further notes that it is important to recognize that formatting data for the computer is different for Q than for R factor analysis. That is, when R is employed, persons form the rows and items form the columns; while in Q, items form the rows and persons form the columns. Thus, factor loadings are correlation coefficients representing the degree to which each individual's entire Q-sort correlates with the various factors. Because an individual provided each Q-sort, factor loadings reflect persons rather than single items. Each factor is interpreted conceptually using both inductive and deductive reasoning. The inductive approach requires the investigator to set aside the theory underlying the study and the Q-sort blueprint and allow an understanding of the factor to emerge spontaneously from the data. While factors may be examined deductively as well to ascertain whether or not the interpretation of the factor bears a resemblance to the investigator's original conceptualization, Dennis cautions us to bear in mind that the important concern is with the dimensions of the phenomenon as characterized by the subjects (Dennis, 1985, pp. 12–15). Further, Nunnally and Bernstein (1994) note that Q design concerns clusters of people, that each factor is a prototypical person defined by his or her pattern of responses, and that the correlations among actual people specify to what extent they are mixtures of the various types.

QMETHOD, a factor analysis program (Atkinson, 1992), is a valuable resource for analyzing the results of a Q-sort that is available at no cost at http://www.rz.unibw-muenchen.de/~p41bsmk/qmethod/. This software program provides statistical summaries that can be used to differentiate factors chosen for study in two forms: 1) the Z-score value for each statement on each factor, and 2) the average Q-sort value for each statement which resulted from the original responses provided by respondents.

RELIABILITY AND VALIDITY

Intrarater reliability is of concern when the same individual is asked to sort the same set of items on two or more occasions. As with all cases when this type of reliability is employed, it is important to ascertain that nothing occurred in the interval between the sortings to influence responses. Interrater reliability is paramount when two or more subjects respond to the same items on one or more occasions. Specific procedures for determining these two types of reliability are discussed in chapter 5.

Because of the concern that the selection of items adequately represents the domain or universe of interest, the determination of content validity is paramount when the Q-sort technique is used. In addition, depending upon the purpose for the measure, construct and/or criterion-related validity may be of equal concern. Specific procedures for obtaining evidence for these types of validity are addressed in chapter 6. Readers are referred to Dennis (1985a) for further discussion of estimating the reliability and validity of Q methodology.

ADVANTAGES AND DISADVANTAGES

In addition to the flexibility Q methodology affords, the fact that the Q-sort has as its unit of analysis items rather than subjects renders it more amenable to experimental control than other methods, such as interviews and rating scales. Because subjects' responses are structured, less social desirability comes into play, the problems of missing data are not applicable, and midpoint, undecided, or neutral responses are virtually nonexistent. Fewer subjects are required than with most other methods, and once the Q-sort is developed and tested, it tends to be less time consuming and less costly to administer than most other methods for the measurement of attitudes. In fact, the control inherent in the method, its adaptability to a variety of measurement concerns, and the relative simplicity with which it can be administered renders it particularly useful for making interorganizational comparisons (e.g., comparisons among hospitals). In addition to being complete, the data resulting from application of the Q-sort procedure tend to be relatively simple to handle and analyze and tend to demonstrate high reliability.

Disadvantages stem from the fact that the Q-sort, depending upon its scope, can be time consuming to administer. Similarly, if sufficient attention is not given to item selection, validity may suffer. In addition, critics have argued that when subjects are forced to place a predetermined number of closely related items into distinct piles, they may make mechanical rather than conceptual choices simply to complete the procedure. This danger may be minimized, however, by using a four-step procedure such as the one developed by Whiting (1955) or by ensuring that directions are clearly specified and that the subject understands and accepts the importance of the study.

REFERENCES

Andrews, L. W., Daniels, P., & Hall, A. G. (1996). Nurse caring behaviors: Comparing five tools to define perceptions. *Ostomy/Wound Management, 42*(5), 28–37.

Atkinson, J. R. (1992). QMETHOD (computer software program). Kent, OH: Computer Center, Kent State University.

Beck, C. T. (1999). Quantitative measurement of caring. *Journal of Advanced Nursing, 30*(1), 24–32.

Block, J. (1961). *The Q-sort method in personality assessment and psychiatric research.* Springfield, IL: Charles C. Thomas.

Broom, G. M., & Dozier, D. M. (1990). *Using research in public relations: Applications to program management.* Englewood Cliffs, NJ: Prentice-Hall, Inc.

Brown, S. R. (1980). *Political subjectivity: Application of Q methodology in political science.* New Haven, CT: Yale University Press.

Dennis, K. E. (1985). *A multi-methodological approach to the measurement of client control.* Unpublished doctoral dissertation, University of Maryland, Baltimore, MD.

Dennis, K. E. (1985 June 27). *Q-methodology: New perspectives on estimating reliability and validity.* Paper presented at the Measurement of Clinical and Educational Nursing Outcomes Conference, New Orleans, LA. June 27, 1985.

Dunlap, M. S., & Hadley, B. J. (1965). Quasi Q-sort methodology in self-evaluation of conference leadership skill. *Nursing Research, 14*(2), 119–125.

Felkins, P. K., Chakiris, B. J., & Chakiris, K. N. (1993). *Change management: A model for effective organizational performance.* White Plains, NY: Quality Resources.

Fox, D. J. (1976). *Fundamentals of research in nursing.* New York: Appleton-Century-Crofts.

Freihofer, P., & Felton, G. (1976). Nursing behaviors in bereavement: An exploratory study. *Nursing Research, 25*(5), 332–337.

Gargan, J. J., & Brown, S. R. (1993). What is to be done? Anticipating the future and mobilizing prudence. *Policy Science, 26,* 347–359.

Holroyd, E., Yue-Kuen, C., Sau-wai, C., Fung-shan, L., & Wai-wan, W. (1998). A Chinese cultural perspective of nursing care behaviors in an acute setting. *Journal of Advanced Nursing, 28*(6), 1289–1294.

Hulela, E. B., Akinsola, H. A., & Sekoni, N. M. (2000). The observed nurses caring behavior in a referral hospital in Botswana. *West African Journal of Nursing, 11*(1), 1–6.

Kimorita, N., Doehring, K., & Hirchert, P. (1991). Perceptions of caring by nurse educators. *Journal of Nursing Education, 30*(1), 23–29.

Kyle, T. V. (1995). The concept of caring: A review of the literature. *Journal of Advanced Nursing, 21*(3), 506–514.

Larson, P. (1984). Important nurse caring behaviors perceived by patients with cancer. *Oncology Nursing Forum, 11*(6), 46–50.

Larson, P. (1986). Cancer nurses' perceptions of caring. *Cancer Nursing, 9*(2), 86–91.

MacKinnon, D. W. (1958). *An assessment study of Air Force officers, Part I: Design of the study and description of the variables.* Technical report, WADC-TR-58-91, Part I, AS-TIA Document No. AD 152-040. Lackland Air Force Base, Personnel Laboratory, Lackland, Texas.

McKeown, B., & Thomas, D. (1990) *Q methodology.* Newbury Park, CA: Sage Publications.

Meehl, P. E. (1956) Wanted: Good cookbook. *American Psychologist, 11,* 263–272.

Mickey, T. J. (1995) *Sociodrama: An interpretive theory for the practice of public relations.* Lanham, MD: University Press of America, Inc.

Mowrer, O. H. (1953). *Psychotherapy: Theory and research.* New York: Ronald Press.

Nunnally, J. C., & Bernstein, I. H. (1994). *Psychometric theory* (3rd ed). New York: McGraw-Hill, Inc.

Nutt, P. C. (1989). *Making tough decisions.* San Francisco, CA: Jossey-Bass Publishers.

Popovich, K., & Popovich, M. (1996). Use of Q methodology by public relations practitioners for hospital strategic planning. *Journal of Operant Subjectivity,* 17, 40–54.

Rosenthal, K. (1992). Coronary care patients' and nurses' perceptions of important nurse caring behaviors. *Heart and Lung, 21*(6), 536–539.

Stephenson, W. (1953). *The study of behavior: Q technique and its methodology.* Chicago: University of Chicago Press.

Valenta, A. L., & Wigger, U. (1997). Q-methodology definition and application in health care informatics. *Journal of the American Medical Informatics Association, 4*(6), 501–510.

Von Essen, L., & Sjoden, P. (1991). The importance of nurse caring behaviors as perceived by Swedish hospital patients and nursing staff. *International Journal of Nursing Studies, 28*(3), 267–281.

Watson, J. (2000). *Assessing and measuring caring in nursing and health science.* New York: Springer Publishing.

Whiting, J. F. (1995). Q-sort: A technique for evaluating perceptions of interpersonal relationships. *Nursing Research, 4*(2), 70–73.

Whiting, J. F. (1959). Patients' needs nurses' needs, and the health process. *American Journal of Nursing, 59*(5), 661–665.

Widmark-Patersson, V., von Essen, L., & Sjoden, P. (1998). Perceptions of caring: Patients and staff's association to CARE-Q behaviors. *Journal of Psychosocial Oncology, 16*(1), 75–96.

15

Visual Analog Scales

Visual analog scales (VAS) are typically used to measure the intensity, strength, or magnitude of individuals' sensations and subjective feelings and the relative strength of their attitudes and opinions about specific stimuli. The VAS is one of the most popular measurement devices in nursing research and practice, in large part because it is easily administered, even in the critical care environment (Wewers & Lowe, 1990). It is a very common approach to measuring the intensity of pain. Visual analog scales employ a drawn or printed straight line of a specified length, with verbal anchors at each end, to represent a subjective state or stimulus, such as pain (Luffy & Grove, 2003; Tittle, McMillan, & Hagan, 2003; Zimmer, Basler, Vedder, & Lautenbacher, 2003; Collins, Moore, & McQuay, 1997; Adachi, Shimoda, & Usui, 2003; Lundeberg et al., 2001; Stanik-Hutt, Soeken, Belcher, Fontaine, & Gift, 2001; Gupta, Nayak, Khoursheed, Roy, & Behbehani, 2003), dyspnea (Anderson, 1999; Gift & Narsavage, 1998) appetite (Stubbs et al., 2000; Williams, 1988), fatigue (Eller, 2001; Milligan, 1989), nausea (Ward et al., 2002), and mood (Monk, 1989).

Although VAS lines can range from 50–200 mm, typically, a 100-mm line with right-angle stops and anchor phrases at each end is used. It can be drawn either horizontally or vertically; however, the horizontal format is most common. The anchors usually depict extreme states, ranging from absence of the sensation (e.g., "no pain") to maximum intensity (e.g., "worst pain imaginable"). The line can be drawn without any numbers or calibrations, or numbers from 0 to 10 can be placed at equal intervals below it (see Good et al., 2001, p. 237 for an example). The latter variation is sometimes called a numerical rating scale.

The subject is instructed to place a mark on the line to self-report the intensity or quality of his/her perception of the sensation or other quality being experienced. The scale is scored by measuring the distance, usually in millimeters, from the low end of the scale to a specified place on the subject's mark, often the extreme bottom or left margin of the mark. The data are usually treated as being at least interval level. There is controversy about the level of measurement, however. Although some researchers argue that they are ratio level (Burns & Grove, 1987), there is little evidence to suggest that, for example, a score of 40 on a VAS measuring pain represents half the intensity of pain rated as 80, or that ability to judge ratios is the same at all points along the VAS line (Wewers & Lowe, 1990).

Visual analog scores tend to correlate positively with scores on ten-point numerical rating scales or the more easily administered verbal numerical rating scales (e.g., "rate your pain on a scale from zero to ten with zero being no pain and ten being the worst pain imaginable"); and although the VAS is generally considered to be more sensitive (that is, better able to detect small changes over time) (Good et al., 2001), the two types of scales are actually able to detect minimal clinically significant differences in symptom intensity and function that are very similar (Bijur, Latimer, & Gallagher, 2003; Guyatt, Townsend, Berman, & Keller, 1987).

One of the advantages of VAS is that they are relatively easy to construct, administer, and score. The first step in constructing a scale is to decide which dimension of the sensation, state, or attitude is to be measured with the scale. A given VAS can be used to measure only one dimension of a phenomenon at a time; however, some investigators have used several different

VAS to measure different dimensions of a given phenomenon, such as quality of life, simultaneously (Cella & Perry, 1986; Padilla et al., 1983). Good and colleagues (2001) used two different VAS scales to measure the sensation and distress components of pain (see example below). One potential bias that can occur when asking a rater to score multiple VAS simultaneously is the tendency to place the marks at a similar position on each scale, usually near the center (Gift, 1986, 1989). It is not advisable to use one VAS to represent multidimensional phenomena.

Once the dimension to be measured has been determined, the anchors are identified and the scale drawn. As noted above, the most typical format is a 100-mm horizontal line with vertical ends. The anchor phrases are optimally placed beyond the end of the line; however, they are sometimes placed below the vertical mark at the end of the line. With respect to the wording of the anchors, short phrases that are easily understood and clearly depict the extreme ends of a continuum are recommended. Using a line 100 mm in length facilitates scoring. However, lines of varying length have been used. Photocopying the scale can cause small, systematic alterations in the length of the line (Wewers & Lowe, 1990); therefore, printing is preferable to photocopying instruments containing VAS.

The scale is introduced with clearly worded instructions that indicate the dimension to be rated, the time frame, the procedure for recording the response, and sometimes an example. Training and practice sessions may be required for subjects who may have difficulty conceptualizing what the line represents; elderly subjects may require repeated instruction. For some populations, such as children and cognitively impaired adults, a more easily understood visual scale such as a pain thermometer, which is actually a special case of the VAS (Wewers & Lowe, 1990), can be substituted for the traditional line (Taylor & Herr, 2003). In general, however, people do not have a great deal of difficulty using the VAS format, and it has been used successfully even in high-stress settings, such as emergency departments.

The VAS in its traditional form is presented on paper to the subject. It can be handed to the respondent on a clipboard or incorporated as a page on a mailed questionnaire. The data collector may have to mark the scale for subjects who have motor difficulties or are otherwise unable to hold or use a pencil. The subject indicates when to stop, and the data collector marks the line accordingly. Recent developments in technology permitting the use of handheld computers or PDAs for data collection have opened up new possibilities for administering the VAS. Jamison and colleagues (2002) compared electronic and paper modes of administration and found a high correlation between the two (the median of correlations comparing the electronic touch screen and paper VAS ratings was .99 for verbal and .98 for sensory stimuli). Their conclusion was that the computer version of the VAS was valid for pain measurement.

Visual analog scales are scored by measuring the distance of the respondent's mark from the end of the scale in millimeters. Generally the low end is used as the zero point on the scale. To ensure consistency of scoring, rules are established before scoring begins to address such issues as the exact point on the line to be designated zero (e.g., outside or inside the vertical end marker), which border of the respondent's mark will be used, and how the mark will be scored if it falls between calibrations on the ruler. If more than one ruler is being used, they should be compared to ensure that they are identical so that systematic bias can be avoided. Such issues will become less problematic with the shift to computerized administration and scoring.

RELIABILITY AND VALIDITY

Reliability of visual analog scales is most frequently assessed using the test/retest method, and correlations between the two administrations have been moderate to strong; however, Wewers and Lowe (1990) have pointed out that this method of reliability assessment is unacceptable because the phenomena that are rated with VAS tend to be highly dynamic, and are likely to change from day to day or moment to moment. The low coefficient of reliability that would result from applying test/retest reliability assessment to a dynamic characteristic, would be attributable to an actual change in the stimulus, rather than any problem with the scale itself. Good and colleagues (2001) argue that test/retest reliability can be used when the sensation is believed to be quite stable (e.g., chronic pain) or when a short retest interval is used (e.g., 15 minutes). A second problem relates to subjects' recalling their rating on the original test and allowing that to influence the retest rating. The ultimate outcome due to these confounding situations is questionable reliability coefficients. Internal consistency reliability cannot be assessed on one-item measures. Interrater reliability needs to be assessed if scoring is being done by more than one person.

Reliability of the method itself has been assessed in a number of studies. Issues examined have included reproducibility of previous ratings at various points along the line (more accurate at the extremes than in the middle ranges), the length and position of the line, the position of the subject (may be problematic for patients in bed), the visual and motor ability of the subject, and the influence of making previous ratings available to the subject (Wewers & Lowe, 1990).

The validity of visual analog scales has been assessed using several methods, the most common approach being to correlate visual analog scale scores with other measures of the phenomenon. Acceptable levels of concurrent or convergent validity have been substantiated for both affective states and sensations (Bigatti & Cronan, 2002; Bijur, Latimer, & Gallagher, 2003; Gupta, Nayak, Khoursheed, Roy, & Behbehani, 2003; Lundeberg et al., 2001; Good et al., 2001). A contrasted groups approach was used by Good and colleagues (2001) to assess both the construct and discriminant validity of sensation and distress VAS for pain. Discriminant validity using the contrasted groups approach has also been established for some VAS measuring mood and quality of life (Padilla et al., 1983); however, Wewers and Lowe (1990) reported research demonstrating only limited support for discriminant validity when using a multitrait/multimethod approach to assess the convergent and discriminant validity of the VAS as a measure of pain and anxiety in laboring women. Luffy and Grove (2003) in a study of African American children from 3–18 with sickle cell anemia compared the validity, reliability, and preference for three pain measurement instruments. They concluded that for preschool and school-aged children, the FACES scale and the African American Oucher Scale were preferable to the VAS, which was not valid for measuring pain in children.

ADVANTAGES, DISADVANTAGES, AND USES

Visual analog scales' major advantages are their ease of use, acceptance by respondents, sensitivity to subtle fluctuations in levels of the stimulus, and reliability and validity coefficients that are often similar to more time-consuming and complex measures. Because they can be administered rapidly, visual analog scales are often preferable to measures that make greater time and effort demands on ill or busy respondents. Visual analog scales use uncomplicated language and are easily understood by most subjects, although some populations, such as the elderly, children, and those with cognitive limitations may find the VAS too abstract. On the other hand, people who are visually oriented may find it easier to express the magnitude or intensity of a subjective state on a VAS than on more verbally oriented ones. The former may also be easier than numerical scales for people who have difficulty comprehending the meaning and placement of numbers. Compared with measures that require subjects to rate the intensity of their moods, feelings, or sensations on a categorical scale or checklist, visual analog scales do not limit subjects to a limited number of possible responses, but allow them to place their response at any point on the continuum. This feature allows visual analog scales to be more sensitive to subtle changes than categorical scales, because potentially finer distinctions can be made. Disadvantages of visual analog scales include their unidimensionality, problems related to inaccurate reproduction and scoring, and the requirement that they appear in print. Verbally presented numerical rating scales may be easier than the VAS to administer in a clinical setting. They can be used to track changes in the magnitude of a sensation or mood over time; however, the impact of testing effects may compromise validity, particularly if the interval between measurements is short.

REFERENCES

Adachi, K., Shimoda, M., & Usui, A. (2003). The relationship between parturient's positions and perception of labor pain intensity. *Nursing Research, 52*(1), 47–51.

Anderson, K. L. (1999). Change in quality of life after lung volume reduction surgery. *American Journal of Critical Care, 8*(6), 389–396.

Bigatti, S. M., & Cronan, T. A. (2002). A comparison of pain measures used with patients with fibromyalgia. *Journal of Nursing Measurement, 10*(1), 5–14.

Bijur, P. E., Latimer, C. T., & Gallagher, E. J. (2003). Validation of a verbally administered numerical rating scale of acute pain for use in the emergency department. *Academic Emergency Medicine, 10*(4), 390–392.

Burns, N., & Grove, S. K. (2001). *The practice of nursing research: Conduct, critique and utilization*(4th ed.). Philadelphia: Saunders.

Cella, D. F., & Perry, S. W. (1986). Reliability and concurrent validity of three visual analogue mood scales. *Psychological Reports, 59* (2, pt. 2), 827–833.

Collins, S. L., Moore, R. A., & McQuay, H. F. (1997). The visual analogue pain intensity scale: What is moderate pain in millimeters? *Pain, 72*(1–2), 95–97.

Eller, L. L. (2001). Quality of life in persons living with HIV. *Clinical Nursing Research, 10*(4), 401–423.

Gift, A. G. (1986). Validation of a vertical visual analogue scale as a measure of clinical dyspnea. *American Review of Respiratory Disease, 133*(4), A163.

Gift, A. G. (1989). Clinical measurement of dyspnea. *Dimensions of Critical Care Nursing, 5*(4), 210–216.

Gift, A. G., & Narsavage, G. (1998). Validity of the numeric rating scale as a measure of dyspnea. *American Journal of Critical Care, 7*(3), 200–204.

Good, M., Stiller, C., Zauszniewski, J. A., Anderson, G. C., Stanton-Hicks, M., & Grass, J. A. (2001). Sensation and distress of pain scales: Reliability, validity and sensitivity. *Journal of Nursing Measurement, 9*(3), 219–238.

Gupta, R., Nayak, M., Khoursheed, M., Roy, S., & Behbehani, A. I. (2003). Pain during mammography: Impact of breast pathologies and demographic factors. *Medical Principles and Practice: International Journal of the Kuwait University Health Science Centre, 12*(3), 180–183.

Guyatt, G. H., Townsend, M., Berman, L. B., & Keller, J. L. (1987). A comparison of Likert and visual analogue scales for measuring change in function. *Journal of Chronic Diseases, 40*(12), 1129–1133.

Jamison, R. N., Gracely, R. H., Raymond, S. A., Levine, J. G., Marino, B., Herrmann, T. J., et al. (2002). Comparative study of electronic vs. paper VAS ratings: A randomized, crossover trial using health volunteers. *Pain, 99*(1–2), 341–347.

Luffy, R., & Grove, S. K. (2003). Practice applications of research: Examining the validity, reliability, and preference of three pediatric pain measurement tools in African-American children. *Pediatric Nursing, 29*(1), 54–59.

Lundeberg, T., Lund, I., Dahlin, L., Borg, E., Gustafsson, C., Sandlin, L., Rosen, A., Kowalski, J., et al. (2001). Reliability and responsiveness of three different pain assessments. *Journal of Rehabilitation Medicine, 33*(6), 279–283.

Milligan, R. A. (1989). *Maternal fatigue during the first three months of the postpartum period.* Unpublished doctoral dissertation. Baltimore: University of Maryland Baltimore.

Monk, T. H. (1989). A visual analogue scale technique to measure global vigor and affect. *Psychiatry Research, 27*(1), 89–99.

Padilla, G. V., Presant, C., Grant, M. M., Metter, G., Lipsett, J., Heide, F., et al. (1983). Quality of life index for patients with cancer. *Research in Nursing and Health, 6*(3), 117–126.

Stanik-Hutt, J. A., Soeken, K. L., Belcher, A. E., Fontaine, D. K., & Gift, A. G. (2001). Pain experiences of traumatically injured patients in a critical care setting. *American Journal of Critical Care, 10*(4), 252–259.

Stubbs, R. J., Hughes, D. A., Johnstone, A. M., Rowley, E., Reid, C., Elia, M., et al. (2000). The use of visual analogue scales to assess motivation to eat in human subjects: A review of their reliability and validity with an evaluation of new hand-held computerized systems for temporal tracking of appetite ratings. *British Journal of Nutrition, 84*(4), 405–415.

Taylor, L. J., & Herr, K. (2003). Pain intensity assessment: A comparison of selected pain intensity scales for use in cognitively intact and cognitively impaired African American older adults. *Pain Management Nursing, 4*(2), 87–95.

Tittle, M. B., McMillan, S. C., & Hagan, S. (2003). Validating the Brief Pain Inventory for use with surgical patients with cancer. *Oncology Nursing Forum, 30*(2, part 1), 325–330.

Ward, R. C., Lawrence, R. L., Hawkins, R. J., DiChiara, S. E. Biegner, A. R., & Varrhiano, C. A. (2002). The use of nalmefene for intrathecal opioid-associated nausea in postpartum patients. *AANA Journal, 70*(1), 57–60.

Wewers, M. E., & Lowe, N. K. (1990). A critical review of visual analogue scales in the measurement of clinical phenomena. *Research in Nursing and Health, 13*(4), 227–236.

Williams, K. R. (1988). *The expression of hunger and appetite by patients receiving total parenteral nutrition.* Unpublished doctoral dissertation, University of California, San Francisco.

Zimmer, C., Basler, H-D, Vedder, H., & Lautenbacher, S. (2003). Sex difference in cortisol response to noxious stress. *The Clinical Journal of Pain, 19*(4), 233–239.

16

Magnitude Estimation Scaling

Magnitude estimation scaling is used to measure the perceived magnitude of stimuli in a comparative context. It was originally developed to measure the intensity or strength of physical stimuli. More recent applications have gone beyond rating the strength of stimuli to asking subjects to rate the complexity or quality of stimuli or to express their relative preference for one stimulus over another. For example, Bettagere and Fucci (1999) asked subjects to rate the quality of tape-recorded and digitized speech sentences; and Fucci, McColl, Bond, and Stockmal (1997) asked subjects to rate 11 languages according to their degree of similarity to the subject's native language. Although the most common use of magnitude estimation scaling is to rate physical stimuli, such as auditory sounds, social stimuli can be rated as well. For example, Sullivan-Marx and Maislin (2000) asked subjects to rate the relative work values of three Current Procedural Terminology (CPT) codes commonly encountered in primary care office practice.

The most common approach to magnitude estimation scaling is that subjects rate the magnitude of a stimulus relative to one of standard strength. For example, subjects might be asked to rate the magnitude of several different pain-inducing stimuli (e.g., electric shocks that vary in intensity) by comparing each to a standard (a shock of mid-range intensity). Numbers are assigned by the subject to each stimulus to reflect its proportional relationship to the standard. Usually scores are calculated for the stimuli, rather than for the subjects rating them; however, comparisons are sometimes made between groups of subjects. For example, Sullivan-Marx and Maislin (2000) compared nurse practitioners' and physicians' ratings of the work

values for three CPT codes. For detailed information the reader is referred to Duncan (1984), Gescheider (1988), Lodge (1981), Sennott-Miller, Murdaugh, and Hinshaw (1988), and Sennott-Miller and Miller (1987).

Magnitude estimation scaling was originally developed in the field of psychophysics. In pioneering work, S.S. Stevens (1953, 1955, 1957, 1975) studied the relationship between the magnitude of a physical stimulus (a sound or a light) and subjects' perceptions of its magnitude. The relationship was determined to be that average magnitude estimates (reflecting perceived magnitude) are approximately a power function of the intensity of a stimulus. Individuals are believed to apply a two-step process in estimating the magnitude of physical stimuli: sensation followed by cognition (Gescheider, 1988).

In magnitude estimation scaling a standard stimulus is first identified and assigned a value. The standard stimulus can be identified by the researcher, or the subject can be asked to identify an average stimulus from a list. The standard stimulus is then assigned a value. Again, this value is usually predetermined by the investigator, but sometimes is set by the subject. In the latter case, because each subject uses his or her personal scale, calibration between persons is virtually impossible. When numerical estimation is being used, the value assigned to the stimulus is usually an easily comprehended and multiplied number, such as 10 or 100. Once the standard is established, the subject is presented with a series of randomly ordered stimuli, and asked to estimate the strength or magnitude of each in proportion to the standard.

In the classical psychophysical experiments, physical stimuli of varying magnitudes were administered and subjects were instructed to estimate their relative magnitudes. Physical stimuli, such as audiotaped samples of speech or other sounds, or even food samples that differ in a quality such as sweetness, are currently being used in fields such as discrimination psychology, perception psychology, and psychoacoustics (e.g. Ellis & Pakulski, 2003; Bettagere & Fucci, 1999; Ellis, 1999; Fucci, McColl, & Petrosino, 1998; Fucci, Petrosino, McColl, Wyatt, & Wilcox, 1977). In behavioral science and nursing research, narrative or verbal stimuli that represent psychological or social phenomena are used. An example is the work of Sullivan-Marx and Maislin (2000), who chose as a stimulus the work value of a particular CPT code. The work value reflects the time required and intensity of work involved in carrying out the procedure that is assigned the code. The CPT code descriptors and associated vignettes are the stimuli, and each subject is instructed to rate work value for the CPT code in comparison to a reference procedure that was chosen by the investigators to be germane to primary care practice, hence familiar to nurse practitioners and physicians. Alternatively, the subject might be asked to select from a list the task that she or he believes to be of average difficulty. This task is then assigned a numerical value of 10. The other stimuli would then be presented in random order, and subjects asked to rate their response to each in proportion to the standard stimulus. A task perceived to be one quarter as time consuming and intense as the reference service would receive a score of 2.5, and one that took twice as long would receive a score of 20.

Scores are typically analyzed for specific stimuli across subjects, with a mean, median, or geometric mean of subjects' ratings computed for each stimulus (in the above example, each CPT code). According to Lodge (1981), the geometric mean (the antilog of the mean of the logs of the subjects' numerical responses) is the most appropriate measure of central tendency to use with magnitude estimation data. More commonly in nursing, arithmetic means are compared. Magnitude estimation scales generally yield curvilinear data that, when plotted logarithmically, yield linear relationships that can be analyzed using least-squares statistical

procedures. Experts disagree as to whether magnitude estimation scaling results in ratio- or interval-level data (Lodge, 1981; Duncan, 1984).

USES, ADVANTAGES, AND DISADVANTAGES

Magnitude estimation scaling has been used not only to study psychophysical questions related to sensations, but also to study psychological and sociological phenomena. Some uses in the psychosocial realm have included comparative ratings of the difficulty of tasks, the ambiguity of language, the seriousness of criminal offenses, the scaling of social status, the strength of political or social opinion, and occupational prestige. An important advantage of magnitude estimation scaling, when compared with categorical scaling, is that it forces the subject to make proportional comparisons, rather than simply rank ordering or categorizing stimuli according to the perceived strength of a given stimulus. The data are therefore believed to reflect finer distinctions. Moreover, magnitude estimation scales are deemed superior to categorical scales, because they can be used to specify the form of functional relationships and to determine the rate and impact of change (Kent, 1989; Lodge, 1981; Sennott-Miller & Miller, 1987). It should be noted, however, that there is potential for confusion, because the term *magnitude estimation* is sometimes used to refer to a rating procedure that is different from the one described here. Instead the rater is asked to assign a value that reflects the magnitude of a given stimulus, but no explicit directions are given to generate the ratings by comparing them with a specified standard.

Magnitude estimation scaling is not an easy technique for subjects to use. Because it requires abstract and complex thinking, it is inappropriate for some subjects, such as those who are ill, experiencing stress, have difficulty comprehending instructions, or are of limited intelligence. Although a number of studies have revealed that respondents of average intelligence seem to be able to estimate the perceived magnitude or strength of difficult stimuli, subjects must be carefully trained and given the opportunity for practice exercises. Instructions must be very clearly written with considerable detail.

RELIABILITY AND VALIDITY

Reliability assessment in magnitude estimation scaling is generally accomplished using the test/retest procedure, and coefficients between 0.78 and 0.99 have been reported in nursing research (Sennott-Miller & Miller, 1987). Memory bias and response bias are less of a problem with this measurement technique than with some others because subjects are required to make multiple judgments regarding multiple stimuli, which are presented in random order. Nevertheless, Gescheider (1988) noted the potential for some response bias related to the sequential effects of the stimuli, the instructions given to subjects, the tendency toward centering responses, and the stimulus- and response-equalizing bias.

Validity has been a major focus of those developing magnitude estimation scales. One concern has been whether the methods of psychophysics could legitimately be adapted to psychosocial phenomena. Much validation activity has examined "how well the psychophysical responses of subjects can be predicted from theories of sensory and cognitive processes" (Gescheider, 1988, p. 170), that is, from the power law. Results are mixed, and some investigators such as Ward, Armstrong, and Golestani (1996), have found inconsistency "with the metatheory on which modern psychophysical scaling practice is based" (p. 793). Other validation has included comparisons between the use of magnitude estimation, category rating and ordinal scales (e.g., Guirardello & Sousa, 2000), and cross-modality matching, where magnitude estimation approaches are compared with other response modalities, such as drawing lines of varying length and using a dynamometer to measure handgrip strength. The validity of any measure involving magnitude estimation scaling is contingent on subjects' comprehension of, and ability to carry out, the instructions. This type of scaling should be considered when comparative matching of the strength of selected sensations, tasks, or opinions is required; however, its applicability to nursing problems and many of the populations of interest to nurses is limited.

REFERENCES

Bettagere, R., & Fucci, D. (1999). Magnitude-estimation scaling of computerized (digitized) speech under different listening conditions. *Perceptual and Motor Skills, 88*(3, pt. 2), 1363–1378.

Duncan, O. D. (1984). *Notes on social measurements: Historical and critical.* New York: Russell Sage Foundation.

Ellis, L. W. (1999). Magnitude estimation scaling judgments of speech intelligibility and speech acceptability. *Perceptual and Motor Skills, 88*(2), 625–630.

Ellis, L. W., & Pakulski, L. (2003). Judgments of speech intelligibility and speech annoyance by mothers of children who are deaf or hard of hearing. *Perceptual and Motor Skills, 96*(1), 324–328.

Fucci, D., McColl, D., & Petrosino, L. (1998). Factors related to magnitude estimation scaling of complex auditory stimuli: Aging. *Perceptual and Motor Skills, 87*(3, pt. 1) 836–838.

Fucci, D., McColl, D., Bond, Z., & Stockmal, V. (1997). Magnitude-estimation scaling of complex auditory stimuli: Native and non-native languages. *Perceptual and Motor Skills, 85*(3, pt 2), 1468–1470.

Fucci, D., Petrosino, L., McColl, D., Wyatt, D., & Wilcox, C. (1997). Magnitude estimation scaling of the loudness of a wide range of auditory stimuli. *Perceptual and Motor Skills, 85*(3, pt. 1), 1059–1066.

Gescheider, G. A. (1988). Psychophysical scaling. *Annual Review of Psychology, 39*, 169–200.

Guiradello, E. deB., & Sousa, F. A. (2000). Measurement of the care directed by nurses: Comparison between three psychophysical methods. *Revista Latino-Americana de Enfermagem, 8*(3), 108–114.

Kent, V. (1989). *Measurement issues in the use of scaling techniques: Visual analog scales, multidimensional scaling and magnitude estimation scales.* Unpublished manuscript.

Lodge, M. (1981). *Magnitude scaling: Quantitative measurement of opinions.* Beverly Hills, CA: Sage Publications.

Sennott-Miller, L., Murdaugh, C., & Hinshaw, A. S. (1988). Magnitude estimation: Issues and practical applications. *Western Journal of Nursing Research, 10*(4), 414–424.

Sennott-Miller, L., & Miller, J. L. L. (1987). (1987). Difficulty: A neglected factor in health promotion. *Nursing Research, 36*(5), 268–272.

Stevens, S. S. (1953). On the brightness of lights and loudness of sounds. *Science, 118*(3072), 576.

Stevens, S. S. (1955). The measurement of loudness. *Journal of the Acoustical Society of America, 27,* 815–829.

Stevens, S. S. (1957). On the psychophysical law. *The Psychological Review, 64*(3), 153–181.

Stevens, S. S. (1975). *Psychophysics: Introduction to its perceptional, neural and social prospects.* New York: John Wiley & Sons.

Sullivan-Marx, E. M., & Maislin, G. (2000). Comparison of nurse practitioner and family physician relative work values. *Journal of Nursing Scholarship, 32*(1), 71–76.

Ward, L. M., Armstrong, J., & Golestani, N. (1996). Intensity, resolution and subjective magnitude in psychophysical scaling. *Perception and Psychophysics, 58*(5), 793–801.

17

Guidelines for Writing Multiple-Choice Items

Karen L. Soeken

Good tests don't just happen! It takes hard work to create a good test. Any test is only as good as the items (questions) on the test. Multiple-choice items have been criticized on the grounds that they tend to test only at the knowledge or recall level. Unfortunately, this criticism is more reflective of the item writer than the item format. Multiple-choice items can test at the application level if they are carefully constructed. In fact, they are the most widely used type of item on certification examinations that test at the application level. Item writing has been described as "a rather demanding exercise in creative writing" (Thorndike, 1982) and as more art than science. "Just as there can be no set of formulas for producing a good story or a good painting, so there can be no set of rules that guarantees the production of good test items" (Wesman, 1971). Writing good items requires a combination of "soundness of values, precision of language, imagination, knowledge of subject matter and familiarity with examinees" (Wesman, 1971). No matter how hard writers try to produce quality items, an estimated 40% do not work as the writer intended (Haladyna, 1994). Given the use of multiple-choice items in the classroom and on certification exams, it is useful to review the guidelines for writing them.

As noted in chapter 4, multiple-choice items consist of a stem followed by choices known as responses, options, or alternatives. One option is *correct* or *best* and the others are referred to as *distractors* or *foils.* Their role is to appear plausible to the less knowledgeable examinee, while the more knowledgeable examinee recognizes them as incorrect. Some general guidelines can be offered for constructing both the stem and the set of options:

1. Base the item on sound, significant ideas. Avoid testing trivial material and using "trick" items.
2. The item must have a clear correct or best answer. Do not ask for opinion.
3. Phrase items so that content rather than form determines the answer. For example, if the item contains double negatives or complicated sentences, then it assesses only test-taking skills and reading ability.
4. The vocabulary and difficulty of the item should reflect the group being tested. Items testing measurement concepts as part of an undergraduate nursing research course, for example, would not use the same vocabulary as items testing measurement concepts in a doctoral level course.
5. Items must be kept independent of one another so that the answer to one does not depend on giving the correct answer to another. Sets of items about a case scenario can be an effective way of testing as long as the items themselves are independent.

WRITING THE STEM

Stem Guideline #1

The stem should include all the information the examinee needs to select the correct option. The stem is the most important part of an item because it poses the problem and serves as the stimulus for the response. In a quality item the stem will include all the information the examinee needs to select the correct or best option. One quick check on the clarity and completeness of a stem is to cover the options and try to anticipate the answer. If one has to read the options to determine what is being asked, then the stem is either not clearly written or it is incomplete. Examinees should not have to read the options to figure out what is being asked.

Either a completion format or a question format can be used for the stem. Be aware that the completion format can increase test anxiety if the examinee has to try each option with the stem to determine the correct or best option. If the completion format is used, place the blank near the end of the stem. Also, the completion format can result in an ambiguous stem. For these reasons, the question format is preferred. Compare these two stems and decide which more clearly states the problem:

Completion Format	*Question Format*
The consistency of responses is reflected in the _____ of the test.	Which measurement property reflects the consistency of responses?
A. generalizability	A. generalizability
B. believability	B. believability
C. reliability	C. reliability
D. validity	D. validity

Stem Guideline #2

Word the stem positively. Avoid stems such as "Which of the following is NOT true?" or "All of the following are true EXCEPT:" In one study of 200 nursing students, the reliability was significantly lower for items that were negatively worded, and the scores were artificially high when compared with questions requiring a true/false response (Harasym, Doran, Brant, & Lorscheider, 1993). It is easy to see why this is true. An examinee might recognize the exception or the false option and not know that all the other options are true. For example:

All of the following are measures of reliability EXCEPT:

A. coefficient alpha
B. coefficient of stability

C. omega coefficient
D. coefficient of determination

There may be times when it is appropriate and even necessary to use an "except" item. For example, it might be important to test whether a student knows which intervention should not be used with a patient with a specific condition. As a general rule, however, one should use "except" items and negative wording sparingly in order not to confuse examinees.

Stem Guideline #3

Include as much information as possible in the stem and as little as possible in the options. More difficult items tend to have longer stems and shorter, more discriminating options. For example, if you want to test the definition of measurement error, you should not use "What is measurement error?" as the stem. Rather, give the definition in the stem and present several similar terms as options. This guideline also means that if words need to be repeated in each option, they can be moved out of the options and put in the stem. In the following example, the word "validity" has been incorporated in the stem rather than repeated in each option:

What type of validity is assessed when the scores from two measures of the same variable are correlated?

A. Concurrent
B. Construct
C. Content
D. Predictive

Stem Guideline #4

Avoid "window dressing" or unnecessary wording. There may be times when it is important to include extraneous information in order to test the examinee's ability to sort out what is important. For example, a stem may include more lab values than necessary so that the examinee is required to know which values are important in deciding what action to take next for a patient. As a rule, though, unnecessary information merely increases the reading time and can be deleted without affecting clarity. For example:

> There are several types of objective items that can be written for a classroom test to assess student learning. Each type has strengths and weaknesses that must be considered by the item writer. Which of the following is a type of objective item?
>
> A. case study
> B. essay
> C. multiple choice

This item could easily be rewritten without the extraneous information, as follows:

> Which of the following is a type of objective item for classroom tests?
>
> A. case study
> B. essay
> C. multiple-choice

WRITING THE OPTIONS

It goes without saying that one of the options should clearly be correct or best, and options should be grammatically correct and consistent with the stem. Items can be made more difficult by having options that are similar. Two other guidelines for writing the options are very important: distractors should be plausible, and options should not provide clues for test-wise examinees.

Option Guideline #1

Use as many distractors as plausible. Multiple-choice items generally contain anywhere from 3–5 options from which the examinee selects the correct or best option. A good distractor (incorrect option) is one that is selected by less knowledgeable examinees, so it is important that distractors be plausible. Some recommend using 4 or 5 options while others recommend using as many distractors as plausible. Empirical evidence suggests there is no difference in the discrimination or item difficulty of comparable 3- and

5-option items (Owen & Froman, 1987). Having more options per item tends to increase the reliability of a test, but only if the distractors are plausible. Unfortunately, in most cases, it is difficult for writers to develop four plausible distractors.

Haladyna and Downing (1993) examined items on three standardized multiple-choice tests and found that about two-thirds had only one or two effective distractors, leading them to recommend that 2- or 3-option items be used rather than 4- or 5-option items. For some items, only three options are possible. For example:

> How does increasing the number of items on a test tend to change the reliability of a test?
>
> A. decreases it
> B. has no effect
> C. increases it

More recently other researchers examined the effect of eliminating nonfunctioning distractors (Cizek, Robinson, & O'Day, 1998). They found increased reliability, decreased testing time, and increased validity of score interpretation when nonfunctioning distractors were removed. Given that the plausibility of distractors is more important than the number of distractors, there is no advantage to having the same number of options for each item (Frary, 1995).

Option Guideline #2

Construct options that are uniform in content, length, and grammatical structure. Often item-writers try to ensure that no one will argue with the correct or best answer so more information or technical detail is added to that option. However, differences in content, length, and structure can often serve as a clue for the wise test taker.

Option Guideline #3

Avoid using "all of the above" or "none of the above" as an option. Item-writers sometimes use these options when they cannot think of another plausible option. However, there are difficulties with each option. Consider the following item:

What is the capital of Missouri?

A. Rolla
B. Columbia
C. Kansas City
D. None of the above

Test-takers may answer the item correctly by knowing that the first three choices are not the capital without knowing what is the capital. The item asks examinees to select the correct response to the question and yet the options fail to provide the correct response. There is no advantage to this approach. There is one exception: if the item requires computation, then "none of the above" can serve as a plausible option.

A similar problem exists with items that include the option "all of the above" as in the following item:

Which of the following reflect reliability?

A. Alpha coefficient
B. Coefficient of stability
C. Generalizability coefficient
D. All of the above

Test takers who recognize that two of the first three options are correct will probably select option D, which is the correct response. Do they really know that all three are coefficients of reliability? In both instances—where "none of the above" and "all of the above" are options—the score for an individual would be artificially inflated.

Option Guideline #4

Do not include specific determiners or absolute qualifiers in the options. Sometimes item-writers include terms like all, none, always, never, etc. in an option to make the option clearly incorrect. Test-wise students often can use this clue when they are not certain of the correct answer.

Option Guideline #5

Avoid overlapping options. Such items may have more than one correct option and could even have all correct options. Consider this example:

An acceptable level of reliability for research purposes is:

A. $> .60$
B. $> .70$
C. $> .80$
D. $> .85$

In summary, prior to using the multiple-choice items you have constructed, review them against the guidelines. Check the grammar, punctuation, spelling, and sentence structure. (Interestingly, incorrect options tend to have more grammar and spelling errors than the correct option since more attention is paid to the correct option.) Have you avoided cluing in the stem and/or options? Is there unnecessary wording? Are items independent of one another—that is, does answering one item correctly depend on having answered another correctly? Using a case scenario with several items can be an effective strategy, but only if the items are independent of one another. Finally, remember that item writing is more art than science. The best way to learn to write quality items is to follow the old adage: practice, practice, practice!

REFERENCES

Cizek, G. J., Robinson, K. L., & O'Day, D. M. (1998). Nonfunctioning options: A closer look. *Educational and Psychological Measurement, 58*(4), 605–611.

Frary, R. B. (1995). More multiple-choice item writing do's and don'ts. *Practical Assessment, Research & Evaluation, 4*(11). Retrieved from http://edresearch.org/pare/getvn.asp?v=4&n=11

Haladyna, T. M., & Downing, S. M. (1993). How many options is enough for a multiple-choice test item? *Educational and Psychological Measurement, 53*(4), 999–1010.

Haladyna, T. M. (1994). *Developing and validating multiple-choice items.* Hillsdale, NJ: Lawrence Erlbaum Associates.

Harasym, P. H., Doran, M. L., Brant, R., & Lorscheider, F. L. (1993). Negation in stems of single-response multiple-choice items. *Evaluation & the Health Professions, 16*(3), 342–357.

Owen, S. V., & Froman, R. D. (1987). What's wrong with three-option multiple choice items? *Educational and Psychological Measurement, 47*(3), 513–522.

Thorndike, R. L. (1982). *Applied psychometrics.* Boston: Houghton Mifflin.

Wesman, A. G. (1971). Writing the test item. In R. L. Thorndike (Ed.), *Educational measurement* (2nd ed., pp. 99–111). Washington, DC: American Council on Education.

18

Measurement of Physiological Variables Using Biomedical Instrumentation

Kathleen S. Stone and Susan K. Frazier

Researchers and clinicians are interested in capturing a comprehensive view of the health and health alterations of their subjects and patients. Health as defined by the World Health Organization comprises three domains: medical or physiological, social, and psychological (World Health Organization, 1995). Researchers and clinicians are interested in measuring the physiological, social and psychological well being of their subjects and patients in order to determine the effectiveness of nursing interventions (Figure 18.1).

While clinicians are at the forefront of utilizing physiological measures to monitor the

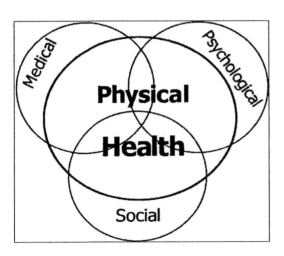

FIGURE 18.1   World Health Organization's Venn diagram of physical health and the associated dimensions of medical (physiological), psychological and social components.

progress of their patients, researchers have not readily incorporated physiological outcome variables in their research. The National Institute of Nursing Research (NINR) conducted a portfolio analysis of the 141 funded nursing research grants in 1988 and reported that 35 grants (25%) included the measurement of physiological variables (Cowan, Heinrich, Sigmon, & Hinshaw, 1993; Sigmon, 1993). NINR held its Biological Task Force meeting in 1990 and invited nurse researchers, nurse physiologists, pharmacologists, and exercise physiologists to develop strategies to enhance the use of cutting-edge physiologic measurements and techniques in nursing research (Sigmon, 1993). In 1991, Cowan developed a 10-year plan to enhance the educational opportunities and research training of nurse researchers to learn biomedical instrumentation and measurement techniques to capture physiological data. Recommendations included increasing the content on physiological measurement techniques in doctoral nursing programs (Cowan, Heinrich, Sigmon, & Hinshaw, 1993). The Molecular Biology Nursing Research Task Force Meeting was held in 1992 to recommend strategies to facilitate the incorporation of genetics into nursing clinical practice and research (Sigmon, 1993).

The Human Genome Project completed a draft of the entire human genome sequence that was published in *Nature* (International Human Genome Sequencing Consortium, 2001) and *Science* (Venter, Adams, & Myers, 2001) in February 2001. The clinical application of genetic technology is becoming a reality. Researchers are beginning to include genotyping and cellular genetic expression in their research programs. The National Coalition for Health Professional Education in Genetics (NCHPEG) has issued a set of competencies that mandates new directions for nursing education and research (Jenkins et al., 2001). Most recently, Dr. Patricia Grady, Director of the National Institute of Nursing Research, established the Summer Genetics Institute (SGI) to train selected nurse researchers, doctoral students, and advanced practice nurses in the techniques necessary to perform genomic research (Grady, 2003). In addition, a postdoctoral training program funded by the National Institute of Nursing Research was established at the University of Iowa in 2000 (Williams, 2002). Clinicians and researchers will be required to learn new measurement techniques to meet the future challenges of genomics as applied to the clinical and research arena.

This chapter provides an introduction to the principles of physiological measurement using biomedical instrumentation. An overview of biomedical instrumentation will be presented, since bioinstruments are the tools used to measure physiological variables. The major classes of physiological measurement including biophysical and biochemical will be addressed. Techniques to measure electrical activity, pressures, gases, lung volumes, temperature, metabolism, cellular products, and nucleic acids including DNA and RNA will be presented.

BIOMEDICAL INSTRUMENTATION

Biomedical instruments are electrical devices that measure physiological variables. Researchers and clinicians can make visual (cyanosis, edema, or Cheyne-Stokes breathing) or auditory (heart sounds) assessments of their subjects and patients that provide valuable data regarding health status. However, observations are limited by the senses of the observer, are subject to interpretation, and yield repeatable quantitative measures with difficulty. Actual measures of blood oxygen levels, respiratory volumes and patterns, and electrocardiographic and echocardiographic

analysis of the heart using biomedical instrumentation provide more definitive quantitative measures. Biomedical instrumentation extends the human senses by monitoring very small changes in physiological variables. Biomedical instrumentation then amplifies, conditions, and displays the physiological variables so that it can be sensed visibly or audibly, or displayed numerically. For example the electroencephalogram measures milli-volt changes in the electrical activity of the brain, amplifies the signal to volts, and displays the signal on an oscilloscope, graphic recorder, magnetic tape, or computer.

CLASSIFICATION OF BIOMEDICAL INSTRUMENTS

There are two of classes of biomedical instruments, *in vivo* and *in vitro*.

In Vivo

Instruments that are applied directly within or on a living organism (human or animal) are classified as in vivo. In vivo instruments can also be further classified as *invasive* or *noninvasive*. Invasive biomedical instruments require the breaking of the skin or the entrance into a body cavity for the application of the recording device. For example, arterial blood pressure can be invasively monitored by placing a polyethylene catheter directly into the brachial or femoral artery and attaching the catheter to a strain gauge pressure transducer. A noninvasive biomedical instrument uses the skin surface for the application of the recording electrode. An electrocardiogram or electroencephalogram can be obtained by placing a surface recording electrode on the chest or scalp respectively. When conducting research, the method of measuring physiological variables (invasive versus noninvasive) should be considered. Biomedical human subjects committees who review grant proposals are responsible for evaluating the risks to the subjects (human or animal) relative to the measurement technique. For example, there are known risks associated with invasive physiological monitoring of arterial blood pressure including blood loss, blood clotting, a decline in blood flow to the dependent limb, and infection. Non-invasive indirect automated oscillometric blood pressure monitoring may be used to determine blood pressure indirectly. The blood pressure cuff cycles every 2–3 minutes to monitor blood pressure intermittently. Bridges has described the controversy regarding direct versus indirect measurement of blood pressure relative to reliability and validity (Bridges, 1997). In choosing between the two techniques, one must consider the importance of direct versus indirect measurement, continuous versus intermittent measurement, the overall accuracy of the measure, as well as the risk to the subject. Consequently, the researcher must be cognizant of the risks associated with each alternative measurement method and is required to address the risk benefit ratio in grant proposals.

In Vitro

In vitro biomedical instrumentation requires the application of the measuring device outside of the subject. Neurohormones including norepinephrine, epinephrine, cortisol, or their breakdown products can be measured in blood, urine, or saliva using radioimmunoassay. The samples are obtained from the subject, preserved, and later analyzed outside of the subject using a biomedical instrument. While there is less risk to the subject using an in vitro biomedical instrument, consideration should be given as to whether a direct measure of the neurohormone is needed from a blood specimen as opposed to a breakdown product measured in urine or saliva. While the risks associated with venipuncture are minimal when performed properly and according to guidelines, the total amount of blood removed (for example, in neonates) may be an issue. Research subjects are often more likely to participate if the sampling technique is less invasive. For example, in smoking cessation studies, carbon monoxide, a byproduct of cigarette smoke, can be measured directly in blood by using an in vitro biomedical instrument called gas chromatography or co-oximetry, and indirectly in exhaled air by using an ecolyzer.

Care must be taken to prevent contamination when obtaining a sample to be measured using an in vitro biomedical instrument. Contamination could alter the results of the measurement. The sample may be obtained in a specimen container with preservative. Each type of sample (i.e., blood, or amniotic fluid) may require different types of preservatives. Once the sample has been obtained, cell and fluid separation may be necessary and can be performed using centrifugation. Centrifuges spin the sample at high rates of speed and cause the heavier cells to fall to the bottom of the container and the fluid or supernatant to rise to the top. The cells or the supernatant may be stored separately by removing the supernatant using a pipette in measured aliquots. The samples may then be refrigerated for later analysis.

CLASSIFICATION OF PHYSIOLOGICAL VARIABLES MEASURED BY BIOMEDICAL INSTRUMENTATION

There are numerous physiological variables that can be measured using biomedical instrumentation. The clinician or advanced practice nurse in the clinical setting, including hospitals, outpatient clinics, community, nursing home facilities, or home settings, frequently monitor physiological variables to assess the health status of their patients. Diabetic patients, for example, use home blood glucose monitoring 3–4 times per day to guide insulin administration. These data can be stored in the memory of the glucose monitor and can be downloaded into a home computer and printed out for the patient or downloaded during the outpatient clinic visit. The advanced practice nurse will order a hemoglobin A1c blood test to determine overall blood glucose control during the past three months. These data can be used for clinical monitoring of the patient or for research purposes to determine the effectiveness of a nursing intervention to enhance glycemic control.

Telehealth initiatives supported by the National Institute of Nursing Research will expand patient home monitoring using biomedical instruments. Biomedical instruments can send real-time videos of wounds, transmit vital signs from sensors sewn in a shirt, or send lung spirometry values via the telephone to monitor chronic lung disease patients and lung transplant patients (Frantz, 2003).

Physiological variables can be classified by body system (cardiovascular, respiratory, reproductive, etc.) or by type of biophysical or biochemical parameter being measured. Table 18.1 lists the classification of physiological variables by the biophysical or biochemical parameter being measured. When physiological variables are classified by this method, the type of biomedical instrument used to measure the variable naturally follows. For example, pressures measured in arteries, veins, lungs, esophagus, bladder, and uterus can all be measured using biophysical strain gauge transducers. Gases from the lungs and blood can be measured by the same category of biochemical biomedical instruments.

BIOMEDICAL INSTRUMENTATION MEASUREMENT SCHEMA

Figure 18.2 presents the components of the organism-instrument schema.

Subject

The majority of nursing research studies are conducted in human subjects who have been selected based upon specific clinical and demographic characteristics. Some research questions cannot be measured in human subjects due to the level of risk to the subject or due to the type of biomedical instrument that must be applied or inserted. For ethical reasons the research may need to be conducted in an animal model. The investigator needs to choose the most appropriate animal model that most closely reflects the characteristics of a human subject. There are a number of established animal models that can be used by nurse researchers. Collaboration with a veterinarian or a medical researcher can assist the nurse researcher in choosing the most appropriate model so that the findings generated by the research can be applicable in humans.

Stimulus

The experimental stimulus may arise naturally or may be administered as in nursing care procedures or interventions. In nursing care studies, the stimulus may result from the clinical environment as noise or light. The circadian rhythm of a patient may be significantly altered by hospitalization in both neonates and adults, particularly in the intensive care unit. Monitoring the stimulus (noise in decibels, and light in watts) and the physiological outcome variables: (neurohormone levels, sleep using electroencephalography, and movement using wrist actigraphy) can provide valuable insight into the physiological effect of hospitalization. A multicomponent

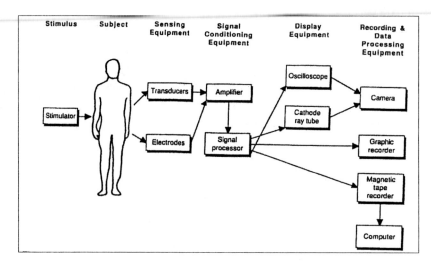

FIGURE 18.2   Components of the organism-instrument system.

TABLE 18.1   Categories of Physiological Variables Detected by Biomedical Instruments

Categories	Variables
Electrical Potentials	• Heart — electrocardiogram (ECG) • Brain — electroencephalogram (EEG) • Muscle — electromyogram (EMG)
Pressures	• Arteries — systolic and diastolic arterial pressure and mean arterial pressure (MAP) • Veins — central venous pressure (CVP) • Lungs — intra-airway (P_{aw}) , and intrapleural pressure • Esophagus — esophageal pressure (E_{os}) • Bladder — degree of distention determined by pressure in the bladder • Uterus — uterine activity determine by monitoring pressure in the uterus • Brain — intracranial pressure (ICP)
Mechanical Waves	• Heart — heart sounds • Ears — sound waves
Gases	• Blood — arterial concentrations of oxygen (P_aO_2), carbon dioxide (P_aCO_2), and carbon monoxide (CO) • Lungs — oxygen, carbon dioxide, nitrogen, and carbon monoxide
Temperature	• Core • Surface • Ear
Cellular Products	• Hormones • Cellular proteins and enzymes • Cytokines
Nucleic Acids	• DNA • RNA

biopsychosocial intervention in African Americans to facilitate blood pressure control can serve as a stimulus and can be monitored by the use of oscillometric blood pressure readings and by electronically monitored pill count (Scisney-Matlock et al., 2000).

The stimulus or nursing intervention can be manipulated by altering the intensity, duration, or frequency. Endotracheal suctioning, a common nursing care procedure, can be altered by increasing or decreasing the intensity (mmHg of mercury of vacuum), the duration of exposure (5–10 seconds), and the frequency (every 4 hours).

SENSING EQUIPMENT

A biomedical instrument is an electrical device that responds to changes in electrical output. Ohm's law expresses the relationship between voltage, current, and resistance:

Voltage = Current **x** Resistance

The majority of biomedical instruments measure changes in voltage. However, the physiological variables that are to be measured include electrical potentials, pressures, mechanical waves, gases, and temperature. Therefore, a transducer is required to sense the change in the physiological variable. A transducer is a device that converts one form of energy, such as pressures, into an electrical output in volts that is proportional to the phenomenon of interest. There are many different types of transducers including an electrode to measure electrical activity in the heart, a displacement transducer to measure pressures, a Doppler used to measure mechanical sound waves in a blood vessel, a pulse oximeter to measure oxygen saturation, and a thermister to measure temperature.

A displacement transducer to measure pressure will be discussed to illustrate the principle of a tranducer. The most common pressure transducer is a statham displacement transducer. The transducer is placed outside the subject's body and is connected to the subject by a polyethylene catheter placed in either an artery or a vein. The catheter is attached to pressurized tubing filled with fluid. Special pressurized tubing is required to prevent dampening of the pressure wave signal. The pressurized tubing is then connected to a fluid-filled dome that covers the surface of the sensing diaphram of the statham transducer (Figure 18.3).

With pulsatile blood flow in the blood vessel, the sensing diaphragm is displaced alternately inward and outward at a distance that is proportional to the degree of pressure change within the vessel. The sensing diaphragm is connected by a wire to a bonded or semiconductor strain gauge. Stretching of the wire causes a change in the electrical resistance of the wire. In this biomedical instrument the current remains constant. Hence the change in the electrical resistance of the wire results in a change in voltage that is detected by the biomedical instrument according to Ohm's law described above.

Temperature can be measured with the use of a thermister. A thermister is a thin wire whose resistance changes as the temperature changes. In a cold environment, the resistance in the wire increases, while in a warm environment the resistance decreases. A thermister can measure temperature changes in the blood in the pulmonary artery using a pulmonary artery (Swan-Ganz) catheter, on the skin surface, or in a body cavity (rectum, bladder, or uterus).

Not all biomedical instruments measure changes in voltage. For example a Clark-type oxygen polarographic electrode uses a chemical reaction (reduction) to measure oxygen partial pressure. Blood oxygen diffuses through a semipermeable membrane and equilibrates in a solution of potassium chloride. The solution is exposed to a polarizing voltage of 600–800 millivolts that is held constant. The subsequent reaction produces a current flow at the cathode surface of the electrode. The current change in milliamps is detected by the bioinstrument. The current change is proportional to the partial pressure of oxygen in the electrolyte solution. The biomedical instrument then displays the current change numerically on the front panel as the partial pressure of oxygen (PaO_2).

When using a transducer, a number of confounding variables must be addressed in order to assure the validity, accuracy, and reliability of the data obtained. Blood pressure must be measured consistently against a standard reference plane, that is, the right atrium of the heart. This reference site is determined with the subject in the supine position. The right atrium is fixed at a point at the fourth intercostal space along the midaxillary line. The pressure transducer's balancing port is positioned using a level so that it is horizontal to the subject's right atrium (Figure 18.4). Leveling of the transducer is important, since for each inch (2.5 cm) of difference between the balancing port and the right atrium, the blood pressure varies 2 mmHg.

All transducers must be zeroed and calibrated. It is essential that the voltage or current be set to zero at baseline before any measurement is made. For a displacement transducer, the balancing port of the dome is opened to the atmosphere to expose the sensing diaphragm to the atmospheric pressure and the voltage is set to zero on the biomedical instrument. The displacement transducer is then calibrated by applying a known pressure in either millimeters of mercury (mmHg) or in centimeters of water

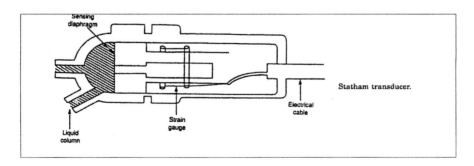

FIGURE 18.3   Statham displacement transducer.

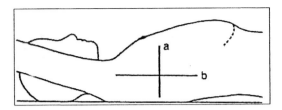

FIGURE 18.4 Determination of the phlebostatic axis in the supine subject. Line *a* represents the fourth intercostal space, and line *b* is the midaxillary line.

(cm H_2O). Centimeters of water pressure are used when greater sensitivity is required. The known values are applied in equally spaced intervals, for example, 50, 100, 150, and 200 mmHg to determine that the output voltage is linear and proportional to the applied pressure. An oxygen electrode is zeroed by exposing the Clark-type polarographic electrode to a solution with no oxygen and then to a known oxygen solution using a low and high value. The calibration is then repeated automatically every 30 minutes to 1 hour throughout the day since this type of electrode experiences electrical drift.

SIGNAL CONDITIONING EQUIPMENT

The output signal from the transducer is usually in millivolts or milliamps. An electrical amplifier is required to increase the output to volts or amps to drive the display unit (oscilloscope, graphic recorder, or computer). The majority of display units require a 5- to 10-volt output. The amount of voltage or current required can be obtained from the instrument manual. The amplification of the signal is referred to as "increasing the gain". Occasionally the electrical signal will include noise or artifact. Electrical noise may be the result of 60-cycle Hz from the environment as the result of alternating current (AC). Electrical noise can be eliminated by grounding, or reduced by using an electrical filter. Artifact may arise from muscle movement as with an electrocardiographic (ECG) signal. Artifact can be separated, diluted, or omitted by adjusting the electrical filter or sensitivity control on the biomedical instrument.

DISPLAY EQUIPMENT

Display equipment converts the electrical signals into visual (cathode ray oscilloscope, graphic recorder, or computer) or auditory (Doppler, or a beeping sound) output so that the human senses can perceive the information.

Cathode Ray Oscilloscope

An oscilloscope is a voltage meter that measures voltage versus time. An oscilloscope has the advantage that the beam of electrons generated from the cathode (electron emitter) has very little inertia and is therefore capable of rapid motion. Some physiological phenomena occur so rapidly (action potential in a neuron, or electrical activity in the heart muscle) that it can only be displayed on an oscilloscope screen. The beam of electrons interacts with the phosphor screen to produce a physiological waveform (Figure 18.5). An oscilloscope interfaced with a computer allows for the physiological waveform to be stored or entered as a numerical value into an Excel™ spreadsheet. In the clinical setting, these data can be recalled for further review or analysis. In addition, the data can be trended over hours, days, or weeks. The data can also be displayed as histograms. This clinical information can serve as a rich source of data for example to examine the circadian rhythm of cardiac alterations in the critical care setting.

Graphic Recorders

The graphic recorders used in the clinical setting to display physiological data are generally curvilinear recorders. A curvilinear recorder has a significant limitation when used for research purposes. The display system of a curvilinear recorder uses an inking system in which the pen moves in an arc and produces a display on curvilinear recording paper. It is not possible to obtain an exact value of the physiological parameter being measured using a curvilinear recorder. In contrast, a rectilinear recorder uses an inking pen that moves in a linear mode (vertical) that produces an exact value. When the graphic recorder is calibrated

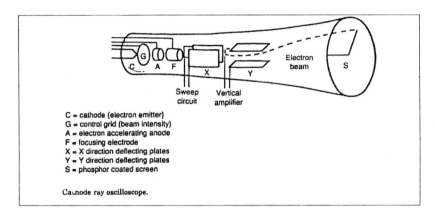

C = cathode (electron emitter)
G = control grid (beam intensity)
A = electron accelerating anode
F = focusing electrode
X = X direction deflecting plates
Y = Y direction deflecting plates
S = phosphor coated screen

Cathode ray oscilloscope.

FIGURE 18.5   Cathode ray oscilloscope.

against a known value, for example, mmHg, exact blood pressure values can be obtained (Stone & Frazier, 1999)

Graphic recorders may use a traditional inking pen that is water-based, or imbed the ink into specialized paper. A water-based ink may be subject to smearing or, when in contact with water, may be removed from the paper. An alternate method is the use of a thermal array recorder that uses a heat stylus (pen). The heated pen, as it moves along a waxed recording paper, produces a black tracing. It should be noted that the tracing produced using a thermal pen and waxed paper can fade over time.

Data can be stored permanently on a magnetic tape. A Holter monitor records 24-hour electrocardiographic (ECG) data and stores it on a cassette tape (Figure 18.6). The tape is then removed from the Holter monitor and is inserted into an interface box. The data from the tape is then uploaded onto the hard drive of a computer. Specialized software is used to analyze the data for heart rate, rhythm, and heart rate variability.

The majority of physiological data can now be acquired and displayed using a computer. National Instruments and Gould Corporation have developed integrated systems that include

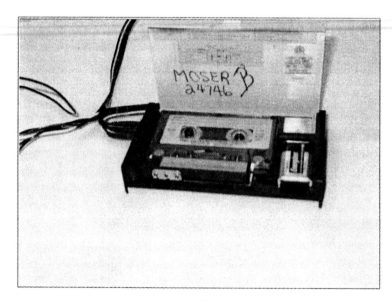

FIGURE 18.6   Holter monitor with recording tape.

preamplifiers, signal conditioning equipment, and the computer for the display of data. The pre-amplifiers are specific for each type or category of data, including electrical potentials, pressures, lung volumes, and temperatures. Specialized software, pre-programmed or programmable, is available to acquire and store the data automatically into an Excel™ spreadsheet or to an SPSS output file. The software packages allow for operator visualization of the data and hand selection of specific areas of the data for further analysis.

The characteristics of biomedical instruments are listed in Table 18.2. The specific characteristics of the biomedical instrument can be obtained from the manufacturer's operator manual or by contacting the research and development department of the manufacturer. It is important when purchasing a biomedical instrument that the characteristics of the instrument match the physiological variable of interest. For example, does the instrument measure in the range of interest (0–250 mmHg, for example) and is it sensitive enough to accurately capture the data? The characteristics of the measurements are listed in Table 18.3 and address the issues of validity, accuracy, precision, and reliability.

The major classes of physiological measurement including biophysical and biochemical will be discussed in the order presented in Table 18.1. While a comprehensive discussion of all of the available measurement techniques is beyond the scope of this chapter, the topics to be addressed were chosen based upon general applicability to both clinicians and researchers.

MEASUREMENT OF ELECTRICAL POTENTIALS

Electrophysical measurements provide data about voltage changes that occur during depolarization and repolarization of tissues like those in the heart and nervous system. These voltage changes are transmitted to the surface of the body and detected through electrodes that contain a conductive solution (Figure 18.7).

The electrocardiogram (ECG) is the most common type of electrophysical measurement.

TABLE 18.2   Characteristics of Biomedical Instrumentation

Characteristics	Examples
Range of an instrument, is the complete set of values that an instrument can measure	Scale to measure weight from 0–100 grams Heart rate monitor from 1 to 250 beats per minute Thermometer from 0 to 60°C
The frequency response of an instrument, which indicates the capability of the instrument to respond equally well to rapid and slow components	Measuring the action potential of a neuron requires equipment with a fast response time, as the total time for an action potential is in milliseconds. This type of physiological phenomenon requires a cathode ray oscilloscope for the measurement. The response time of the instrument is rapid because there is no inertia in the beam of electrons. A graphic recorder cannot be used to measure a neural action potential because the frequency response is too slow. The inertia of the pen as it moves across the graph paper results in a slow response time.
Sensitivity of an instrument, which is the degree of change in the physiological variable that the instrument can detect	One instrument might weigh material within one tenth of a gram (0.1 g), where as another instrument might weigh the same material within one hundredth of a gram (0.01 g), with the latter instrument being the more sensitive.
Specificity of an instrument is the capability of the instrument to measure the desired variable of interest	The blood gas analyzer is specific for the measurement of oxygen and carbon dioxide in a blood sample. This same equipment is not able to measure oxygen and carbon dioxide in an exhaled breath.

(continued)

TABLE 18.2   Characteristics of Biomedical Instrumentation (Continued)

Characteristics	Examples
Stability of an instrument, which is the ability to maintain a calibration over a given time interval.	Over time, biomedical instruments frequently lose calibration, called "drift." It is important that a biomedical instrument maintain calibration because the reliability of the data is dependent on an accurate measure. The instruction manual normally specifies the stability of the instrument over time. The manual also indicates how often the manufacturer recommends recalibration. Because loss of calibration, or "drift," is common among biomedical instruments, it is important to check the calibration before, during, and after an experiment to ensure the reliability of the data.
Linearity of the instrument, which is the extent to which an input change is directly proportional to an output change.	For every one degree of actual change in a subject's temperature, there is a one-degree change recorded on the thermometer.
Signal-to-noise ratio of an instrument, which indicates the relationship between the amount of signal strength and the amount of noise or artifact.	The higher the signal-to-noise-ratio, the less the artifact.

Appropriate ECG electrode placement is essential to detect accurate electrocardiographic changes. Figure 18.8 displays the appropriate placement of electrodes using a 12-lead system. The voltage changes are filtered and amplified to produce characteristic waveforms that can be printed and examined, or digitized and analyzed, by computer algorithms.

This detection of voltage changes that occur in heart muscle provides information about the transmission of the wave of depolarization and repolarization that precedes and stimulates cardiac muscle contraction. The electrocardiogram is a graphic display of voltage versus time. The p wave of the ECG reflects atrial depolarization, the QRS reflects ventricular depolarization, and the T wave is ventricular repolarization (Figure 18.9). An electrocardiogram provides direct data about cardiac conduction and rhythm, and indirect information about cardiac structures and blood supply. The electrocardiogram can also provide indirect information about autonomic nervous system tone.

Heart rate is modulated by the autonomic nervous system through its effect on the pacemaker of the heart, the sinoatrial node. The

TABLE 18.3   Characteristics of the Measurements obtained by Using Biomedical Instruments

Characteristics	Definitions
Validity	The extent to which the biomedical instrument measures the actual parameter of interest (for example, the validity of an arterial blood pressure measurement can be determined by the typical characteristics of the arterial pressure wave that validates the correct placement of the arterial catheter)
Accuracy	The degree to which the parameter sensed by the instrument reflects the actual value
Precision	The discriminatory power of the instrument (that is, the smaller the change sensed, the greater the precision of the instrument)
Reliability	The accuracy of the measurement over time

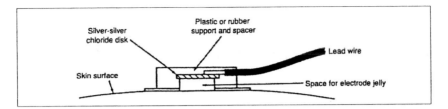

FIGURE 18.7   Diagram of a floating type skin surface electrode.

electrocardiogram may be analyzed to provide information about the balance between sympathetic and parasympathetic influences upon heart rate by examining the sequential distances between R waves (Figure 18.10).

Heart rate variability analysis may be performed in the time domain or the frequency domain. Time domain analyses provide a number of measures that identify the mean time between heartbeats in milliseconds, the standard deviation of this time, and other derived measures based on these two. Frequency domain analysis employs power spectral analysis to decompose the electrical signal into the sum of sine waves with different amplitudes and frequencies, i.e., this technique breaks down the

cardiac signal into its frequency components and quantifies them based on their intensity or power. This method permits differentiation of sympathetic and parasympathetic activity (Figure 18.11).

Investigations of heart rate variability have identified that increased sympathetic tone and reduced heart rate variability is associated with mortality in a number of disease states (Galinier et al., 1999; Hedman, Poloniecki, Camm, & Malik, 1999; Van Boven et al., 1998). Further analyses of standard electrocardiogram may provide additional important information.

Continuous ST-segment monitoring provides a reliable assessment of myocardial ischemia in patients and subjects with acute coronary

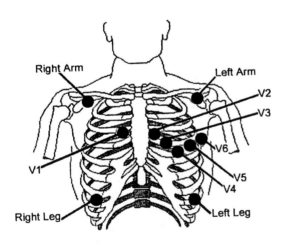

FIGURE 18.8   Standard electrode placement for a 12-lead electrocardiogram. Electrode position for the V leads include: V_1, at the fourth intercostal space right sternal border; V_2 at the fourth intercostal space left sternal border; V_3, halfway between V_2 and V_4; V_4, at the fifth intercostal space left midclavicular line; V_5, at the fifth intercostal space anterior axillary line; V_6, at the fifth intercostal space midaxillary line.

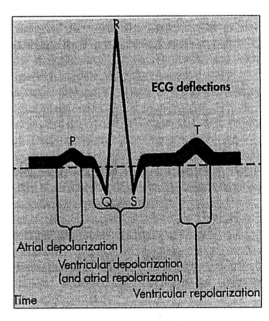

FIGURE 18.9   Electrocardiogram of the heart. The p wave reflects atrial depolarization, the QRS reflects ventricular depolarization, and the T wave reflects ventricular repolarization.

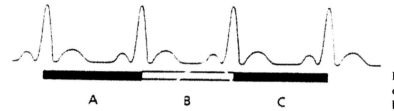

A   B   C

FIGURE 18.10   R-R intervals of the electrocardiogram marked by segments A, B, & C.

syndromes. While a 12-lead electrocardiogram is the standard technique to assess alterations in the ST-segment it only provides a single, one-time snapshot of the myocardium. Continuous ST-segment monitoring provides the opportunity to monitor myocardial physiology during periods of normal function and during ischemia.

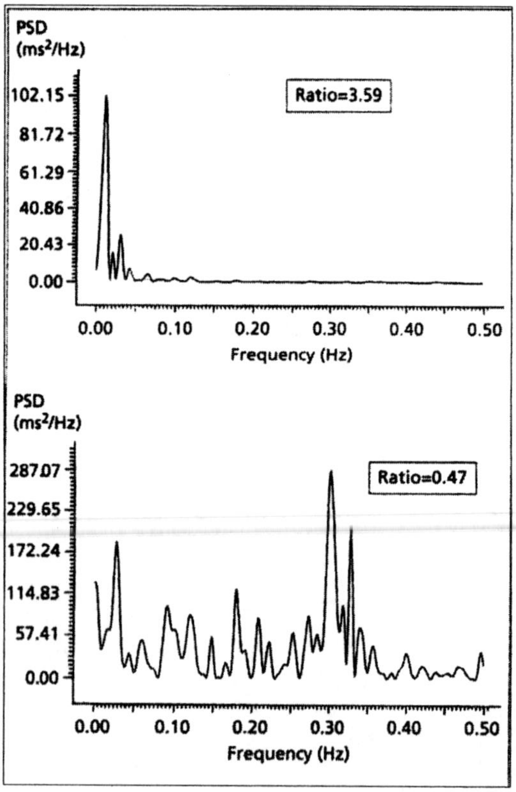

The ECG is more sensitive than patient's symptoms for detecting ischemia. Eighty to ninety percent of ischemic events detected by ECG are not associated with clinical symptoms (Drew et al., 1998; Crater et al., 2000). Alterations in the ST-segment, either elevation or depression, are independent predictors of myocardial infarction or cardiac death. The recommended ST-segment analysis point is 60 ms (0.06 sec.) beyond the J point (Drew & Krucoff, 1999) (Figure 18.12). It is recommended that alarms to alert the clinician or researcher should be programmed to activate with 1–2 mm deviation above or below the baseline indicating ischemia. Continuous ST-segment monitoring can be used to detect ischemia in subjects with acute coronary syndromes in emergency departments, during cardiac catheterization, in the intensive care unit, or in the telemetry unit (Leeper, 2003a). Continuous ST-segment monitoring has

FIGURE 18.11   Power spectral analysis of heart rate variability. The upper figure illustrates a subject with increased sympathetic tone as represented by the large peak in the very low frequency less than 0.04 Hz. The lower figure illustrates a normal subject with normal heart rate variability with both sympathetic and parasympathetic tone seen across the range of frequencies.

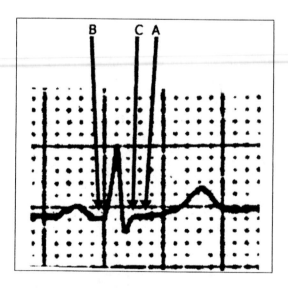

FIGURE 18.12   Reference points for ST-segment analysis. *A* is the recommended point of 0.06 seconds after the J point.

been used to monitor the effectiveness of fibrinolytics, during the monitoring of acute closure of coronary vessels following angioplasty, post-myocardial infarction, weaning (Chatila et al., 1996: Srivastava et al., 1999) and endotracheal suctioning (Bell, 1992).

Signal averaged electrocardiography (SAECG) is a technique that permits analysis of small segments of a standard ECG waveform like the T wave and provides a more detailed evaluation of the spatial and temporal differences of the electrocardiographic waves (Zabel et al., 2000). Small segments of electrocardiographic data are amplified and then filtered. These signals are then averaged by computer algorithm. Late potentials, i.e., low amplitude signals, have been found using this technique. These low amplitude signals have been found to be associated with serious cardiac rhythm disturbances and sudden cardiac death in a number of investigations (Hohnloser, Klingen-heben & Zabel, 1999; Klein, Auricchioa, Reek & Geller, 1999; Okin et al., 2002)

Electrical potentials generated by neurons provide information about central nervous system function. The frequency and amplitude of electrical potentials is captured by skin electrodes that contain conductive solution. These potentials are filtered and amplified and may be digitized, printed, and analyzed. The electroencephalogram (EEG) provides information about cerebral metabolism and neurotransmitter function. Normal cerebral electrical activity is variable and responsive to external stimulation. This is a common measure in studies of sleep (Parthasarathy & Tobin, 2002; Resnick et al., 2003). EEG data may be collected to examine cerebral responses to illness or injury (Wallace, Wagner, Wagner, & McDeavitt, 2001) or to evaluate the response to drugs like sedatives or anesthetic agents (Rhoney & Parker, 2001).

EEG technology is the basis for the Bispectral Index, a technology that is used clinically to monitor arousal and depth of sedation in the operating room and critical care units (Arbour, 2000; DeDeyne et al., 1998). This EEG based measure assigns a numeric value from 0 (absent electrical activity) to 100 (normal awake state) based on computer analysis of one channel of EEG and electromyographic evaluation of the muscles of the forehead.

MEASUREMENT OF PRESSURES, FLOW, AND HEMODYNAMICS

The measurement of arterial blood pressure may be obtained either indirectly, using a blood pressure cuff, or directly, by the placement of a polyethylene catheter in an artery. The oscillometric (cuff) indirect method of measuring arterial blood pressure is based upon flow-induced oscillations in the arterial wall as compared with the direct method that measures pressure directly in the vessel. As previously discussed, Ohm's law (Pressure = Flow **x** Resistance) also expresses the relationship between pressure, flow, and resistance. A positive relationship exists between pressure and flow when resistance is constant. However, when evaluating arterial pressure it must be appreciated that resistance in the vascular bed does not remain constant and is influenced by perfusion requirements, autonomic nervous system tone, and vasoactive medications. Hence, there may be differences in indirect versus direct arterial pressure measurements based upon physiological changes in the vascular bed (Bridges, 1997).

A key to accurate oscillometeric indirect arterial blood pressure measurement is the use of the correct size cuff and proper use of the blood pressure cuff. The optimal ratio of the width of the bladder of the blood pressure cuff to the circumference of the arm is 0.4 in that the bladder width is 40% of arm circumference. Figure 18.13A illustrates that if the cuff is correctly positioned at the midpoint of the upper arm and wrapped around the arm, that the end of the cuff should fall in the range marked D. If the bladder is too wide or greater than 40% of arm circumference, then the cuff will fall to the left of D and underestimate the pressure. If the bladder is too narrow or less than 40% of arm circumference the cuff will be to the right of D overestimating pressure.

There are a number of confounding variables that may result in error. These include not wrapping the cuff snugly enough (one finger under the cuff), expressing the air out of the cuff bladder before application of the cuff, a kinked hose, or not supporting the arm at heart level. Anatomical and physiological variables in the subject can also influence accuracy such as

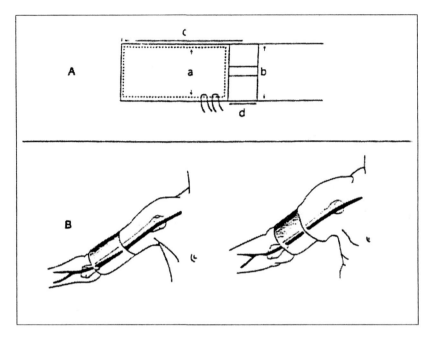

FIGURE 18.13   Sizing of blood pressure cuff and associated problems. *A* **illustrates the sizing of the cuff.** *B* **illustrates problems associated with inappropriate cuff size. In the drawing on the left, the bladder width is correct for the arm so that with the bladder inflated the brachial artery is compressed. In the drawing on the right, the bladder width is small for the arm and the full cuff pressure cannot be applied to the brachial artery.**

talking, arm motion, seizure activity, shivering, an obstruction in the vessel limiting flow, or alterations in heart rhythm (Bridges, 1997).

Direct arterial blood pressure monitoring is accomplished by the insertion of a polyethylene catheter directly into the artery that is then attached by pressurized tubing to the fluid-filled dome of a statham displacement transducer. The transducer must then be zeroed and calibrated against a column of mercury. Referencing the transducer to the right atrium at the phlebostatic axis, as discussed earlier in the chapter, must be completed before taking pressure measurements. The pressure transducer then senses the pressure pulse generated by the contraction of the left ventricle. Vasodilation or vasoconstriction of the vascular bed will alter the arterial blood pressure reading resulting in lower or higher readings respectively. When blood flow stops an end pressure occurs in the vessel and will cause the systolic arterial blood pressure reading to be falsely high by 2–10 mmHg. If the pressures appear to be dampened then the fast-flush technique should be performed to assess the dynamic response characteristics of the system (Bridges, 1997).

When choosing which method is preferable, either oscillometric or direct arterial cannulation, consideration must be given to the invasive nature of arterial cannulation. The risks associated with the procedure include blood loss, hematoma, occlusion of the vessel, and infection.

A frequently employed hemodynamic monitoring technology to assess pressures and cardiac status is the pulmonary artery catheter (PAC). This catheter is a multiple lumen, balloon, flow-directed catheter. Two of the catheter lumens are interfaced with a statham transducer to measure central venous pressure (CVP) or right atrial pressure (RAP) and pulmonary artery pressure (PAP). The catheter system is also interfaced with a thermodilution cardiac output computer. The catheter is inserted into the jugular vein and directed to the right atrium of the heart. The balloon is then inflated and the flow of blood floats the catheter into the right ventricle and out into the pulmonary artery until the tip of the catheter is wedged in the small vessels of the lower lobe of the lung. In the absence of mitral valve dysfunction, the pulmonary artery occlusion pressure (PAOP) with the balloon inflated is reflective of left ventricular end-diastolic pressure. Four centimeters from the tip of the catheter is a thermister that measures blood temperature. With the injection of 10 cc's of either room temperature or iced injectate (D_5W) at end-expiration a thermodilution cardiac output curve can be obtained. The cardiac output computer integrates the area under the thermodilution curve to calculate cardiac output (Figure 18.14).

More recently, a modified pulmonary artery catheter has become available for continuous measurement of right ventricular end-diastolic volume (RVEDV) as an indicator of cardiac preload. The catheter contains a thermal filament 10 cm in length located approximately 14 cm to 25 cm from the tip of the PAC. The thermal filament emits pulses of thermal energy as the indicator of the changing temperature of the blood. A relaxation waveform is generated based on a repeating on/off input signal. Data are collected throughout the respiratory cycle (Figure 18.15).

Volumetric parameters can be obtained using this catheter and include stroke volume (SV), right ventricular end-diastolic volume (RVEDV), right ventricular end-systolic volume (RVESV), and right ventricular ejection fraction (%). All volumes can be indexed to body surface area. These values are invaluable as clinical indicators in the treatment of patients with trauma, sepsis, acute respiratory distress, cardiac surgery, pulmonary hypertension, and heart failure. The modified PAC allows for the measurement of filling volumes in addition to the traditional filling pressures (Leeper, 2003b).

Noninvasive hemodynamic and thoracic fluid status can now be measured using impedance cardiography. Impedance cardiography technology uses four external electrodes that are applied on either side at the base of the neck and at the level of the xiphoid process at the midaxillary line (Figure 18.16).

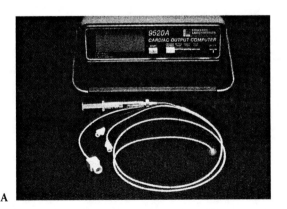
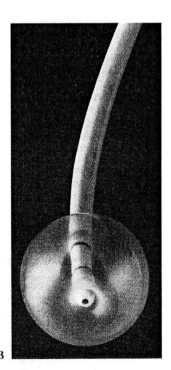

FIGURE 18.14 **Pulmonary artery catheter and cardiac output computer (A) and flow directed catheter with the balloon inflated (B).**

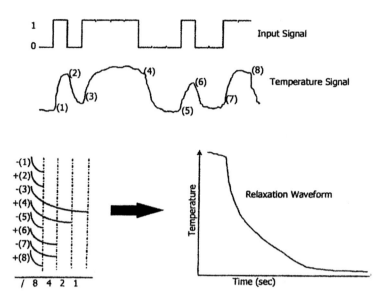

FIGURE 18.15   Right ventricular volumetric measurements. The filament emits pulses of thermal energy as the signal. The relaxation waveform is generated to resemble the thermodilution washout decay curve with the standard pulmonary artery catheter. The waveform is based on repeating on/off input signal and is generated by accumulating the temperature change for each off and on segment of the input signal.

A high-frequency, low-amplitude current is generated through the electrodes to measure electrical resistance changes in the thorax. Impedance (Z) changes occur due to variations in blood volume and flow velocity in the

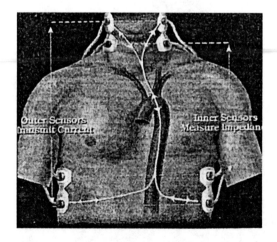

FIGURE 18.16   Placement of the electrodes for impedance cardiography measurements. Four dual electrodes are placed on opposite sides at the base of the neck and at the level of the xiphod process at the midaxillary line.

ascending aorta during systole. Impedance to the electrical current decreases during systole as blood volume and flow velocity increases, while impedence increases during diastole. Baseline impedence (Zo), pulsatile impedance/time (dZ/dT) (the change in thoracic impedence per unit time), and the electrocardiogram (ECG) are used to calculate cardiac stroke volume, cardiac output, and contractility. When compared with invasive PAC intermittent thermodilution, the correlation coefficients range from r = 0.86–0.93 (Lasater & VonRueden, 2003). A unique aspect of impedance cardiography is the measurement of thoracic fluid (Zo) including interstitial, intravascular, or intraalveolar fluid which reduces impedance to electrical current flow. Increased fluids and electrolytes in the fluid decreases the impedance to current flow. In patients with heart failure, Zo has been found to correlate closely with chest radiographic findings. Zo values less than 19 ohms are reported to have 90% sensitivity and 94% specificity (Milzman, Hogan, & Han, 1997). Impedance cardiography is useful for outpatient management of patients with congestive heart failure and to determine the effectiveness of diuretics, angiotension-converting enzyme (ACE) inhibitors, and beta blockers (Lasater & Von Rueden, 2003).

A minimally invasive method of monitoring hemodynamics is Doppler cardiography. Continuous real-time Doppler-based hemodynamic assessment can be obtained by an esophageal Doppler catheter inserted to a depth of approximately 35–40 cm from the teeth. The tip of the esophageal catheter rests near T5-T6 where the esophagus is parallel to the descending aorta (Figure 18.17).

Esophageal Doppler monitoring produces a two-dimensional physiologic waveform consisting of velocity of pulsatile blood flow in the descending aorta, and time. The esophageal catheter directs a beam of ultrasound waves at red blood cells flowing through the descending aorta. The frequency of the reflected ultrasound waves caused by the moving red blood cells provide a real-time display of blood velocity against flow time. The waveform allows for the derivation of cardiac output, stroke volume, and a qualitative indicator of preload, afterload, and contractility. The normal physiologic waveform is triangular and comprises beginning systole, peak systole, and end systole (Figure 18.18).

The waveform changes associated with preload, afterload, and contractility are illustrated in Figure 18.19.

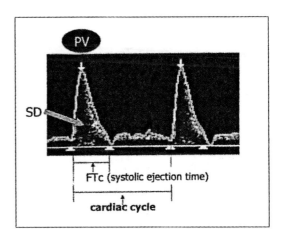

FIGURE 18.18 Waveform obtained from the Doppler esophageal probe. PV = peak velocity; FTc = flow time corrected; SD = stroke distance.

The width of the waveform base, expressed as flow time corrected (FTc) may be altered by changes in preload. A narrow base is reflective of hypovolemia. Afterload is indicated by the width and the amplitude of the waveform. A narrow waveform with a decreased amplitude is indicative of an increase in afterload. A wide waveform and increased amplitude is seen with afterload reduction. The peak velocity is a marker of contractility and can be visualized by the amplitude of the waveform (Turner, 2003). This technology is available in the emergency department, operating room, post-anesthesia care, and critical care areas. Esophageal Doppler

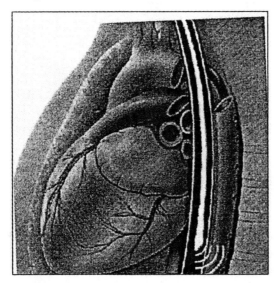

FIGURE 18.17 Doppler esophageal probe placement.

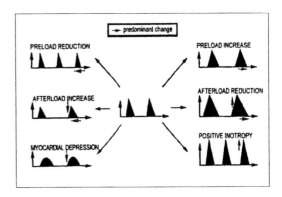

FIGURE 18.19 Esophageal Doppler waveforms illustrating preload, afterload, and myocardial contractility or inotrophy.

monitoring has been used intraoperatively to enhance fluid optimization. Use of this technique is contraindicated in coarctation of the aorta, pathology of the esophagus, or coagulopathies (Turner, 2003).

MEASUREMENT OF GASES

Determination of the partial pressures of gases like oxygen and carbon dioxide can be obtained by analysis of blood concentrations of individual gases and evaluation of transcutaneous measurements of oxygen and carbon dioxide, pulse oximetry, capnography, and regional carbon dioxide evaluation. Gas measurements are commonly used as a variable in studies that investigate cardiopulmonary status during illness or following injury (Kharasch, Vinci, Hirsch, Cranley & Coates, 1994) and during interventions like endotracheal suctioning and ventilator weaning (Banasik & Emerson, 2001; Cordero, Sananes, & Ayers, 2001; Grap, Glass, Corley, & Parks, 1996; Mohr, Rutherford, Cairns, & Boysen, 2001). Gas concentrations are also frequently evaluated in studies of shock (LeBuff, Decoene, Pol, Prat, & Vallet, 1999; Miller, Kincaid, Meredith, & Chang, 1998).

Arterial Blood Gases

Arterial blood gas sampling and evaluation allows calculation of total gas content in the blood and, in combination with cardiac output data, evaluation of gas delivery (Blonshine, Foss, Mottram, Ruppel, & Wanger, 2001). Most commonly, blood oxygen concentration, the partial pressure of oxygen (PO_2), is measured by a Clark-type polarographic electrode, which uses a chemical reaction (reduction) to measure oxygen partial pressure. The oxygen electrode contains a membrane through which oxygen from the blood sample diffuses and equilibrates in a solution of potassium chloride. This solution is exposed to a polarizing voltage of 600–800 mV, and the subsequent reaction produces a current flow at the cathode surface of the electrode. This current is linearly proportional to the partial pressure of oxygen in the electrolyte solution (Figure 18.20).

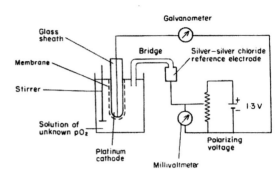

FIGURE 18.20 Diagram of a polarographic oxygen electrode.

The partial pressure of carbon dioxide (PCO_2) is typically measured by a Stow-Severinghaus electrode, which contains two separate chambers separated by a semipermeable membrane. One chamber of this electrode is for the blood sample. The second chamber contains a pH electrode surrounded by a buffer solution of sodium chloride and bicarbonate. The carbon dioxide from the blood sample freely diffuses through the membrane and into the buffer solution until equilibration. Changes in carbon dioxide concentration alter the pH of the buffer solution, and the pH electrode detects this change. This pH change is proportional to the concentration of carbon dioxide (Figure 18.21).

Transcutaneous Measurement of Gases

Oxygen and carbon dioxide concentrations may also be evaluated noninvasively by a transcuta-

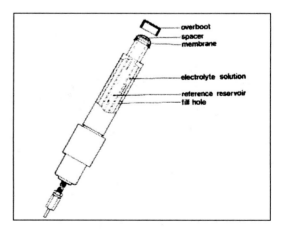

FIGURE 18.21 Carbon dioxide electrode.

neous method. Human skin releases small amounts of both oxygen and carbon dioxide and a combination Clark-type polarographic oxygen electrode and a Stow-Severinghaus carbon dioxide electrode may be used to measure these concentrations as previously described. For this technique, electrodes are attached to the skin in an area where good contact between the electrode membrane and skin occurs. The electrode heats the skin exposed to the electrode to 44°C to produce maximum vasodilation and blood flow. Measures are made following a 15-minute skin warming period. Transcutaneous values of oxygen ($TcPO_2$) and carbon dioxide ($TcPCO_2$) are positively correlated with arterial values in many studies ($TcPO_2$ r = 0.87, $TcPO_2$ r = 0.96) (Wimberley, Frederiksen, Witt-Hansen, Melberg, Friis-Hansen, 1985; Rithalia, Farrow, & Doran, 1992).

Oxygen Saturation

Oxygen saturation, the proportion of hemoglobin sites bound with oxygen molecules, is measured from an arterial blood sample (SaO_2), from pulse oximetry (SpO_2) or from an indwelling catheter placed in the pulmonary artery (SvO_2). With each of these measures, hemoglobin molecules are exposed to red and infrared light by a light-emitting diode. Hemoglobin bound to oxygen (oxyhemoglobin), absorbs more infrared light and hemoglobin without oxygen molecules, (deoxyhemoglobin) absorbs more red light. Once the light passes through the hemoglobin molecules, a light-receiving sensor determines the proportion of red and infrared light received and calculates the proportion of oxyhemoglobin in the sample.

Blood samples are exposed to up to five wavelengths of light in the laboratory setting using a co-oximeter. The use of a co-oximeter also allows accurate measurement of dysfunctional hemoglobin like methhemoglobin (heme iron oxidized to the ferric state) and carboxyhemoglobin (hemoglobin bound to carbon monoxide).

Pulse oximetry uses a sensor containing the light-emitting and light-receiving diodes placed on a finger, toe, foot, hand, earlobe, or bridge of nose (Avant, Lowe, & Torres, 1997). The light-emitting portion of the sensor is placed on one side of an area with a pulsating arterial bed, and the light-receiving diode is placed so that it will receive the light once it has traversed the pulsatile bed. Typically, pulse oximetry uses two wavelengths of light and provides a measure of the proportion of available hemoglobin that is oxygenated. Dysfunctional hemoglobins are not detected by pulse oximetry.

Oxygen saturation of pulmonary artery blood or mixed venous oxygen saturation (SvO_2) is performed with a specialized fiberoptic pulmonary artery catheter (Gawlinski & Dracup, 1998). The catheter contains one optic fiber to emit the red and infrared lights and a second to detect the light that reflects from the hemoglobin molecules. The saturation is determined by the absorption of red and infrared light by the exposed hemoglobin molecules.

Capnography

Capnography, the measurement of carbon dioxide concentration in exhaled gas, may be an invasive or noninvasive measure. Exhaled gas may be sampled via an invasive artificial airway like an endotracheal tube, or noninvasively from nasal prongs. Gas may be sampled either by mainstream or sidestream technique. With mainstream sampling, the measurement sensor is placed at the proximal tip of the artificial airway and exposed to the gas as it is expired from the respiratory tract. With sidestream sampling, exhaled gas is collected from the proximal end of an artificial airway or nasal prongs and diverted through a sampling tube to the analyzer located in the monitor. Regardless of sampling technique, either infrared spectography or mass spectography is used to analyze the gas sample and measure carbon dioxide concentration.

Infrared spectography is the most common method of analysis for capnography (Raemer & Philip, 1990). Carbon dioxide selectively absorbs infrared light in the 4.3 micrometers wavelength. Exhaled gas is exposed to infrared light and the selective absorbance of this wavelength of light is proportional to the concentration of carbon dioxide in the gas. With mass spectography, the gas sample is aspirated into a high-vacuum chamber. The gas is exposed to an electron beam that fragments the gas. Following fragmentation, the ions contained in the gas are accelerated by an electric field into a chamber with a magnetic field located at right angles to the stream of ionized gas. Here molecules are separated based on their mass to charge ratio and the concentration of gas components like carbon dioxide is determined.

Regional Carbon Dioxide Measurement

Evaluation of carbon dioxide concentration in localized tissue affords a measure of tissue blood flow (Ivatury et al., 1996). Carbon dioxide accumulates during periods of reduced tissue blood flow. Thus, an increase in tissue carbon dioxide may be used to evaluate the adequacy of perfusion in selected tissue beds. The measurement of gastric carbon dioxide (gastric tonometry) and sublingual carbon dioxide are two techniques currently in use in research and clinical practice.

Gastric tonometry provides a close estimate of gut carbon dioxide concentration (Gomersall et al., 2000; Huang, Tsai, Lin, Tsao, & Hsu, 2001). This technique requires placement of a modified nasogastric tube that contains a gas permeable balloon on the distal end of the catheter. To measure gastric carbon dioxide, the balloon is filled with air that remains in place for a ten minute period. During this dwell time, carbon dioxide diffuses freely into the balloon and equilibrates with the local tissue carbon dioxide levels. At the end of ten minutes, the balloon air is withdrawn and carbon dioxide concentration is commonly measured by infrared spectroscopy as previously described. Bicarbonate ion concentration may be used in conjunction with the gastric carbon dioxide value to calculate the intramucosal pH (pHi). There is an integral negative relationship between the gastric carbon dioxide and intramucosal pH; as carbon dioxide increases, pHi decreases. The calculation of the gap between arterial and gastric carbon dioxide may provide more relevant data about tissue perfusion. There should be little difference (<10 mmHg) between gastric and arterial carbon dioxide [P(g-a)CO$_2$]. However,

as perfusion is reduced this difference will increase in size due to poor regional perfusion.

Sublingual capnometry provides a measure of carbon dioxide concentration for proximal esophageal tissue in the sublingual area (Marik, 2001; Weil et al., 1999). Prior investigations demonstrated that increased sublingual carbon dioxide occurred in conjunction with increases in esophageal and gastric carbon dioxide (Jin et al., 1998; Povoas et al., 2000). With this technique, a disposable, microelectrode sensor is placed in the sublingual space for five minutes or less. This sensor is connected to a fiberoptic cable that conveys information from the sensor to an analyzer. When the sensor is placed in the sublingual space, carbon dioxide freely diffuses through the sensor and into the fiberoptic cable. This cable is coated with a fluorescent dye that is permeable to and reacts with carbon dioxide. The dye emits light in proportion to the concentration of carbon dioxide present, and this light is used to calculate the concentration of carbon dioxide present. Sublingual carbon dioxide is well correlated with gastric carbon dioxide (r = 0.86) and has been found to have a 100% positive predictive value for shock (Weil et al., 1999).

MEASUREMENT OF PULMONARY VOLUMES AND GAS FLOW

Measurement of pulmonary volumes and gas flow provides specific information about lung function. Pulmonary volumes and capacities, and gas flow rates, are commonly used to assess the degree of obstructive or restrictive lung disease prior to study or in response to some intervention (Carter et al., 2002; Ferreira et al., 2003; Hilbert, Choukroun, Gbikpi-Benissan, Guenard, & Cardinaud, 1998).

Static pulmonary gas volumes are not influenced by gas flow. These volumes are most commonly measured by a spirometer and include tidal volume, inspiratory and expiratory reserve volumes, inspiratory capacity and vital capacity. A spirometer will provide a direct measure of ventilated gas volume that may be presented as a graphic display of volume over time called a spirogram (Figure 18.22).

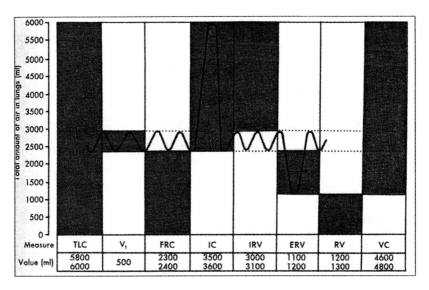

Measure	TLC	V_t	FRC	IC	IRV	ERV	RV	VC
Value (ml)	5800 6000	500	2300 2400	3500 3600	3000 3100	1100 1200	1200 1300	4600 4800

FIGURE 18.22   Spirogram of lung volumes.

A spirometer may be classified as a volume displacement or flow sensing spirometer. With a volume displacement spirometer, exhalation of a volume of gas most commonly displaces a bell in a water tank an equivalent volume (Figure 18.23).

With other volume displacement spirometers, exhalation of gas moves a piston or a bellows, and that movement is transformed into the equivalent volume of gas. Flow sensing spirometers primarily measure gas flow and use this value to calculate simultaneous volume by integration of the flow signal. Flow sensors measure the rate of gas flow by detection and analysis of a pressure drop across a resistance pneumotach (Figure 18.24), detection of cooling of a heated wire (anemometer), or by calculation using the rotation of a turbine blade. This type of spirometer has the ability to integrate the flow and volume data simultaneously and produce a flow volume loop that provides additional data about pulmonary status. Although spirometry provides important information

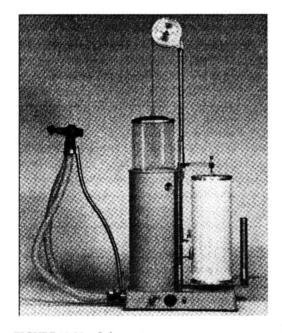

FIGURE 18.23   Spirometer.

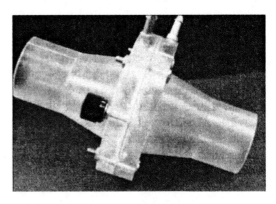

FIGURE 18.24   Pneumotachometer.

about many lung volumes and gas flows, measurement of other volumes like functional residual capacity, total lung capacity, and residual volume require other techniques.

Functional residual capacity, residual volume and total lung capacity must be measured indirectly. These gas volumes are most commonly measured by the use of a helium dilution technique or body plethysmography. With the helium dilution technique, the subject breathes a known volume of gas that contains a small, known concentration of helium for three to five minutes. At the direction of the investigator, the subject exhales gas down to residual volume (exhales as much as possible) and the investigator measures the concentration of helium in the volume of gas. This known concentration volume of gas is used to calculate the residual volume. The subject is requested to perform a vital capacity maneuver (maximal inspiration following a maximal expiration) and the calculated residual volume is added to the vital capacity to provide the total lung capacity. Clearly, the individual must be able to fully cooperate and participate for this technique to provide useful data.

Body plethysmography uses Boyle's law to calculate total lung volume. The individual is placed in a sealed chamber and requested to breathe through a mouthpiece. During this ventilation, a shutter obstructs the mouthpiece and the individual attempts to ventilate against the closed gas pathway. Contraction of the diaphragm reduces intrathoracic pressure and with an increase in chest size, the volume and pressure in the sealed chamber are altered. The differences in pressure and volume in the sealed chamber are used to calculate total lung volume. This method also provides a measure of airway resistance to gas flow (Figure 18.25).

MEASUREMENT OF TEMPERATURE

The body temperature of an individual is the result of a dynamic balance between heat production and heat loss. Body temperature measurements may be made from a number of sites: oral, axillary, rectal, skin, pulmonary artery, and bladder. Body temperature is often used as a

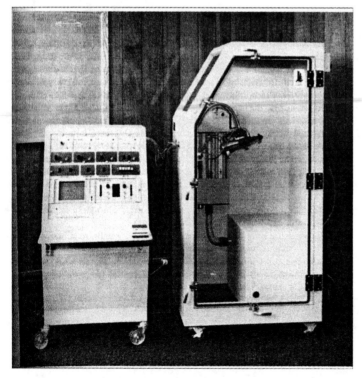

FIGURE 18.25   Body plethysmograph.

variable in studies of neonates (Bosque, Brady, Affonso, & Wahlberg, 1995).

Body temperature may be evaluated by a thermistor, infrared detector, or less commonly, a liquid in glass thermometer. Thermistors are located at the distal end of a probe. This type of device is found in the distal tip of a pulmonary artery catheter or in an electronic thermometer. The electrical resistance in the thermistor is altered in proportion to body temperature. This change in electrical resistance is converted to temperature and displayed. Infrared thermometers evaluate body temperature by detection of infrared emissions from the tympanic membrane, skin, or axilla. Infrared thermometers measure body temperature by quantifying radiant body heat loss in the form of infrared heat rays. Liquid in glass thermometers consist of a solution (usually alcohol) in a bulb connected with a glass column marked with the appropriate measurement scale. When the bulb area is exposed to body temperature, the solution heats, expands, and moves into the column. Once the solution equilibrates with body temperature, the solution expansion ceases and body temperature is indicated by the location of the solution on the measurement scale.

MEASUREMENT OF METABOLISM

Metabolism refers to the total energy expended by all chemical reactions in the body. The measurement of energy expenditure permits an investigator to evaluate individual metabolic responses to illness and injury and to determine metabolic responses to interventions like weaning from mechanical ventilation or inclusion of specific nutrients in feedings (Brandi et al., 1999; Petros & Engelmann, 2001; McClave et al., 2001). Estimates of caloric requirements and energy expenditure have been approximated for decades by the use of established equations like the Harris-Benedict equation. However, this equation was based on normal, healthy young individuals in the early twentieth century and has been found to overestimate actual energy expenditure by as much as 15% (Frankenfield, Muth, & Rowe, 1989; Glynn, Greene, Winkler, & Albina, 1999).

Metabolism may be quantified by calorimetry, a technique that measures the energy released from the individual's total chemical reactions (Bursztein, 1989). Heat production from chemical combustion is a constant and is proportional to the rate of chemical reaction. Thus, a measure of the heat produced by an individual may be used to quantify metabolism. Direct calorimetry, the most valid measure of energy expenditure, involves direct measurement of an individual's heat dissipation. To make metabolic measures using direct calorimetry, an individual is placed in a closed metabolic chamber for a minimum of 24 hours and instructed to perform certain activities, in addition to eating regular meals and sleeping. The heat released from the individual's body during these activities provides data about the individual's energy expenditure and is used to calculate energy expenditure. This technique requires specialized facilities and is expensive and time consuming.

Metabolic measures are more typically made using indirect calorimetry (Flancbaum, Choban, Sambucco, Verducci, & Burge, 1999). This technique is based on the fact that the chemical combustion of 1 calorie requires precisely 208.06 milliliters of oxygen. Thus, oxygen consumption is directly associated with energy expenditure. Oxygen consumption (VO_2), carbon dioxide production (VCO_2), and minute ventilation (V_E) are used in the calculation of resting energy expenditure (REE), the amount of calories required for a specified period of time by an individual. Indirect calorimetry may be performed in the laboratory setting or in a clinical site using equipment that is either separate from or integrated into a mechanical ventilator or a bedside monitor (McArthur, 1997; Headley, 2003). The individual is interfaced with the calorimetry equipment either through a mouthpiece, facemask, canopy, or specialized attachment to an endotracheal tube. These devices permit precise evaluation of the volumes of inspired and expired gases. The concentration of oxygen and carbon dioxide are determined typically by spectroscopy as previously described. Oxygen consumption is calculated as the difference between inspired and expired oxygen concentration, while carbon dioxide production is determined by subtracting the inspired concentration of carbon dioxide from the expired concentration. Both values are multiplied by the minute ventilation and then entered into a Weir equation for the calculation of resting energy expenditure.

MEASUREMENT OF CELLULAR PRODUCTS

The level of cellular synthesis of proteins like cytokines, hormones, and neurohormones often provide important data for investigations (Furukawa et al., 2003; Jessup, Horne, Yarandi, & Quindry, 2003). These products may be measured using a variety of techniques that include chromatography, electrophoresis, immunohistochemical staining, and enzyme-linked immunosorbent assay (ELISA).

Chromatography is a process that separates the components of a sample and permits identification and quantification of a selected substance. There are many different forms of chromatography including, liquid, gas, gas-liquid, and ion-exchange. Within each sample to be separated each component has different chemical, electrical, and physical properties. The sample is exposed to a bed or column. The substrate in the bed or column called the stationary phase is specifically selected based on its ability to attract the substance to be quantified. As the sample is passed over the bed or through the column, the substance to be measured is attracted to the specific components of the substrate and this attraction permits quantification. In gas chromatography, a carrier gas is used to transport the sample. The sample is passed over the separating column and the rate at which the sample passes through the column is detected by a heat sensing device called a kathrometer. Each component of the sample separates out at differing rates and amounts producing a series of waveforms for each component, and the area under the waveform reflects the amount of the component in the sample.

Electrophoresis is a technique that uses an electrical field to separate proteins within a sample. A substrate or gel is inoculated with the sample. An electrical field is then established

and proteins are attracted to either the positive or negative end of the field. The attraction of the molecules is dependent upon the charge and the molecular weight of the molecule. Thus, some proteins will be attracted to the positive end of the field, the anode and others to the negative end of the field or the cathode. The degree of attraction will also influence the result by its effect on the speed of movement of the proteins. This technique allows identification of multiple proteins within a sample.

Immunohistochemical staining may be used to identify cytokines and requires careful selection of a specific antibody for the cytokine of interest. The sample may be incubated with an antibody for a specified time period, and then stained with a chromogenic solution. The stain is attracted to the antibody that is bound to the cytokine and produces a color change that affords the investigator the ability to observe and quantify using a microscope. Antibodies may also be coupled to molecules of fluorescent dye and introduced into a tissue sample. There the antibody dye molecules bind with the protein of interest. Inspection of fluorescent molecules under a microscope provides a means to identify the protein.

Radioimmunoassays (RIAs) use a competitive binding technique. The protein of interest is labeled with radioactivity. These radioactive molecules are added to a sample that contains specific antibodies to the protein along with a known quantity of the same protein that has not been radiolabeled. These proteins competitively bind with antibodies and the amount of free protein and protein bound to antibody is determined. A number of determinations are made with different amounts of radiolabeled and free protein. The concentrations of labeled and free protein are plotted to form a standard curve. Then the sample with the unknown concentration of protein is mixed with radiolabeled antigen and antibody. The unknown proteins in the sample competitively bind with the antibodies and the results are compared with the standard curve previously prepared to determine the concentration of the protein.

Enzyme-linked immunosorbent assays (ELISA) are immunodiagnostic assays that use an immune reaction to measure specific proteins. A solid support medium is coated with an antibody that is specific for an antigenic site on the protein of interest. These antibodies bind with the protein. In a sandwich type assay, a detector antibody is then added. The detector antibody binds to the previously formed antigen-antibody complex. Once this "sandwich" is formed the addition of a substrate that activates a specific enzyme will generate a signal proportional to the concentration of the antigen/protein of interest. ELISA is the easiest, most accurate, and most sensitive method for the quantification of cytokine protein levels. The sandwich type assay technique is used, and monoclonal or polyclonal anticytokine antibodies are conjugated to one of a number of available enzymes. The assays must also take into account the species specificity of the cytokine being analyzed, for example, human versus mouse (Cooper & Broxmeyer, 1989).

MEASUREMENT OF NUCLEIC ACIDS

The human genome contains large amounts of deoxyribonucleic acid (DNA) that contains the code for controlling all aspects of embryogenesis, development, growth, metabolism, and reproduction. There are about 50,000 genes encoded in the DNA that make up the chromosomes in the nucleus of the cell. The double-stranded DNA serves as the code or the template for the production (transcription) of the single-stranded messenger RNA or ribonucleic acid. Messenger RNA contains the instructions for the production of proteins (translation) in the cell cytoplasm at the ribosome of the endoplasmic reticulum. Advances in the understanding of molecular genetics has facilitated the development of revolutionary new technologies that have permitted the analysis of normal and abnormal genes and the detection and diagnosis of genetic diseases.

Molecular geneticists had to overcome two fundamental obstacles in order to study the molecular basis of hereditary disease. The first challenge was to produce a sufficient quantity of either DNA or RNA to permit analysis. Hence, molecular cloning techniques were developed.

The second challenge was to purify the sequence of interest from all other segments of DNA or RNA. Polymerase chain reaction (PCR) can selectively amplify a single molecule of DNA or RNA several billion times in a few hours (Nussbaum, McInnes, & Willard, 2001).

Molecular Cloning

The process of molecular cloning is the transfer of a DNA sequence into a single cell of a microorganism so that as it grows in culture it reproduces the DNA. A significant advance in molecular biology occurred in the 1970s with the discovery of bacterial restriction endonucleases or restriction enzymes. These bacterial enzymes are capable of recognizing specific double-stranded sequences in the DNA and cleaving the DNA at specific recognition sites. For example *Escherichia coli* RY 13 or *Eco*RI recognizes the specific six base-pair sequence 5'-GAATTC-3' in the double-stranded DNA molecule. The enzyme cleaves the DNA by placing a nick on each strand between the G and the adjacent A. More than 1,000 restriction enzymes have already been identified (Figure18.26).

A vector is a DNA molecule that can auto-replicate in a host cell such as bacteria or yeast so that the DNA can be isolated in its pure form. Generation of the desired number of identical copies (clones) of a particular DNA sequence by a bacteria or other cell is called recombinant DNA technology. Plasmids are circular, double-stranded DNA molecules that replicate extrachromosomally in bacteria or yeast. Another commonly used vector is a bacteriophage lambda, which is a bacterial virus with a relatively large double-stranded DNA molecule. The *E.coli* cell is infected with the lambda virus and the human DNA sequence so that cloning of DNA pieces can be accomplished. Other vectors include the cosmid and bacterial artificial chromosomes (BACs) and the yeast artificial chromosome (YAC) that can carry large (100–300kb) inserts of human DNA. The purpose of molecular cloning is to isolate a particular gene or DNA sequence to allow further study. A set of clones of bacteria or yeast that contain a vector into which a fragment of DNA has been inserted is called a library.

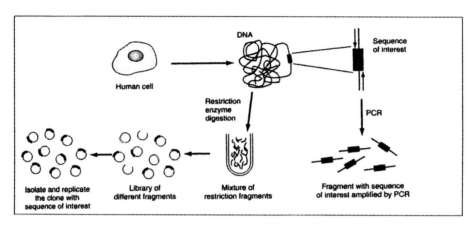

FIGURE 18.26   **Molecular cloning and the polymerase chain reaction (PCR).**

Following cloning to produce a sufficient quantity of the DNA sequence of interest, the next step is to analyze the DNA fragment.

Southern Blotting

The Southern blotting technique is the standard method for analyzing the structure of the DNA cleaved by the restriction enzymes. DNA is first isolated from a human cell usually a lymphocyte obtained from a blood sample using venipuncture. DNA cannot be extracted from a mature red blood cell since they are nonnucleated cells. Samples can also be taken from cultured skin fibroblasts, amniotic fluid, or chorionic villus cells of the placenta for prenatal screening. The cloned DNA fragments are then separated on the basis of size by agarose gel electrophoresis. The small DNA fragments move through an electric field and are separated based on size and charge. The separated DNA segments are then stained with a fluorescent DNA dye such as ethidium bromide causing the DNA fragments to appear as a smear of fluorescing material. The Southern blotting technique allows one to find and examine the one or two DNA fragments of interest. The now single-stranded DNA fragments are transferred from the gel to a nylon filter paper by blotting hence the name Southern blotting. A radioactively labeled piece of cloned DNA is used to identify the DNA fragments of interest. The radioactively labeled probe and the filter are incubated to allow DNA base pairing. After washing to

remove unbound probe, the filter is exposed to x-ray film to reveal the position of the one or more fragments to which the probe hybridized (Figure 18.27) (Nussbaum, McInnes, & Willard, 2001).

The best probe to use for detection of a particular single base mutation is a synthetic oligonucleotide because it is shorter in length and is more sensitive to one single base-pair mismatch. An allele-specific oligonucleotide (ASO) can be used to detect deletions or insertions of a single base.

Northern Blotting

RNA analysis is performed by the counterpart of Southern blotting called Northern blotting. DNA restriction enzymes cannot be used for RNA. RNA transcripts can be identified and are then separated by gel electrophoresis followed by transferring to nylon filters (blotting). The filter is then incubated with a denatured, radiolabeled probe. After washing, the filter is exposed to x-ray to permit visualization.

Polymerase Chain Reaction

The polymerase chain reaction (PCR) can selectively amplify a single molecule of DNA or RNA in a few hours. PCR is an enzymatic amplification of a fragment of DNA. Repeated cycles of heat denaturation, hybridization of the primers, and enzymatic DNA synthesis results in exponential amplification. PCR can also be applied

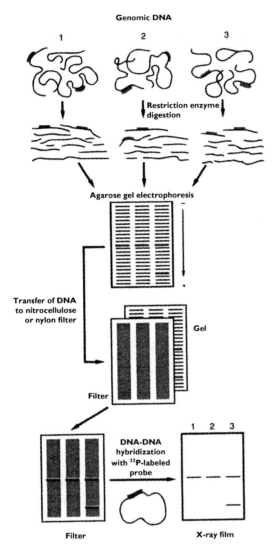

Genomic DNA

Restriction enzyme digestion

Agarose gel electrophoresis

Transfer of DNA to nitrocellulose or nylon filter

Gel

Filter

DNA-DNA hybridization with ^{32}P-labeled probe

Filter

X-ray film

FIGURE 18.27   Southern blot procedure for DNA analysis.

to the analysis of small samples of RNA in a procedure called reverse transcriptase PCR. A single-stranded cDNA is synthesized from the mRNA by reverse transcriptase. The PCR primers are then added along with the DNA polymerase.

PCR is an extremely sensitive technique. It allows for the detection and analysis of specific gene sequences without cloning or Southern or Northern blotting. Analysis can be performed from a single cell from a hair root, from sperm obtained from a vaginal sample from a rape victim, or from a drop of dried blood at a crime scene.

In Situ Hybridization

Probes can be hybridized to DNA contained within chromosomes and immobilized on a microscope slide. This process is called in situ hybridization. The cells must be in metaphase when the chromosomes are visible and are aligned in the middle of the nucleus of the cell. The DNA is denatured and fixed into place on the microscope slide. A fluorescent dye is applied and the slide is exposed to a wavelength of light that excites the fluorescent dye. This process is called fluorescence in situ hybridization (FISH). FISH is used widely in diagnostic clinical cytogenetics as well as gene mapping.

Another FISH technique is spectral karyotyping (SKY). Twenty-four different chromosome painting probes, one for each of the 24 human chromosomes, is used. Each chromosome is separated out by size and banding characteristics using fluorescence-activated chromosome sorting. Each chromosome is represented by a probe with its own spectrum of wavelengths of fluorescence. A computer assigns each chromosome a specific color which is used to identify the chromosome.

Western Blotting

Genes direct protein synthesis by the coding of mRNA from DNA. The analysis of both normal and abnormal gene function requires an examination of the protein encoded by the normal or mutant gene of interest. Western blotting is used to obtain information on the size and the amount of mutant protein in cell extracts from patients with genetic diseases. Proteins isolated from cell extracts are separated by polyacrylamide gel electrophoresis and then transferred to a membrane. The membrane is then incubated with antibodies that recognize the protein to be analyzed. This antigen-antibody reaction can then be detected by a second antibody against the first, which has been tagged with a detectable fluorescent, histochemical, or radioactive substance. Figure 18.28 is an example of a Western blot to detect the muscle protein dystrophin in patients with X-linked muscular dystrophy.

With the rapid advances in the development of technologies to clone and separate DNA and

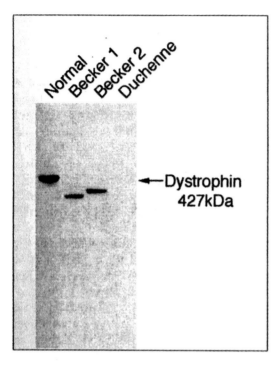

FIGURE 18.28 Western blot demonstrating the presence or absence of muscle protein Dystrophin in subjects screened for muscular dystrophy.

RNA, it is important that nurses keep abreast of these latest technologies in the measurement of nucleic acids and incorporate them in their programs of research. Nurses may become familiar with these technologies through a Web-based educational program (University of Cincinnati), participation in the Summer Genetics Institute (SGI), or through doctoral or postdoctoral work. Nurses are encouraged to work collaboratively with cytogeneticists to incorporate these technologies into nursing research.

REFERENCES

Avant, M., Lowe, N., and Torres, A. (1997). Comparison of accuracy and signal consistency of two reusable pulse oximeter probes in critically ill children. *Respiratory Care, 42*(7), 698–704.

Arbour, R. (2000). Using the bispectral index to assess arousal response in a patient with neuromuscular blockade. *American Journal of Critical Care, 9*(6), 383–387.

Banasik, J. L., & Emerson, R. J. (2001). Effect of lateral positions on tissue oxygenation in the critically ill. *Heart Lung, 30*(4), 269–276.

Bell, N. (1992). Clinical significance of ST-segment monitoring. *Critical Care Nursing Clinics of North America, 4*(2), 313–323.

Blonshine, S., Foss, C. M., Mottram, C., Ruppel, G., & Wanger, J. (2001). Blood gas analysis and hemoximetry. *Respiratory Care, 46,* 498–505.

Bosque, E. M., Brady, J. P., Affonso, D. D., & Wahlberg, V. (1995). Physiological measures of kangaroo versus incubator care in a tertiary-level nursery. *Journal of Obstetric, Gynecologic, and Neonatal Nursing, 24*(3), 219–226.

Brandi, L. S., Santini, L., Bertolini, R., Malacarne, P., Casagli, S., & Baraglia, A. M. (1999). Energy expenditure and severity of injury and illness indices in multiple trauma patients. *Critical Care Medicine, 27*(12), 2684–2689.

Bridges, E. J. (1997). Direct arterial vs. oscillmeteric monitoring of blood press: Stop comparing and pick one (a decision-making algorithm). *Critical Care Nurse, 17*(3), 58–72.

Buraztein, S. (1989). *Energy metabolism, indirect calorimetry, and nutrition.* Baltimore: Williams & Wilkins.

Carter, R., Holiday, D. B., Grothues, C., Nwasuruba, C., Stocks, J., & Tiep, B. (2002). Criterion validity of the Duke Activity Status Index for assessing functional capacity in patients with chronic obstructive pulmonary disease. *Journal of Cardiopulmonary Rehabilitation, 22*(4), 298–308.

Chatila, W., Ani, S., Guaglianone, D., Jacob, B., Amoateng-Adjepong, Y., & Manthouss, C. (1996). Cardiac ischemia during weaning from mechanical ventilation. *Chest, 109*(6), 1577–1583.

Cooper, S. H., & Broxmeyer, H. E. (1989). Measurement of IL-3 and other hematopoietic cytokines. *Current Protocol in Immunology, 6*(4), 20, Supplement 18.

Cordero, L., Sananes, M., & Ayers, L. W. (2001). A comparison of two airway suctioning frequencies in mechanically ventilated, very-low-birthweight infants. *Respiratory Care, 46*(8), 783–788.

Cowan, M. J., Heinrich, M. L., Sigmon, H., & Hinshaw, A.S. (1993). Integration of biological and nursing sciences: A 10-year plan to enhance research and training. *Research in Nursing and Health, 16*(1), 3–9.

Crater, S., Taylor, C. A., Maas, A. C. P., Loeffler, A. K., Pope, J. E.,& Drew, B. J. (2000). Real-time application of continuous 12-lead ST-segment monitoring: 3 case studies. *Critical Care Nursing, 20*(2), 93–99.

DeDeyne, C., Struys, M., Decruyenaere, J., Creupelandt, J., Hoste, E., & Colardyn, F. (1998). Use of continuous bispectral EEG monitoring to assess depth of sedation in ICU patients. *Intensive Care Medicine, 24*(12), 1294–1298.

Drew, B. J., Pelter, M. M., Adams, M. G., Weng, S., Chou, T. M., & Wolfe, C. C. (1998). 12-lead ST-segment monitoring vs. single-lead maximun ST-segment monitoring for dectecting ongoing ischemia in patients with unstable coronary syndromes. *American Journal of Critical Care, 7*(5), 355–363.

Drew, B. J., & Krucoff, M. W. (1999). Multilead ST-segment monitoring in patients with acute coronary syndromes: A consensus statement for healthcare professionals. *American Journal of Critical Care, 8*(6), 372–388.

Ferreira, C. A., Stelmach, R., Feltrin, M. I., Filho, W. J., Chiba, T., & Cukier, A. (2003). Evaluation of health-related quality of life in low-income patients with COPD receiving long-term oxygen therapy. *Chest, 123*(1), 136–41.

Flancbaum, L., Choban, P. S., Sambucco, S., Verducci, J., & Burge, J. C. (1999). Comparison of indirect calorimetry: The Fick method and prediction equations in estimating the energy requirements of critically ill patients. *American Journal of Clinical Nutrition, 69*(3), 461–466.

Frankenfield, D. C., Muth, E. R., & Rowe, W. A. (1998). The Harris-Benedict studies of human basal metabolism: History and limitations. *Journal of the American Dietary Association, 98*(4), 439–445.

Frantz, A. K. (2003). Current issues related to home monitoring. *AACN Clinical Issues, 14*(2), 232–239.

Furukawa, F., Kazuma, K., Kawa, M., Miyashita, M., Niiro, K., Kusukawa, R., et al., (2003). Effects of an off-site walking program on energy expenditure, serum lipids, and glucose metabolism in middle-aged women. *Biological Research for Nursing, 4*(3), 181–192.

Galinier, M., Pathak, A., Fourcade, J., Andriodias, C., Curnier, D., Varnous, S., et al., (2000). Depressed low frequency power of heart rate variability as an independent predictor of sudden death in chronic heart failure. *European Heart Journal, 21*(6), 475–482.

Gawlinski, A., & Dracup, K. (1998). Effect of positioning on SvO$_2$ in the critically ill patient with a low ejection fraction. *Nursing Research, 47*(5), 293–299.

Glynn, C. C., Greene, G. W., Winkler, M. F., & Albina, J. E. (1999). Predictive versus measured energy expenditure using limits of agreement analysis in hospitalized obese patients. *Journal of Parenteral and Enteral Nutrition, 23*(3), 147–154.

Gomersall, C. D., Joynt, G. M., Freebairn, R. C., Hung, V., Vuckley, T. A., & Oh, T. E. (2000). Resuscitation of critically ill patients based on the results of gastric tonometry: A prospective, randomized, controlled trial. *Critical Care Medicine, 28*(3), 607–614.

Grady, P. (2003). The future arrives: Genetic research initiatives of NINR. *Nursing Outlook, 51*(2), 90.

Grap, M. J., Glass, C., Corley, M., & Parks, T. (1996). Endotracheal suctioning: Ventilator vs. manual delivery of hyperoxygenation breaths. *American Journal of Critical Care, 5*(3), 192–197.

Headley, J. (2003). Indirect calorimetry: A trend toward continuous metabolic assessment. *AACN Clinical Issues, 14*(2), 155–167.

Hedman, A. E., Poloniecki, J. D., Camm, A. J., & Malik, M. (1999). Relation of mean heart rate and heart rate variability in patients with left ventricular dysfunction. The *American Journal of Cardiology, 84*(2), 225–228.

Hilbert, G., Choukroun, M. L., Gbikpi-Benissan, G., Guenard, H., & Cardinaud, J. P. (1998). Optimal pressure support level for beginning weaning in patients with COPD: Measurement of diaphragmatic activity with step-by-step decreasing pressure support levels. *Journal of Critical Care, 13*(3), 110–118.

Hohnloser, S. H., Klingenheben, T., & Zabel, M. (1999). Identification of patients after myocardial infarction at risk of life-threatening arrhythmias. *European Heart Journal, 1*(suppl C), C11–C20.

Huang, C. C., Tsai, Y. H., Lin, M. C., Tsao,T. C., & Hsu, K. H. (2001). Gastric intramural PCO2 and pH variability in ventilated critically ill patients. *Critical Care Medicine, 29*(1), 88–95.

International Human Genome Sequencing Consortium. (2001). Initial sequencing and analysis of the human genome. *Nature, 409*(6822), 860–921.

Ivatury, R. R., Simon, R. J., Islam, S., Fueg, A., Rohman, M., & Stahl, W. M. (1996). A prospective randomized study of end points of resuscitation after major trauma: Global oxygen transport indices versus organ-specific gastric mucosal pH. *Journal of the American College of Surgeons, 183*(2) 145–154.

Jenkins, J., et al., (2001). Core Competency Working Group of the National Coalition for Health Professional Education in Genetics (NCHPEG). Recommendations of core competencies in genetics essential for all health professionals. *Genetic Medicine, 3*(2), 155–158.

Jessup, J. V., Horne, C., Yarandi, H., & Quindry, J. (2003). The effects of endurance exercise and vitamin E on oxidative stress in the elderly. *Biological Research for Nursing, 5*(1), 47–55.

Jin, X., Weil, M. H., Sun, S., Tang, W., Bisera, J., & Mason, E.J. (1998). Decreases in organ blood flows associated with increases in sublingual PCO_2 during hemorrhagic shock. *Journal of Applied Physiology, 85*(6), 2360–2364.

Kharasch, S. J., Vinci, R. J., Hirsch, E., Cranley, W., & Coates, E. (1994). The routine use of radiography and arterial blood gases in the evaluation of blunt trauma in children. *Annals of Emergency Medicine, 23*(2), 212–215.

Klein, H., Auricchioa, A., Reek, S., & Geller, C. (1999). New primary prevention trials of sudden cardiac death in patients with left ventricular dysfunction. *American Journal of Cardiology, 83*(5B), 91D–97D.

Lasater, M., & Von Rueden, K. T. (2003). Outpatient cardiovascular management utilizing impedance cardiography. *AACN Clinical Issue, 14*(2), 240–250.

LeBuffe, G., Decoene, C., Pol, A., Prat, A., &

Vallet, B. (1999). Regional capnometry with air-automated tonometry detects circulatory failure earlier than conventional hemodynamics after cardiac surgery. *Anesthesia and Analgesia, 89*(5), 1084–1090.

Leeper, B. (2003a). Continuous ST-segment monitoring. *AACN Clinical Issues, 14*(2), 145–154.

Leeper, B. (2003b). Monitoring right ventricular volumes. *AACN Clinical Issues, 14*(2), 208–219.

Marik, P. (2001). Sublingual capnography: A clinician validation study. *Chest, 120*(3), 923–927.

McArthur, C. (1997). Indirect calorimetry. *Respiratory Care Clinics of North America, 3*(2), 291–307.

McClave, S. A., Lowen, C. C., Kleber, M. J., Nicholson, J. F., Jimmerson, S. C., McConnell, J. W., et al., (1998). Are patients fed appropriately according to their caloric requirements? *Journal of Parenteral and Enteral Nutrition, 22*(6), 375–381.

Miller, P. R., Kincaid, E. H., Meredith, J. W., & Chang, M. C. (1998). Threshold values of intramucosal pH and mucosal-arterial CO_2 gap during shock resuscitation. *Journal of Trauma, 45*(5), 1868–1872.

Milzman, D., Hogan, C., & Han, C. (1997). Continuous noninvasive cardiac output monitoring quantifies acute congestive heart failure in the emergency department. *Critical Care Medicine, 25*(1, suppl.), A47.

Mohr, A. M., Rutherford, E. J., Cairns, B. A., & Boysen, P. G. (2001). The role of dead space ventilation in predicting outcome of successful weaning from mechanical ventilation. *Journal of Trauma, 51*(5), 843–848.

Nussbaum, R. L., McInnes, R. R., & Willard, H. F. (2001). Tools of human molecular genetics. In *Thompson and Thompson genetics in medicine* (6th ed.). Philadelphia: W.B. Saunders.

Okin, P. M., Devereux, R. B., Fabsitz, R. R., Lee, E. T., Galloway, J. M., & Howard, B. V. (2002). Principal component analysis of the T wave and prediction of cardiovascular mortality in American Indians: The Strong Heart Study. *Circulation, 105*(6), 714–719.

Parthasarathy, S., & Tobin, M. J. (2002). Effect of ventilator mode on sleep quality in critically ill patients. *American Journal of Respiratory and Critical Care Medicine, 166*(11), 1423–1429.

Petros, S., & Engelmann, L. (2001). Validity of an abbreviated indirect calorimetry protocol for measurement of resting energy expenditure in mechanically ventilated and spontaneously breathing critically ill patients. *Intensive Care Medicine, 27*(7), 1164–1168.

Povoas, H., Weil, M. H., Tang, W., Moran, B., Kamohara, T., & Bisera, J. (2000). Comparison between sublingual and gastric tonometry during hemorrhagic shock. *Chest, 118*(4), 1127–1132.

Raemer, D. B., & Philip, J. H. (1990). Monitoring anesthetic and respiratory gases. In C. E. Blitt (Ed.), *Monitoring in anesthesia and critical care medicine* (2nd ed., pp. 373–386). New York: Churchill Livingston.

Resnick, H. E., Redline, S., Shahar, E., Gilpin, A., Newman, A., Walter, R., et al. (2003). Diabetes and sleep disturbance: Findings from the Sleep Heart Health Study. *Diabetes Care, 26*(3), 702–709.

Rhoney, D. H., & Parker, D. (2001). Use of sedative and analgesic agents in neurotrauma patients: Effects on cerebral physiology. *Neurological Research, 23*(2-3), 237–259.

Rithalia, S. V. S., Farrow, P., & Doran, B. R. H. (1992). Comparison of transcutaneous oxygen and carbon dioxide monitors in normal adults and critically ill patients. *Intensive and Critical Care Nursing, 8*(1), 40–46.

Sigmon, H. D. (1993). Answering critical care nursing questions by interfacing nursing research training, career development, and research with biologic and molecular science. *Heart and Lung: The Journal of Critical Care, 22*(4), 285–288.

Scisney-Matlock, M., Algase, D., Boehm, S., Coleman-Burns, P., Oakley, D., Rogers, A. E., et al. (2000). Measuring behavior: Electronic devices in nursing studies. *Applied Nursing Research, 13*(2), 97–102.

Srivastava, S., Chatila, W., Amoateng-Adjepong, Y., Kanagasegus, S., Jacob, B., & Zarich, S. (1999). Myocardial ischemia and weaning failure in patients with coronary artery disease: An update. *Critical Care Medicine, 27*(10), 2109–2112.

Stone, K. S., & Frazier, S. K. (1999). Biomedical Instrumentation. In Mateo and Kirchoff (Eds.), *Using and conducting nursing research in the clinical setting* (2nd ed., pp. 243–255). Philadelphia:W.B. Saunders.

Turner, M. A. (2003). Doppler-based hemodynamic monitoring. *AACN Clinical Issues, 14*(2), 220–231.

Van Boven, A. J., Crijns, H. J., Haaksma, J., Zwinderman, A. H., Lie, K. I., & Jukema, J. W. (1998). Depressed heart rate variability is associated with events in patients with stable coronary artery disease and preserved left ventricular function. *American Heart Journal, 135*(4), 571–576.

Venter, J. C., et al. (2001). The sequence of the human genome. *Science, 291*(5507), 1304–1351.

Wallace, B. E., Wagner, A. K., Wagner, E. P., & McDeavitt, J. T. (2001). A history and review of quantitative electroencephalography in traumatic brain injury. *Journal of Head Trauma and Rehabilitation, 16*(2), 165–190.

Weil, M. H., Nakagawa, Y., Tang, W., Sato, Y., Ercoli, F., Finegan, R., et al. (1999). Sublingual capnography: A new noninvasive measurement for the diagnosis and quantitation of severity of circulatory shock. *Critical Care Medicine, 27*(7), 1225–1229.

Williams, J. K. (2002). Education for genetics and nursing practice. *AACN Clinical Issues: Current Issues in Genetics, 13*(4), 492–500.

Wimberley, P. D., Frederiksen, P. S., Witt-Hansen, J., Melberg, S. G., & Friis-Hansen, B. (1985). Evaluation of a transcutaneous oxygen and carbon dioxide monitor in a neonatal intensive care department. *Acta Paediatrica Scandinavica, 74*(3), 352–359.

World Health Organization Quality of Life Assessment (WHO-QOL) (1995). Position paper. *Social Science Medicine, 41*(10), 1403–1409.

Zabel, M., Acar, B., Klingenheben, T., Franz, M. R., Hohnloser, S. H., & Malik, M. (2000). Analysis of 12-lead T-wave morphology for risk stratification after myocardial infarction. *Circulation, 102*(11), 1252–1257.

19

Uses of Existing Administrative and National Databases

Meg Johantgen

Researchers across disciplines are increasingly relying on existing data sources to examine health issues. The increasing computerization of health information, decreasing costs of storage, increasing analytical tools and techniques, and the constraints on collecting primary data have propelled the use of such data. Existing data sources include both administrative data—data collected for reasons other than research—and data developed for other targeted studies or for surveillance. Utilizing existing data is particularly desirable because it is relatively cheap (compared with primary data collection), covers large samples, is often longitudinal, and is not intrusive to subjects.

Despite these advantages, technical and methodological barriers make using existing data particularly challenging. The fundamental issues relate to the fact that the data were not developed and collected to answer the researcher's questions. Traditionally, researchers conceptualize their research study and develop a methodology that is consistent with the conceptualization. The research design, the sample, the measures, and the proposed analyses are intimately linked to the research aims. Using existing data places constraints on all aspects of the research. The designs are most often correlational or quasiexperimental. Study subjects must be selected from the data by inclusion and exclusion criteria that are defined with existing data. Researchers may have to rely on measures developed by and for others that may not be consistent with their conceptualization or study sample. Analyses are constrained by the level of

existing data and potential bias in some data elements. Researchers must be aware of how the ideal conceptualization and measures vary from what is possible with existing data. This puts burden on users to know their data, conduct iterative preliminary analyses to be more confident of reliability and validity issues, and to summarize findings acknowledging the potential limitations.

This chapter provides an overview of common sources of existing data, including the types of information that are included and the limitations of that information when used for research. Selected sources of existing health data are summarized in Appendix B for illustrative purposes. Issues in working with these data are discussed, with particular emphasis on reliability and validity, and what can be done to address these concerns.

EXISTING HEALTH DATA

Existing health data can be broadly divided into two categories: secondary data and administrative data. While the use of any data not collected specifically for a research study (e.g., primary data) might be referred to as secondary data, a distinction is made here between data that was collected for surveillance or another research study (secondary data) and data not collected for research purposes (administrative data).

Secondary data allow analysis of hypotheses and relationships that may not have been examined in the original study. This approach is efficient since planning for and collection of data is eliminated, but it is also challenges the researcher to understand the original researcher's conceptualizations and methodological choices. A good example of secondary data that have been used to address health issues relevant to nursing are the surveys from the National Center for Health Statistics (NCHS), Centers for Disease Control and Prevention (CDC). These data sets, developed for surveillance and research, provide important information to guide actions and policies related to the health of people in the United States. The need to measure varied aspects of health, to be representative of target populations, and to cover diverse types of health conditions and health services, imposes strong methodological rigor on the surveys. Moreover, these studies employ well-developed definitions, and strict data collection procedures, and are ongoing. The National Health Interview Survey, for example, is used to monitor progress for several of the Healthy People 2010 indicators (NHIS, 2003).

A second broad category of existing data is administrative data, most often resulting from the administration of services and programs. A frequently used source of administrative data in health care is claims for services such as physician visits, prescription drug use, and hospitalization. Federal and state governments and health care insurers are the primary holders of these data. The first edition of Iezzoni's (1994) book on risk adjustment in measuring health outcomes identified three major sources of frequently used data: administrative data, medical record information, and patient-derived data. The later edition of this book (1997) acknowledges that boundaries between these data sources have been blurred due to patients entering their own clinical health data into computers, electronic medical record expansion with large data repositories, and increasing inclusion of patient outcomes.

As with secondary data, researchers using administrative data do not have to bear the expense of primary data collection. Yet, the advantages extend beyond the researcher's efficiency and include the ability to cover entire systems of care or populations rather than segments (e.g., by payer, organization, etc.). Large data sets allow an examination of infrequent outcomes and have adequate power to detect differences. Many administrative data bases also have additional advantages such as the ability to examine changes over time and to link to other data sets representing other explanatory variables (e.g., organizational and geographic attributes). This is particularly important in studying outcomes where a systems approach is desirable. However, administrative data are, by definition, collected for reasons other than research. The purposes and procedures for collecting that data may have inherent sources of bias. Therefore, there is a greater onus on the researcher to understand what the data represent—and what they do not represent.

TYPES OF DATA

Secondary and administrative data sources represent varied levels of data, extent of information, and ability to link to other data sources. To organize selected examples of existing data, the taxonomy adapted by Paul, Weiss, and Epstein (1993) from the Agency for Health Care Policy and Research Report to Congress (1991) is used. The categories in this taxonomy include:

Clinical/epidemiological data
- Disease registries
- Epidemiological surveys

Administrative data
- Claims/encounters
- Providers of services
- Certifications and surveys

Sociodemographic data
- Vital statistics and census results
- Health resources

Selected sources of existing health data are summarized using these categories in Appendix B.

It should be noted that much of the existing data do not reflect what nurses do. The clinical data in current administrative data sets are primarily represented by diagnoses, procedures, and equipment codes—most often those that are related to reimbursement or other reporting requirements. Despite these limitations, these data have been used to develop outcome measures, some of which are considered "nurse-sensitive". Relationships between nurse staffing and these outcomes have been examined in acute care (Aiken, Smith, & Lake, 1994; Kovner & Gergen, 1998; Blegen & Vaughn, 1998; Needleman, Duerhas, Maltke, Stewart, & Zelevinsky, 2002) and in long term care (Johnson-Pawlson & Infeld, 1996; Harrington, Zimmerman, Karon, Robinson, & Beutel, 2000). Other information systems have the potential to provide valuable data about nursing, but barriers remain such as the complexity of health languages, the lack of electronic data capture of nursing care, and poorly integrated information systems. National and international efforts to document nursing assessments, interventions, and outcomes are evident (Charters, 2003), but there is no consensus.

TYPES OF INFORMATION

While existing databases vary considerably, common data elements can be summarized under four categories: patient demographics, clinical diagnosis and treatment, organizational characteristics, and geographic characteristics. The definitions and coding of these variables, however, varies considerably. Table 19.1 illustrates common coding systems seen in administrative data. With the standardization of coding of health care transactions required through the Health Insurance Portability and Accountability Act (HIPAA) of 1996, data comparability should improve when the data are generated for health care transactions. However, current data present a challenge to researchers who must deal with inconsistent identifiers and categories.

TABLE 19.1 Coding Seen in Existing Health Data

Name	Description
Diagnoses International Classification of Diseases, 9th Revision, Clinical Modification (ICD-9-CM)	Diagnoses, supplementary classifications representing factors influencing health status (V-codes) and environmental events that may have contributed to adverse events (E-codes)
Procedures/Services International Classification of Diseases, 9th Revision, Clinical Modification (ICD-9-CM)	Procedures performed in inpatient settings
Current Procedural Terminology (CPT)	Procedures performed in clinics, radiology and laboratory settings
Healthcare Common Procedure Coding System (HCPCS)	Items, supplies and nonphysician services not covered CPT codes
Pharmacy National Drug Codes (NDC)	Universal product identifier for human drugs
Occupation Standard Occupational Codes (SOC)	Codes to classify jobs on the basis of work performed, required skills, education, training, and credentials
Organizations Standard Industrial Codes (SIC)	Four digit code to represent employer type
North American Industry Classification System (NAICS)	Six-digit hierarichical coding system to represent employer type
Location/Geography Federal Information Processing Standards (FIPS)	Codes for a variety of geographic entities including county, metropolitan statistical area, place, and state
Metropolitan Statistical Area (MSA)	Codes to identify an area according to population, allowing designation of how rural or urban

Demographics

Demographic elements are measured in various ways. This includes both the definition of the measure and the coding when the variable is nominal. Age, gender, and marital status are collected in most person-level data. While there is some variation in categories, the data can most often be used with little reassignment. The coding of race and ethnicity is much more inconsistent and controversial. While many acknowledge that it is important to measure race, they also agree that it is not clear what race represents—culture, genetics, socioeconomic status, or some combination. Self-reported versus observer-reported race were also known to affect data quality. To address some of these concerns, the standards for coding race and ethnicity changed with the 2000 Census to include multiple race categories (Sondik, Lucas, Madans, & Smith, 2000; Mays, Ponce, Washington, & Cochran, 2003). Other government and private data collectors have adopted these standards but concerns remain about what race represents, how it should be coded, and how it should be used in research (Nerenz, Bonham, Green-Weir, Joseph, & Gunter, 2002).

Continuous demographic variables may be collapsed to categories that may not be consistent across data sets. Income, for example, may be collected as actual income but collapsed to ordinal categories for data release. These income categories vary widely and researchers may need to further collapse them based on the distribution of the data, the research design, or the comparisons that are to be made. Reporting ordinal or categorical data is likely to become more

common with increased concerns for patient confidentiality. Age, for example, is not a protected element, but using age in combination with other elements in the file (e.g., location of care, procedures, diagnoses, etc.) may allow identification of an individual in a data set. Thus, age is released only in aggregate categories in some databases.

Other demographic data may be represented by codes. The most common way to classify worker occupation type has been the Standard Occupational Classification (SOC) codes. The SOC system classifies occupations on the basis of work performed, required skills, education, training, and credentials. The codes were revised in 2000 to provide more detail in the computer, engineering, health, and science occupations. Table 19.2 illustrates the codes that represent occupations related to nursing. If text is used rather than a coding system, workers need to be categorized by hand. For example, many text descriptions of job titles could be categorized as "nurse's aide". These titles often include abbreviations (e.g., NA), official certification titles (e.g., Certified Nursing Assistant), or common institutional names for these workers (Aide).

Clinical Data

Much of the clinical data in surveys and administrative data are represented by diagnoses, procedures, and services provided. The International Classification of Diseases, Ninth Revision, Clinical Modification (ICD-9-CM) is used for coding diagnoses in most databases. Three-, four-, and five-digit codes, organized by body system, reflect increasing specificity. For

TABLE 19.2   Standard Occupational Classification (SOC) Codes Representing Nursing

Code	Description
29-1000	Healthcare Practitioners and Technical Occupations
29-1110	Registered Nurses
29-2660	Licensed Practical and Vocational Nurses
31-0000	Healthcare Support Occupations
31-1010	Nursing, Psychiatric, and Home Health Aides
31-1011	Home Health Aides
31-1012	Nursing Aides, Orderlies, and Attendants
31-1013	Psychiatric Aides

example, Table 19.3 illustrates the ICD-9-CM diagnosis code for diabetes. The fourth digit represents the manifestations (e.g., ketoacidosis, coma, and circulatory disorders) and the fifth digit representing the type of diabetes (Type 1, Type 2). The ICD-9-CM procedure codes are used for coding of inpatient procedures and are four-digit codes organized by body system. Table 19.4 illustrates the ICD-9-CM procedure codes for breast excisions. Note that the codes reflect an increasing extent of breast removal, but it may represent differences in how a surgeon classifies a lumpectomy from a quadrant resection. Coders are instructed to code to the highest specificity possible, but a nine in the fourth position often indicates a less specific category. To code clinical diagnoses, procedures, drugs, and other medical services appropriately, it is necessary to have a good working knowledge of medical terminology and the coding systems used. Transforming verbal descriptions of diseases, conditions, and interventions into numerical representations is complex and should not be done without training.

While diagnoses and procedures are usually coded with consistent coding systems due to reimbursement methodologies, and while coding clinics and reference books emphasize rules, coding error remains a major concern. Iezzoni (1997) provides several examples to illustrate the practical difficulties. The first is a lack of clarity of what the correct diagnosis code should be. A patient presenting to the emergency room with decompensation of chronic lung disease could legitimately be coded as chronic obstructive lung disease (491.2), chronic bronchitis (491.9), emphysema (492.8), acute bronchitis (466.0), or respiratory failure (492.8). The second difficulty is how diagnoses are selected, recorded, and ordered. It is likely that physicians become knowledgeable of the common codes used in their practice and fit patient conditions to the known codes. Even how the patient relates their medical history can influence coding as they are likely to report "old" diagnoses. The ordering of diagnoses is also crucial in settings where it affects payment. Yet, it is not always clear what the principal diagnosis should be, particularly when patients have multiple chronic illnesses. For example, a patient admitted for postobstructive pneumonia related to lung cancer may be assigned a pneumonia code or a lung cancer code. Researchers using these data should consult with clinicians if there are questions about coding practices.

In addition to ICD-9-CM codes, other data elements may be used to reflect patient condition. Hospital discharge data have several variables that are commonly used to assess risk or other outcomes: source of admission (e.g., emergency room, home, physician's office, etc.), type of admission (e.g., emergent, urgent, elective), and disposition (e.g., routine, to home care, died, etc.). Differences in coding have been found across states (Coffey, Ball, Johantgen, Elixhauser, Purcell, et al., 1997) and across hospitals, reflecting inconsistencies in emphasis or interpretation. While the HIPAA transaction

TABLE 19.3 Diabetic Diagnoses Coding in ICD-9-CM

ICD-9-CM Code	ICD-9-CM description
250.0	Diabetes mellitus without mention of complications
250.1	Diabetes with ketoacidosis
250.2	Diabetes with hyperosmolarlity
250.3	Diabetes with other coma
250.4	Diabetes with renal manifestations
250.5	Diabetes with ophthalmic manifestations
250.6	Diabetes with neurological manifestations
250.7	Diabetes with peripheral circulatory disorders
250.8	Diabetes with other specified manifestations
250.9	Diabetes with unspecified complication

TABLE 19.4. Excisional Breast Procedures Coding in ICD-9-CM.

ICD-9-CM Code	ICD-9-CM description
85.0	Mastotomy
85.11	Closed breast biopsy
85.12	Open breast biopsy
85.19	Breast diagnostic procedure not elsewhere classified
85.20	Breast tissue destruction not otherwise specified
85.21	Local excision of breast lesion
85.22	Quadrant resection of the breast
85.23	Subtotal mastectomy
85.24	Excision of ectopic breast tissue
85.25	Excision of nipple
85.41	Unilateral simple mastectomy
85.42	Bilateral simple mastectomy
85.43	Unilateral extended simple mastectomy
85.44	Bilateral extended simple mastectomy
85.45	Unilateral radical mastectomy
85.46	Bilateral radical mastectomy
85.47	Unilateral extended radical mastectomy
85.48	Bilateral extended radical mastectomy

standards will establish consistent coding standards, variations in diligence in assigning these codes in organizations may result in continued bias within and across organizations.

Researchers must be familiar with the structure and limitations of the codes used in their research study. Many codes influence reimbursement and may be inherent sources of bias. Diagnosis and procedure codes are particularly crucial as they are used to select the study sample, to control for comorbidities, and to identify outcomes.

With more than 13,000 ICD-9-CM diagnosis codes, several aggregations of codes create new data elements. For example, hospital discharge data are "grouped" using the diagnosis related groups (DRG) algorithm as part of the hospital prospective payment system. Researchers can use this aggregated grouping to include or exclude patients from their sample, to examine variations in costs, and to measure case mix. Other aggregations of ICD-9-CM codes have been developed to represent clinically meaningful categories (Agency for Healthcare Research and Quality, 2003), to assign patient severity (Averill, Goldfield, Hughes, Muldoon, Gay, et al., 2003), or to measure comorbidities (Elixhauser, Steiner, Harris, & Coffey, 1998). All of these are dependent on the original coding that is done at the time of care.

Organizational Characteristics or Identifiers

It is often desirable to examine organizational characteristics, particularly in outcome studies. This necessitates the inclusion of the characteristics themselves or identifiers to link to the characteristics. If organizational or provider identifiers are required for calculating reimbursement, the linkage identifiers are generally good. However, there are still concerns because organizations merge, close, or change their character, making longitudinal analyses challenging. The Medicare provider number used to identify individual health care organizations is particularly useful to link files. For example, when using the minimum data set (MDS) from long-term care, the Medicare provider number is on the patient file and on the file representing organizational characteristics (the Centers for Medicare and Medicaid Services (CMS) Online

Survey Certification and Reporting database (OSCAR)). Likewise, hospital discharge records can be linked to the organizational characteristics represented in the CMS Prospective Payment Impact File. This file reflects the information needed to calculate hospital reimbursement rates (e.g., teaching intensity, case mix index, hospital type, etc.) and can be downloaded from the CMS website (CMS, 2003). The American Hospital Association (AHA) Annual Survey Database includes a broader array of hospital characteristics, including specific services offered, number and type of employees, and types of affiliations.

Linking the organizational databases to individual records depends on the use of a common identifier. When administrative data are collected primarily for aggregate reporting of utilization, there may be little attention to identifiers. In some state workers' compensation files, for example, the name of the individual organization is not important; instead, reports are aggregated to the type of organization. The name of the employer may be identified in a text field and the text may represent abbreviations, corporate names, or outdated names. Attempting to assign a single organization name and determine a common identifier can be tedious. Coding systems for employers such as Federal Employer Identification Number (FEIN) exist, but are not used consistently.

The Standard Industrial Code (SIC) and, the National Council on Compensation Code (NCCI), or both, may be use to identify type of organizations. The SIC is a four-digit numeric code that allows the selection of employer type. For example, the first three digits of SIC code 805 reflects nursing homes. The fourth digit reflects the type of home: 0 = nursing and personal care facilities, 1 = skilled nursing facilities, 2 = intermediate care facilities, 9 = nursing and personal care not elsewhere classified. All four digits are needed to select specific industries. The NCCI includes over 600 codes intended to cover workplace exposure. As of January 1, 2002, all Federal statistical data were required to be published using the North American Industry Classification System (NAICS). NAICS was jointly developed by the United States, Canada, and Mexico to better represent the range of industries in these countries. A six-digit hierarchical coding system is used. The first two digits represent 20 broad categories, with increasing specificity down to the six-digit level. Table 19.5 illustrates coding for the hospital and nursing home sector.

Geography

For many research aims, geographic characteristics are important to analyze. For example, hospital zip codes can be used to define market

TABLE 19.5 Hospital and Nursing Home Codes Represented in the North American Industry Classification System (NAICS)

NAICS Code	NAICS Description
62	Health Care and Social Assistance
621	Ambulatory Health Care Services
622	Hospitals
6221	General Medical and Surgical Hospitals
6222	Psychiatric and Substance Abuse Hospitals
6223	Specialty (except Psychiatric and Substance Abuse) Hospitals
623	Nursing and Residential Care Facilities
6231	Nursing Care Facilities
6232	Residential Mental Retardation, Mental Health and Substance Abuse Facilities
6233	Community Care Facilities for the Elderly
623312	Homes for the Elderly
6239	Other Residential Care Facilities

areas, and patient zip code information can be used to examine referral patterns, access to services, and community needs. Zip code or geographic area files that include data reflecting characteristics of that zip code can be purchased. For example, the median income of the zip code and its population density may be used to construct proxies of socioeconomic status. County-level statistics are not as specific as zip codes but they are less constrained by privacy concerns and provide needed elements. The Federal Information Processing Standards (FIPS) codes uniquely identify various jurisdictions such as place, county, state, and metropolitan statistical area (MSA). A county code uniquely identifies every county in the U.S. and may be placed in person-level administrative data in lieu of zip code. FIPS county codes can be linked to the Area Resource File (ARF), a database containing more than 6,000 variables for each county in the U.S., including economic indicators, health professions supply, health facility numbers and types, population characteristics, and environment (Quality Resource Systems, n.d.). Since zip code is considered protected health information under HIPAA privacy regulations, (DHHS, 2003) requests for this element must be clearly justified.

ACCESS TO DATA

Access to large existing health care data has both technical and privacy barriers. Until the past few years, access to these data sets required expert technical data management skills since the large and complex files had to be loaded, often from tapes, and stored on a mainframe computer. Many of these data sets are now available on CD-ROM and can be managed on a local area network (LAN). Data may be supplied in a particular software format (e.g., SAS, SPSS) or may be in ASCII form with programs allowing the user to load only the needed data. Some data sets are released through downloads while large and proprietary data may need to be purchased. The Inter-university Consortium for Political and Social Research (ICPSR) (http://www.icpsr.umich.edu/index-medium.html), a not-for-profit organization that serves member colleges and universities, maintains data sets and provides access to archives of social science data (ICPSR, 2003).

While the increasing accessibility makes data management easier, research teams must include individuals with experience manipulating these data. Just as important are individuals who are knowledgeable of the technical aspects of data preparation such as imputation, formats, and sampling. Documentation provided with data can vary in breadth and quality. Documentation and technical reports, formerly requiring several notebooks, are now stored in electronic, hyperlinked files. Users must read the documentation thoroughly to make sure that they are conducting appropriate analyses and not misrepresenting findings. This is perhaps the greatest difference in using data where researchers have control over the definitions and measures that are used. With administrative data, users must consistently consider how their conceptualization might differ from what the documentation details.

The burden of assuring patient privacy has been heightened by the recent enactment of the HIPAA privacy and data access regulations. While organizations, state and federal agencies, and individual providers have always been concerned with maintaining patient confidentiality, the regulations include very specific language related to release of patient data for research purposes. Systems have been developed to review data requests using federally mandated definitions. Data requests may undergo legal and ethical reviews. The fundamental approach is that researchers should request and receive the smallest reasonable amount of information that will allow them to answer the research questions. This is the "minimum necessary" requirement. Furthermore, data should be deidentified as quickly as possible and securely stored with limited access.

METHODOLOGICAL ISSUES WITH EXISTING DATA

Considering that the researcher must often fit available data to the study conceptualization, there are multiple concerns related to internal and external validity. Fundamentally, the researcher must understand what the data represent and consider how this will affect the proposed study. Database documentation and technical reports must be reviewed thoroughly prior to design and throughout the study. The inability to design a study to fit the conceptualization has implications for every area of methods—database selection, study design, sample selection, reliability, and validity of measures, analyses, and conclusions.

APPROPRIATENESS OF DATABASE

While it may seem obvious, one of the basic questions is to determine if the data are appropriate to answer the research questions. Many questions cannot be answered with existing data sources. For example, most data sets have little information about the decision making process that was used in determining a course of treatment. While many correlational studies seek to determine what factors influenced a particular outcome, the ability of the factors to explain the outcome is usually low. Researchers must be knowledgeable about the primary data elements but also about the elements that will be used for sample inclusions and exclusions, statistical controls, and data quality assessment. A good source of information about what is possible is other studies that have used the data to ask similar questions. In addition to published studies, project reports, technical summaries, and database staff should be consulted prior to developing a proposal.

STUDY DESIGN

Some of the earliest users of existing data were health service researchers studying hospital costs and markets. In the late 1980s, an increasing focus on health care outcomes led to the creation of the Agency for Health Care Policy and Research (AHCPR) and a program of research on outcomes, effectiveness, and appropriateness of health care services. This research program was diverse and resulted in concur-

rent data development, advances in analyses, improved linkages among databases, as well as effectiveness studies.

The medical effectiveness studies use a variety of research designs ranging from randomized controlled trials to descriptive/correlational studies. They may include both primary data collection and secondary analyses of existing data. In most studies, there is no attempt to alter the procedures or course of treatment; rather outcomes of groups are compared. Case control or cohort designs may also be used, particularly when there is longitudinal data as in the national health surveys. While the experimental designs clearly provide the stronger level of evidence, they are not feasible or practical for some studies. Nonexperimental and quasiexperimental studies provide an alternative and are generalizable to broader populations, treatments, and situations. For these reasons, many medical effectiveness studies use observational approaches that rely on existing data sources. Even with stronger designs and improved measures, there is healthy skepticism about making definitive assessments of effectiveness. Causal inferences are difficult since the timing of events is often hard to pinpoint, and extraneous factors influencing outcomes are numerous and difficult to assess.

Existing data are also used to meet operational needs of programs or organizations. For example, hospitals and health insurers must project service demand, conduct surveillance, and monitor cost and utilization. While the motivation for conducting these analyses is different from research, the same methods are often used. Likewise, many public health evaluation activities utilize the same methods but are often not considered research. Considering that these evaluations use case-control or cohort designs, conduct complex statistical analyses, and are published in peer-reviewed journals, it is difficult to distinguish them from research (Amoroso & Middaugh, 2003).

MEASUREMENT

Many existing surveillance databases and national surveys include embedded measures of depression, activities of daily living, or functional status. When scaled variables are used, researchers must assess the reliability and validity using the approaches defined in this book. However, the majority of elements in existing databases are not scaled variables, but nominal measures. The measures may be purely labels (e.g., social security number) or they may involve issues of classification—defining whether objects fall in the same or different categories with respect to a given attribute. For classification, rules are needed to guide decisions about whether objects are equivalent or not equivalent. Equivalence means that two objects have a critical property in common (Nunnally & Bernstein, 1994). In some instances, these decision rules are clear (e.g., male, female) while in others (e.g., race), the rules are difficult to determine and apply, and may be dependent on social norms. Even with highly developed coding systems like ICD-9-CM, there are multiple opportunities for error. More often, the rules under which the data were defined, collected, and categorized are not known or fully understood.

RELIABILITY

The reliability of administrative data generally reflects the reproducibility of the data—collected by different methods, by different persons, and at different sites. Some of the elements in administrative data represent observed events that can be clearly classified with nearly universal understanding (e.g., died). When these events are important for reimbursement or outcome evaluations, the likelihood that they will be classified correctly is even greater. It is possible to examine other variables in the same data set to check the reliability (e.g., consistency of death with cardiac arrest diagnosis, intensive care use, etc.). However, there are other variables that are less easy to categorize, such as those that are based on a subjective assessment. The reason for a health visit, for example, may be recorded based on a receptionist's note, the patient's words, or the physician's judgment. Finding another variable in the data set to check reliability is not likely. If there are multiple waves of data collection, it is possible to assess reliability, although it may be confounded with true change (Campbell, 1996).

From the time of designing the data collection protocols to the actual entry of data into the computer, there are many potential areas for error. For example, new procedures and technologies are often performed before they are added to the diagnosis and procedure coding systems. Alternate legal codes are often used, but may not represent the exact procedure that was done. In this instance, the classification rules are flawed, which results in inaccurate information. Another major source of error in health claims data is inadequate documentation. The physician may not clearly describe the procedure, the coder may not be able to read or understand what the physician wrote, or the code that is closest to the existing code may be used. Other problems with the ICD-9-CM codes themselves have been described and include the inability to distinguish clinically dissimilar diagnoses because of inherently imprecise codes, the lack of definitions for codes, or the availability of nonspecific codes as alternatives to more precise codes (Romano & Luft, 1992).

Whenever possible, the results found with analyses of existing data should be compared with other sources of the same information. Results obtained may be compared with measures from other time periods, or data from other sources. This "benchmark" data may not represent the exact population studied, but should be close. For example, rates of disease may be benchmarked with another data source. When individual data in electronic claims are compared with other sources for the same individual (e.g., medical records), it is referred to as a reabstraction study. For example, researchers in California compared electronic discharge abstracts to medical records and found that blood transfusions, treadmill tests, EKGs, and inhalation therapy were coded with less than 50% sensitivity (defined as the percentage of cases with the procedures coded in medical records) (Romano & Luft, 1992). Reliability should also be assessed at different levels of analysis, depending on what is known about the potential sources of error. For example, percentage agreements may be reported by hospital, by physician, or by patient subgroups. Unfortunately, reabstraction studies are expensive and often only a sample of records can be done.

Categorical data elements may be employed in an algorithm to create other categorical variables, such as DRGs. Scaled measures may be created from the categorical data through the use of original data elements such as comorbidities, risk of mortality, and functional status. Researchers should consult the literature to understand how others have used these scaled data and reliability assessments should be done during the analyses.

Data elements that represent labels may also be sources of error. For example, social security numbers and telephone number are labels with no inherent definitions for categories or mathematical properties. Yet, these variables are also subject to error from multiple sources. They may be recorded wrong initially, or may be recorded with extra or missing digits, as a result of keystroke error. Data analyses can identify extra or missing digits through algorithms that search for codes that do not meet defined specifications. However, when data are collected incorrectly in the first place or there are data entry coding problems, identifying these errors is difficult and most often they go undetected.

problem. A good example is the measurement of complications with ICD-9-CM data. While there are codes that represent complications (primarily the 990-999 ICD-9-CM diagnosis codes), and rules for how these are to be used, physicians may not use them out of fear of malpractice or of being identified as providing poor quality of care. Incorrect diagnoses may be entered on a medical record or provisional diagnoses may be disproved but left on the record.

An obvious—but costly—approach to dealing with validity problems is to use different measures and different methods to assess the same attribute. This might mean prospectively collecting data on the same patients represented in the administrative data or using other sources of information. This would be more realistic in the health surveys where questions can be asked in different ways within the same survey. Electronic edits and corroborating measures may also be used to assess validity. For example, if cardiogenic shock were an assigned diagnosis, a one-day length of stay would only seem likely if the patient died.

VALIDITY

Validity in administrative data reflects how closely the data correspond to the researcher's conceptualization and the needs of the study. For many data elements in existing data, the definitions and coding rules have already placed constraints on what is really desirable for study purposes. For example, reported family income may be used to compute measures of socioeconomic status. Yet, the measure itself may not be defined to take into account the number of people in the household. Moreover, the actual reported amount may have been coded into ordinal categories to protect privacy. Thus, the ability of income to truly represent socioeconomic status is further compromised.

Identifying criterion measures for variables in administrative data is particularly difficult. The medical record, while considered the gold standard, may be missing important information. The old adage in health care, "if it is not documented, it did not happen," reflects this

ANALYSES

In light of the multiple sources of bias, it is apparent that researchers using existing data must conduct adequate analyses to be assured that the findings are accurate and the conclusions are not overstated. Extensive preliminary analyses are essential. This iterative process seeks to identify outliers, wild codes, and other data irregularities. Data quality assessments seek to identify the sources and extent of missing data. But, more specific to existing data, potential sources of bias must be uncovered. Descriptive findings may be compared with other elements within the database or to outside benchmark data. Once the preliminary assessments are done, then decisions must be made about how to deal with these issues. Data elements may be dropped, recoded, or transformed. Missing data may be imputed. Research questions may need to be changed. And all of this should be done before beginning the principal analyses.

SUMMARY

Researchers have access to massive amounts of data. Data quality is improving. Techniques to analyze data have expanded. Yet, there are many challenges that must be met when using existing data. Making sure that the data are appropriate for the question is fundamental. Becoming knowledgeable about the data and the potential problems must be done in the early stages of a study. A detailed review of the documentation and technical documentation is time consuming but will help shape the study design. Researchers must utilize their fundamental knowledge of research methodology to design the best study possible—despite the potential sources of bias. Finally, when discussing findings, language should be specific, limitations must be acknowledged, and findings should not be overstated.

REFERENCES

Agency for Health Care Policy and Research (AHCPR). (1991). *Report to Congress: The feasibility of linking research-related data bases to federal and non-federal medical administrative data bases* (AHCPR Publication No. 91-0003). Rockville, MD: Author

Agency for Healthcare Research and Quality (AHRQ). (2003, July). *Clinical classifications software (ICD-9-CM) summary and download.* Retrieved September 10, 2003, from http://www.ahcpr.gov/data/hcup/ccs.htm

Aiken, L. H., Smith, H. L., & Lake, E. T. (1994). Lower medicare mortality among a set of hospitals known for good nursing care. *Medical Care, 32*(8), 771–787.

Amoroso, P. J., & Middaugh, J. P. (2003). Research vs. public health practice: When does a study require IB review. *Preventive Medicine, 36*(2), 250–253.

Averill, R., Goldfield, N., Hughes, J., Muldoon, J., Gay, J., Mccullough E., et al. (2003). *What are APR-DRGS? An introduction to severity of illness and risk of mortality adjustment methodology.* Retrieved September 10, 2003, from http://multimedia.mmm.com/mws/mediawebserver.dyn?qqqqqq&8iBEqKUrq1UrqqqMBgaLPdU8U-

Blegen, M. A., & Vaughn, T. (1998). A multisite study of nurse staffing and patient occurrences. *Nursing Economics, 16*(4), 196–203.

Campbell, R.T. (1996). Measurement models and survey research: Reliability and validity matters. In R. Warnecke (Ed.), *Health survey research methods conference proceedings* (AHCPR Pub. No. 96-1013) (pp 41–43). Rockville, MD: Agency for Health Care Policy and Research.

Centers for Medicare and Medicaid Services (CMS). (2003, September 5). *CMS files for download for medicare payment systems.* Retrieved September 10, 2003, from http://cms.gov/providers/pufdownload/default.asp

Charters, K. (2003). Nursing informatics, outcomes, and quality improvement. *AACN Clinical Issues, 14*(3), 282–294.

Coffey, R. C., Ball, J. K., Johantgen, M. E., Elixhauser, A., Purcell, P., & Andrews, R. M. (1997). The case for national health data standards. *Health Affairs, 16*(3), 58–72.

Elixhauser, A., Steiner, C., Harris, D. R., & Coffey, R. M. (1998). Comorbidity measures for use with administrative data. *Medical Care, 36*(1), 8–27.

Harrington, C., Zimmerman, D., Karon, S. L., Robinson, J., & Beutel, P. (2000). Nursing home staffing and its relationship to deficiencies. *Journals of Gerontology Series B-Psychological Sciences & Social Sciences, 55B*(5), S278–287.

Health Insurance Portability and Accountability Act (1996) Administrative Requirement. 45 CFR part 162.

Iezzoni, L. I. (Ed.). (1994). *Risk adjustment for measuring health care outcome.* Chicago, IL: Health Administration Press.

Iezzoni, L. I. (Ed.). (1997). *Risk adjustment for measuring health care outcome* (2nd ed.). Chicago: Health Administration Press.

Inter-university Consortium for Political and Social Research (ICPSR). (2003, August 27). Retrieved September 10, 2003, from http://www.icpsr.umich.edu/index-medium.html

Johnson-Pawlson, J., & Infeld, D. L. (1996). Nurse staffing and quality of care in nursing facilities. *Journal of Gerontological Nursing, 22*(8), 36–45.

Kovner, C., & Gergen, P. (1998). Nurse staffing

levels and adverse events following surgery in U.S. hospitals. *Image, 30*(4), 315–321.

Mays, V. M., Ponce, N. A., Washington, D. L., & Cochran, S. D. (2003). Classification of race and ethnicity: Implications for public health. *Annual Review of Public Health, 24*, 83–100.

National Health Interview Survey (NHIS). (2003, August 23). Retrieved September 10, 2003, from http://www.cdc.gov/nchs/nhis.htm

Needleman, J., Duerhaus, P., Mattke, S., Stewart, M., & Zelevinsky, K. (2002). Nurse-staffing levels and the quality of care in hospitals. *New England Journal of Medicine, 346*(22), 1715–1722.

Nerenz D. R., Bonham V. L., Green-Weir. R., Joseph, C., & Gunter, M. (2002). Eliminating racial/ethnic disparities in health care: Can health plans generate reports? *Health Affairs, 21*(3), 259–263.

Nunnally, J. C., & Bernstein, I. H. (1994). *Psychometric theory* (3rd ed.). New York: McGraw-Hill, Inc.

Paul, J. E., Weis, K. A., & Epstein, R. A. (1993). Data bases for variations research. *Medical Care, 31*(Supp. 5l), YS96–102.

Quality Resource Systems Inc. (n.d.). Retrieved September 10, 2003, from http://www.arfsys.com/

Romano, P. S., & Luft, H. S. (1992). Getting the most out of messy data: Problems and approaches for dealing with large administrative data sets. In M. L. Grady (Ed.), *Medical effectiveness research data methods* (AHCPR Pub. No. 92-0056) (pp. 57–75). Rockville, MD: Agency for Health Care Policy and Research.

Sondik, E. J., Lucas, J. W., Madans, J. H., & Smith, S. S. (2000). Race/ethnicity and the 2000 census: Implications for public health. *American Journal of Public Health, 90*(11), 1709–1713.

U.S. Department of Health & Human Services (HHS). (2003, August 4). *Medical privacy—National standards to protect the privacy of personal health information.* Retrieved September 10, 2003, from http://www.dhhs.gov/ocr/hipaa/.

20

Collecting Sensitive Information

Greater emphasis on an individual's right to privacy, concomitant with legislation aimed toward ensuring an individual's privacy such as the Health Insurance Portability & Accountability Act (HIPAA) that is discussed in chapter 24 have increased the challenges facing nurses and other health care professionals studying sensitive issues. Sensitive information usually focuses on personal and/or social topics of a nature likely to evoke strong emotional responses from subjects, such as embarrassment, humiliation, fear, stigma, guilt, anger, vulnerability, pain, stress, and/or anxiety. While there are some topics, such as the sudden violent death of a loved one, criminal behavior, and life-threatening illness that are generally identified as sensitive topics, there are other topics such as abortion, drug abuse, and controversial political activities that may be viewed as more or less sensitive depending upon the specific attributes of the subjects and/or the context in which the information is sought. Lee (1993) points out that large groups of respondents experience research on sensitive topics as threatening because it is intrusive to their privacy and may result in sanctions for deviant behavior or unwanted scrutiny, as in the case of organizational research.

ISSUES IN COLLECTING SENSITIVE INFORMATION

While each measurement effort in which sensitive information is sought will give rise to a unique set of concerns, there are several issues that are germane to most, and hence worthy of consideration here. Most subjects, when asked to respond to measurement methods seeking sensitive information from them, tend to refuse to participate more often than those from whom nonsensitive information is solicited. Subjects may just be too emotionally distressed to make a decision whether or not to respond, or they may, because of other factors, not have the time or emotional energy to participate, as in the case of an individual who has a spouse with a life-threatening illness or who has experienced a sudden death in the recent past. Refusal to participate may, in part, be a function of the timing of the measurement effort. That is, during certain stages of an intense emotional life experience, subjects may simply be unable and/or unwilling to deal with the sensitive topic. They may view participation as too threatening or they may not consider participation worth the risk to them. Hence, efforts to collect sensitive information tend to have higher nonresponse rates than other efforts.

Similarly, higher attrition rates characterize such measurement efforts in that subjects will agree to participate, but when actually faced with responding to sensitive information will experience feelings such as embarrassment, lowered self-esteem, and/or fear of appearing abnormal, and will withdraw their participation. Similarly, subjects who agree to participate, when actually faced with responding, may experience reluctance to describe their thoughts, feelings, and/or behavior openly and instead, consciously or unconsciously, provide evasive, false, and/or socially desirable responses.

There are also concerns relative to the investigator trying to collect sensitive data. Depending upon the type of measurement method employed, the investigator may experience, to a greater or lesser extent, the feeling of intruding into subjects' personal lives, anxiety, uncertainty, and/or self doubt when trying to get subjects to participate and/or encouraging them to continue. Similarly, the investigator may need to come to grips with his or her own preconceived attitudes toward the sensitive topic and how to handle them while conducting the measurement effort. Other challenges to the investigator include maintaining confidentiality, researcher detachment, and objectivity; avoiding overidentification with subjects; and determining what information may be too personally sensitive to seek and/or record. Cowles (1988) presents a cogent article discussing issues in qualitative research on sensitive topics that is worthy of attention.

For all these reasons, when preparing for the collection of information that may be sensitive, the investigator needs to consider thoroughly the range of possible emotions that his or her subjects may demonstrate and the kinds of problems they may engender for both the subjects and the investigator within the context of the specific measurement effort. On this basis, the investigator then may select and employ strategies and techniques for the collection of sensitive information that are likely to be successful in dealing with the issues described above, and that are most likely to result in a reliable and valid measurement effort. Readers are referred to the work of Stevens (1994), Chavez, Hubbell, Mishra, and Valdez (1997), Juarbe (1998), Lesjak, Hura, and Ward (1999), and Bernhard (2001) who further address problems encountered by subjects and investigators in their work collecting sensitive information.

STRATEGIES AND TECHNIQUES

In addition to ethical considerations and HIPAA requirements addressed in chapter 24 that must be taken into account, there are other strategies and techniques that are especially useful for dealing with the difficulties encountered in collecting sensitive information. Regardless of the specific measurement method employed, the probability of higher response rates and of lower attrition rates is greater if the following actions are undertaken by the investigator:

1. Anonymity of respondents is assured
2. Confidentiality of responses is maintained
3. Only the most significant and relevant information is sought and that fact is reflected in the items
4. Information that may be too personally sensitive is avoided
5. Items in paper-and-pencil measures are sequenced or ordered from less to more sensitive, and when more personal methods such as interviews are employed there is flexibility to direct responses in and out of sensitive areas as necessary
6. The amount of time allotted to respond is flexible and takes into consideration the respondents' potential for fatigue, difficulty in focusing on sensitive items, and the need to express emotions
7. Provision is made to stop data collection temporarily, if necessary, to accommodate respondents' emotional needs
8. The frequency of data collection allows participants psychological and/or emotional recovery time
9. The time of day when data is collected is appropriate for subjects meeting their other needs and demands
10. Procedures for dealing consistently with respondents' emotional responses, if and when they occur, are devised prior to the collection of data
11. Guidelines for when, if, and how to intervene, if necessary, are devised prior to data collection
12. Only information relevant to the measurement purpose is included in the measure, and decisions are made regarding what information is too sensitive to record prior to data collection
13. Procedures are derived prior to data collection for how the investigator will maintain objectivity and detachment consistently across respondents
14. Provision is made for enabling the investigator to recognize and deal with his or her own emotional responses to the sensitive topic, before and during the conduct of the measurement effort.

Measurement tools and methods that incorporate strategies and techniques for collecting sensitive information are exemplified in the work of McFarlane, Greenberg, Weltge, and Watson (1995), Feldhaus and colleagues (1997), Campbell, Soeken, McFarlane, and Parker (1998), Goodman, Dutton, and Bennett (2000), and Campbell, Sharps, and Glass (2001). Strategies and techniques for minimizing socially desirable responses are discussed in chapter 25. Several measurement techniques discussed in Part III are especially useful in collecting sensitive information. They include interviews, questionnaires, observations, and Q-sorts. Another technique developed specifically for the collection of sensitive information is the randomized response technique (RRT).

The randomized response technique was developed for the express purpose of increasing response rates and eliminating evasive or dishonest responses to sensitive items (Warner, 1965; Buchman & Tracy, 1982; Musch, Bröder, & Klauer, 2001). A basic tenet of this approach to data collection is that subjects are more willing to respond to sensitive items in a truthful manner if they are certain that their responses cannot be directly attributed to them. Originally, the technique was developed to estimate accurately and without bias the frequency of single, stigmatizing characteristics while enabling the respondent to preserve his or her self-image.

In the simplest case, RRT is employed in the following manner. The purpose of the measurement is to estimate the prevalence of a sensitive phenomenon, such as elder abuse, incidents of tax evasion, theft, rape, intimate partner violence, or AIDS, in a specified population. In a one-on-one interview, each subject is given a randomization device such as a coin, die, spinner, colored sphere, ball, or card. Each subject is instructed to use the device to respond in a certain manner depending upon the outcome. For example, the subject might be instructed to flip a coin and to respond "yes" to the investigator if he or she obtains "heads" or has a history of elder abuse. If a respondent answers "yes," it is not certain whether he or she has abused an elder or simply obtained heads on the coin flip. Thus, the respondents' anonymity is preserved. That is, the investigator does not know what question the subject is actually responding to and merely records the answer to a random question.

Based on various stochastic relations between the questions and the response, it is possible to obtain estimates of parameters in the aggregate. For example, if 60 of 100 subjects respond "yes," it can be assumed that 50% of the 100 correspond to "heads" on the coin flip, regardless of whether or not the subject has abused an elder. The surplus 10 reflect those subjects who obtained tails on the flip of the coin, but have abused an elder. Further, since one can assume that 50 subjects received tails on the coin flip, 10 of those 50, or 20%, is an estimate of the prevalence of elder abuse. Clearly, the 20% prevalence for those obtaining tails should exist as well for those obtaining heads on the coin flip. Thus, of the total 100 subjects, one can estimate that 20 have abused elders. Again, it should be emphasized that it is impossible to ascertain which of the 60 who responded "yes" are the elder abusers. Since only aggregate estimates are possible, not only are respondents protected, but many ethical concerns regarding the solicitation of sensitive information are minimized as well.

Warner (1965) developed the original approach to obtaining randomized responses, now known as the *related-question method*, that employs dichotomous response variables, where an estimate of the proportion possessing some sensitive attribute (e.g., elder abuse) is desired. With the aid of a randomizing device that is concealed from the investigator and that follows a Bernoulli distribution with known parameters, each respondent is instructed to answer "true" or "false" to a question or its converse, depending on the outcome of the randomizing device. For example:

I have abused an elder.
I have not abused an elder.

Using probability rules, the overall probability of an affirmative response is then determined. This first effort to develop the RRT was followed by a myriad of research activities designed to make statistical improvements in the method, primarily due to concern with the large standard error and resulting low power of Warner's method and/or to compare the utility of employing RRT relative to other more conventional methods.

Horvitz, Shah, and Simmons (1967), concerned that Warner's (1965) approach tends to evoke suspicions on the part of subjects that there is a way of mathematically determining their true status because both alternatives are sensitive, suggested a modified approach, referred to as the *unrelated-question method,* in which an innocuous alternative question is combined with the sensitive question. For example:

I have abused an elder. (Sensitive)
I watch the 6 p.m. TV news. (Nonsensitive)

Two samples are then employed with respective probabilities of selecting the sensitive question, and appropriate rules of probability are applied to estimate the desired proportion.

In an attempt to further preserve the anonymity of respondents as well as introduce greater precision and efficiency into the procedure, several others have suggested alternative approaches. Boruch (1971) designed a *forced response method,* also known as the *contamination RRT,* and Moors (1971) suggested a *two-sample approach* in which the second sample is used exclusively to estimate the nonsensitive parameter; that is, a nonsensitive alternative is employed in the first sample, and the nonsensitive question alone is used directly in the second sample. Similarly, Folsom, Greenberg, Horvitz, and Abernathy (1973) proposed a two-sample approach employing two nonsensitive alternatives. As in Moors's (1971) approach, the nonsensitive parameters are estimated directly, and as in the approach of Horvitz, Shah, and Simmons (1967) both samples are still employed for estimating the parameter of the sensitive question. That is, in the first sample, the sensitive question is combined with one of the nonsensitive questions and a randomization process, and the other nonsensitive question is asked directly. The placement of the nonsensitive question is reversed in the second sample. That is, in the first sample, subjects might be instructed to respond to a randomized pair depending on the flip of a coin and then to answer a nonsensitive question directly. For example:

Have you abused an elder? (Heads)
Do you watch the 6 p.m. TV news? (Tails)
Do you own a car? (Direct)

In the second sample, the same procedure would be employed, but the placement of the nonsensitive questions would be reversed. For example:

Have you abused an elder? (Heads)
Do you own a car? (Tails)
Do you watch the 6 p.m. TV news? (Direct)

The affirmative response probabilities are estimated from the sample proportions using probability rules.

Greenberg, Kuebler, Abernathy, and Horvitz (1977) extended the technique to quantitative measures. In their approach, the subject would be instructed to answer one of two questions, depending on the outcome of a randomized procedure. For example:

How many times in the past 12 months have you abused an elder? (Sensitive)
How many times in the past 12 months have you watched the 6 p.m. TV news? (Nonsensitive)

Warner (1971), and Liu and Chow (1976) proposed alternatives using multiples added to the true value on the sensitive question and known distributions on the sensitive response, respectively.

Clark and Desharnais (1998) noted that with RRT it is possible that an unknown proportion of respondents does not answer as directed by the randomizing device, thus resulting in an underestimation of the frequency of the sensitive behavior. To address this concern they developed a method to determine the proportion of those whom they referred to as "cheating" respondents. Their method combines survey techniques with an experimental approach based on a between-subject manipulation of the applying random probabilities and computation of a confidence interval for the true value of the frequency of sensitive behaviors. They contend that if the rules of RRT are being followed, as determined through testing, this method makes it possible to determine the exact frequency of a socially undesirable, embarrassing, or criminal behavior of interest.

Musch, Bröder, and Klauer (2001) employed this cheating detection technique in an experimental study conducted using a Web-based survey to determine the frequency of tax evasion. Results demonstrated greater readiness to admit tax fraud when RRT was employed, as compared with a conventional survey.

Readers interested in RRT review articles emphasizing statistical developments and procedures are referred to Fox and Tracy (1986), Chaudhuri and Mukerjee (1988), Antonak and Levneh (1995), and Tracy and Mangat (1996). Readers with advanced statistical background who are interested in more technical articles describing the most recent RRT statistical developments are referred to the work of Singh, Joander, and King (1996), Singh, Horn, and Chowdhuri (1998), Singh, Singh, and Mangat (2000), Tracy and Singh (1999), Singh and Tracy (1999), and Singh (2002).

Studies undertaken to compare different RRTs and other methods for collecting sensitive information (Horvitz, Shad, & Simmons, 1967; Lamb & Stem, 1978; Beldt, Daniel & Garchia, 1982; Wimbush & Dalton, 1997; Van der Heijden, Van Gils, Bouts, & Hox, 1998, 2000) have resulted in contradictory findings regarding whether different RRTs performed better than direct questioning, self-administered questionnaires, telephone interviews, computer assisted self-administered interviews, and/or face-to-face interviews. Lensvelt-Mulders and Hox (2000) conducted a meta-analysis of RRT comparative studies to assess which RRTs produced the most valid results and to compare the performance of RRTs with other more conventional data collection methods across existing studies. They found that in the two unrelated questions RRT demonstrated the most evidence for validity and that RRT produced more valid population estimates for sensitive topics relative to other data collection methods.

Considerations to be made when selecting a randomized response technique include the following:

- Whether the phenomenon of interest is dichotomous or quantitative in nature

- The respondent's ability to understand the approach; that is, more complicated approaches are less appropriate for less sophisticated and/or less educated subjects
- The potential that a given approach is more likely to minimize respondent skepticism

It should be noted that, generally, the respondent will feel more comfortable with a design as the chance of having to respond to the sensitive question decreases. That is, if a very large portion of the affirmative responses are to the nonsensitive question, then responding truthfully to the sensitive question will appear safe or nonjeopardizing for those who, in fact, possess the sensitive attribute (Fox & Tracy, 1980).

Further, in the absence of definitive findings from studies undertaken to validate results of RRTs with external criteria (Umesh & Peterson, 1991), readers who employ RRT in their research and measurement efforts are advised to stay abreast of developments in RRT, to exercise caution in how the technique is used in the absence of best practice guidelines, and to undertake rigorous investigations seeking evidence for validity within the context of their work.

REFERENCES

Antonak, R. F., & Livneh, H. (1995). Randomized response technique: A review and proposed extension to disability attitude research. *Genetic-Social, and General-Psychology-Monographs, 121*(1), 97–145.

Beldt, S. F., Daniel, W. W., & Sarchia, B. S. (1982). The Takahasic-Sakasegawa randomized response technique: A field test. *Sociological Methods and Research, 11*, 101–111.

Bernhard, L. A. (2001). Lesbian health and health care. In D. Taylor and N. F. Woods (Eds.), *Annual Review of Nursing Research*, (Vol. 19 pp. 145–177). New York: Springer Publishing.

Boruch, R. F. (1971). Assuring confidentiality of responses in social research: A systematic analysis. *American Psychologist, 26*(4), 413–430.

Buchman, T. A., & Tracy, J. A. (1982). Capsules

and comments: Obtaining responses to sensitive questions: Conventional questionnaire vs. randomized response technique. *Journal of Accounting Research, 20*(1), 263–271.

Campbell, J. C., Sharps, P. W., & Glass, N. E. (2001). Risk assessment for intimate partner violence. In G. F. Pinard and L. Pagani (Eds). *Clinical assessment of dangerousness: Empirical contributions* (pp. 136–156). New York: Cambridge University Press.

Campbell, J. C., Soeken, K. L., McFarlane, J., & Parker, B. (1998). Risk factors for femicide among pregnant and nonpregnant battered women. In J. C. Campbell (Ed.), *Empowering survivors of abuse: Health care for battered women and their children* (pp. 90–97). Thousand Oaks, CA: Sage.

Chaudhuri, A., & Mukerjee, R. (1988). *Randomized response: Theory and techniques.* New York: Marcel Dekker.

Chavez, L. R., Hubbell, F. A., Mishra, S. I., & Valdez, R. B. (1997). Undocumented Latina immigrants in Orange County, California: A comparative analysis. *International Migration Review, 31*(1), 88–107.

Clark, S. J. & Desharnais, R. A. (1998). Honest answers to embarrassing questions: Detecting cheating in the randomized response model. *Psychological Methods, 3*(2), 160–168.

Cowles, K. V. (1988). Issues in qualitative research on sensitive topics. *Western Journal of Nursing Research, 10*(2), 163–179.

Feldhaus, K. M., Koziol-McLain, J., Amsbury, H. L., Norton, I. M., Lowenstein, S. R., & Abbott, J. T. (1997). Accuracy of 3 brief screening questions for detecting partner violence in the emergency department. *Journal of American Medical Association, 277*(17), 1357–1361.

Folsom, R. E., Greenberg, B. G., Horvitz, D. G., & Abernathy, J. R. (1973). The two alternative questions randomized response model for human surveys. *Journal of the American Statistical Association, 68*, 525–530.

Fox, J. A., & Tracy, P. E. (1980). The randomized response approach applicability to criminal justice, research, and evaluation. *Evaluation Review, 4*(5), 601–622.

Fox, J. A., & Tracy, P. E. (1986). *Randomized response: A method for sensitive surveys.* Beverly Hills: Sage Publications.

Goodman, L. A., Dutton, M. A., & Bennett, M. (2000). Predicting repeat abuse among arrested batterers: Use of the danger assessment scale in the criminal justice system. *Journal of Interpersonal Violence, 15*(1), 63–74.

Greenberg, B. G., Kuebler, R. R., Abernathy, J. R., & Horvitz, D. G. (1977). Respondent hazards in the unrelated question randomized response model. *Journal of Statistical Planning and Inference, 2*, 53–60.

Horvitz, D. G., Shah, B. V., & Simmons, W. R. (1967). *The unrelated question randomized response model* (pp. 65–72). In Proceedings of the Social Statistics Section of the American Statistical Association.

Juarbe, T. C. (1998). Cardiovascular disease-related diet and exercise experience of immigrant Mexican women. *Western Journal of Nursing Research, 20*(6), 765–782.

Lamb, C. W., & Stem, D. E. (1978). An empirical validation of the randomized response technique. *Journal of Marketing Research, 15*(4), 616–621.

Lee, R. M. (1993). *Doing research on sensitive topics.* London: Sage Publications.

Lensvelt-Mulders, G., & Hox, J. (2000 October 3–6). *Meta-analysis of randomized response research: 35 years of validation studies.* Paper presented at Fifth International Conference on Social Science Methodology, Cologne, Germany.

Lesjak, M., Hua, M., & Ward, J. (1999). Cervical screening among immigrant Vietnamese women seen in general practice: Current rates, predictors, and potential recruitment strategies. *Australian and New Zealand Journal of Public Health, 23*, 168–173.

Liu, P. T., & Chow, L. P. (1976). A new discrete quantitative randomized response model. *Journal of American Statistical Association, 71*, 72–73.

McFarlane, J., Greenberg, L., Weltge, A., & Watson, M. (1995). Identification of abuse in emergency departments: Effectiveness of a two-question screening tool. *Journal of Emergency Nursing, 21*(5), 391–394.

Moors, J. J. A. (1971). Optimization of the unrelated question randomized response model. *Journal of the American Statistical Association, 66*, 627–629.

Musch, J., Bröder, A., & Klauer, K. C. (2001). Improving survey research on the World Wide Web using the randomized response technique. In U. D. Reips and M. Bosnjak (Eds.), *Dimensions of internet science* (pp. 179–192). Lengerich, Germany: Pabst Science Publishers.

Singh, S. (2002). A new stochastic randomized response model. *Metrika, 56,* 131–142.

Singh, S., Horn, S., & Chowdhuri, S. (1998). Estimation of stigmatized characteristics of a hidden gang in finite population. *Australian and New Zealand Journal of Statistics, 4,* 291–297.

Singh, S., Joarder, A. H., & King, M. L. (1996). Regression analysis using scrambled responses. *Australian Journal of Statistics, 38*(2), 201–211.

Singh, S., Singh, R., & Mangat, N. S. (2000). Some alternative strategies to Moor's model in randomized response sampling. *Journal of Statistical Planning and Inference, 83,* 243–255.

Singh, S., & Tracy, D. S. (1999). Ridge regression using scrambled responses. *Metron, 57,* 147–157.

Stevens, P. E. (1994). Lesbians' health-related expressions of care and non-care. *Western Journal of Nursing Research, 16*(6), 639–659.

Tracy, D. S., & Mangat, N. S. (1996). Some developments in randomized response sampling during the last decade: A follow-up of review by Chaudhuri and Mukherjee. *Journal of Applied Statistical Science, 4,* 147–158.

Tracy, D. S., & Singh, S. (1999). Calibration estimators for randomized response sampling. *Metron, 57,* 47–68.

Umesh, U. N., & Peterson, R. A. (1991). A critical evaluation of the randomized response method. *Sociological Methods and Research, 20*(1), 104–138.

Van der Heijden, P. G. M., Van Gils, G., Bouts, J., & Hox, J. (1998). A comparison of randomized response, CASAQ, and direct questioning: Eliciting sensitive information in the context of social security fraud. *Kwantitatieve Methoden, 19,* 15–34.

Van der Heijden, P. G. M., Van Gils, G., Bouts, J., & Hox, J. (2000). A comparison of randomized response, CASI, and face to face direct questioning: Eliciting sensitive information in the context of welfare and unemployment benefit. *Sociological Methods and Research, 28*(4), 505–537.

Warner, S. L. (1965). The linear randomized response model. *Journal of the American Statistical Association, 66,* 884–888.

Warner, S. L. (1971). The linear randomized response model. *Journal of the American Statistical Association, 60,* 63–69.

Wimbush, J. S., & Dalton, D. R. (1997). Base rate for employee theft: Convergence of multiple methods. *Journal of Applied Psychology, 82,* 756–763.

21

Selection and Use of Existing Instruments

During the past two decades there has been an incredible increase in the number of instruments developed to measure nursing phenomena and an increased number of published reports of instrument development. As a result, a large repertoire of instruments is now available for use in research and practice. It is sometimes difficult to choose the most appropriate instrument, or even to decide whether it would be preferable to develop a new tool. On the one hand, it is generally much less costly and time-consuming to use existing instruments than to expend the effort necessary to develop and adequately test a new measure. In addition to the pragmatic advantage, the use of existing instruments is beneficial from a knowledge building perspective. It allows systematic comparisons to be made across time and space, and among different populations, because characteristics are being measured in the same way. Use of existing tools and devices provides an ever-increasing database for evaluating the properties of the instruments themselves, and allows information about a particular concept or variable to accumulate.

Conversely, nurses may discover, after extensive search of the literature, that there are no instruments that measure a particular concept or variable. They may also find that existing instruments simply are not adequate because of their conceptual basis, poor psychometric properties, inappropriateness for nursing settings or specific populations of interest, or inadequate testing. In such instances, it is often necessary to develop a new tool or substantially modify an existing one. There is clearly a need for nurses to continue to develop and report the results of testing sound measures for use in nursing,

particularly regarding concepts, processes, and outcomes for which measures are nonexistent or inadequate.

It is the view of the authors that when existing instruments are appropriate for nursing measurement, they should be used in preference to developing new ones. Therefore locating, evaluating, using, and reporting the use of existing instruments are vitally important activities, which should be carried out with attention to the same principles of sound conceptualization and measurement that underpin the tool development process.

LOCATING EXISTING INSTRUMENTS

The process of measurement begins with conceptualizing the phenomenon, concept, or problem of interest, and determining the measurement framework that is appropriate. These steps are preliminary to actually searching for existing instruments, because they help define some of the parameters and boundaries of the search process.

The process of locating instruments generally begins in the library or the computer. Suggestions to facilitate library and database searches for instruments include the following: (1) search computerized databases by using the name of the instrument or key words or phrases; (2) generalize the search to the specific area of interest and related topics (research reports are particularly valuable); (3) search for summary articles describing, comparing, contrasting and evaluating the instruments used to measure a given concept; (4) search journals, such as the

Journal of Nursing Measurement, that are devoted specifically to measurement; (5) examine computer-based and print indices, and compendia of instruments developed by nursing and other disciplines (see examples in Appendix A); and (6) examine copies of published proceedings and abstracts from relevant scientific meetings. Although computer searches have revolutionized the process of locating possible measures of a given concept, it is advisable to add at least one other search strategy. It is often very helpful to consult colleagues who are currently conducting related research and are abreast of the most recent literature. Research-focused professional meetings provide fruitful opportunities for discussing measures and for learning about recent developments.

EVALUATING EXISTING INSTRUMENTS

Once potential instruments have been located, they should be carefully evaluated in light of the purpose for which they are to be used. This is a process that requires sophistication in the concepts of measurement and cannot be conducted superficially or with a strong bias toward a particular discipline. For example, an instrument's availability, previous widespread use, and purported ability to measure a concept or variable of interest are not sufficient to legitimize its use for a given nursing measurement activity. Likewise, the fact that an instrument has been developed within the context of another discipline does not automatically exclude it from consideration.

Evaluating the adequacy of any existing instrument requires that consideration be given to its purpose, conceptual basis, development, and psychometric properties. It is critical that the potential borrower or user of the instrument obtain the information necessary to evaluate these features. Despite the increase in publications about instrument development and the requirement that the process of instrument development be described in research reports, the needed information for a thorough evaluation may not be readily available and may require active search by the potential user. It may be advisable to establish personal contact with the instrument's developer and others who may have used it. Although time consuming, obtaining such information before selecting an instrument helps to prevent problems and dilemmas that result from the use of inappropriate or psychometrically inadequate measures and that cannot be rectified after the measure has been employed. Major considerations when evaluating existing tools for use in nursing measurement are considered briefly below. They serve to highlight the information that tool developers have a responsibility to provide about their work.

Purpose

Every measurement instrument is developed for a purpose, whether or not it is explicitly revealed by the developer. The purposes for which the tool was originally developed need not be identical to those for which it is being evaluated, but they should be congruent. For example, a tool developed to measure employee satisfaction for a research study could be employed subsequently by nursing service administrators to assess reasons for employee turnover. Since the purpose for which an instrument is developed is inherently linked to its content and format, it is important that the instrument as a whole and individual items be scrutinized carefully in light of its intended use in particular settings and for particular populations.

Stated Aim of the Instrument

Instruments are developed with one of several goals in mind (e.g., description, diagnosis, screening, selection, prediction). Each of these goals requires different information. For example, a tool developed to provide descriptive information about the mood states of patients with newly diagnosed diabetes may be too imprecise to be used for diagnosing depression.

Measurement Framework

As detailed in chapter 4, norm- and criterion-referenced measures are developed and interpreted differently for different purposes, and should not be used interchangeably. Availability of norms for the former type of measure is an important consideration in instrument selection.

Population

A measure is developed for a particular population and is specific to individuals or groups with given characteristics, such as age, educational or reading level, culture, ethnicity, previous life experiences, and health status (including specific pathologic conditions). As a result, tools often cannot be used for different types of populations without considerable modification.

Setting

An instrument may be designed for use in a particular setting such as a hospital, school, industry, or home, and cannot easily be transferred to another context. The setting may also influence other measures, such as interviews and questionnaires, that require the subject to take a given environment or context into account in formulating responses. For example, an instrument designed to measure patients' perceived control in the intensive care setting would probably be inappropriate for use in a long-term care facility.

Time Perspective

All instruments have an inherent time orientation. Some take only the present into account, while others require recall of past events or projection into the future. It is important to ascertain the extent to which a given instrument may be oriented toward short-term versus long-term conditions or situations, and to estimate the ability of the intended population to adjust their thinking accordingly.

Conceptual Basis for the Instrument

Inherent in every instrument are assumptions about the nature of the entity being measured and how it relates to other concepts. These may be explicitly stated by the developer or may have to be inferred. Every instrument reflects a particular perspective and conceptual mapping

which must be evaluated in terms of its congruence with the views of the potential user. Many instruments that are useful in nursing measure complex concepts, such as stress, anxiety, social support, coping, communication, role, nursing, and health, which have been conceptualized from many different theoretical perspectives. Depending upon the perspective being used, the instruments developed to measure the same concept may differ considerably in the dimensions that are highlighted.

A major consideration in evaluating an existing instrument is the degree of fit between the current conceptualization and that which guided the development of the tool. In addition to ascertaining that underlying assumptions are compatible, important points in assessing the degree of fit include the following: (1) whether the entity to be measured is conceptualized as static or dynamic; (2) whether the entity is conceptualized objectively, subjectively, or both; and (3) the extent to which the original conceptualization includes those aspects or dimensions of meaning that are deemed essential in the situation for which it is being evaluated. A common problem is that the instrument chosen to measure a given concept is not conceptually congruent with the investigator's perspective and theoretical definition of that concept, so validity is compromised and findings cannot be interpreted adequately. The only way to eliminate this problem is to define the meaning domain explicitly and evaluate the domains of existing instruments in that light. Information concerning the conceptual basis and domain of an existing instrument is often available in works written or cited by the developer, in compendia that describe measurement tools, and in review articles and texts that compare theoretical perspectives related to a given concept.

Psychometric Properties

Reliability and validity are fundamental considerations when evaluating an existing instrument for potential use, a point which has been emphasized repeatedly throughout this book. Also important for many kinds of instruments are considerations of sensitivity and specificity. Information about the psychometric properties of any instrument should be obtained and evaluated before the tool is selected for use. A thorough assessment requires that the potential user take into account the procedures that were used to develop the instrument, as well as those that were used to assess its psychometric properties, not only at the time of development, but also in subsequent applications. Consider the types of reliability and validity assessed and the specific populations and conditions of administration for which data have been reported, recognizing that psychometric properties may change under different conditions. Evaluation should take into account: (1) the number and currency of estimates; (2) the diversity of conditions for which estimates have been reported; (3) the nature of the samples from which data were obtained; (4) the degree of similarity between the situation for which the instrument is being evaluated and those for which psychometric data are available; and (5) the appropriateness of the procedures used to assess reliability, validity, specificity, and sensitivity, given the type of instrument and its intended use. Psychometric properties are viewed in light of the purposes for which the tool will be used, including the degree of precision and accuracy that is necessary. For example, considerably more measurement error can be tolerated in an exploratory study than is acceptable in a randomized test of an intervention or a clinical diagnostic tool.

Despite the recent emphasis on the importance of using sound measurement principles and reporting the results of psychometric assessments, there remain significant gaps in the literature. Often reliability and validity are not reported, or are reported for much earlier administrations of the measure. Where data are not reported, the tool developer should be contacted personally.

In addition to psychometric properties and congruence of conceptualization and purpose, some pragmatic aspects of potential instruments need to be considered: (1) the cost, time, and any special requirements or arrangements involved in purchase, administration, and scoring; (2) the demands made on potential subjects; and (3) whether it is possible to secure permission to use the instrument for the intended purpose. After careful review of the above fea-

tures it is often possible to identify one or more existing tools that are acceptable. If more than one instrument appears to be satisfactory, then, all else being equal, the one with the best psychometric performance should be selected.

If existing tools require modifications, such as changes in wording or the addition or deletion of items, then a new instrument has been created. Therefore, previous estimates of psychometric properties and previously established norms are inapplicable, and re-evaluation must be carried out.

USE AND REPORTING

The use of existing instruments entails considerable legal and ethical responsibility on the part of the user. Printed research instruments are subject to protection under copyright law. An increasing number of investigators who develop instruments to measure nursing phenomena are immediately securing copyright for them. Some developers market and sell their instruments, whereas others allow them to be duplicated without charge. The tool developer may own the copyright, or it may be held by an organization, such as a publishing company or university. Permission must be secured from the copyright owner to duplicate and use an existing tool beyond what is considered to fall under the doctrine of fair use. Even when an instrument is not legally protected by copyright, professional ethics dictate that, if possible, permission be secured before duplicating and using it.

Fair use is a legal principle which states that "portions of copyright materials may be used without permission of the copyright owner provided the use is fair and reasonable, does not substantially impair the value of the materials, and does not curtail the profits reasonably expected by the owner" (Owen, 1987, p. 33). Under this doctrine a teacher can make a copy of an instrument for personal use; however, making multiple copies for distribution to students would be problematic without securing permission from the holder of the copyright. Copy services that duplicate packets of materials for sale to students are careful to secure permission to do so. Likewise, publication of multiple copies of a copyrighted instrument for use with subjects in a research study would be precluded unless permission were secured from the copyright holder. The assistance of an attorney should be sought to clarify any issues regarding possible copyright infringement. However, the most appropriate rule of thumb is to secure permission before duplicating, modifying, or using an existing tool.

Permission to use a given instrument for a specific purpose should be requested and secured from the developer and the copyright holder in writing. Correspondence related to the transaction should be kept on file as a legal record of attention to the provisions of copyright law, and credit should be given in writing on the instrument itself and in related publications. When an instrument is a modification of an existing instrument, credit should be given to the original instrument's developer. When an existing instrument is used, any instructions or conditions specified by the developer must be followed. These may include specifications regarding subjects, procedures for administration, scoring and interpretation, requirements for computer scoring, or requirements for sharing information obtained or problems encountered. The importance of adhering to predetermined procedures in the use of standardized instruments was emphasized in chapter 7. Adherence to specified procedures is equally important with nonstandardized measures if comparisons will made with established norms.

Although previously gathered psychometric information may have been secured for an existing instrument, its properties in a different sample are essentially unknown. Thus, the psychometric properties of the instrument should be reassessed with each sample. When the sample or setting differs considerably from previous applications, it is advisable to pretest the tool and calculate reliability and validity statistics using the pretest data. The statistics should be recalculated concurrently with use of the instrument and reported.

Reporting the use of existing instruments to the developer and copyright holder (where appropriate), as well as to the scientific and professional community as a whole, are important considerations. Even when the developer does not require feedback following use of an instrument, it is desirable to communicate the results of having used it, particularly if any problems were encountered. It is particularly important to communicate (1) any difficulties encountered in administration, calibration, scoring and interpretation; (2) the results of psychometric testing; (3) frequency distributions that might have implications for establishing or modifying norms; and (4) any suggestions for modification or future applications. Such feedback is useful, because it helps improve the tool and affects its ultimate utility.

The user of an existing instrument has responsibility to share information about the tool's properties and its potential utility to the scientific community. Any modifications should be detailed explicitly and resulting psychometric data shared. Failures as well as successes also are important. The finding that an instrument demonstrated low reliability or validity when used with a particular population or setting, or that problems were encountered with its use, are vital to preventing future problems and encouraging needed modification.

REFERENCES

Owen, S. (1987). Copyright law: How it affects your hospital and you. *Journal of Nursing Administration, 17*(10), 32–35.

22

Internet Data Collection

The Internet has opened up important possibilities for data collection. When done correctly, the Internet can offer researchers international access, fast interaction with respondents, and almost complete automation of data collection and data management (Joinson, 1999). However, the ease and accuracy of data collection will be influenced by the nature of the data (i.e., qualitative versus quantitative), the computer proficiency of the researcher and respondents, and the sophistication of the available computer hardware and software.

Successful data collection over the Internet will need to address the following issues: (a) developing an Internet data collection protocol that adequately addresses the needs of the investigator while taking advantage of the benefits the Internet offers; (b) ensuring that data collected over the Internet are reliable and valid; (c) converting paper-and-pencil data collection methods for the Internet; (d) making Internet data collection useful and easy for respondents and researchers; and (e) ensuring that data collected using quantitative and qualitative approaches are of high quality (Strickland et al., 2003).

COLLECTING QUANTITATIVE DATA OVER THE INTERNET

Survey data and empirical data for most quantitative studies such as psychological studies or health assessments, can be collected over the Internet (Senior & Smith, 1999). Use of existing paper-and-pencil questionnaires is common over the Internet since they tend to consist of structured, close-ended questions. Questionnaires are particularly convenient for use over the Internet since they can be easily posted to newsgroups, and e-mail lists, e-mailed directly to participants (Sheehan & McMillan, 1999), or placed on a Web site or gopher site for download (Lakeman, 1997; Strickland et al., 2003). It is quite common for existing measurement instruments to be adapted for use over the Internet. It is important for such questionnaires and the data collection methods to be: (a) appropriately revised to address the aims or purposes of the data collection protocol, (b) reliable and valid, (c) adaptable for Internet data collection, and (d) practical for respondents and the researcher. In addition, the Internet protocol needs to ensure the quality of data collected. It is often necessary to modify the format of existing questionnaires for use on the Internet.

Before initiating data collection over the Internet, a detailed and thorough protocol for data collection needs to be carefully delineated. The steps necessary to successfully place each survey questionnaire on the Internet and to download data must be integrated into the protocol. Specification of variables for which data are required is essential, and they should be individually linked to a data collection form or questionnaire that is appropriate for the target population. A sound Internet data collection protocol will consist of the following: (a) details of how potential participants will be screened to ensure that Internet data collection is appropriate, (b) specifications regarding how respondents will be oriented and gain access to the data collection Web site, (c) approaches for generation of respondent identification numbers that are linked to each data source, (d) safeguards to ensure that respondent confidentiality will be maintained over the Internet, (e) details of when and in what order respondents should complete each questionnaire, (f) notation of how and in what form Internet data will be retrieved for analysis, and (g) specification of how Internet data will be permanently removed from the Web site. The involvement of an information services specialist who is informed about the research protocol and who has experience with setting up Web sites for data collection is crucial for the development of an Internet data collection protocol that allows data to be easily entered and downloaded, and kept secure and confidential (Strickland et al., 2003).

Instruments that have prior evidence that they have metric properties of high quality should be selected for Internet data collection. The investigator also must consider whether the Internet is a good forum for collecting the data that is required for each measure, and if this approach is likely to influence the quality of the data obtained. In most situations, questionnaires and forms that have been reliable and valid for self-report using paper-and-pencil methods will also be reliable and valid for completion over the Internet. However, this is not always the case. It is ideal to assess the reliability and validity of questionnaires that are placed on the Internet site prior to using them in a major Internet study. When questionnaires have formats amenable to internal consistency reliability assessment, the alpha reliability coefficient needs to be calculated once data have been collected. If the internal consistency is poor, this would be an indication that the data are either not reliable or lack insufficient variability. In either case, it would not be a good indication that the questionnaire is ready for use over the Internet.

When questionnaires and forms are complicated or have confusing formats, they may present special problems for the Webmaster to place on an Internet site. In addition, they are also likely to be difficult for respondents to complete accurately. If reliable and valid quantitative data are to be collected over the Internet, it is necessary for respondents to have the computer skills to navigate the Internet. In addition, they need to have the reading skills required to understand information on the Web site, particularly the questionnaires placed on the Web site.

Data fraud, data generalizability, and self-selection bias (Smith & Leigh, 1997) are other issues that may affect the validity of Internet data. If the proper safeguards are not established

on the Web site, it is possible that some individuals could complete the questionnaires multiple times. To prevent this from happening, software can be set up to identify the domain address of each respondent so that multiple sets of responses from the same Web address can be identified and deleted from the database. Data fraud and duplicate data collection could also be avoided by first screening participants and then issuing a login name and password. The Web site could be cued to invalidate the password after each questionnaire is completed.

The development of HTML made it possible for respondents to complete questionnaires over the Internet for interactive documents, or "forms". With HTML it is now possible to place questionnaires and forms on the Internet, that are visually and functionally identical to conventional questionnaires. Respondents can check questionnaire boxes, radio buttons, and text-entry boxes with ease and minimal chance of error (Houston & Fiore, 1998). In most cases, directions for forms and questionnaires will need to be made compatible for use on the Internet. For example, changes would need to be made so respondents can easily check and change their responses if they desire. Prompts need to be included that encourage completion of all items unless intentionally left blank. Special links between forms also may be required.

Questionnaires can be placed on the Internet in a manner to reduce errors and missing data by integrating approaches for analyzing responses prior to final acceptance to eliminate errors and inconsistencies in responses (Houston & Fiore, 1998), embedding answer reliability checks in questions, and using forced-choice answers for questionnaires or rating scales (Szabo & Frenkl, 1996), along with an option that notes that an item was intentionally unanswered. When questionnaires have been carefully designed for Internet data collection, it has been shown that there are fewer missing data (Stanton, 1998).

If a longitudinal study is being conducted, the Internet data collection protocol must integrate the timing of data collections. In this regard the communication of data collection points to the participants is particularly important. An approach to remind study participants to complete follow-up data collections at the scheduled times will need to be set up. In addition to reminders for timed data collections, it may be necessary to continuously remind participants to completely finish their Internet questionnaires at a specific data point when they are completing questionnaires at their leisure. To accomplish this, e-mail reminders can be linked to the Web site. It may be necessary to get postal addresses as well as e-mail addresses of respondents since they may use public computers and may not have access to their own personal computer.

The most effective data collection protocols are easy and practical for respondents and for the investigator. Data collection instruments are most practical for respondents when they are accessible, appropriate for the population that will complete them, easy to understand and complete, simple, and not burdensome (Strickland, 1997). This is also applicable when data are collected over the Internet. In the best circumstances, questionnaires and forms should not be above the fifth-grade reading level and should consider the health and capabilities of the target population. The mental or physical limitations of potential respondents that are likely to compromise Internet data collection are a consideration. Young children and ill or frail patients may find Internet data collection too challenging, although Fleitas (1998) found that chronically ill children accommodated to Internet data collection very well. The amount of energy and time required for completion of data collection over the Internet can also interfere with the quality of data collected since high demands could increase the dropout rate (Strickland, 1999). However, the issue of fatigue can be addressed if respondents can return to the Web site and complete questionnaires at their leisure. If this method is used, a mechanism to remind respondents to return to the Web site to complete questionnaires will be required to prevent an increase in missing data.

Access to a computer may be a practical barrier to participation for some potential respondents in studies that involve Internet data collection. As noted above, access to the Internet is often available through public libraries, but respondents must be willing to travel to another site to participate in the study.

The costs associated with the collection of data over the Internet will include the computer equipment and software, the technical expertise of an information services specialist, and support personnel to assist with monitoring the Web site. However, these expenses may be offset by the fact that Internet data collection offers the ability to download questionnaires and forms directly into data management programs, which can greatly reduce cost. If the Internet survey uses a standardized instrument that is usually purchased, there will be a cost associated with obtaining approval to place it on the Web site as well as for scoring. Although data collection over the Internet may be more costly in regards to purchasing equipment and computer expertise, and setting up the Web site, it is likely to be less costly in regards to recruiting and contacting participants, and data management, particularly when a study requires a large sample (Fawcett & Buhle, 1995; Kelly & Oldham, 1997; Wilmoth, 1995). Since the Internet has the advantages of reduced cost, global access, and real-time data collection (Kelly & Oldham, 1997), the human effort required and the financial cost of data collected will be greatly reduced in most cases. Therefore, the potential sizes of clinical and survey studies that can be practically implemented are greatly increased.

When the quality of the data collected within a study is good, the quality of the overall study is improved. Lack of adequate computer skills among study participants can threaten the quality of an Internet study. Some individuals who decide to participate in an Internet study may not have adequate computer skills to navigate the Internet to even get to the Web site. It is also possible that they may not have some of the basic skills required to respond to questionnaires and forms on the Web site. Training of respondents would increase the adeptness of the process of Internet data collection, and may need to be done in real time. It is becoming more common for clinical data to be collected over the Internet. Therefore, clinicians also need to be trained to directly enter data into the Internet database to increase data quality. Real-time data entry by clinicians can reduce transcription errors and "semantic errors as the clinicians managing the patients are directly entering data themselves" (Kelly & Oldham, 1997).

Maintaining the quality of research data can be challenging when large clinical data sets are being compiled. It will be necessary to carefully and continuously record, collate, validate, and enter data into a database (Kelly & Oldham, 1997). Audit and progress charting can be facilitated by data collected over the Internet, which can ensure the quality and completeness of study data. Descriptive statistical reports can be regularly, efficiently, and effectively generated from Web site data throughout the study period to monitor study progress. These reports should include the number of respondents, percentage of respondents completing questionnaires at each data collection point, and the amount and nature of missing data. Internet questionnaire completion results in less risk of coding errors and easy downloading of data for use with other software programs for validation, reliability checks, and analysis. As noted previously, other strategies for ensuring data quality include: (a) encouraging participants to complete all questions and questionnaires through the integration of Web site prompts, (b) ensuring that participants have completed questionnaires at the proper time by monitoring the Web site frequently, and (c) using data generated within the study to assess instruments with scales for internal consistency reliability. It should be noted that an important aspect of Internet data quality is that data collected over the Internet are less likely to be affected by social desirability and inhibition than data collected via paper-and-pencil methods (Im & Chee, 2003).

COLLECTING QUALITATIVE DATA OVER THE INTERNET

Qualitative data collection over the Internet requires that the process adhere to the philosophy of the approach used. Prior to selecting the Internet as a means for data collection, the researcher should weigh the benefits of Internet data collection in relation to whether the Internet will allow the research process to remain true to the philosophy of the qualitative approach. In some qualitative studies it is possible that all the data required for the study could be collected over the Internet. This could be the case with many phenomenological studies, which focus on the meaning of one's lived experience (Morse & Field, 1995), where individual interviews are usually done. Qualitative focus groups may also be appropriate. Moloney, Dietrich, Strickland, and Myerburg (2003) used online discussion boards as virtual focus groups in a study of perimenopausal women with migraines. Other qualitative approaches may only be amenable to having part of the required data collected over the Internet. The grounded theory approach is a good example, since part of the data collected could be obtained over the Internet and because this approach often combines techniques such as interviews, observations, and record reviews. On the other hand, since the ethnographic approach focuses on studying behaviors from within the culture, the Internet may not be highly amenable to use for data collection.

Although one could argue that telephone data collection has more advantages than Internet data collection for qualitative data, the Internet has the advantage over telephone interviews of costing less than telephone contact, particularly when subjects are from other states or geographic regions. Clearly, an advantage of Internet data collection is that respondents can be recruited nationally or internationally, if appropriate, with little additional costs. Therefore, the Internet can afford an investigator access to respondents who would not have been available for recruitment locally. However, there are some caveats that need to be considered when respondents are recruited over the Internet. First, demographic and screening data must be carefully obtained to ensure that respondents are part of the desired target population. In addition, geographic location and culture need to be considered because these could be important factors in the nature of the experience communicated by the respondent (Strickland et al., 2003).

Real-time Internet data collection is now available in today's highly technological society. Also known as synchronous communication, real-time Internet data collection can occur with the respondent providing responses verbally and in writing. When the real-time data collection format is used, open-ended questions can be submitted to the Web site in advance or at the time that the computer interaction occurs. In either case real-time data collection requires the interviewer and respondent to schedule a time for the subject to respond in real time so that both the researcher and the respondent are available simultaneously. When the respondent types in the responses to the questions, they appear on the interviewer's screen instantly. Therefore, the interviewer can clarify confusing written comments or probe comments that require further explication at the time the respondent supplies them over the Internet. Real-time Internet data collection can increase the quality of data and provide the interviewer with more control over the data collected. This approach is likely to keep the respondent engaged and focused on the topic, thus enhancing the possibility that answers will be provided to the researcher's probes or clarifying questions.

When real-time voice capabilities are desired, more sophisticated computer equipment and programs are required. The cost of data collection will be higher with voice exchange capabilities than without it because the researcher must have a live microphone. If there is a need for verbal interchange between the researcher and respondent, then the respondent also must have a microphone. In either case the respondent will need a computer system with an active speaker so that probes and clarifying questions from the researcher can be heard. In addition, real-time computer data collection requires a high-speed Internet connection and computer processor. Since fewer people possess this type of equipment, this limits the potential number of study participants (Lakeman, 1997).

Asynchronous communication may be the preference for some qualitative studies. In this approach, the investigator would prepare open-ended questions to which the respondents would provide answers over the Internet in written form at a later convenient time. Asynchronous Internet data collection requires the researcher to review the respondent's comments after they have been entered at the Web site. The qualitative researcher will need to check the Web site frequently so that clarifying questions and probes can be provided in response to the subject's answers to the original set of open-ended questions. Hence, probes and clarifying questions also are submitted at a later time. A major disadvantage of asynchronous Internet data collection is that it is easy for the respondent not to respond at all or to only provide partial answers to the information requested. Respondents may also wander off the topic rather than providing information relevant to the study. In this situation, the researcher has less control over the data collection process.

In conclusion, Internet data collection offers many advantages, but also has some disadvantages. Researchers must carefully consider their needs in light of the challenges and benefits it can present. In that regard, Strickland and colleagues (2003) offer some general guidelines for researchers who are considering the incorporation of the Internet into their research methods.

1. The investigator needs to keep fairly tight control of the study, carefully screening potential participants to verify their appropriateness for the study, and, where possible, providing individual passwords that can be used only to a limited extent.

2. It may also be helpful to consider mixing use of the Internet with other approaches to communication. For example, screening might be done by phone to establish a relationship with the participant and diminishing the possibility of fraud. In a study that spans several weeks or months, it is helpful to occasionally "check in" with participants by phone to see how they are doing with responding to the Internet data collection protocol.

3. Both the researcher and participants may find that conducting interviews or discussion groups online is rewarding and convenient. However, this experience may be time consuming for the researcher, and may require a major time commitment from the research staff and the participants.

4. It is important to have computer consultation and contact information readily available, unless the researchers themselves are expert in computer usage. Glitches often occur (as when a questionnaire will not advance to the next page, or error messages appear for no

apparent reason), and someone needs to address them quickly to minimize participant frustration and study attrition.

5. Potential respondents who do not own personal computers can be directed to use public library computers. Although public library computers represent a feasible way for individuals to participate in Internet research, this method requires a greater commitment by researchers and participants.

Although data collection over the Internet has many potential advantages, its use should be weighed in relation to its disadvantages given the particular situation for which data are collected. Careful consideration should be given to the purposes of the data collection, the nature of the target population, the type of data required, the availability of computer resources, and the degree to which reliable and valid data can be collected with the intended protocol before a final decision is made regarding use of the Internet for data collection.

REFERENCES

Fawcett, J., & Buhle, E. L. (1995). Using the Internet for data collection: An innovative electronic strategy. *Computers in Nursing, 13*(6), 273–279.

Fleitas, J. (1998). Computer monitor—Spinning tales from the World Wide Web: Qualitative research in electronic environment. *Qualitative Health Research, 8*(4), 283–292.

Houston, J. D., & Fiore, D. C. (1998). Online medical surveys: Using the Internet as a research tool. *M.D. Computing, 15*(2), 116–119.

Im, E., & Chee, W. (2003). Issues in Internet research. *Nursing Outlook, 51*(1), 6–12.

Joinson, A. (1999). Social desirability, anonymity, and Internet-based questionnaires. *Behavioral Research Methods, Instrumentation, & Computers, 31*(3), 433–438.

Kelly, M. W., & Oldham, J. (1997). The Internet and randomised controlled trials. *International Journal of Medical Informatics, 47*(1–2), 91–99.

Lakeman, R. (1997). Using the Internet for data collection in nursing research. *Computers in Nursing, 15*(5), 269–275.

Moloney, M. F., Dietrich, A. S., Strickland, O. L., & Myerburg, S. (2003). Using Internet discussion boards as virtual focus groups. *Advances in Nursing Science, 26*(4), 274–286.

Morse, J. M., & Field, P. A. (1995). *Qualitative research methods for health professionals.* Thousand Oaks, CA: Sage Publications.

Senior, C., & Smith, M. (1999). The Internet. . . . A possible research tool? *Psychologist, 12*(9), 442–444.

Sheehan, K. B., & McMillan, S. J. (1999). Response variation in e-mail surveys: An exploration. *Journal of Advertising Research, 39*(4), 45–54.

Smith, M. A., & Leigh, B. (1997). Virtual subjects: Using the Internet as an alternative source of subjects and research environment. *Behavioral Research Methods, Instrumentation & Computers, 29*(4), 496–505.

Stanton, J. M. (1998). An empirical assessment of data collection using the Internet. *Personnel Psychology, 51*(3), 709–725.

Strickland, O. L. (1997). Challenges in measuring patient outcomes. *Nursing Clinics of North America, 32*(3), 495–512.

Strickland, O. L. (1999). The practical side of measurement. *The Behavioral Measurement Letter, Behavioral Measurement Database Service, 6*(1), 9–11.

Strickland, O. L., Moloney, M. F., Dietrich, A. S., Myerburg, S., Cotsonis, G. A., & Johnson, R. V. (2003). Measurement issues related to data collection on the World Wide Web. *Advances in Nursing Science, 26*(4), 246–256.

Szabo, A., & Frenkl, R. (1996). Considerations of research on Internet: Guidelines and implications for human movement studies. *Clinical Kinesiology, 50*(3), 58–65.

Wilmoth, M. C. (1995). Computer use and nursing research. Computer networks as a source of research subjects. *Western Journal of Nursing Research, 17*(3), 335–338.

23

Computer-Based Testing

Louise S. Jenkins

Computers have touched nearly every area of life, and measurement is not an exception. Innovative strategies, rapid and highly complex computational capability, ever-increasing capacity for storage of information, and undreamed of economy and accessibility are among the characteristics that affect the measurement process. In this chapter, two topics are addressed: (1) computer simulation; and (2) computer-based testing, which encompasses a discussion of computerized fixed testing as well as computer adaptive testing.

COMPUTER SIMULATION

Early uses of computer simulation involved using the computer to carry out a series of statistical trials using the Monte Carlo method (Nunnally & Bernstein, 1994). Today advanced graphical and acoustical simulation are realities, so there are a variety of ways in which computer simulation can be used, including interventions in research studies and providing options for teaching and learning experiences that may also include evaluation of learner outcomes.

In some cases, a simulation is designed for a single purpose while in others, purposes are combined. DxR Clinician (DxR Development, 2001) is an example of patient simulation software that offers case learning experiences with virtual patients, as well as evaluation capability. Advanced-practice nursing graduate students and medical students use these simulations to develop competence working through specified virtual-patient cases. Faculty can use these sim-

ulations to evaluate student clinical decision-making and care management skills. The clinical competency exam information is controlled through CCX Software (DxR Development, 2001) that is made up of four utilities. In the first utility, faculty have the option of creating or editing an existing case, as well as setting the grading criteria. In the second utility, students gather data from their patient that can involve interviewing and examining the patient, as well as ordering laboratory tests for which results are available and need to be interpreted. Students then make a differential diagnosis and develop a plan of care for managing the patient. The third utility allows the faculty to evaluate the record of student interactions with the virtual patient in assessment and patient care planning. The fourth utility handles results from an individual student over multiple cases or groups of students, or performance on a single case or group of cases.

Strengths of computer simulations such as these include: (1) the consistency of case or simulation presentation is assured, thus strengthening the evaluation process; (2) there is an opportunity for the faculty to create or edit scenarios as well as determine the criteria for grading; (3) students have the opportunity to compare their answers with the evaluation criteria, as well as be informed of cost aspects of the laboratory work they have ordered; and (4) student performance records can be captured in workable formats for comparison across virtual patient cases and students. Costs of the simulation software and computer equipment are the major limitations.

In addition, as seen in the section that follows, computer simulations are being used in other aspects of the measurement process. Examples include work with large data sets to compare different types of testing, such as computer adapted testing, with traditional assessment methods.

COMPUTER-BASED TESTING

As noted by Ruiz, Fitz, Lewis, and Reidy (1995), computer-based testing is a very broad term which encompasses a variety of types of tests having in common only that a computer is used in administration of the test/measure. The two major types of tests are *fixed* and *adaptive,* which are discussed below.

Aside from use in the administration of tests, computers are frequently used in various phases of the measurement process including test development, formatting, scoring and reporting, and test/item evaluation. Various software products are available for use in test preparation as well as administration, scoring, estimating reliability and validity, and allowing for different types of item analysis. These software products range from relatively simple to very complex in purpose, capability, and cost.

An example of relatively simple software is a test construction kit providing various types of item shells (e.g. multiple choice, matching, true/false, and cloze sentences) and formatting, available via shareware at http://www.shareup.net/Home-Education/Teaching-Tools/Test-Construction-Kit-review-6354.html (JCG Software, n.d.) at a nominal cost. Some products are designed to perform a particular function such as scoring or creating gradebooks. Examples of more sophisticated products for various aspects of testing such as item banking and item analysis are offered (http://www.assess.com/) by companies such as Assessment Systems Corporation (n.d.). More comprehensive packages provide complete testing systems, some of which are appropriate for online testing. As complexity and capability increase, cost also rises and can be considerable. In selecting software for use in computerized testing—whether test construction, administration, or scoring—the type of testing for which it is appropriate, fixed or adaptive, is an important consideration. Particular care must be exercised in selecting software for aspects of the measurement process, such as item analysis, that are consistent with the parameters included in the model for computer adaptive testing.

Fixed Computer Testing

The original form of computerized testing, as well as the most frequently used form today, is the fixed form. The term "fixed" reflects the static nature of presentation of measures in test administration. In the earliest forms of fixed computer testing, and often in early stages of using an instrument, existing paper-and-pencil measures are formatted for presentation to the respondent on the computer. Current usage of the term fixed computer testing implies that the test/measure is uniformly presented to each respondent. The test is presented to each respondent in exactly the same way, i.e., with the same items, the same number of items, and the same order. Thus, each respondent has a uniform testing/response experience. A lay example of fixed computer testing used in many states in the United States is the examination for a driver's license. Fixed computer testing may serve as an alternate method of administration for a paper-and-pencil examination such as the newly initiated, computer-based certification examinations for family nurse practitioner and adult nurse practitioner candidates offered by the American Academy of Nurse Practitioners (2003).

Since this static presentation has potential for breaches in test security or, in the case of other measures, response set or other types of measurement error, some software allows for use of the domain-sampling model. This process allows for sampling of a fixed number of items with equal characteristics (e.g., difficulty level) from a larger pool of items. Each respondent receives an alternate form of the test/measure with a different group of questions presented in a different order, thereby limiting exposure to any set of items and responses.

Computer Adaptive Testing

Building on the premise that the ideal form of testing uses items at precisely the right difficulty level for the individual respondent (Lord, 1980), computer adaptive testing (CAT) utilizes the ever-increasing capability of the computer to administer automated testing that is tailored to the individual. CAT is sometimes referred to as individualized, response-contingent, branched, sequential item testing, or programmed testing (Halkitis & Leahy, 1993).

Most (Nunnally & Bernstein, 1994) CAT draws on item-response theory (IRT) that is overviewed in chapter 3. IRT theory centers on the item as it considers observed performance of the respondent on an item and item difficulty. (McHorney, 1997). Assumptions of IRT include: (1) the ability or attribute being assessed by CAT is unidimensional; (2) responses to items are independent of each other; and (3) correctly guessing a response is not possible.

Basic components of CAT include an IRT model, a large item pool, an established starting point at which the first item is presented to the respondent, specification of how items will be selected for presentation to the respondent, and a scoring schema. In addition, a set of "end rules" must be created by which it can be determined that the computer has obtained sufficient information from a respondent to meet the designated performance criteria and, thus, to end the testing period. (Halkitis & Leahy, 1993)

The IRT model selected for CAT can contain one or more parameters considering the item and the respondent; these models can be visualized in item characteristic curves (ICC) representing the underlying mathematical equations as described in chapter 3. While other models exist (e.g., the graded response, partial credit models, and the rating scale model), the most commonly used models are: (1) the single-parameter (Rasch) model which addresses item difficulty; (2) the two-parameter model which adds item discrimination; and (3) the three-parameter model which adds the chance of correctly guessing a response to an item (Hays, Morales, & Reise, 2000).

A large item pool, typically numbering several hundred items depending on the nature and purpose of the CAT, is required. This pool must be adequate to allow for calibration and selection of items according to the model selected. Items must be subjected to extensive preliminary testing in a norming procedure, as well as to estimate parameters such as difficulty level and/or ability to discriminate among various levels of performance or amount of the attribute being considered.

In CAT, items are presented to the respondent one at a time. The starting point in CAT, or first item presented to a respondent, is typically of moderate difficulty. Upon response, each item is scored and the next item is selected for presentation adapting to the level of the individual's previous response. Each question presented must be answered to allow the respondent to continue through the test. Generally, correct responses initiate the subsequent presentation of a more difficult item, while incorrect responses initiate an item that is easier than the previous item. This process continues until a preset performance criterion is reached. End rules can include factors such as a minimum and maximum number of items to be presented to the respondent, the amount of time that has passed, and/or that a specified level of precision has been reached in estimating performance of the respondent (Halkitis & Leahy, 1993).

This process means that number and sequence of items presented in CAT is individually tailored, or adapted, to responses. The sequence of items is not fixed. Individual respondents may be exposed to a different selection and number of items. Depending on respondent performance to each item, CAT has the potential to be an alternative to the longer assessments of fixed tests where all respondents respond to the same number of questions regardless of their performance level. Scores are based on which, not how many, test questions are answered correctly. (Tonidandel, Quinones, & Adams, 2002). CAT offers a very different paradigm than that of fixed testing or other types of measures built on classical measurement theory, where each test is its own yardstick and reliability and validity are not generalizable across populations, applications, or testing situations. In CAT, the large item pool places item scores on a common metric. (McHorney, 1997)

CAT has two major purposes: (1) to estimate ability; or (2) to classify respondents as to whether they meet prespecified criteria. Along with content from various areas of the test/instrument, these purposes are key in the process by which the computer selects items for presentation to respondents. In the first case, to estimate ability by ranking level of proficiency, the first item presented to the respondent is of moderate item difficulty. If answered correctly, the computer next selects a more difficult item. If answered incorrectly, the computer next selects a less difficult item. This process is iterative, allowing for ongoing evaluation of responses to items by the computer (which determines which items are presented to the respondent) until sufficient information is obtained to ascertain the ability of the respondent, at which point the test ends. (Ruiz, Fitz, Lewis, & Reidy, 1995) A widely used example of CAT to estimate ability is the Graduate Record Examination (Educational Testing Service, 2003).

When the purpose is to classify the respondent, e.g., "pass" (ready to practice) or "fail" (not ready to practice), according to predetermined criteria, the items in the pool from which the computer selects have evidence of being good discriminators between respondents in different categories. In this case, the set of items presented to an individual respondent is of comparable difficulty to that of other respondents (Ruiz, Fitz, Lewis, & Reidy, 1995). Examples of CAT to classify respondents include the National Council Licensure Examination (NCLEX), administered since 1993 to nursing school graduates (Halkitis & Leahy, 1993; Jones-Dickson, Dorsey, Campbell-Warnock, & Fields, 1993), to determine eligibility for licensure, and certification examinations by specialty groups such as the Council on Certification of Nurse Anesthetists (Bergstrom, 1996).

In describing how CAT works, the National Council of State Boards of Nursing (http://www.ncsbn.org/public/testing/info_cat.htm) likens the process to administration of an oral exam by an educator in that responses to each question suggest what the content and number of subsequent questions will be. There are approximately 1500 items with known item difficulty ranging from easiest to hardest in the NCLEX item pool. Each respondent is presented with a minimum of 15 "tryout" items which do not count in their score. These are practice items that are tracked to determine difficulty level across administrations of the test and may eventually be added to the item pool. The minimum number of items presented on the NCLEX is 75 and the maximum number is 265. The goal is to administer test items covering the test plan content to the point where respondents are getting about 50% correct, which reflects ability level; passing candidates answer 50% or more of the difficult questions correctly while failing candidates answer about 50% of easier questions correctly. There are three aspects to the stop rule: (1) the ability level is within the 95% confidence interval of either meeting or not meeting the passing standard; (2) the respondent has been presented with the maximum number of items allowed; or (3) the respondent has run out of time to complete the test (a maximum of 5 hours is allowed). This ability level is then compared with the passing standard to determine the outcome of the test. The passing standard is periodically adjusted to reflect level of ability for competent practice by entry-level licensed registered nurses.

Respondent skills needed for CAT are different from those needed in paper-and-pencil testing, or in fixed-format computerized testing. For example, in preparing nursing students for the NCLEX, faculty may wish to facilitate this transition by moving away from sequencing of a set of related items to a more independent-item format. Practice with computer-based testing is also facilitative (Halkitis & Leahy, 1993). Computer skills needed by CAT respondents are typically minimal such as being able to use the tab key, the space bar, and the enter key. In the NCLEX examination, respondents are offered a tutorial in how to navigate the examination format with minimal computer skills.

BENEFITS AND CHALLENGES IN USING CAT

The two benefits of CAT cited most frequently are greater efficiency (Weiss, 1985) and greater precision in measurement with a personalized test (Ruiz, Fitz, Lewis, & Reidy, 1995). While CAT is most feasible with large numbers of respondents, there is evidence of its potential utility in individualized testing in classroom and clinical settings. Using data from 621 medical students, Kreiter, Ferguson, and Gruppen (1999) demonstrated how item banks could be used to transition to CAT for in-course assessment. With a 200-item bank, they found that the precision of measurement was comparable to a paper-and-pencil fixed test with approximately half the number of items on the traditional test. They note the size of their item bank should be extended and that there was a clear need for adding items with higher difficulty levels. However, since in-course content is not static with continuing revisions and addition of new knowledge, there is some doubt that CAT will replace traditional testing in the classroom (Nunnally & Bernstein, 1994).

Benefits of CAT cited for the NCLEX test include the economy of items that are not appropriate for the respondent—i.e., in NCLEX the number of easy items presented to respondents with high ability is limited. Further, guessing is minimized by limiting the number of challenging items presented to respondents with low ability (National Council of State Boards of Nursing, n.d.).

A number of potential advantages of using IRT are cited by Hays, Morales, and Reise (2000), who suggest that in the future self-reported health outcomes could possibly be measured using CAT. These advantages include the ability to: (1) obtain more comprehensive and accurate evaluation of item characteristics; (2) assess group differences in item and scale functioning; (3) evaluate scales containing items with different response formats; (4) improve existing measures; (5) model change; and (6) evaluate person fit. They also note the biggest practical problem in applying IRT, and possibly CAT, lies in the available software products that are complex and challenging to learn, as well as use. Additionally, these factors contribute to the generally high cost of such software.

An advocate for the future use of CAT in measuring health outcomes is McHorney (1997). She points to the economic benefits of not having to administer, score, and analyze health questionnaires, the potential for presenting respondents with items at their ability level rather than boring or frustrating them with items below or above their level, and, in particular, the capability for immediate feedback on scores.

Ware, Bjorner, and Kosinski (2000) generally endorse the use of CAT as a way to facilitate comparison of results across individual assessments, as well as across diverse populations. A further goal is to make more practical health assessment measures accessible, as well as to increase the ability to identify those people whose health status indicates that they might benefit from treatment. This group reports in detail an example of patients with headaches giving attention to IRT model selection, item pool calibration, empirical validity, and norm-based scoring. Their results reflect the significant time savings resulting from use of CAT and support their call for more practical applications of IRT and CAT, and greater simplicity of software required in their use.

In a laboratory study comparing different rating techniques, 112 raters used both a CAT rating as well as two traditionally formatted rating instruments to evaluate the performance of six office workers in videotaped simulations. Results showed that the precision of the CAT rating was superior to the other methods and was accomplished with a smaller number of items than on the traditionally formatted instruments. Participants perceived the CAT rating to be acceptable, more accurate, and better able to differentiate between levels of performance than other formats. On the other hand, participants also found CAT to be somewhat harder to understand (Borman et al., 2001).

Two other reports, both using computer simulation, point to the potential for use of CAT in clinical applications. Gardner, Kelleher, and Pajer (2002) found that a CAT simulation required an average of five fewer questions than a fixed computerized version of a standard measure used with parents as respondents to screen for mental health problems in children. Dijkers (2003) found that a CAT simulation was significantly more time efficient than the traditional mode of assessment of patients with spinal cord injury using a widely used measure of functional status, the Functional Independence Measure (FIM). Further, results of the CAT simulation closely approximated the results from traditional assessment. Both of these studies had very large numbers of respondents at 21,150 (Gardner, Kelleher, & Pajer, 2002) and 5969 (Dijkers, 2003) and offer a demonstration of the economy of secondary analyses and the use of computer simulation in selected studies of aspects of the measurement process.

There are other factors related to IRT that are identified as potential limiting factors in its use for CAT. Among these factors, related to measurement of generic health outcomes, are: (1) many generic concepts are not unidimensional; (2) the ordered continuum of IRT items is very different from the more traditional, Likert-type response format; (3) time and complexity are factors in test development; (4) a large number of respondents is required for modeling of the test; (5) a large item pool is required; and (6) the resulting tests created would be generic since each would be individualized to the respondent (as opposed to the more proprietary approach common today) (McHorney, 1997). Extensive resource commitment is needed to support the development of CAT. Nunnally and Bernstein (1994) note that clear advantages to classical testing methods, which are robust, remain.

SUMMARY

Computer-based testing is a rapidly developing area of measurement. The information offered here about major types of computer-based testing is essential to understanding the rapid advances that are taking place. A comparison of selected aspects of fixed and adaptive testing is provided in Table 23.1.

REFERENCES

American Academy of Nurse Practitioners, (2003). Computer based testing initiated. *American Academy of Nurse Practitioners Certification Program NewsBriefs*. Retrieved July 20, 2003, from http://aanp.org/NR/rdonlyres/erecuu5rbrffb5mph6llsfwmory53m

TABLE 23.1   Comparison of Selected Characteristics of Computer-Based Tests/Measures

Characteristics	Fixed	Adaptive
Presentation	Same for each respondent	Tailored to responses of each individual
Number of Items	Preestablished and same for each respondent	Varies depending on responses of each individual; Maximum and minimum number predetermined
Items	Same for each respondent; Selected by test developer	Varies—selected by computer
Item Selection	Prior to test administration	Ongoing during test administration
Order of Items	Same for each respondent	Varies—selected by computer
Evaluation of Respondent Performance/Scoring	At conclusion of test	After each item and at conclusion of test
Respondent Mobility Within Test/Measure	Total—can respond in any order	Must respond to each item to move on to next item

c4z6aoaw3u7umrv57o2g2qqwwozj52csniddv 4khba5tkzsbtbn5kqc5ubq3g/Final+Certification+Newsletter+2003.pdf.

Assessment Systems Corporation (n.d.). Retrieved July 30, 2003, from http://www.assess.com/

Bergstrom, B. (1996). Computerized adaptive testing for the national certification examination. *Journal of the American Association of Nurse Anesthetists, 64*(2), 119–124.

Borman, W., Buck, D., Hanson, M., Motowidlo, S., Stark, S., & Drasgow, F. (2001). An examination of the comparative reliability, validity, and accuracy of performance ratings made using computerized adaptive rating scales. *Journal of Applied Psychology, 86*(5), 965–973.

Dijkers, M. P. (2003). A computer adaptive testing simulation applied to the FIM instrument motor component. *Archives of Physical Medicine and Rehabilitation, 84*(5), 384–393.

DxR Development. (2001). *DxR Clinician.* Retrieved July 30, 2003, from http://www.dxrclinician.com/

Educational Testing Service. (2003). *Graduate Record Examination 2003–2004: Guide to the use of scores.* Retrieved July 30, 2003, from ftp://ftp.ets.org/pub/gre/994994.pdf

Gardner, W., Kelleher, K., & Pajer, K. (2002). Multidimensional adaptive testing for mental health problems in primary care. *Medical Care, 40*(9), 812–823.

Halkitis, P., & Leahy, J. (1993). Computerized adaptive testing: The future is upon us. *Nursing & Health Care, 14*(7), 378–385.

Hays, R., Morales, L., & Reise, S. (2000). Item response theory and health outcomes measurement in the 21st century. *Medical Care, 38*(9), II28–II42.

JCG Software. (n.d.). *Test Construction Kit.* Retrieved July 30, 2003, from http://www.shareup.net/Home-Education/Teaching-Tools/Test-Construction-Kit-review-6354.html

Jones-Dickson, C., Dorsey, D., Campbell-Warnock, J., & Fields, F. (1993). Moving in a new direction: Computerized adaptive testing (CAT). *Nursing Management, 24*(1), 80, 82.

Kreiter, C., Ferguson, K., & Gruppen, L. (1999). Evaluating the usefulness of computerized adaptive testing for medical in-course assessment. *Academic Medicine, 74*(10), 1125–1127.

Lord, F. M. (1980). *Applications of item response theory to practical testing problems.* Hillsdale, NJ: Lawrence Erlbaum Associates.

McHorney, C. (1997). Generic health measurement: Past accomplishments and a measurement paradigm for the 21st century. *Annals of Internal Medicine, 127*(8), 743–750.

National Council of State Boards of Nursing. (n.d.). *Computerized Adaptive Testing.* Retrieved July 30, 2003, from http://www.ncsbn.org/public/testing/info_cat.htm

Nunnally, J. C., & Bernstein, I. H. (1994). *Psychometric theory* (3rd ed.). McGraw Hill.

Ruiz, B., Fitz, P., Lewis, C., & Reidy, C. (1995). Computer-adaptive testing: A new breed of assessment. *Journal of the American Dietetic Association, 95*(11), 1326–1327.

Tonidandel, S., Quinones, M., & Adams, A. (2002). Computer-adaptive testing: The impact of test characteristics on perceived performance and test takers' reactions. *Journal of Applied Psychology, 87*(2), 320–332.

Ware, J., Bjorner, J., & Kosinski, M. (2000). Practical implications of item response theory and computerized adaptive testing. *Medical Care, 38*(9), II73–II82.

Weiss, D. J. (1985). Adaptive testing by computer. *Journal of Consulting and Clinical Psychology, 53*(6), 774–789.

Part IV

Special Issues

24

Ethical Issues

The nursing profession has taken very seriously the importance of ethical considerations in research and practice. Standards, codes, and guidelines designed to assure ethical practice and protection of patients and research subjects have been established and updated by professional and specialty organizations. Examples include the American Nurses' Association's Code of Ethics with Interpretive Statements (2001), the ANA Position Statement on Ethics and Human Rights (1991), and the American Association of Critical Care Nurses' (2002) statement on ethics in critical care research. Despite the existence of such guidelines and increased attention in the literature, complex ethical issues in measurement remain, in part due to rapid changes in the health care environment and technology, such as increased use of the Internet for primary data collection in research (e.g., Im & Chee, 2002) and the implementation of privacy protections mandated by the Health Insurance Portability and Accountability Act (HIPAA), specifically the Privacy Rule issued by the Department of Health and Human Services in 2002 and implemented April 14, 2003 (see Title 45 Code of Federal Regulations, parts 160 and 164, which may be obtained and guidance provided at the HHS Office for Civil Rights Web site at http://www. hhs.giv/ocu/hipaa).

The purpose of this section is to call attention to some of these issues, recognizing that there are no simple solutions. While an exhaustive discussion is beyond the scope of this book, responsibilities of the nurse to clients or subjects, to colleagues, and to the scientific and professional community will be highlighted. Readers desiring a more detailed treatment of ethical dimensions of measurement and research should consult comprehensive sources such as Levine (1986), Beauchamp and Childress (2001), and Beauchamp and Walters (2003).

ETHICAL ISSUES RELATED TO MEASUREMENT OF HUMAN SUBJECTS

Most of the ethical issues regarding measurement of human subjects have been addressed in connection with biomedical and social research. Following World War II and the Nuremberg trials, which called attention to abuses in human experimentation, there has been ongoing activity to assure ethical and humane treatment of human and animal subjects in research. Guidelines are provided in such well-known documents as the Nuremberg Code of 1947 and the 1964 Declaration of Helsinki; in the codes of professional organizations such as the American Nurses' Association, American Medical Association, American Dental Association, American Psychological Association, American Sociological Association, American Hospital Association, American Political Science Association, American Anthropological Association, and American Personnel and Guidance Association (for information about these guidelines and reprints of some of the codes see Beauchamp and Walters, 2003, and Levine, 1986); and in published requirements for research funded by the U.S. Department of Health and Human Services (2001b) (see Title 45 Code of Federal Regulations, Part 46, available at http://ohrp.osophs. dhhs.gov/humansubjects/guidance/45cfr46.ht). The guidelines address multiple aspects of research, and hence include, but are broader in scope than, the measurement considerations that represent the focus of the following discussion. They should be consulted and followed by any nurse proposing to engage in research involving human subjects.

Three basic, comprehensive ethical principles provide the foundation for the guidelines, recommendations, and standards that have been designed to provide for the rights and well-being of human subjects in measurement and research: respect for persons, beneficence, and justice (National Commission for the Protection of Human Subjects of Biomedical and Behavioral Research, 1978). The principle of respect for persons includes the conviction that all persons should have autonomy or self-determination, and that those whose autonomy is reduced because of age, illness, or incapacity are entitled to protection. This principle is particularly important for underpinning subjects' rights to informed consent. The principle of beneficence refers not only to the duty not to harm others (nonmaleficence) but also to the duty to maximize potential benefits and minimize possible risks associated with the research or measurement procedure. It provides important underpinnings for subjects' rights to protection from harm and for analyzing the ratio of potential risks to benefits. The principle of justice refers to the obligation to treat individuals equally and fairly; it underpins selection of research subjects and research designs.

In accordance with these basic ethical principles, researchers are obliged to recognize and protect the basic rights of subjects in measurement activities. Important ethical dimensions of measurement activities include informed consent, refusal to participate or withdrawal without recrimination, privacy, confidentiality, anonymity, and protection from harm. Measurement-related issues and responsibilities for each of these areas will be addressed.

Informed Consent

Informed consent applies to many types of patient-professional interaction. It can be said to occur if a patient or research subject who has substantial understanding of what he or she is being asked to do, and is not being controlled or coerced to do so by others intentionally,

authorizes a professional to do something (Beauchamp & Childress, 2001). Essential elements of informed consent are (1) competence of the subject to consent (a precondition), (2) disclosure of information, (3) the subjects understanding of the information being disclosed, (4) volition or choice in the consent, and (5) authorization of consent. While the professional's provision of information is important, equal emphasis is placed on the ability of the subject to understand and consent (Beauchamp & Childress, 2001). To try to assure the subject's self-determination, that is, to protect autonomous choice, the subject must be competent to comprehend information and make decisions, be fully informed of and comprehend what is involved, and agree freely to participate before measurement can be carried out.

As detailed in the DHHS policy on human subjects research (U.S. Department of Health and Human Services, 2001b) the information provided to the potential subject includes:

(1) a statement that the study involves research, an explanation of the purposes of the research and the expected duration of the subject's participation, a description of the procedures to be followed, and identification of any procedures which are experimental; (2) a description of any reasonably foreseeable risks or discomforts to the subject; (3) a description of any benefits to the subject or to others which may reasonably be expected from the research; (4) a disclosure of appropriate alternative procedures or courses of treatment, if any, that might be advantageous to the subject; (5) a statement describing the extent, if any, to which confidentiality of records identifying the subject will be maintained; (6) for research involving more than minimal risk, an explanation as to whether any compensation and an explanation as to whether any medical treatments are available if injury occurs and, if so, what they consist of, or where further information may be obtained; (7) an explanation of whom to contact for answers to pertinent questions about the research and research subjects' rights, and whom to contact in the event of a research-related injury to the subject; and (8) a statement that participation is voluntary, refusal to participate will involve no penalty or loss of benefits to which the subject is otherwise entitled, and the subject may

discontinue participation at any time without penalty or loss of benefits to which the subject is otherwise entitled (45 CFR 46.116a).

It should be underscored that the provision of information does not necessarily ensure comprehension by potential subjects. Comprehension can be heightened by carefully wording the information provided, gearing the information to the subject's reading and comprehension level, encouraging potential subjects to ask questions, and asking subjects to voice their understanding and interpretation of what will be required before consent can be assumed to be secured. Im and Chee (2002) point out that research subjects in Internet studies may actually have more opportunity to ask questions and self-determine their participation than those in more traditional quantitative approaches to measurement, such as surveys.

Although the obligation to assure informed consent has been universally accepted, it raises a number of issues. One example of a hotly debated topic is how much information to disclose. Several attempts have been made to establish standards of disclosure. However, the various standards (e.g., professional, reasonable person, and subjective standards) have problems associated with them (see Beauchamp & Childress, 2001). The combined standard is to disclose whatever information a reasonable person placed in the subject's position would need to know in order to make an autonomous decision, but to make modifications based on an assessment of the unique needs and desires of the individual subject.

These standards, while helpful, do not resolve the problem that providing information to potential subjects about the measurement activity may serve to alter the outcomes of the measurement. For example, if a subject is aware in advance that his or her behavior will be observed for a given purpose, he or she may not display usual behavior, but modify actions during the observation period. Proposed solutions to the problems are themselves laden with issues. One suggestion is to provide the required explanation in a debriefing session immediately after data are gathered; however, ex post facto information does not really provide for informed consent and subjects can become embarrassed

and angry. Another suggestion is to provide only general information to subjects initially, eliminating detailed explanations until after measurement is complete. While some reactivity to measures may be eliminated in this way, the information provided before measurement should be sufficient to provide a basis for decision making, and the elements of voluntary participation and free withdrawal should be stressed. Deception and coercion must be avoided. In the research context, the Institutional Review Board that is charged with assuring that the rights of human research subjects are protected may be willing to approve a consent procedure that does not contain all of the above elements of informed consent, provided that "(1) the research involves no more than minimal risk to the subjects; (2) the waiver or alteration will not adversely affect the rights and welfare of the subjects; (3) the research could not practicably be carried out without the waiver or alteration; and (4) whenever appropriate, the subjects will be provided with additional pertinent information after participation" (U.S. Department of Health and Human Services, 2001b, Section 46.116d).

Another difficult issue surrounding informed consent is ensuring the rights of individuals who have limited ability to comprehend or who are unable to do so because they are ill, incapacitated, naive, frightened, or lack facility with language or familiarity with terminology. Informed consent clearly depends on effective communication that takes into account varying abilities of individuals to comprehend and process information, as well as their experiential background and culture. It is also important to avoid information overload, and to allow time for subjects to make their decisions.

Nurses attempting to secure informed consent for measurement and research may often encounter subjects whose ability to comprehend is limited. Examples include children, the mentally retarded, the mentally ill, the critically ill, and the unconscious patient. Although consent has generally been secured from a surrogate (e.g., a relative or guardian), a number of questions have been raised regarding these populations that need vigilant protection. Specific guidelines have been established for children

(U.S. Department of Health and Human Services, 2001b, Sections 46.401–409). Parents or guardians must be informed of the implications of participation, and a signed consent must be secured. If possible, the child's assent should be secured as well, particularly if the child is over the age of assent, which Federal guidelines suggest to be 7 years of age. The child's maturity and psychological state should be taken into account, and the child provided a simplified consent form. Adolescents between 13 years of age and the state-defined legal age should sign a regular adult consent form, but must have it countersigned by a parent.

In the case of adults who are unable to give informed consent because of illness or incapacity, the situation is complex. The American Association of Critical Care Nurses (2002) recommends that proxy consent can be considered when benefit clearly outweighs risk. According to Woods (1988) the surrogate should be someone who understands "the potential patient's values, beliefs, and preferences well enough to accurately substitute his or her own judgment for the patient's" (p. 91), and should act in the best interest of the patient. Individuals able to give consent include legal guardians, a designated health surrogate, or legal next of kin (American Association of Critical Care Nurses, 2002). Permission to conduct measurement activities with these potentially vulnerable subjects should never be assumed simply because the relative or guardian does not raise specific objections.

Individuals who are members of captive audiences are at risk of having their right to informed consent compromised because the element of self-determination may be in question. The examples most frequently encountered in nursing are hospitalized patients, students, and employees. The ultimate example, of course, is prisoners, for whom special provision is made in Federal guidelines (see U.S. Department of Health and Human Services, 2001b, 45 CFR 46.301-306). The major problem is that these individuals may perceive pressure to comply with requests to participate in measurement activities or research and may acquiesce even though they do not really wish to do so. The perceived pressure may be due to status and power differentials between potential subject and the investigator, the promise of rewards, or concern that failure to participate will jeopardize the subject's condition or position. Whether such captive subjects should even be asked to participate and whether, even if they are told that a genuine choice exists, they will perceive participation to be completely voluntary presents a dilemma. Some IRBs require that researchers request employees who are being asked to participate as subjects in research being carried out at their institution complete an additional form as part of the consent procedure.

In the measurement contexts other than research, there may be instances in which the individual may accurately perceive limited freedom of choice regarding measurement activities. For example, once having signed a general consent form, the hospitalized patient is often assumed to be willing to acquiesce to a considerable number of measurement activities, including invasive laboratory procedures, only the most potentially dangerous of which usually require special consent assurance. The American Hospital Association's Patient's Bill of Rights (1992) indicates that the patient has the right to receive information necessary to give informed consent before the start of any procedure or treatment; however, the extent to which such information is actually communicated for relatively routine procedures is questionable. There have been many instances in the past when patient information in hospital records has been used for research purposes without the patient's knowledge or consent. This practice has been severely curtailed by provisions of the HIPAA Privacy Act discussed below.

The student who has voluntarily enrolled in an educational program is the recipient of many measurement activities undertaken to evaluate attainment of competencies and content mastery, as well as evaluation of the educational program. Such activities are a routine part of the educational environment, and failure to participate may have negative consequences for the student. In the research, clinical, and program evaluation contexts, it is essential to provide a genuine choice, to provide as complete information as possible, and to avoid applying subtle pressures to which captive subjects are susceptible. In the educational and administrative contexts, at the very least, potential subjects should be informed before entering the situation (i.e., before enrolling in an educational program or taking a position) about the measurement-related expectations and the consequences of nonparticipation.

Refusal or Withdrawal

A generally accepted ethical position is that research subjects should be free to refuse to participate or withdraw from participation without recrimination or prejudice. The ability to refuse or withdraw is necessary to ensure that consent to participate in a measurement activity is given voluntarily. As noted previously, potential research subjects should be informed of this right at the time their informed consent is solicited, and subtle pressures to participate should be avoided. Special attention is required to ensure that no negative consequences stem from refusal or withdrawal from research-related measurement activities. This includes actions to prevent negative attitudes directed toward the subject. In the clinical, educational, and administrative contexts, the individual has a right to refuse or withdraw from measurement activities; however, there may be negative consequences to this action. The individual should be informed of the consequences before the decision is made whether to participate.

Privacy

The principle of privacy, which is related to the principles of respect for persons and beneficence/nonmaleficence, also has many implications for measurement. Although defined in a variety of ways, the right to privacy asserts essentially that an individual should be able to decide how much of himself or herself (including thoughts, emotions, attitudes, physical presence, and personal facts) to share with others. Measurement activities are designed to yield information about individuals or groups and usually involve at least some intrusion into an individual's life and activities. They are therefore in potential violation of this basic right unless care is taken. It is also important is to assure that the information shared or revealed by the individual is not used in a way that will cause harm.

Three major points regarding privacy should be borne in mind. First, individuals and cultural groups differ in the extent to which they are willing to divulge specific kinds of information, to whom, and under what conditions. For example, a client may be willing to reveal information about sexual behavior to a nurse or physician in a one-on-one interview in a therapeutic context, but unwilling to answer the same questions on a survey research questionnaire or in a group setting. Some sensitive or potentially damaging topics such as drug use, alcohol use, sexual behavior, or family relationships might be willingly discussed by some individuals, but not by others, for a variety of reasons which cannot always be anticipated. Given the social, cultural, and situational relativity with which privacy is defined, it is necessary that every effort be made to understand the social and cultural values of potential subjects and that no prior assumptions be made that a given measurement activity, even a particular question or item on an instrument, will be universally acceptable. Rather, each subject has a right to know in advance what information is to be gathered and how it will be used. In addition, the subject should be able to negotiate in advance which audiences have a right to know the information. Subjects must have the right to refuse to answer any questions or otherwise reveal information that they deem private.

Second, the nurse, by virtue of being an accepted and generally trusted health care provider, often receives information from and about clients that they would not ordinarily reveal to a nonprofessional. The nurse's unique status in relation to clients should be recognized and care be taken that it not be used to the client's disadvantage. Any intent to share the information with others should be explicitly revealed to the client in advance and permission received. Information gathered in a care-giving context should not be used for other purposes (e.g., research) without the client's permission. The HIPAA privacy rules discussed below are very explicit about the care that must be taken to assure the privacy of individuals' health information.

Third, measurement procedures differ in the extent to which they are likely to compromise the subject's privacy. The most serious questions have been raised about those procedures that allow measurement without the subject's knowledge or active involvement (e.g., unobtrusive measures, observation, content analysis of records, or covert tape recordings) and those that may encourage the subject to reveal more information than intended (e.g., in-depth interviews and psychological tests). The former are problematic in that they invalidate the subject's right to decide what to reveal. The latter pose problems, because they remove some of the subject's ability to control the content revealed. Coercion (overt and subtle) and deceit should be avoided. Further, data should be handled, interpreted, and shared carefully, with attention to potential privacy violations. In longitudinal research involving repeated measures, privacy is especially difficult to maintain. Particularly in situations in which the subject may inadvertently reveal more than intended or in which the information gathered might have negative consequences (e.g., cause others to alter their opinion of the subject), it is advisable to check with the individual before sharing any information with others. The section of this book concerning collection of sensitive data from subjects also addresses some ethical dimensions and suggested techniques related to the issue of privacy.

HIPAA's Implications for Measurement and Research

The Health Insurance Portability and Accountability Act (HIPAA) privacy regulations took effect on April 14, 2003. These provisions, which require health care organizations and providers to protect the privacy of patient information, underscore the importance of privacy in the measurement context, and constrain the communication and use of individual patient health information in both practice and research. In essence, they extend and supplement the *Common Rule,* the set of standards for federal agencies that fund research involving human subjects. The Common Rule standards regarding ethical conduct of research are monitored and enforced by institutional review boards. The

HIPAA privacy rules do not replace these Common Rule standards, but supplement them. A brief overview of the privacy provisions of HIPAA, particularly as they pertain to research, is included here. For more detailed information, the reader is referred to the Department of Health and Human Services, Office for Civil Rights-HIPAA Web site; it addresses the national standards to protect the privacy of personal health information and can be found at (http://www.hhs.gov/ocr/hipaa/privacy.html). A discussion of the implications of the HIPAA Privacy Rule for institutional review boards can be found in NIH publication Number 03-5428 (National Institutes of Health, 2003). Other helpful resources for the nurse researcher and clinician include Frank-Stromborg (2003), Olsen (2003), Connor, Smaldone, Bratts, and Stone (2003), and Woods and Stockton (2002) for the American Council on Education. One of the very important consequences of HIPAA for measurement and research is that it has greatly heightened awareness of the importance of patient privacy, and the ease with which privacy can be violated.

Although HIPAA was directed primarily toward insurers, health care clearinghouses, and health care providers who transmit any health information in electronic form (they are termed *covered entities*), it does have important implications for much nursing research. Researchers are not necessarily covered entities unless they also provide care and transmit health information electronically for insurance claims; however, if researchers are employees of a hospital, health insurer, or other covered entity, they probably will have to comply with that entity's HIPAA privacy policies. In many cases, schools of nursing are required to comply with the HIPAA privacy policies of the covered entity institutions with which they have clinical affiliations. A researcher may also be impacted by HIPAA if he or she uses data provided by a covered entity. The law applies to *protected health information* (PHI), which is a subset of *individually identifiable health information* (IIHI). IIHI is any information about an individual's physical or mental health, the health care provided to him/her, and that which identifies the individual (Olsen, 2003). "With certain exceptions, *individually identifiable health infor-*

mation becomes PHI when it is created or received by a covered entity" (National Institutes of Health, 2003, p. 1).

HIPAA privacy regulations impact nursing research when researchers must access data from a covered entity (e.g., from the patient's medical record), when the researcher creates individually identifiable health information in the course of the study (e.g., in a clinical trial or other intervention research), and when disclosing data (e.g., when sharing data with another researcher). Access to IIHI is monitored by the covered entity and is subject to HIPAA guidelines (unless explicitly excluded). For example, HIPAA pertains only to information gathered about living persons, and does not apply to information that has been deidentified. Deidentification is the process by which all identifiers have been removed, including names, addresses, dates (birth date, admission date, etc.), telephone numbers, e-mail addresses, social security numbers, patient ID numbers, photographic images, etc. (See U.S. Department of Health and Human Services, 2001a, and Olsen, 2003). Access to IIHI is permissible if the data set is limited and the researcher has a data use agreement with the covered entity.

According to Woods and Stockton (2002), once implemented in 2003, the HIPAA privacy rules dictate that "a health care provider may only use or disclose protected health information (PHI) for treatment, payment, and health care operations purposes. For all other purposes, including clinical research, the health care provider must obtain a written authorization from the individual, unless an exception applies" (pp. 1–2). It is also possible for the researcher to obtain a waiver to authorization requirement from an IRB or privacy board.

In the event that the patient is being asked for an authorization to use PHI for research purposes, the authorization may be included as part of the informed consent or may be a separate document. The authorization must contain the following core elements: the description of the information to be used or disclosed, the name of the person or class of persons authorized to make the request for information use, the name of the person or class of persons to whom the covered entity may make the requested

use of information, a description of each purpose of the requested use, an expiration date that relates to the individual or the purpose for the use or disclosure, and the individual's signature and date. The authorization must include information about the individual's right to revoke it, and should not be a condition for receipt of treatment (Woods & Stockton, 2002). Many IRBs provide templates to investigators for authorization forms that include all necessary information.

Criteria for IRBs or privacy boards to waive the requirement of authorization are:

1. The use or disclosure of PHI involves no more than a minimal risk to the privacy of individuals, as demonstrated by a plan to protect the identifiers, a plan to destroy the identifiers (unless there is research or health justification), and adequate written assurances that the PHI will not be inappropriately reused or disclosed to any other person or entity unless legally required or as part of a HIPAA compliant disclosure.

2. The research could not practicably be conducted without the waiver.

3. The research could not practicably be conducted without the PHI.

When the measurement activity results in the creation of new health information data, the subject must authorize the use of the information. The subject must be given explicit information about the groups or individuals with whom the information might be shared, and permission secured. Researchers who are involved in multidisciplinary and multisite studies, and/or who may want to share the data with colleagues and students, must conform to HIPAA regulations. The researcher is also responsible for tracking any further disclosures of the data through waiver of authorization and for informing the patient of those disclosures. These regulations underscore the importance of maintaining contact information about research subjects in case later tracking is necessary.

Confidentiality-Anonymity

Closely related to the principle of privacy and included in the provisions of HIPAA, is the ethical assertion, reflected in the codes of professional associations, that the anonymity of subjects be preserved whenever possible and that information that would allow identification of the subject be held in confidence by the professional. This right not only protects the subject but also has the important measurement implication of increasing the likelihood that responses will be more truthful and complete (i.e., more valid) than if anonymity and confidentiality cannot be ensured. Complete anonymity of subjects is possible in a few types of measurement activities, such as mailed questionnaires; but even in such instances it may be impractical to promise complete anonymity, because follow-up of nonrespondents would be precluded. Generally the principle of anonymity has been operationalized in research by ensuring that subjects will not be identifiable in public reports by name or any other defining characteristics. As noted in the above discussion of HIPAA, deidentification of patient data is becoming more common to allow their use in research. In nonresearch contexts the right to anonymity may be difficult or impossible to ensure under certain conditions, such as when measurement data about a client are needed for assessment, diagnosis, and intervention, or instances in which data about a particular student or employee are used to evaluate performance. The degree to which anonymity can or cannot be ensured should be made clear to the subject prior to initiating the measurement. Promises of anonymity should never be given unless they can be guaranteed. The right to confidentiality means that the subject should have the right to assume that information yielded by measurement activities will not be made available to others without prior consent. The specific right-to-know audiences who will have access to the information should be specified to the subject. For example, measurement data recorded on a hospitalized patient's record are appropriately available only to those hospital personnel who must have access to the information to provide care and cannot be legitimately obtained by others without the patient's consent, the removal of identifying information, or waiver of authorization requirements.

In addition to highlighting responsibilities of the nurse regarding informed consent and care in the handling and reporting of data, the HIPAA privacy rules have clarified some of the difficult questions that previously surrounded implementation of the right to confidentiality. For example, the rules are explicit about the conditions under which data collected in research can be shared or used for other purposes (see Woods & Stockton, 2002; Connor, Smaldone, Bratts & Stone, 2003; Olsen, 2003). Additionally, the HIPAA privacy rules limit the PHI that may be disclosed to law enforcement officials (see Frank-Stromborg (2003) for a discussion of the practice implications of HIPAA).

Risks and Benefits, and Protection From Harm

The ethical principle of beneficence (and the related principle of nonmaleficence) asserts the obligation not to do harm, to maximize potential benefits, and to minimize potential harm resulting from the measurement or research. This principle is highly compatible with nursing's norms, since nursing as a profession is dedicated to enhancing the health and well-being of human beings. It may seem self-evident that professional ethics underscore the importance of preventing or minimizing potential risks to subjects, regardless of the context for measurement. However, it is necessary to realize that all measurement activities involve possible risks and benefits which, although they may not be fully known in advance, must be anticipated and evaluated before deciding how to design a measurement tool or device and whether to initiate the measurement activity. Researchers who conduct clinical trials of medications, devices, procedures, and intervention protocols must give serious consideration to assessing the associated benefits and risks, some of which may be life-threatening.

Before proceeding with the discussion of weighing risks and benefits in measurement, it is necessary to define some frequently used terms. In the Belmont Report (National Commission for the Protection of Human Subjects of Biomedical and Behavioral Research, 1978), risk is defined as "the possibility that harm may occur" and benefit is "something of positive value related to health or welfare" (p. 15). Benefits are conceptualized to accrue to individuals (e.g., subjects) and to society as a whole. The risk-benefit ratio expresses the relation of all anticipated risks and human costs to all known and anticipated benefits. It is based on a risk and benefit assessment procedure which is described later in this chapter. Minimal risk is defined as the degree of risk that is normally encountered in everyday life or in routine medical or psychological examination and treatment. When the risks of a given research or measurement procedure are more than minimal or exceed potential benefits, the procedure is generally not justified. For a discussion of assessing benefits and risks in clinical trials see Spilker (1991).

Risk Associated With Measurement

In assessing risks associated with measurement, it is necessary to consider those that may result from the measurement procedure itself and those that may result from the way in which the results of measurement are used. The most readily apparent risks of measurement procedures are those that are associated with physical harm. The physiologic measures employed by nurses generally involve little danger to the subject, because they are minimally invasive. This does not preclude the possibility that seemingly routine and innocuous measures may involve possible risks, particularly with subjects who are very ill. For example, withdrawal of blood for a laboratory test may introduce infection or cause pain; repeated blood pressure monitoring may cause pain or vascular problems; or an improperly maintained or operated polygraph EKG recorder could result in an electric shock. While relatively unlikely and largely preventable, such risks are inherent in some nursing measurement activities and should be acknowledged and minimized.

Less obvious, but equally important, are psychological risks potentially associated with many of the measurement activities commonly employed in nursing. A measurement instrument or activity may inadvertently expose the subject to stress resulting from loss of self-esteem, generation of self-doubt, embarrassment, guilt, disturbing self-insights, fright, or concern about things of which the subject was previously unaware. For example, an instrument measuring parent-adolescent relations may include items that cause the parent to worry about aspects of the relationship or the adequacy of specific parenting behaviors; a measure that requests factual information or recall of specific events may embarrass a subject who is not able to respond; or psychological inventories may provide the subject with insight into aspects of personality or interpersonal relationships that alter previous self-perceptions and cause distress. While most measurement-related sources of psychological harm are inadvertent, potential measures and items should be assessed carefully in light of their capacity for exposing subjects and their families to psychological risk. In some types of measurement, social risk may be involved.

A related consideration that the nurse needs to assess honestly is the extent to which planned measurement activities will make demands on the subject's time and energy, or the patient burden that it involves. Given the importance of obtaining multiple measures of a given concept, it is easy to lose sight of the time that may be involved in a subject's completing several instruments. Demanding requirements may result in unwillingness to participate in measurement activities, or in withdrawal, fatigue, and anger, which may ultimately compromise reliability and validity. Measurement procedures should be designed to minimize disruption and should be feasible, realistic, and possible to carry out with reasonable effort. They should also not involve financial costs to subjects.

Some measurement procedures, such as measuring heart rate changes after exercise, impose energy requirements that may be risky to some clients. The amount of time and energy required to complete planned measurement activities and the condition and situation of the potential subject should be taken into account, recognizing that different types of measures impose different demands. For example, busy individuals such as employees and mothers of young children may be unable to participate in time-consuming measurement procedures such as in-depth interviews. Subjects who are ill or under stress are particularly vulnerable to fatigue and should not be expected to engage in lengthy sessions or physically demanding activities. Unrealistic or impractical demands on subjects should be avoided, even if it means sacrificing optimal measurement practices. Subjects should always be informed in advance of the time and energy requirements involved and their special needs taken into account in planning and scheduling measurement activities.

Individuals or groups may experience harm that results not from the measurement procedure itself, but from the way in which the results of measurement are interpreted and used. One of the most important social risks encountered by subjects is being labeled negatively as a result of measurement. A number of cognitive and personality measures, even some physiological measures, are designed to produce scores to which labels may be assigned (e.g., normal, abnormal, hypertensive, paranoid, obsessive-compulsive, gifted, neurotic, antisocial, other-directed). Some clearly have negative connotations. Whether or not the measurement results and labels are actually communicated to the subject, those that cast an individual or group in a negative light when communicated to others may have deleterious consequences.

Use of measurement information to label subjects is problematic, particularly given considerations of measurement error and bias inherent in instruments. Unless individual and cultural differences are expressly taken into account in procuring and interpreting measurement data, a given conclusion or label, whether negative or positive, can be unwarranted. Many frequently used instruments such as intelligence tests, attitude scales, personality inventories, and behavioral checklists are culturally biased and are inappropriate for some subpopulations, including those minority groups who are currently receiving considerable research attention because of health disparities. For example, instruments measuring mother-infant attachment frequently incorporate behavioral indicators that reflect American, White, middle-class behavioral patterns and have not been sufficiently well-tested to establish their validity with other cultural and socioeconomic populations. Even

some physiologic measures such as the Apgar measure of the health status of a newborn has questionable validity for non-Whites. Using unmodified tools and undifferentiated norms for potentially biased measures can result in inaccurate interpretation and erroneous, unjustified interpretations and labels. Full and frank disclosure of measurement information requires that the limitations of tools and procedures be made explicit to aid in interpretation.

In many instances measurement information is used as the basis for decisions that may profoundly influence a subject's life. Examples include admissions decisions in educational programs, employment decisions, and decisions about the desirability or efficacy of a particular nursing intervention. In such instances there is invariably some degree of risk to the subject because of the possibility of inaccurate interpretation. Although it cannot be eliminated completely, risk can be minimized through carefully scrutinizing reliability and validity of measures, using only defensible information sources and disclosing relevant information about their credibility, using multiple indicators, and interpreting scores in the light of measurement.

Risk-Benefit Ratio

Since it is impossible to remove all possibility of risk from measurement activities, it is necessary to evaluate the degree of potential risk in relation to the potential benefits which will accrue to the subject or society as a result of the activity. As noted above, the risk-benefit ratio expresses the relationship of all anticipated risks and human costs to all anticipated and future benefits. To compute a cost/benefit ratio, it is necessary for the researcher or measurement expert to: (1) consider all possible consequences (negative and positive) of the measure; (2) ascertain whenever possible the types (physical, psychological, social) and degree of risks involved to the subject and to society on the basis of previous empirical evidence or preliminary data; (3) identify and, if possible, quantify possible benefits to the subjects and to society; and 4) consider how the risk-benefit ratio for a given procedure or activity may change over time as additional information is accrued and plan accordingly to reassess periodically (Levine, 1986; Spilker, 1991).

Some potential benefits of measurement activities for subjects include increased knowledge about one's health, understanding of oneself or one's relationships to others, acquisition of new information, increased awareness of available options, opportunity to express one's views or opinions, perceived prestige related to having been selected to participate, and having the opportunity to contribute to a worthwhile undertaking. Some measurement activities result in no potential benefits to the subject directly, but are beneficial to society in that they contribute to knowledge and understanding of health-related phenomena and the ultimate improvement of health care. All known risks and benefits must be communicated to subjects as the basis for informed consent and every effort must be made to eliminate or minimize risks and maximize benefits. An activity should not be undertaken if benefits do not justify the risks.

Risk to the Researcher

It is possible to expand the conceptualization of risk to encompass that which may be experienced by the researcher. Nurses who engage in measurement may themselves incur some personal risk. The nurse is potentially liable if found to be acting in violation of institutional policies or subjects' rights, or inflicting any psychological, social, or physical harm in the process of gathering, interpreting, and reporting measurement data. Peer review of planned measurement activities, accomplished through such mechanisms as IRBs, is helpful in identifying potential human rights violations and ensuring that appropriate precautions are taken. Also helpful are the guidelines of professional associations and government. Such mechanisms protect not only the subject but also the investigator, and should be viewed as a valuable resource. These mechanisms, however, do not prevent nurse researchers from experiencing guilt or self-doubt about measurement in which some risk is involved. It should be noted that violation of HIPAA privacy rules also places the researcher at risk, so training about the rules and strategies to assure that they are followed is essential.

Personal risk can also be incurred in the process of gathering measurement information from subjects. For example, data collection in some settings (e.g., dangerous neighborhoods, hospital units with high infection rates) and with some populations of interest to nurses (e.g., drug addicts, combative patients) may result in physical harm unless proper precautions are taken. Psychological problems can result from repeatedly being used as a sounding board for subjects' problems, repeatedly being exposed to depressing situations, or undertaking personally unrealistic time and energy demands related to measurement. While all such risks cannot be eliminated, every effort should be made to minimize them. Clinical agencies that employ nurses are beginning to take steps to acknowledge and protect the rights of nurses who are expected to participate in medical or nursing research by, for example, developing policies that ensure the right to refuse to become involved in any research activity deemed unsafe or unethical. Such steps might include nursing input in the design of clinical trials, mandating that nurses be included as members of IRBs, defining the procedures to be used in identifying vulnerable subjects, and securing informed consent.

In summary, protecting the rights of subjects is a basic consideration in planning and undertaking any measurement activity. The nurse has the responsibility to become informed about and adhere to existing policies and guidelines that help guarantee those rights. Only a brief and superficial overview of ethical considerations in measurement has been provided. Since many ethical issues related to nursing measurement remain open to considerable controversy, the nurse who is unsure of the ethical and risk-related consequences of a given activity is well-advised to consult others before proceeding. Potential resources include ethicists, lawyers, measurement experts, and medical and nursing personnel, including IRB members. Another valuable resource is the growing body of literature in philosophy, nursing, medicine, and other fields which address ethical issues.

ETHICAL ISSUES IN RELATION TO THE SCIENTIFIC AND PROFESSIONAL COMMUNITY

Throughout this book, emphasis has been placed on the importance of adhering to sound measurement principles in the development, selection, and use of instruments and devices to measure variables of interest to the nursing community. Ethical problems result when unsound measurement practices are used. Improper use of instruments or use of those with questionable psychometric properties not only poses potential risks to subjects but also represents misuse of subjects' and nurses' time. It also has important consequences for nursing knowledge and practice. Inadequate measurement has the potential to produce useless or erroneous information which, if accepted uncritically as fact, can have a negative impact on the knowledge upon which it is based. The nurse engaged in measurement has the ethical responsibility to apply sound principles at every stage of the measurement process and to disclose fully any violation of these principles in using or reporting measurement information. Likewise, the consumer of measurement information (i.e., the reader of research reports or the decision maker) is responsible for scrutinizing the procedures used in the light of sound measurement principles and evaluating and using findings conservatively.

Development of measures, regardless of how sound and sophisticated they may be, does little to advance professional knowledge and practice, unless information about them is disseminated. Hence, it is argued that it is an ethical responsibility to make instruments and information about them available to others (nurses and those from other disciplines) via publication and presentations. The developer of an instrument should honestly and accurately report the way in which it was developed, tested, and used, providing all relevant psychometric data and acknowledging its known limitations and flaws, so that potential users can make informed judgments about its utility and correctly interpret resulting data. Data about extraneous or confounding variables that may influence subjects' scores should be reported as well.

Questions can be raised regarding the point in the development and testing of an instrument when it is appropriate to share information about it with others. On the one hand, premature reporting before the instrument has been sufficiently tested to ascertain its properties in different situations may overestimate its potential value and provide insufficient information to allow reasonable evaluation by possible users. On the other hand, inordinate delay in reporting the availability of an instrument precludes its use by others and may impede the accumulation of data about its properties, much of which can be furnished by others using the tool. After a tool has been developed, pretested, revised, and used at least once, there is generally sufficient information to legitimize reporting its availability, provided the state of its development and testing is made explicit and appropriate cautionary statements are included. The instrument should be neither underrated nor oversold. The standard is to provide sufficient data for informed evaluation by others.

Users of existing instruments also have ethical responsibilities. The most obvious requirements, which unfortunately are not always followed, are to obtain permission for intended use of the tool and to give credit to the developer when reporting its use. These requirements should be met whether an instrument is used in its original form or modified. The user is obliged to report to the developer and others the results of use and any problems encountered. Instrument development is frequently undertaken as a collaborative activity in which each individual plays an active role based on particular areas of expertise in order to produce a high-quality instrument. In addition to clearly defining roles and responsibilities, collaboration requires that professional ethics and norms be considered in assigning credit for the ultimate product and related publications. Guidelines for acknowledging contributions and awarding credit should be agreed upon before collaboration begins.

Measurement instruments and activities are important aspects of nursing research, practice, education, and administration. Thus, information about and derived from them constitutes an essential part of nursing knowledge which the nurse has an obligation to share and use according to accepted scientific and professional ethics.

REFERENCES

American Association of Critical Care Nurses. (2002). *Statement on ethics in critical care nursing research.* Aliso Viejo, CA: Author.

American Nurses Association (ANA). (2001). *Code of ethics for nurses with interpretive statements.* Retrieved March 25, 2004, from http://nursingworld.org/ethics/chcode.htm

American Nurses Association (ANA). (1991). *Position statement: Ethics and human rights.* Retrieved March 25, 2004, from http://nursingworld.org/readroom/position/ethics/etethr.htm

American Hospital Association (AHA). (1992). *A patient's bill of rights.* Retrieved March 24, 2004, from http://www.hospitalconnect.com/aha/about/pbillofrights.html

Beauchamp, E. L., & Childress, J. F. (2001). *Principles of biomedical ethics* (5th ed.). New York: Oxford University Press.

Beauchamp, T. L., & Walters, L. (Eds.). (2003). *Contemporary issues in bioethics* (6th ed). Belmont, CA: Wadsworth.

Connor, J. A., Smaldone, A. M., Bratts, T., & Stone, P. W. (2003). HIPAA in 2003 and its meaning for nurse researchers. *Applied Nursing Research, 16*(4), 291–293.

Frank-Stromborg, M. (2003). They're real and they're here: The new federally regulated privacy rules under HIPAA. *MEDSURG Nursing, 12*(6), 380–385, 414.

Im, E-O., & Chee, W. (2002). Issues in protection of human subjects in Internet research. *Nursing Research, 51*(4), 266–269.

Levine, R. J. (1986). *Ethics and regulation of clinical research* (2nd ed.). Baltimore, MD: Urban & Schwarzenberg.

National Commission for the Protection of Human Subjects of Biomedical and Behavioral Research (1978). *Belmont Report: Ethical principles and guidelines for research involving human subjects.* DHEW Publication No. (05) 78-0012. Washington, DC: U.S. Government Printing Office.

National Institutes of Health (NIH). (2003). *Institutional review boards and the HIPAA privacy rule* (NIH Publication No. 03-5428). Washington, DC: Government Printing Office.

Olsen, D. P. (2003). HIPAA privacy regulations and nursing research. *Nursing Research, 52*(5), 344–348.

Spilker, B. (1991). *Guide to clinical trials.* Philadelphia: Lippincott-Raven.

U.S. Department of Health and Human Services. (2001a). Code of Federal Regulations, 45 CFR, Parts 160 and 164. *Standards for privacy of individually identifiable health information—The HIPAA privacy rule.* Retrieved March 24, 2004, from http://www.hhs.gov/ocr/hipaa

U.S. Department of Health and Human Services. (2001b). Code of Federal Regulations, 45 CFR, Part 46. *Protection of Human Subjects.* Retrieved March 24, 2004, from http://ohrp.osophs.dhhs.gov/humansubjects/guidance/45cfr46.htm

U.S. Department of Health and Human Services, Office for Civil Rights. (2003). *Medical privacy—National standards to protect the privacy of personal health information.* Retrieved March 24, 2004, from http://www.hhs.gov/ocr/hipaa/privacy.html

Woods, G. W., & Stockton, L. L. P. (2002). *Impact of the HIPAA privacy rule on academic research.* American Council on Education. Retrieved March 24, 2004, from http://www.acenet.edu

Woods, S. L. (1988). Informed consent in research and the critically ill adult. *Progress in Cardiovascular Nursing, 3*(3), 89–92.

25

Other Measurement Issues

This chapter addresses selected measurement issues that threaten the reliability and validity of the measurement effort. Topics include: social desirability, process and outcome measurement, measuring state and trait characteristics, cross-cultural measurement, and triangulation. In most cases, if sound measurement principles are carefully employed, along with the strategies and techniques discussed in this chapter, the researcher will be well-positioned to resolve these issues and thus, increase the likelihood that results will be reliable and valid.

SOCIAL DESIRABILITY

Social desirability is usually defined as the tendency of individuals to project favorable images of themselves during social interaction. Social desirability is a potential concern in interpreting responses to socially related measures, especially affective self-report measures (Strosahl, Linehan, & Chiles, 1984; Nunnally & Bernstein, 1994; Krosnick, 1999), personality measures (Bentler, Jackson, & Messick, 1971; Otto, Lang, Magargee, & Rosenblatt, 1988; Hogan & Nicholson, 1988; Johnson & Fendrich, 2002), and surveys (Phillips, 1972; Krause, 1985; Krosnick & Chang, 2001; Dillman et al., 2001). Social desirability is a response set that influences how one responds to a measure (Cronbach, 1949; Edwards, 1957; Rorer, 1965; Gillis & Jackson, 2002). A *set* according to Rorer (1965) "connotes a conscious or unconscious desire on the part of the respondent to answer in such a way as to produce a certain picture of himself" (p. 133). A *response set* is the tendency on the part of the respondent to consistently respond differently to test items from how he or she would respond if the content were presented in

a different form (Cronbach, 1949). Hence, a response set is determined by the format of the measure (Berg, 1961; Rorer, 1965).

A *socially desirable response* is defined as a favorable response to an item with a socially desirable value, or as an unfavorable response to an item with a socially undesirable value (Edwards, 1957; Berg, 1961; Nunnally & Bernstein, 1994). Sensitive questions are especially prone to socially desirable responses. The reasons for this are that (1) content is often perceived as an invasion of respondents privacy; (2) there is the risk of disclosure of their answers to third parties; and (3) answers might be perceived as socially undesirable (Tourangeau, Rips, & Rasinski, 2000). Thus, it is essential that items on measures be scrutinized both a priori and empirically to ascertain if there is anything about them (e.g., wording or format) that might cause subjects to respond to them in a socially desirable manner rather than on the basis of item content. In addition, Nunnally and Bernstein (1994) note that social desirability varies as a result of the context in which measurement occurs, using as an example that individuals seen in a psychotherapeutic setting would tend to find it more appropriate to endorse self-descriptive questions about pathology than would individuals in an employment setting (p. 315).

STRATEGIES FOR MINIMIZING SOCIALLY DESIRABLE RESPONSES

During the selection and/or development phase of instrumentation, the investigator should consider how the respondent is likely to think about each item when responding to the measure of interest. In this regard, Klockars (1975) found that when a forced-choice format is employed, social desirability may be minimized by giving respondents two socially desirable options rather than one socially desirable and one socially undesirable option. This would serve to remove the evaluation dimensions from the ratings of the phenomenon of interest, that is, by requiring the respondent to choose between pairs of items matched for social desirability. Knowles (1988) notes that when an individual has to consider the same general issue repeatedly across the items in a multi-item, single-dimension measure, there is a tendency toward polarization of the respondent's judgment on the issue, and for the addition of cognitions consistent with the subject's judgment about the issue that allows the individual to reinterpret evidence to be consistent with his or her judgment. He further notes that item formats such as direct questions that require greater depth of processing tend to generate more thoughts and more polarized answers. Thus, he concludes the probability of socially desirable responses is increased when the respondent is required to repeatedly respond to closely related items in a single dimension scale. Babad (1979) cautions that the investigator needs to be sensitive to the suggestibility or influence of the information within the item on the response. For example, providing a scenario and then asking an individual to respond to an item on the basis of how he or she would react in the situation described, is likely to induce a socially desirable response since the respondent may be influenced by the information given in regard to what would put him or her in the most favorable light. Gibson, Wermuth, Sorensen, Menicucci, and Bernal (1987) note that socially desirable responses may be minimized when a single measure is employed with multiple sources to corroborate the results. Similarly, McCrae (1986) notes that multiple methods of measurement may also be employed in this regard. Nunnally and Bernstein (1994) caution that to the extent that there are tendencies to respond in a socially desirable manner, measures may tend to correlate because they share social desirability variance (p. 315). Becker (1976) found that requiring subjects to indicate their names and social security numbers on response sheets biased their responses to an item in a measure, whereas requiring a social security number did not bias their response. He concluded from his work that the less subjects believe there is a potential for identification of their responses, the less social desirability is likely to come into play. Hence, anonymity, since it decreases subjects' concern for social approval and/or awareness that others will evaluate their responses and know who it was that responded, also tends to minimize the probability of social desirability.

Other actions that may be taken by the developer to reduce the potential for social desirability include:

1. Using "do guess" directions when multiple-choice measures are employed
2. Wording directions as clearly and concisely as possible to avoid ambiguity and to ensure that each subject responds with the same response set
3. Avoiding item formats that use fixed-response alternatives such as true/false and yes/no
4. Using items with a general rather than a personal referent
5. Designing measures whenever possible that assess multiple dimensions of a phenomenon rather than only one dimension
6. Avoiding any words or actions that might communicate to subjects that the investigator would positively or negatively value certain responses
7. Recognizing that certain approaches to measurement have more or less probability of eliciting socially desirable responses and accordingly selecting a method in situations where social desirability is expected to more likely occur (e.g., mailed questionnaires have a lower probability of producing socially desirable responses than do telephone interviews or personal face-to-face interviews (which have the highest probability of the three)
8. Employing a measure of social desirability as a covariate in order to statistically control the social desirability response set (Dillman, 1978; Bochner & Van Zyl, 1987; Fowler, 1984; Furnham, 1986; Hays &

Ware, 1986; Nunnally & Bernstein, 1994; Ethier, Poe, Schulze, & Clark, 2000; Gillis & Jackson, 2002).

Other strategies proposed for minimizing social desirability are The Bogus Pipeline Technique (BPL) (Jones & Sigall, 1971), Randomized Response Techniques (RRT) (Van der Heijden & Van Gils, 1996), computer-assisted interviewing (CAI) and audio computer-assisted self-interview (CASI) (Leeuw, Hox, & Snijkers, 1998; Aquillino, Wright, & Supple, 2000), and computer-assisted randomized response (CARR) (Boeije & Lensvelt-Mulders, 2002). The Bogus Pipeline Technique allows for control of a portion of the variance in experimental situations attributable to socially desirable responding. Essentially, the subject is convinced that a "physiological monitoring device" is capable of assessing the truth or falsehood of their responses. The subject is instructed that any deviation from accuracy in responding can be detected by the investigator through the apparatus attached to the respondent. Millham & Kellogg (1980) note that, in this way, the results obtained represent a subject's response "uncontaminated by many of the biases that obscure paper and pencil measures" (p. 447). Studies such as one conducted by McGovern and Nevid (1986) have not supported this contention. The Randomized Response Technique (RRT), designed by Warner (1965), has as its purpose to increase the subject's willingness to truthfully answer questions of a sensitive or socially undesirable nature. The basic assumption underlying this approach is that the respondents believe that their responses cannot be directly linked to them. When RRT is employed, an individual's response to a sensitive question remains unknown alleviating concerns with privacy invasion and a population estimate of the sensitive topic is computed. Using a logistic regression approach allows for the sensitive behavior estimates to be linked to explanatory variables (Maddala, 1983; Scheers & Dayton, 1988; Van der Heijden & Van Gils, 1996).

Gupta (2002), comparing RRTs with personal interview surveys involving sensitive questions and the Bogus Pipeline Technique, found that RRTs were at least as effective in reducing social desirability as the BPL, while being less intrusive. More specific information regarding the Randomized Response Technique is provided in chapter 20 where the collection of sensitive data is discussed.

The survey and interviewing literature suggests that the use of computer-administered surveys on highly sensitive topics minimizes or eliminates the effects of social desirability (Taylor, 2000) even when humanizing features such as voice are employed (Dillman et al., 2001). For this reason, there has been increased use of computer-assisted interviewing especially use of Web-based surveys (Couper & Nicholls, 1998) and computer-assisted self-interviewing (CASI) methods, whereby the respondent interacts directly with the computer to answer questions. For example, when the audio CASI method is employed, the respondent listens to the questions read over headphones using a digitized voice and enters the responses into the computer. Studies comparing CAI and audio CASI to other data collection methods have found a reduction in social desirability bias relative to surveys administered by an interviewer and a paper-based self-administered approach (Tourangeau & Smith, 1998; Turner et al., 1998a; Turner et al., 1998b).

On the other hand, in the field of human-computer interaction, a basic premise under investigation is that humanizing cues, such as voice, in a computer interface can result in responses similar to those in human-to-human interaction (Nass, Fogg, & Moon, 1996; Fogg & Nass, 1997; Nass, Moon, & Carney, 1999).

MEASURES OF SOCIAL DESIRABILITY

In addition to the a priori actions to minimize the probability of socially desirable responses that may be taken by the investigator during the instrument selection and/or development stage of the measurement process, the extent to which this response set exists also may be investigated empirically during the reliability and validity testing phase of the measurement effort. Several tools and methods for measuring social desirability have been developed for this purpose.

Edwards (1957) developed the first such measure, The Edwards Social Desirability Scale, based upon his belief that social desirability scale values of personality statements can be obtained by various psychological scaling methods in order to obtain a scale value for any personality statement on a single dimension, the social desirability-undesirability dimension, relative to other personality statements. His basic premise is that if one knows the position of a statement on the social desirability continuum, one can predict, with a high degree of accuracy, that the statement does describe the respondents (p. 3). When his measure is employed, one obtains for each personality statement, a social desirability scale value. The more favorable the social desirability response of an item, the greater the likelihood of its endorsement under standard test-taking instructions. On the basis of the resulting values one is able to detect the extent to which social desirability comes into play and hence the credibility that can be attributed to the resulting scores (Edwards, 1957, 1970). Studies providing information regarding the use of Edward's scale, including reliability and validity data, are discussed in Edwards (1957, 1970), Millham and Kellogg (1980), and Carstensen and Cone (1983).

Viewing, as a limitation of the Edwards' scale, the fact that the items were drawn from clinical scales that could be characterized by their pathological content, Crowne and Marlowe (1964) developed the *Marlowe-Crowne Social Desirability Scales,* which are designed to include items that are culturally appropriate and yet untrue of virtually all people and that have minimal pathological or abnormal implications (p. 22). They based their scales on the premise that people describe themselves in favorable or socially desirable terms in order to achieve the approval of others. They view social desirability as a response style or personality trait rather than a response set. When administering their scale, they note that little concern needs to be given to the testing situation as a social context that might influence the subject's need to give a socially desirable response. Factors that could influence how an individual responds were identified as (1) the need to attain success in academic, social-recognition,

or competitive business situations; (2) the need to win approval and affection from others; and (3) dependence needs, such as help, protection, and succorance. If it is important for a subject to gain approval, deny inadequacies, obtain dependency gratifications, or achieve recognition or status, the investigator would anticipate that the individual's responses to items would tend to serve these aims (Crowne & Marlowe, 1964). The Marlowe-Crowne scales have been widely used. Johnson and Fendrich (2002) conducted a study to investigate the validity of the Marlowe-Crowne scale. Findings from their study supported the original conceptualization of social desirability as a personality trait. Additional information regarding reliability and validity is reported in the literature by Jacobson, Berger, and Milham (1970), Phillips (1972), Hogan and Mookherjee (1980), Holden and Mendonca (1984), Strosahl, Linehan, and Chiles (1984), Ellis (1985), Helmes and Holden (1986), and O'Grady (1988). Short forms of the Edwards scale and the Marlowe-Crowne scale have been developed and tested for reliability and validity (Reynolds, 1982; Silverstein, 1983; Ray, 1984).

The *Multi-Dimensional Social Desirability Inventory* was developed by Jacobsen, Kellogg, Cauce, and Slavin (1977), who contend that social desirability is a multidimensional construct. Their instrument is essentially a social approval inventory that is designed to assess factors that comprise the assumed need for approval. The measure comprises four scales of 17 items each. The scales are (1) attribution of positive traits, (2) attribution of negative traits, (3) denial of positive traits, and (4) denial of negative traits. Scores on each scale provide a measure of the extent to which the subject accepted or denied traits differing in social desirability value. In addition to their own studies of the inventory, reliability and validity information has been reported by Jacobson, Brown, and Ariza (1983), and Kral (1986).

Measures of social desirability have been employed both a priori and a posteriori in the development of measures of sensitive topics. For example, to address concerns regarding social desirability response bias in scores resulting from items on a newly developed self-report measure prior to development of the new measure, the Marlowe-Crowne Social Desirability Scale (SDS), (Crowne & Marlowe, 1964) could be used to scrutinize and remove items from the developing measure that correlate with items on the SDS prior to construction of the final version of the new measure. In addition, a posteriori statistical techniques could be employed to investigate and control for social desirability in the final version of the new self-report measure. An example of a multicultural specific social desirability scale designed to be employed in concert with the Multicultural Counseling Inventory (MCI) can be found in the work of Sodowsky, Kuo-Jackson, Richardson, and Corey (1998).

According to Nunnally and Bernstein (1994), "preferences for the socially desirable response are a function of (1) level of adjustment, (2) knowledge of one's self, and (3) frankness" (p. 391). One approach to investigating these factors is Watson's (2003) suggestion that, in concert with established measures of social desirability, postadministration interviews be conducted to provide insight into how respondents conceptualize and rate themselves on the measure of interest.

PROCESS AND OUTCOME MEASUREMENT

Process and outcome measurement has become very popular and highly valued in nursing. This trend has come about because of an increased emphasis on investigating the worth of nursing programs and activities in clinical and educational settings, and because nurses have become more interested in understanding the relationship between nursing activities and practice outcomes. In addition, consumers have become more concerned about knowing what they are buying and whether health services purchased will actually improve their health status (Burns & Grove, 2001). Clinicians have become more interested in knowing whether care provided is effective, "with whom it is effective, how much benefit it produces, and whether associated, adverse outcomes occur" (Brown, 2002, p. 317). External pressures to the nursing profession

also have contributed to nursing interest and activity in this area. The nation has come to expect that health care providers document the effectiveness of their care (Strickland, 1995). The passage of the Professional Standards Review Organization (PSRO) legislation (PL 92-603) in 1972 further encouraged interest in process and outcome measurement. This legislation mandated that the quality of medical care financed by federal funds be monitored. Although the legislation was primarily aimed at physicians, it did not exclude other health care providers. Nurses increased their activity in the area of monitoring the quality of nursing care, and this required that measurement of processes and outcomes in nursing be given special attention. In addition to its impact resulting from PSRO legislation, the federal government also stimulated interest in process and outcome measurement by requiring that educational and health care programs that receive federal funding be evaluated. As part of the evaluation of the processes for implementing such programs, nurses were required to focus on measurement of process and outcome variables.

With all of this activity, process and outcome measurement has not proven to be a simple matter. Issues have been raised regarding frameworks that should be used, the approaches to process and outcome measurement, and the meaning of findings. This chapter will address such issues. However, before focusing specifically on measurement of process and outcomes per se, it is necessary to provide definitions of these terms.

Definitions

Process is the manner or approach by which a program or provider delivers services to clients. Outcomes are the outputs or results of the program or the activities of the provider. It is noteworthy that one should be careful not to confuse process/outcome measurement with process/outcome research and evaluation. Process/outcome research involves investigating relationships among process variables or outcome variables in order to make decisions regarding statistical hypotheses and inductive inferences concerning the probable truth or falsity of a research hypothesis. Process/outcome research is conducted primarily to build theory and to add to the knowledge base in an area.

Process/outcome evaluation is a decision-making process by which one examines the manner in which a program or provider delivers services or their outputs and makes judgments about what is done or how well objectives are met. Evaluation of processes and outcomes can be expected to lead to suggestions for action to improve effectiveness and efficiency. Nursing quality of care assessment and nursing audit are examples of process/outcome evaluations.

Process/outcome measurement relates to how a specified process or outcome is operationalized, that is, quantified or classified. Measurement is a part of the research process and the evaluation process, but is not synonymous with either.

Process Measurement

The term "process" by its very nature is dynamic, and it projects a sense of movement and fluidity. This quality makes the measurement of a particular process quite challenging. However, the approach to operationalizing a process follows the same basic principles as for measurement of most other variables. Since measurement should be based on how a variable is conceptualized, this indicates that the measurement of process must consider its dynamic quality. The specific process that is the focus of measurement should be clearly defined in a manner that captures the essence of its characteristics. Within nursing, specific nursing interventions or programs are common processes that are the focus of measurement. Interventions are any therapies that are designed to improve a client's health condition toward desired health outcomes and may include treatments, procedures, or other actions implemented by providers to and with clients (Sidani & Braden, 1998).

The determination of the conceptual framework for the process is one of the first essential steps in the development of a reliable and valid measurement approach. The conceptual framework or conceptual model on which a process is based determines the variables that should be selected and studied within the process itself to ensure the quality of its implementation, as well as the outcome variables that need to be assessed to determine the effectiveness or efficacy of the process (Strickland, 1995; 1997). Since most processes are not unitary phenomena, a number of concepts may be required for the formulation of a sound definition . Each concept in the framework must be defined and the relationships between key constructs identified. Previous descriptive research can be used to help identify constructs that are likely to account for large amounts of variance in the intervention, whether the intervention should be targeted for a specific population or setting, and aid in the identification of outcome variables that are most likely to be affected by the intervention. Related previous intervention studies can be examined to ascertain intervention doses, and attributes of effective interventions included in other experimental investigations (Conn, Rantz, Wipke-Tevis, & Maas, 2001). The level of specification or generality of the intervention also is important because underspecified conceptual frameworks can lead to the lack of identification of constructs that are important to address within the intervention, while overspecification can introduce unimportant constructs and make operationalization of the intervention unnecessarily burdensome. Specification errors in the conceptual framework can lead to an invalid measurement procedure. When formulating a conceptual framework for a process, such as a nursing intervention, specification errors can arise from three sources: (1) underspecification (missing key variables) or overspecification (including extra variables); (2) inaccurate or incomplete definitions of the key variables; and (3) inaccurate identification of the relationships among the key variables (Atwood, 1980, p. 105).

The conceptual framework for an intervention should also give some guidance relative to whether a single or bundled intervention should be designed. The study of some phenomena may require bundled or multiple interventions. "Bundled interventions are appropriate when a multidimensional problem is located in a conceptual framework that suggests combining multiple interventions" (Conn, Rantz, Wipke-Tevis,

& Maas, 2001. p. 437). A limitation of bundled interventions is that it may be difficult to interpret the effects of the various components of the intervention. However, use of a factorial design where individual interventions can be assessed for the effectiveness of components can address this issue (Piantadosi, 1997).

Another important issue related to operationalizing interventions is the degree to which they can be designed to be patient-centered or to fit the individual needs of clients and still maintain their measurement integrity. Patient-centered care focuses on respect for and integration of individual differences when delivering patient care. Clearly, standardized interventions are much easier to test than patient-centered interventions since the needs of individual patients vary. The assessment of patient-centered interventions are important to measure and test to clarify the situations in which such interventions are likely to be the least or most effective. However, a concern that has been raised regarding outcomes from patient-centered intervention studies is that they often result in small effect sizes (Lauver, et al., 2002). As patient-centered studies are implemented in the future, it will be necessary to carefully document variations in different patient interventions within such studies in order to elucidate differences in effect sizes.

The dose of interventions is another issue in developing interventions. Even when the content of an intervention is appropriate, if it is delivered in insufficient doses then the potential effectiveness can be obscured. Decisions related to dose of an intervention also include those regarding duration of delivery over hours, days, weeks, or months. Increasing treatment doses can make a psychosocial nursing intervention more robust. However, increasing treatment dose needs to be carefully considered in relation to demands placed on participants since this could lead to high subject attrition. Testing intervention dose may also be the focus of study (Conn, Rantz, Wipke-Tevis, & Maas, 2001), as was done by Rothert and associates (1997) who studied empowerment of menopausal women by varying dose by offering one group only written materials, another group written materials and didactic information, and yet another group written materials, didactic information, and additional activities.

The most common conceptual frameworks used in nursing to facilitate process specification and outcomes assessment are: (a) the structure-process-outcome framework, (b) the condition-focused or disease-focused model, and (c) the sequential model (Strickland, 1995). Within the structure-process-outcome framework the inputs, prerequisites, or structures for patient care are identified, along with the processes (interventions) and outcomes (outputs). These components are studied in relation to each other. In the condition-focused or disease-focused model, clinical conditions or diagnoses are identified for a specific patient population, and nursing treatments or interventions for the conditions are designed to specifically address identified symptoms and problems along with expected results. Outcome variables are selected based on the expected results as indicators of the efficacy or effectiveness of the intervention. The sequential model is used in situations where specific stages or phases of a condition or disease can be identified, for example, pregnancy or cancer. Symptoms and health problems associated with each stage are identified, interventions are designed to address the specific problems, and expected outcomes of the interventions are identified and measured (Strickland, 1995).

Once the conceptual framework of the process has been delineated, the blueprint or specific approach to measurement is developed. The measurement approach should address the key variables that are included in the conceptual framework; therefore, several variables or dimensions may be included in the measurement process. If the nursing process model were used as the conceptual framework for measuring the process of nursing care, one would include assessment, planning, implementation, and evaluation as key components in the measurement.

For the most part, measurement of process in nursing has been approached conceptually in two ways: by focusing on the services or care provided by the nurse, and by focusing on the services or care received by the client. In addition to a well-developed and explicit conceptual framework for the intervention, operationalization of an intervention involves developing a detailed written protocol that includes (1) the protocol's purpose, (2) the equipment, materials and resources required to conduct the intervention, (3) a step-by-step description of the procedures to be followed during implementation, (4) a timeline for implementation, (5) the persons responsible for implementing the protocol and their characteristics, training, and qualifications, (6) the manner by which the intervention is to be delivered, such as by telephone, mail, printed materials, internet, or in person, and (7) the person(s) responsible for evaluating whether the intervention is conducted according to the written protocol. A well-written protocol and training of those who conduct it are necessary to ensure that the persons who implement it do so consistently (reliably) and accurately (validly) (Strickland, 1997).

When process measurement is conducted during process evaluation, criteria or standards are specified which describe the nature and, when appropriate, the events that should occur in the process and the expected interaction of activities and participants involved in the process. The criteria serve as the basis for making judgments regarding the adequacy of the process. In developing criteria, one seeks to specify the important aspects of the process in measurable terms. For example, the process criteria for nursing care on a specified nursing unit might include the following:

- Comatose patients will be repositioned every 2 hours.
- A psychiatric nurse specialist will assess each patient having an alteration in body image.

Process criteria for a nursing education program might include:

- Admission criteria and procedures are closely followed.
- Students are provided opportunities to evaluate the curriculum.
- Faculty members involve students in their research activities.

Several types of measurement methods are amenable to measuring processes and included among these are observation, interviews, diaries, record audit, focus groups, and questionnaires. Tools that employ the branching technique are particularly useful when the nature of the process involves several interrelated steps that are dependent upon each other, such as with measurement of the process of decision making. The branching technique provides several options or choices along the way at various stages of the process. The option selected will determine other situations or options that will be presented to the subjects. Hence, the various available options, if selected, subsequently provide different situations or options in a sequential manner similar to the branches of a tree. However the extent to which decision-making processes used by human beings are invariant across tasks has been questioned (Corcoran, 1986). This indicates that the process of decision making is highly contingent on the complexity of the task, which has a major implication for measurement.

Because of the complexity of most processes and the number of key variables that may be involved, multiple measures can increase the reliability and validity of results. Therefore, use of multiple measures in process measurement is encouraged.

A major concern related to process measurement is that the act of measuring the process may alter the process and, thereby, the subsequent findings. This issue might not be crucial during process evaluation in which information obtained may be intentionally used for making decisions for change. Clearly, process measurement can give clues to corrective action and provide a means for elucidating consequences of certain actions. However, this problem could be a severe limitation to research studies that require the measurement of process variables. In any case, efforts should be made to conduct measurements as unobtrusively as possible.

Outcome Measurement

A major issue for nurses regarding outcome measurement is that of selecting appropriate outcomes for study. In a given situation, a wide array of variables may be appropriate for outcome measurement. As with process measurement, in most instances there is no single concept that is likely to adequately represent the outcomes of a particular intervention or process. Therefore, the outcomes selected must be based on, and be consistent with, the conceptual framework that is being considered. In other words, the outcomes selected must be meaningful and salient to the focus of the investigation. If the focus of the study is concerned with health state, then the appropriate outcome variables should relate to health state. If the basic problem is conceptualized in terms of cognitive phenomena, then appropriate cognitive outcomes should be selected.

Clinical outcomes that are discussed in the general nursing literature frequently are limited to the consideration of disease status, symptoms, and function. However, several recent books that focus on nursing outcomes have become available, which reflect the broadening range of outcomes that have evolved in nursing (Waltz & Jenkins, 2001; Strickland & DiIorio, 2003a, 2003b). Clinical outcomes in the research literature often deal with a single psychosocial variable rather than including several psychosocial, cognitive, and physiologic variables. Outcome measurement should include a variety of client states and behaviors, such as level of satisfaction with care knowledge of illness, and compliance with the prescribed health regimen. Since nursing views humans as biopsychosocial beings, key outcome variables in those areas should be selected which relate to the framework under consideration. The study of several key outcome variables and their relationships with each other and the intervention will provide more information and will more likely further develop the knowledge base regarding the phenomenon of interest than a single outcome variable.

When the interest is on evaluating the outcomes of a process such as an educational program or health care program, the focus might be on assessing outcomes of provider behaviors, the influence of the program on provider and client attitudes, or the impact of the program's services within a specified geographic area. When programs are assessed, the objectives or goals of the program are the primary outcome criteria. Outcome criteria are used to make judgments regarding the effectiveness of a process or program. An outcome criterion or standard can be considered valid if it is an accurate statement of the following:

1. Something that should or should not occur in the status of the patient (or client)
2. The level at which it should occur
3. The point in time at which it should occur
4. Something that is expected to occur in good measure as a result of the care (or process), which is to be assessed (Bloch, 1980, p. 71)

Patient care goals should be formulated in such a manner that they can serve as the outcome criteria for assessing the quality of the process of nursing care provided to an individual patient (Strickland, 1995). Examples are:

- The patient will care for the colostomy without assistance prior to discharge.
- The patient will lose 10 pounds within 6 months.

Another issue that causes concern about the selection of outcomes is that most outcomes are influenced by many factors beyond those that are the focus of study. A client's attitudes, behaviors, health state, or knowledge may be influenced by care or services received from other providers. It is difficult to select outcomes that can be solely attributed to any one factor, such as nursing care or a particular health care program or educational program. However, in most instances it is possible to select outcomes that can be related temporally to the intervention or process that is the focus of investigation. Temporally relating variations in outcomes to the expected sources of such changes supports the validity and usefulness of the outcome selected. Thus, timing of measurements is important. Outcomes are selected that are expected to respond to the type of action, intervention, or process that is conducted. The prevention and healing rate of decubitus ulcers is an example of an outcome that would be expected to respond to nursing care. Another related issue is that nursing addresses, to a great extent, subtle pyschosocial problems. The impact of nursing on the client's state may be difficult to measure, because psychosocial variables often are difficult to measure.

As with the measurement of process variables, the use of multiple measures of outcome variables can provide more support for reliability and validity. Interviews, questionnaires, record audits, direct observation, and use of laboratory data are among the various approaches that may be employed for the measurement of outcomes and for the assessment of quality of care. However, it should be noted that record audit will not provide reliable and valid indicators unless measurement or the method of recording data is reliable and valid. Whereas certain information on a record, such as temperature readings or results of laboratory tests, may be highly reliable and valid, others, such as behaviors learned by the client for self-care, may not be adequately documented. Strickland (1995, 1997) has identified several important points that should be considered in the selection and measurement of outcomes of care:

1. They should be conceptually appropriate and compatible with the conceptual framework of the intervention or program.
2. They should represent the full conceptual model of the intervention or program.
3. Variables should have an effect size to allow adequate statistical power given the sample that is selected or that is available.
4. Intended and unintended outcomes should be selected, since planned and unplanned outcomes may occur from any intervention. The investigator needs to be aware of potential unintended outcomes and measure them.
5. Positive and potentially negative outcomes should be selected based on expected results from the intervention.
6. Outcomes should be important to clients.
7. Longitudinal assessments of outcomes need to carefully consider timing of the data collection to reflect the most important and relevant time points for the expression of outcomes, selection of measures that are sensitive to small changes in the variables studied, and the selection of variables that represent intermediate outcomes that may be precursors to longer-term outcomes.

There also are several client-related measurement issues that need to be considered during outcome measurement. These include (1) the impact of comorbidity on outcomes, which could mask the impact of the intervention; (2) the fact that some variables are characterized by periodicity and circadian rhythms, which could influence measurements taken; and (3) population subsets may respond differently for certain outcomes. In addition, outcome measurements need to be feasible and practical to use, and compatible with the age, education, gender, and cultural backgrounds of clients.

Finally, qualitative approaches can be very useful to aid in outcomes assessment. Data collected using qualitative approaches can also clarify findings obtained from quantitative measures. Chinn and Kramer (1999) suggest that several types of quality-related outcomes are particularly suited for planning deliberative validation of theoretic relationships. Among them are qualitative data to assess the scientific competence of nurses, functional outcomes, satisfaction of nurses, and quality of care perceived by those who receive care.

MEASURING STATE AND TRAIT CHARACTERISTICS

Most attributes that are measured are conceptualized as stable or exhibiting little variation over time. However, in the real world a number of attributes can and do vary from moment to moment and day to day. Those attributes that are conceptualized as being stable with little variability are referred to as *trait* characteristics. State attributes are conceptualized as dynamic and changeable over relatively short periods of time and from one situation to another. In essence, while traits are more enduring characteristics, states are more temporary and fleeting in nature (Knapp, Kimble, & Dunbar, 1998).

Trait Attributes

A trait description provides a statistical summary of the attribute of interest over many situations. Scores on a trait measure for an attribute represent the probability that an individual will react in a defined way in response to a defined class of situations or stimuli (Cronbach, 1970). For example, if assertiveness were conceptualized as a trait, one would be interested in the typical or usual assertiveness level. If a trait measure of assertiveness indicated that a nurse is assertive, this does not mean that the nurse is assertive in all situations. No one is 100% assertive or 0% assertive. It only implies that the nurse is assertive in most situations. The nurse might be very nonassertive in interactions with her supervisor, and the trait score would not reflect this difference in assertiveness level for this particular situation.

Conceptualization of attributes of individuals as traits is deeply embedded in Western languages. Most adjectives that are used to characterize people are descriptive traits, for example, honest, happy, shy, thrifty, liberal, healthy, hypertensive, or hyperactive. Three assumptions underlie trait conceptualizations:

1. Behavior is habitual within individuals. A person tends to exhibit consistent reactions over a range of similar situations.
2. Different individuals vary in the frequency and degree of any type of behavior or response.
3. Personalities have some degree of stability (Cronbach, 1970).

Traits, therefore, economically describe broad characteristics of phenomena. Measurement of trait attributes focuses on significant variation in general behavior over a wide range of situations and does not consider specific behaviors or responses in specific situations.

State Attributes

Since the 1960s there has been concern about the lack of emphasis on situational specificity in measurement (Anastasi, 1976). In the area of personality assessment, much criticism has been leveled regarding the conceptualization of attributes as general, ubiquitous styles. There has been a tendency to reject personality description in terms of broad traits (Bandura, 1969; Goldfried & Kent, 1972; Mischel, 1969, 1973). This type of criticism has been provided with regard

to all traits; however, there is higher cross-situational consistency and temporal stability of cognitive as compared with noncognitive attributes (Anastasi, 1976).

Individuals exhibit situational specificity for many attributes. A particular situation may elicit a specific attribute or behavior quite differently from another situation. For example, a person might be calm during a physical examination if there has been no indication of potential problems, but may on another occasion be highly anxious during a physical examination if there are signs of illness. Similarly, a person who cheats on income taxes might be scrupulously honest in money matters with business associates. Hence, there is a person-by-situation interaction in the exhibition of many attributes, i.e., a person may exhibit an attribute differently in different situations.

State attributes reflect the variability of phenomena over rather short periods of time and from situation to situation. For example, the concept of pain for the most part is considered as a state in nursing and measured from the state perspective because it fluctuates over time. A nurse may have good reason for wanting to measure how an attribute changes from time to time, or from one situation to another. For example, a nurse might want to know under what circumstances a patient's blood pressure increases or decreases, or whether it changes in response to treatment. Within this context, blood pressure would be conceptualized as a state attribute. Many physiological variables that are observed within nursing clinical settings are conceptualized as state characteristics, since such variables are measured to assess responses to illness or treatment over time. Nurse researchers often study state attributes within the realm of their investigations. There may be an interest in studying the effects of a mood-altering drug on the anxiety and depression levels of clients, for example. Hence, the focus of measurement of state attributes is on the nature of a particular attribute at a particular time or in a particular situation. Phenomena are perceived as possessing the potential for having an affinity to time and situation, and the aim of measuring state attributes is to detect the state of phenomena at a given moment or in a given situation. It is common for state attributes to be measured with visual analog scales, such as is often done with pain (Good et al., 2001). A specific concept may be conceptualized either as a trait or state. For example, Speilberger, Gorsuch, Luchene, Vagg, and Jacobs (1983) have conceptualized anxiety as a trait and a state characteristic. Trait and state measures of anxiety have been developed for adults (Speilberger, Gorsuch, Luchene, Vagg, & Jacobs, 1983; Kulik, Mahler, & Earnest, 1994) and for children (Baker-Ward & Rankin, 1994). A measure of trait anxiety would be used in a study when the researcher is concerned about understanding how one's general personality level of anxiety might be associated with or influences some other variable. The state measure of anxiety would be used when the researcher is concerned about how some particular situation, such as being in labor while having a baby, influences anxiety. Grimm (1989) has conceptualized hope as having state and trait characteristics in that one has a general level of hope and a level that fluctuates from situation to situation, such as during the trajectory of cancer. On the other hand Hinds (1988) has conceptualized hopefulness as a state phenomenon, i.e., a dynamic internal state that may be influenced by external factors. The manner in which the attitude is conceptualized and used will determine whether it should be measured as a trait or state.

Implications for Measurement

Conceptualization of an attribute as either a trait or state has implications for how a measurement tool is constructed, how a measurement procedure is conducted, how a device is used, and how reliability and validity are assessed. Consider that state characteristics are conceptualized as dynamic and changeable, while trait attributes reflect typical responses. A device designed to measure a state attribute must possess the sensitivity and precision to detect changes over time. On the other hand, a tool designed to measure a trait attribute should consistently measure the attribute over long periods of time given the same measurement circumstances.

The usual trait inventory is phrased in a manner to obtain information about a person's life style or typical behavior, and it does not elicit information regarding present state or state at a particular moment. When tools are constructed to obtain information on a subject's state, questions are framed in terms of the present moment or a limited time period of interest, such as "Are you tense?" This same question framed in terms of a trait attribute would be "Are you usually tense?" The way in which items are framed in a tool affects the information obtained by altering the response set (Cronbach, 1970).

Zuckerman and Lubin (1985) have developed the Multiple Affect Adjective Check List, which measures trait and state mood, specifically, anxiety, depression, and hostility. This questionnaire was developed in two forms: general and today. The general form measures trait mood, and the today form measures state mood. The only difference between the two forms is in the directions to the respondent. The subject is instructed to respond to the general form according to how he generally feels. On the today form the subject is instructed to respond according to how he feels at the moment. The adjective checklists for both forms are identical and are scored by the same keys to arrive at scores for anxiety, depression, and hostility. Retest reliabilities for the trait scale were satisfactorily high, but this was not the case for the state scale, for which temporal stability is not expected. The internal-consistency reliabilities on both forms of the tool at a single testing were high.

For the most part, physiologic phenomena are highly variable, even within the same individual, and often are conceptualized as state attributes. However, there are times when determining whether a physiologic measurement is reflective of a trait or state is important. For example, in the case of blood pressure one would not want to initiate long-term treatment for hypertension unless the client is typically hypertensive. Therefore, it would be important to have a good estimate of the individual's typical or trait blood pressure. If the nurse took the client's blood pressure while he was unusually anxious, the blood pressure reading might be unusually high due to his present emotional state. Hence, the results of the measurement would be a state measurement instead of a trait measurement. The nurse must be clear about the purposes for which a specific physiologic variable is being measured, understand under what conditions such measurements are likely to be most stable and variable, and obtain measurements at times and in situations that will provide the type of data that are most useful.

Since state attributes are changeable from situation to situation and trait attributes are considered relatively stable, this must be given consideration in the assessment of reliability. Given that state measures are not expected to be stable over time, if one did a test-retest reliability assessment and found a high coefficient, then this would be evidence against the reliability of the tool unless the original situation under which the subjects were measured could be replicated. In most situations this is difficult to do. Therefore, test-retest reliability should not be done with state measures unless the point is to show that there is not consistency in the state measure over time. However, internal consistency reliability assessment would be appropriate since the object of this approach to reliability estimation is to determine the level of homogeneity or consistency of the items. One should expect a high internal consistency reliability index for both state and trait measures. Other measures of reliability for a state measure in addition to internal-consistency reliability assessment include parallel forms reliability, and where appropriate, interrater reliability.

When validity is assessed, the approaches that are useful for assessing tools that measure trait attributes also are useful for assessing state measures. Hypothesis testing as a means of construct validation often is employed to support the validity of state measures. For example, a group of subjects might be administered the measure at a time when or in a situation in which the state attribute would be expected to be low and at another time when it would be expected to be significantly higher. If significant differences were found between the measurements over time or from one situation to another in the direction expected, this would support the validity of the tool. For example, in validity assessments of the Multiple Affect Adjective Check List, college students scored significantly higher on the today form of the tool on examination days than on nonexamination days (Zuckerman & Lubin, 1985).

Interpreting State and Trait Measurements

As noted previously, when tools are selected to measure an attribute, care should be taken that the conceptual orientation of the tool be consistent with the purpose for which the tool is used. This is particularly important in terms of whether a state or trait characteristic is the focus of measurement. A nurse would not want to use a tool that measured trait anxiety, for example, when the purpose is to measure state anxiety, or vice versa. Whether state or trait attributes are measured will influence the type of interpretations that can be validly made about the results. If a nurse were interested in the long-term effects of a particular phenomenon, it would be more appropriate to employ a trait measure. The reason for this would be that the nurse is really interested in making interpretations about the influence of the phenomenon on the general responses or behaviors of the subject in terms of that attribute, that is, on the trait expression of the attribute. If, on the other hand, the concern were with the changes that occur within a relatively short time period or in a particular situation, then a state measure would be employed. One cannot assume that changes reflected by a state measure are long lasting. Neither can one assume that lack of change in scores obtained by a trait measure also indicates lack of situational or short-term fluctuations in the attribute. The interpretations that can be appropriately made about trait and state characteristics are directly linked to the nature of the measurement tool and the circumstances under which the measurements are made.

CROSS-CULTURAL MEASUREMENT

Over the last decade, interest in employing measures across cultures has gained significantly in importance. Factors contributing to this trend are (1) the increased awareness of health problems that have a global impact, and the committant rise in cross-cultural research collaborations to address them, and (2) the greater concern with health disparities among subgroups of the population, and the realization that cultural differences in beliefs, traditions, norms, and values of health care providers and clients often serve as a basis for understanding and rectifying these differences.

The focus of this discussion is employing measures across cultures. It is important to note that *cross-cultural* refers to different cultures within one country or between one cultural group and another. *Cross-national* refers to research conducted in more than one country. Cross-national work may not be cross-cultural if the two nations are similar in the phenomenon of interest. Cross-national research is often cross-cultural, but cross-cultural research may or may not be cross-national (Bullinger, Anderson, Cella, & Aaronson, 1993; Corless, Nicholas, & Nokes, 2001).

An example of a cross-cultural research effort is found in the work of Owens, Johnson, and O'Rourke (1999) who studied responses of minority group respondents and members of acculturated immigrant groups to four large health-related surveys. Because this effort was conducted only within the U.S., it is also an example of cross-cultural research that is not cross-national.

Whenever possible, existing measures should be employed in cross-cultural research rather than developing a new instrument or measurement method. When measures are employed and tested over time more substantial evidence for reliability and validity is accrued than is possible within the context of a single study, and the cost of instrumentation is less than when developing and testing a new measure. Use of a tool from one culture to another requires, first and foremost, attention to the cultural relevance of the measure for the cultures for which it is being employed. An existing tool or method when used in measuring a phenomenon in another cultural group for which the tool was not designed often requires translation. An important consideration then is whether the tool can be translated from the *source language* (i.e., the original language of the tool) into the *target language* (i.e., the language into which the tool is to be translated) without losing meaning in the translation process.

Carlson (2000) points out that *translation* means literally changing word-by-word without considering conceptual meaning. When an instrument or measurement method is translated word for word, the result is apt to be an instrument in the target language that has awkward sentence structure and that lacks clear and comprehensible meaning. Further, difficulties in translation result from the fact that in some cases, there are no words within the target language that are equivalent to those in the source language and/or there are no equivalent parts of speech between the two languages. For this reason, in recent years as translation methodology has further developed, the emphasis has shifted from a focus on instrument translation to instrument adaptation. *Instrument adaptation* is the preferred process because, unlike translation, it takes into account conceptual meanings in the source language within the context of the translation process.

The final goal of tool adaptation according to Hambleton (1994) and Sireci (1997) is to maintain construct equivalence and content representation across the two languages. When measures are employed across cultures, several issues that can affect the reliability and validity of the measurement results must be considered and steps must be taken to resolve them. These issues are discussed below.

Cultural Equivalence

A primary issue to be considered in regard to cross-cultural equivalence relates to the concept being measured. *Equivalence* (Van de Vijver & Leung, 1997) refers to the extent to which scores obtained from the same measure when employed in different cultural groups are comparable. One cannot assume that specific concepts or ideas present in one culture are also present and/or have the same meaning in another culture (Brislin, Lonner, & Thorndike, 1973; Hwang, Yan, & Scherer, 1996; Hilton & Skrutkowski, 2002) or that they are readily transferred from one culture to another (Carlson, 2000). For equivalence to be present when measures are employed across cultures, it is necessary to consider equivalence in terms of the meaning of the concepts (e.g., depression) that serve as the basis for the measure's development and to ascertain that they have the same meaning within each of the cultures in which the measure is employed. One way in which this can be accomplished is to pretest the measure with subjects from each of the cultures of interest to ascertain similarities and/or differences in their response patterns. For example, Byrne and Campbell (1999) administered the Beck Depression Inventory to groups of Bulgarian, Canadian, and Swedish subjects and compared the response patterns across groups using the degrees of skewness and kurtosis. They found that the concept of depression among the Swedes differed in that the Swedes were prone to either acquiescent or socially desirable responding, tendencies which they accounted for as a reluctance to openly acknowledge any evidence of weakness in terms of depressive symptoms.

Other examples of efforts to validate conceptual equivalence across cultures can be found in the works of Corless, Nicholas, and Nokes (2001), who examined cross-cultural measurement of quality of life and issues to consider in adapting existing quality of life measures for cross-cultural use, and Chen, Lee, and Stevonson (1995) who studied response styles of East Asian and North American students and concluded that the response patterns of Asian subjects differed in that they tended to be influenced by their beliefs, based on Confucian philosophy, that they should not stand apart from the group. Hwang, Yan, and Scherer (1996) note that successful translation efforts depend upon the concepts being understood in a similar manner within the two cultures. Thus, prior to translation, it is essential to establish cultural equivalency. Within the translation literature, two terms are frequently used in this regard: *emic,* from the word "phonemics" (sounds that occur in only one language), and *etic,* from the word "phonetics" (sounds that occur in all languages). *Emic concepts* refer to ideas and behaviors that are culture specific. Emic concepts do not survive backtranslation aimed at cultural adaptation. *Etic concepts,* on the other hand, refer to ideas and behaviors that are universal. Etic concepts survive backtranslation. During the translation process, an emic concept in the source language becomes an imposed etic in the target language, thus, modifications may be needed for an imposed etic to become an emic concept in the source language, in order to make emic concepts in both languages comparable (Banville, Desrosiers, & Genet-Volet, 2000).

Cultural Bias

A major factor that threatens the validity of cross-cultural measurement is bias. Cultural bias may manifest when the concepts measured differ in meaning across cultural subgroups, that is, when they are not conceptually equivalent, or if the items in the tool differentially represent or underrepresent the concept across cultural subgroups measured, and/or as a result of the measurement method employed, especially in regard to how it is administered.

Specifically, cultural bias can result from poor item translations, inappropriate item content, and/or lack of standardization in administration procedures. Thus, three types of bias are of concern in cross-cultural measurement: construct, method, and item bias. *Construct bias* is a threat to validity when the construct measured is not identical across cultural groups, when there is no associated construct and/or dissimilar behaviors define the construct across culture(s), or when the construct is underrepresented in the instrument or method being employed to measure it. Van de Vijver and Poortinga (1997) identify the following sources of construct bias:

- Differences in the appropriateness of content
- Inadequate sampling of all relevant behaviors
- Underrepresentation of the construct
- Incomplete overlap of the construct across cultures (p. 26).

This threat can be avoided by pretesting the measure with informants representative of the cultures of interest asking them to describe the concept and its characteristic behaviors (Serpell, 1993), or by comparing factor structures of scores across the cultural subgroups. For example, Wilson, Hutchinson, and Holzemer (1997) used a grounded theory approach with an ethnically diverse population of Hispanic, Anglo-American, and African-American people living with advanced HIV, family and significant others, caregivers, and experts in HIV/AIDS, to ascertain their conceptualization of quality of life.

Bias can also result from the method of measurement employed and/or from the manner in which it is administered. For example, Hui and Triandis (1989) found that Hispanics tended to choose extremes on a five-point rating scale more often than did White Americans. Similarly, Iwata, Roberts, and Kawakami (1995) who employed Likert-type scales with a Puerto Rican sample of diabetic patients, and Bernal, Wooley, and Schensul (1997) who compared Japanese and U.S. workers using a depression scale, found differences across cultures in how subjects responded to this method.

Method bias is a function of how members of different cultural groups respond to a specific type of measurement instrument or method. For example, experience with the procedures for responding to a particular type of measure may vary across cultures, and/or communication between an interviewer and interviewee may be adversely affected by language problems when the interview language is the second language of the interviewer. Specific sources of method bias according to Van de Vijver and Poortinga (1997) include:

- Differences in tendency toward social desirability
- Response style differences such as tendency to acquiescence
- Lack of sampling comparability on variables such as age, gender, educational background
- Physical conditions of administration differ
- Familiarity with response procedures differs
- Interviewer effects
- Interviewer-respondent effects such as communication problems (p. 26)

Van de Vijver and Poortinga (1992) note that cross-cultural studies often involve highly dissimilar groups as a result of how subjects are sampled across cultural groups. As a result, groups often differ in background characteristics that may not be relevant to the measurement purpose thus, adversely affecting the validity of resulting scores and their comparability with scores of other groups.

Owens, Johnson, and O'Rourke (1999) in studying responses of minority group respondents and members of acculturated immigrant groups to four large health-related surveys, found higher nonresponse rates among one or more of the minority groups when compared with non-Hispanic White respondents. African-American respondents commonly had higher item nonresponse rates to health questions as did males. In both subject groups they found higher item nonresponse rates among those who had lower incomes, males, and those who were less educated. More educated respondents were more likely to refuse to answer income questions and less likely to answer "don't know" to them. Older respondents were more likely to refuse to answer income questions. They concluded that trends in refusals and "don't know" responses suggested problems with information processing, and social desirability explained differences across cultures. For example, Hispanics refused to answer questions concerned with their social relationships that, based upon well documented importance of family ties and unwillingness to report other than positive interactions with family and friends, led to their higher item nonresponse.

Bias at the item level usually results from cross-cultural differences in the appropriateness of the item content, inadequate item formulation (i.e., when the wording employed is too complex), and inadequate translation. Sources of item bias include:

- Poor item translation
- Inadequate item formulation
- Additional traits or abilities invoked by items
- Incidental differences in appropriateness of the item content such as when the topic of the item is not present in one cultural

group (Van de Vijver & Poortinga, 1997, p. 26).

Bias at the item level is evidenced when subjects of the same ability level who are members of different cultural subgroups differ in their responses to an item(s). This type of bias is referred to as *Differential Item Function* (DIF). The relationship between item format and DIF of translated items has been studied by Angoff and Cook (1988) who found greater DIF in antonym and analogy items and less DIF in sentence completion and reading comprehension items in translating from English to Spanish. Similar findings resulted from the studies of Gafni and Canaan-Yehoshafat (1993) and Beller (1995) who also found that items translated from Hebrew to Russian, demonstrated the most DIF in analogy items and the least DIF in the logic and sentence completion items. In an attempt to understand the causes of DIF with an eye to developing item writing guidelines to minimize DIF in translated items, Allalouf, Hambleton, and Sireci (1999) conducted a study to identify the types of verbal items most likely to display DIF when translated from one language to another, Hebrew to Russian. To detect causes of DIF, they employed two procedures: (1) analysis of DIF direction, i.e. which group performed better on which items and item types, and (2) analysis by translators of the type and content of the DIF items (p. 187). Their findings indicated that 34% of the items demonstrated DIF across languages, and that the most problematic item formats were analogy items (65%), and sentence completion items (45%), respectively. Further, they found that the primary reasons for DIF were changes in word difficulty and item format, differences in cultural relevance, and changes in content (pp. 194–195). DIF is discussed in chapter 6 along with suggested approaches for detecting when it is present in a measure. Other examples of studies of cross-cultural differences in response patterns can be found in the work of Jones and Kay (1992), Iwata, Roberts, and Kawakami (1995), and Lee, Jones, Mineyama, and Zhang (2002).

Strategies for minimizing the effect of method bias include the following:

1. Adverse effects from the presence of a culturally different individual, (such as an interviewer or researcher or data collector) at the time of administration can be minimized by:
   - introducing the individual to respondents and affording them opportunities to become familiar with the individual before the measurement
   - adequately training individuals to perform in a culturally relevant manner and by making them aware of potential adverse effects and how to avoid them
   - statistically assessing the effects a posteriori, employing a procedure such as analysis of covariance using attributes of the individual (e.g., attitudes toward the phenomenon being measured, age, gender, ethnicity) as the covariant
   - conducting postadministration interviews and/or focus groups with respondents to assess these effects
2. Sampling procedures in cross-cultural measurement may result in inclusion of subjects who differ within a specific culture, as well as across cultures, with regard to variables not measured that may affect the phenomenon of interest and hence may have an adverse impact on the measurement results. To avoid such effects, it is important to:
   - consider a priori respondent attributes identified in the literature and in previous studies that potentially may have an impact on how they respond to the measure.
   - undertake a pilot study to investigate the reliability and validity of the measure that includes assessment of differences in the attributes of those selected for inclusion in the sample that may affect the phenomenon under study, and the ability of those selected to respond to the specific method of measurement being employed
3. Bias resulting from the measure method, item format, and/or administration procedure can be reduced by:
   - administering the measure to a sample of respondents from the target group,

and either during or immediately following the completion of the measure, interviewing them regarding their reactions to various attributes of the measure, and/or asking them to explain or interpret their responses to the items included in the measure

- assessing the extent to which the type of measurement method employed influences respondents scores on the measure, using multitrait, multimethod analysis that is discussed in chapter 6
- conducting interviews or focus groups with subjects during pretesting to ascertain their familiarity and/or previous experience with the method of measurement and/or item format to be employed
- undertaking a covariate analysis post-measurement to assess the effect of previous experience on resulting scores

Further, Allalouf, Hambleton, and Sireci (1999) note that differential item functioning (DIF) detection is an important component of test adaptation and, if known, factors affecting DIF should be taken into account before test administration, rather than post hoc, as is now most often the case.

Translation Approaches

Increased awareness of worldwide health problems and the formation of international educational, research, and clinical collaborations to address them, have made the need to develop instruments that can be readily translated into other languages a salient concern. Brislin, Lonner, and Thorndike (1973) proposed the following rules that are still relevant today for developing instruments in English that can be easily translated into other languages:

- Use short, simple sentences of less than 16 words with a single or main idea in each sentence
- Use the active voice, since it is easier to translate, and avoid the passive voice
- Repeat nouns rather than using pronouns
- Avoid metaphors and idioms, because they

are least likely to have equivalent meanings in the target language

- Avoid the conditional mode, i.e. verb forms with would, should, and could.
- Give additional sentences to provide a context for key ideas
- Avoid the use of adverbs and prepositions (i.e. where or when, frequent, beyond, and upper) should be avoided since they do not usually have direct equivalent meanings in other languages.
- Avoid possessive forms since the concept of ownership may not have the same meaning across cultures.
- Use specific terms and avoid general terms
- Avoid words that can generate vague meaning regarding a thing or event (e.g., probably, maybe, or perhaps)
- Avoid sentences that contain two different verbs if those verbs suggest different actions.

Other considerations in employing measures cross-culturally are the reading level required of subjects responding to instruments, and the methods requiring them to read and provide a written response. The Flesch-Kincaid readability index computed for the source language instrument should be determined and should as a rule of thumb be at the grade level of 6 or 7, as is commonly recommended for patient educational materials (Estrada, Hryniewicz, Higgs, Collins, & Byrd, 2000).

Asymmetrical translation (unicentered) refers to translation where the target language remains loyal to the source language. A *unicentered translation strategy* is employed when operational goals are used to examine the cultural distance between groups or the degree of acculturation and the source language group functions as the criteria for interpreting scores of the target group. This strategy allows the target language version to remain loyal to the original.

When the study purpose is to examine cultural differences or acculturation, a symmetrical approach is indicated. *Symmetrical translation* refers to a translation where both source language and target language are open to revision. Both languages are considered equally important and a researcher does not focus on one particular language. *Decentering* is a process used in symmetrical translation. A *decentered translation strategy* is used when the target language is unnatural and/or very different, thus requiring comparative goals to be used to examine the phenomenon across cultures. A decentered translation strategy allows the source and target languages to remain loyal to meanings and allows revision in order to improve meaning and meaning equivalence. Decentered translation is preferred for use with new measures. Werner and Campbell (1970) suggest that instruments should be developed by collaborators from the two cultures. In the decentering process, the researcher reads the backtranslation to identify words and concepts that cannot be well translated and then consults with bilinguals to revise the source language version, a process that continues until evidence for equivalence is obtained. Steps undertaken when a decentered translation strategy is employed include:

- Translation from the source to the target language
- Translation from the target language back to the source language
- Committee review of the translation and backtranslation
- Pretesting for equivalence using appropriate techniques
- Assuring cross-cultural equivalence with regard to content, semantics, technical issues, criteria, and conceptual equivalencies

Backtranslation, a process used to verify a translated version, includes the following:

- The translated version is translated back into the source language
- Psychometric equivalence for original and target versions are assessed using monolingual or bilingual subjects
- A translation error may be influenced by whether the source and target language are similar in structure
- Translation errors can be corrected through the comprehensive processes of translation and backtranslation.

Establishing evidence for reliability and validity is essential for credibility of the measurement results. Comparing the psychometric properties of the source and target language versions provides additional data for assessing equivalence.

Issues addressed earlier in this section that need to be considered and adequately addressed when translation methodologies are undertaken include linguistic adaptation, cultural concepts, and psychometric properties. As noted earlier, when undertaking a translation process, it is necessary to be aware of linguistic differences between the two cultures. Linguistic differences may involve grammatical structures and literal meaning of words. When there are grammatical and structural differences between the source and target languages, the process of translation is more difficult than when there are none. Relevance of the concepts to be measured should be investigated by conducting a review of the literature in the culture in which the translation is to occur to ascertain the importance of the phenomenon in that culture and the extent to which it has been measured and/or researched. Cross-cultural equivalence should be considered by examining the characteristics of philosophy and the written and spoken language, and their congruence or lack thereof within the culture in which the original tool was developed and tested and the culture within which it will be employed.

Psychometric properties of the target language instrument may differ from that of the source language version. Thus, it is imperative that reliability and validity studies of both instruments be undertaken and compared, and that necessary modifications be made in either or both prior to use in research.

Translation Methodologies

One-way translation refers to the use of a bilingual translator who translates the instrument from the source language into the target language. The advantage of one-way translation is that it is simple and inexpensive. The disadvantages are that the translated instruments are solely dependent upon the skill and knowledge of one translator and that the translated instruments are likely to have less evidence for reliability and validity when compared with the original ones.

With *forward translation,* multiple translators work in collaboration to conduct a source-to-target language translation. A second group of translators judge the equivalence of the two versions. Variations of this approach are referred to as "decentering" or "focus group translation" or "translation by committee". An equal value is placed on both languages in each of these approaches. That is, a word in the source language is subject to change in order to more closely approximate the word that is most appropriate to use in the target language. Adaptations of source language cannot be made to standardized measures or copyrighted materials, which is a drawback to the use of these translation strategies. The advantage of translation by committee is that it is less time consuming than backtranslation. Disadvantages stem from the fact that translators who have similar backgrounds may share common cultural perceptions, may be influenced by their peers, and/or be reluctant to criticize each other's work. In addition, the committee may produce an accurate translation, that could, however, be inappropriate for the target population and/or they may not take into account relevant socioeconomic and cultural factors of the target population, thus rendering the translated instrument not applicable.

Backtranslation, also referred to as *double translation,* involves the use of two translators. Working independently, one translates the items from the primary (source) to a second (target) language, and the second translates the items back to the original source language. The two original language versions are compared to identify flaws in the target language version.

In many cases, original items are prepared in a dual language format in which items in the source and target language appear next to each other allowing bilingual responders to double check the understanding of a statement by reading each item a second time in the alternative language, thus, enhancing the understanding of the question by incorporating the best sense derived from each language version. This format also allows for instruments to be completed with the assistance of family or friends who may be at various levels of competency in either language, and who, therefore can also benefit from the immediately available translation.

A key to successful use of this method is the use of translators who are native speakers and readers of the target language. A drawback to the method is that the cultural context in which the translation is imbedded involves the life experience of only two individuals who may share a common world view due to similar backgrounds. Limitations of backtranslation can be minimized by emphasizing instrument adaptation instead of translation (Geisinger, 1994), and by providing explicit instructions to translators regarding inference, wording, and phrasing to enhance conceptual equivalence (Marin & Marin, 1991). It is also desirable to select translators from different backgrounds to avoid the shared world view and to use more than two translators and multiple iterations, even though it is time consuming and expensive. Werner and Campbell (1970) suggest the use of expert panels and multiple translators in multistage backtranslation procedures, including the use of professional translators, monolingual lay people who represent the population of interest, bilinguals with the source language as their first language, and bilinguals with the target language as their first language.

When employing both the forward and backtranslation methods, the selection of translators who are ethnically and culturally representative of the population among whom the method will be employed is a priority consideration, and a translation consensus that incorporates and reflects the complexities of idiomatic language and cultural values is the intended outcome (Carlson, 2000; Sireci, 1997). The following criteria should be taken into account in selecting translators. In both cases, translators should be fluent in both the source and target language and familiar with both cultures (Bontempo, 1993; Twinn, 1997), and should have learned both languages at different times and in different cultures. Source language translators should be knowledgeable about the constructs being measured and how the measure will be used (Geisinger, 1994) while target language translators should not be aware of the intent and concepts underlying the measure (Guillemin, Bombardier, & Beaton, 1993). The background of the translators should be included in the methodological section of reports.

Successful translations from one culture to another are most likely to occur when the following conditions prevail:

- Translators use terms that refer to real experiences that are familiar in both cultures.
- Translators assess that each item developed in the source culture describes a phenomenon that is relevant to the target culture and make the necessary modifications when they are not.
- Each item has the same meaning in the source and target language.
- When necessary, in translating sentences, grammatical changes are made
- In translating idioms, translators recognize differences in meaning and take steps to assure that idioms have equivalent meanings in the two languages.
- The source version and the target version of the instrument are administered in the same manner so that valid comparisons of the findings from the two measures can be made.
- Methods for assessing concepts are comparable between the two cultures in terms of the resulting data.

Evaluative and Psychometric Testing

Translated instruments are usually pretested using three techniques: random probe technique, committee approach, and field testing with bilinguals. When the *random probe approach* is employed:

- A researcher selects a random sample of items from a translated instrument.
- Individuals from the target population are then asked individually to read or listen to each item and paraphrase their understanding of the item.
- An open-ended question such as "What do you think this question asks?" is used for this purpose and individuals verbalize their understanding by answering the question, or individuals are asked to answer each question in the instrument and then asked, "What do you mean?"

- If they cannot justify their responses or their justification is unusual, it suggests that the intent of the question is not being conveyed.
- Responses are expected to closely resemble the source language version, and if discrepancies are found, they are analyzed for mistranslation so changes can be made.

When the *committee approach* is employed:

- Two or more experts review the clarity and linguistic appropriateness of the translated version of an instrument (Geisinger, 1994).
- Experts usually meet face to face and discuss the merits of each item (Brislin, Lonner, & Thorndike, 1973).
- An optimum translation is selected based upon all contributed opinions.

Field testing with bilinguals involves the following:

- Both versions of the instrument are administered to bilingual individuals from the target population, with the intent of detecting possible discrepancies (Guillemin, Bombardier, & Beaton, 1993).
- Subjects are asked to rate each item regarding its equivalence between the source and target versions.
- Items rated low on equivalence or items with discrepancies are revised.
- Item scores of respondents can also be compared with their total scores between the two versions.
- Items with different scores should be examined and retranslated.
- Item and total scores that are highly correlated between the two versions are desirable and suggest that the two versions are likely to be equivalent.
- Item analysis is performed to examine if specific items perform differently on the two versions since total scores may hide inconsistency (Hilton & Skrutkowski, 2002).

Such field testing with bilinguals may not be feasible in all settings because of difficulty in finding representation from the target population. Having bilinguals rate the equivalence of the two versions affords insight into the quality of the translation. On the other hand, bilinguals are used based on the assumption that they represent the monolingual target population. Criticisms of employing bilinguals, however, stem from the fact that they may differ from monolinguals to which the translated instrument will be administered in that they most likely have adopted culture, concepts, norms, and/or values of the second language they mastered (Hilton & Skrutkowski, 2002). Translators whose items are consistently rated low on equivalence may not be qualified to translate the instrument. Herrera, DelCampo, and Ames (1993) suggest the inclusion of representatives of the monolingual source and target populations in field testing. Their approach includes:

- Pretesting and posttesting a source language version of the instrument with the monolingual source population to establish a baseline reliability index.
- Pretesting and posttesting a target language version of the instrument with the monolingual target population to determine the reliability of the translated version with the target population.
- Pretesting and posttesting with two bilingual groups and controlling for administration effects by administering two versions of the instrument in alternative sequences.

Once the final version of the translated instrument is obtained, the psychometric properties of both versions of the tool are tested in the target and source groups employing approaches to determining evidence for reliability and validity discussed in chapters 5 and 6. Examples of evaluative and psychometric testing of translated instruments can be found in Chen, Horner, and Percy (2002), who undertook a study to validate a translated smoking self-efficacy survey for Taiwanese children, and in Haddad and Hoeman (2001), who tested a translated version of an Arabic-language version of an English-language questionnaire.

TRIANGULATION

Triangulation affords a means for combining multiple methods in the study of the same phenomenon (Webb, Campbell, Schwartz, & Sechrest 1966; Denzin, 1970; Haase & Myers, 1988; Kimchi, Polivka, & Stevenson, 1991; Thurmond, 2001). When employed within the context of a given study, it enables one to gain a broader perspective on a phenomenon of interest, reduces the probability of bias, and increases the researcher's ability to interpret the findings with a greater degree of confidence (Jick, 1979; Mitchell, 1986; Breitmayer, Ayres, & Knafl, 1993; Foster, 1997; Thurmond, 2001). Risjord, Dunbar, and Moloney (2002) note that in nursing, triangulation is advocated by many researchers as an important strategy for combining qualitative and quantitative methods in order to provide stronger evidential support for a hypothesis and produce more reliable and highly confirmed results than either method would when used alone (Duffy, 1987; Haase & Myers, 1988; Mitchell, 1986; Shih, 1998).

The basic tenet underlying all approaches to triangulation is that the weaknesses in each method employed are compensated for by the counterbalancing strengths of other methods employed within the same measurement effort. It is assumed that triangulation exploits the assets of each measurement method and neutralizes, rather than compounds, the liabilities of other methods (Campbell & Fiske, 1959; Webb, Campbell, Schwartz, & Sechrest, 1966; Bouchard, 1976; Rohner, 1977). When qualitative and quantitative methods are employed in triangulation, they are conceptualized as complementary rather than opposing perspectives—with neither approach necessarily given precedence over the other. Working in combination with each other in an iterative fashion, they enable the investigator to derive a more complete understanding of the phenomenon under study (Rossman & Wilson, 1985; Mitchell, 1986; Duffy, 1987; Sohier, 1988; Knafl & Breitmayer, 1991; Shih, 1998).

According to Mitchell (1986), four principles must be taken into account whenever triangulation is employed:

1. The problem, the kind of data needed regarding the problem, and the relevance of the problem to the methods chosen must be evident.
2. The strengths and weaknesses of each method employed should complement each other.
3. Methods should be selected on the basis of their relevance to the nature of the phenomenon of interest.
4. The methodological approach employed should be continually monitored and evaluated to ensure that the first three principles are being followed. (pp. 22–23)

Triangulation was first applied by Campbell and Fiske (1959) within the context of their multitrait-multimethod approach, which is discussed and illustrated in chapter 6. More recently, the term triangulation has been used to refer to a variety of approaches to employing multiple methods.

Types of Triangulation

Denzin (1970) identified four different types of triangulation: *data, investigator, theoretical,* and *methodological.* More recently, Kimchi, Polivka, and Stevenson (1999) have suggested a fifth type, *analysis* triangulation.

Data triangulation involves the use of multiple sources of data within the same measurement effort to elicit information regarding the phenomenon of interest. Data sources may vary by person, place, or time. For example, information regarding the phenomenon may be collected from different groups of subjects, in different settings, or during different time periods. Each data source is chosen to represent dissimilar comparison to obtain diverse data regarding the phenomenon. Variances in person, place, and time may serve to increase confidence in the findings according to Fielding and Fielding (1986), because it increases the possibility of revealing atypical data or potential for identifying similar patterns.

When *investigator triangulation* is employed, multiple investigators collect and analyze data in regard to the phenomenon of interest. Denzin (1970) suggests that all investigators should

be experts in the phenomenon and all should be directly involved in the conduct of the effort. This type of triangulation increases the probability of greater reliability in the data collection and analysis because it allows for the comparison among investigators and for the detection of potential bias in reporting, coding, or analysis. When data is confirmed by investigators who have had no prior discussion or collaboration with each other, the findings have greater credibility than when this is not the case (Denzin, 1970). Banik (1993) further notes that an advantage of data triangulation is the nature and amount of data generated for interpretation.

Additional advantages of using investigator triangulation include increased credibility of findings from having a team of investigators who are versed in employing both qualitative and quantitative methods (Duffy, 1987; Connelly, Bott, Hoffart, & Taunton, 1997; Beck, 1997) to keep each other on target (Lincoln & Guba, 1985), thus reducing the potential for bias in data collection, reporting, coding and/or analysis of the data (Denzin, 1970; Mitchell, 1986) and contributing to increased reliability (Banik, 1993), internal validity (Boyd, 2000), and value of the findings (Thurmond, 2001). Examples of this type of triangulation can be found in the work of Breitmayer, Ayres, and Knafl (1993) and Knafl, Breitmayer, Gallo, and Zoeller (1996).

Theoretical triangulation involves the use of multiple perspectives and/or hypotheses regarding the phenomenon of interest within the same measurement effort. This approach, which is similar to the method of multiple working hypotheses referred to by Chamberlin (1965), allows several alternative perspectives, each theoretically different but related enough to be considered together and tested within the same data set. When an accepted hypothesis has been tested against rival hypotheses with the same data set, more confidence can be placed in the results.

Advantages of theoretical triangulation result from the fact that it enables one to test various theories by analyzing findings from a common data set (Boyd, 2000), uses more than one theoretical perspective or hypothesis tending to decrease alternative explanations for a phenomenon (Mitchell, 1986), and provides a broader, deeper analysis of findings (Banik, 1993).

Methodological triangulation, in large part because of the various terms used to describe it in the literature, is often the most difficult type to understand. Specifically, it has been referred to as *multimethod, mixed-method,* and *methods triangulation* (Greene & Caracelli, 1997; Barbour, 1998). Goodwin and Goodwin (1984) note that in some cases methodological triangulation when discussed in the literature, refers to research designs and at other times to data collection methods. Further complicating the issue, according to Thurmond (2001, p. 254), is the fact that some authors discuss methodological triangulation in reference to qualitative and quantitative methods, indicating a paradigmatic connection (Greene & Caracelli, 1997; Barbour, 1998) and others in reference to qualitative and quantitative data collection methods, analysis, and interpretation rather than philosophical viewpoints (Goodwin & Goodwin, 1984). In any case, methodological triangulation involves the use of multiple methods in an attempt to decrease the weaknesses and biases of each method and to increase the potential for counterbalancing the weaknesses and biases of one method with the strengths of the other method(s) (Mitchell, 1986, pp. 19–21).

Within the context of measurement, the interest in methodological triangulation relates to its use as a strategy that employs several different methods or procedures for collecting data within a single measurement effort. This type of triangulation is best exemplified by the multitrait-multimethod approach of Campbell and Fiske (1959). Jick (1979) notes that this type of triangulation is most appropriate when the intent is to study complex concepts with multiple dimensions. This approach to triangulation usually takes one of two forms: within method or between method. The *within-method* approach is most often employed when the phenomenon of interest is multidimensional, in that it uses multiple techniques within a given method to collect and interpret data. It is important to recognize that the within-method approach involves the use of two or more data collection procedures from the same design

method, i.e., qualitative or quantitative (Kimchi, Polivka, & Stevenson, 1991). For example, when the survey method is employed, it might involve the use of multiple scales or indices of the phenomenon or, in the case of a qualitative method like participant observation, the use of multiple comparison groups (Jick, 1979). While the within-method approach allows for assessing the reliability of the data, especially internal consistency, it still uses only one method and, hence, has more potential for bias and threats to validity than do other approaches (Webb, Campbell, Schwartz, & Sechrest, 1966; Jick, 1979).

The *between-method* approach, also referred to as *across-method* triangulation, is more complex and allows for the assessment of external validity, especially convergent validity. Jick (1979) notes that this approach, the most frequently employed, is largely a vehicle for cross validation when two or more methods are found to be congruent and yield comparable data. In contrast to the within-method approach, between- or across-method triangulation employs both qualitative and quantitative methods within the context of the same study (Denzin, 1970; Mitchell, 1986; Kimchi, Polivka, & Stevenson, 1991; Boyd, 2000; Thurmond, 2001). For example, using a combination of a questionnaire and focus groups in the same study or employing an unstructured interview with a Q-sort. A second variation of the between-method approach described by Rossman & Wilson (1985) provides for one type of data (e.g., qualitative) to elaborate findings of another (e.g., quantitative). They advocate this approach because such elaboration may not only add to the credibility of the findings, but provide a different perspective on the same phenomenon as well. For example, one method might be used to generate ideas that are tested by another method, as when researchers employ qualitative methods such as interviews of participants and participant observation to better understand a phenomenon, and then use the results to develop or test quantitative methods such as questionnaires. Likewise, results from the administration of a quantitative method such as a questionnaire might be followed by a qualitative investigation using focus groups to better understand and/or expand upon the findings from the questionnaire. Yet another elaboration of between-method triangulation is referred to as *holistic* or *contextual triangulation,* where the purpose is to identify areas where findings do not converge; that is, to uncover paradox and contradiction rather than to seek confirmatory evidence (Rossman & Wilson, 1985). This approach to triangulation, according to Bargar and Duncan (1990) has the potential to produce a significant alteration in the overall perspective with which the phenomenon as a whole has been viewed. Similarly, Jick (1979) recognizes that it allows qualitative methods to play an important role in eliciting data and to suggest conclusions that might be missed by other methods.

Advantages of methodological triangulation include broader representation of world views that is obtained by combining qualitative and quantitative methods (Lincoln & Guba, 2000), qualitative findings that may help to explain the success of interventions when quantitative findings fail to do so (Polit & Hungler, 1995), and quantitative data that can enhance understanding by revealing outliers or unique individual cases (Duffy, 1987; Hinds, 1989). Examples of methodological triangulation can be found in Burr (1998), Connelly, Bott, Hoffart, and Taunton (1997), Wilson and Hutchinson (1991), and Floyd (1993).

Data-analysis triangulation employs two or more approaches to the analysis of the same set of data. It usually involves using different families of statistical testing or different statistical techniques to determine similarities or to validate data (Kimchi, Polivka, & Stevenson, 1991).

According to Mitchell (1986), "when two or more different examples of a particular type of triangulation are present within a single study, that study is said to be triangulated. For example, a *triangulated study* is any study that has several different data sources, or involves multiple investigators or tests multiple competing hypotheses or includes two or more kinds of data collection methods, such as qualitative and quantitative methods" (p. 19). She further notes that the term *multiple triangulation* refers to studies where two or more types of triangulation are represented.

Analysis of Data Resulting From Triangulation

The primary task in analyzing data from triangulation efforts is to determine whether or not results have converged. Jick (1979), in discussing the difficulties in making such a decision, notes that "if there is congruence, it presumably is apparent. In practice, though, there are few guidelines for systematically ordering eclectic data in order to determine congruence or validity" (p. 607). When analyzing triangulation data, the investigator needs to consider the following:

1. Does each method employed demonstrate reliability and validity in its own right?
2. Should all methods employed in the analysis be given equal weight in terms of importance and usefulness? If not, on what basis should the data be weighted?
3. What will constitute evidence for consistency or congruence of methods? (It is essential to be aware of the fact that while statistical tests can be applied to a particular method, there are no universally accepted methods for describing the statistical significance among methods. The concept of significant differences when applied to qualitative methods does not readily compare with statistical tests of the significance of differences in quantitative methods. Similarly, if convergence or agreement is the concern, is it appropriate to use statistical differences as a criterion or should congruence be assessed using relational techniques such as correlation and regression?)
4. When different methods yield dissimilar or divergent results, how will the investigator reconcile and/or explain the differences?

Useful information may be obtained whether or not there is convergence in results. Where there is convergence, one can place more confidence in the reliability of the results and with the probability that they result from trait, rather than method, variance. Another important variance component not provided for in Campbell and Fiske's (1959) multitrait-multimethod approach is measurement error. Eid, Lischetzke, Nussbeck, and Trierweiler (2003, pp. 38–39) recognize that since Campbell and

Fiske's (1959) original work, multitrait-multi-method and multimethod strategies in general have gained in importance, and for this reason a wide array of multidimensional measurement methods for analyzing trait, method, and measurement error components of such data sets have been developed, including confirmatory factor analysis (CFA) models, covariance components models, and the direct product model (Browne, 1984; Kenny & Kashy, 1992; Millsap, 1995; Wothke, 1995, 1996). Readers interested in a more advanced discussion of these approaches to data analysis are referred to their articles.

When divergence results, it is necessary to consider alternative explanations for the unexpected findings. Jick (1979) states that "Overall, the triangulating investigator is left to search for a logical pattern in mixed-method results. His or her claim to validity rests on judgment, or as Weiss (1968, p. 349) calls it, 'a capacity to organize materials within a plausible framework.' One begins to view the researcher as a builder and creator, piecing together many pieces of a complex puzzle into a coherent whole. . . . While one can rely on certain scientific conventions . . . for maximizing the credibility of one's findings, the research using triangulation is likely to rely still more on a feel of the situation. This intuition and first-hand knowledge drawn from multiple vantage points is centrally reflected in the interpretation process" (p. 608).

In general, the following steps should be undertaken in analyzing the data generated from triangulation:

1. Each method employed should be assessed within the context of the present effort for evidence of reliability and validity in its own right.
2. Data in regard to the phenomenon of interest resulting from each method should be analyzed separately according to accepted principles and practices for that particular type of method.
3. Significant findings from the separate analyses should be identified and examined for obvious convergence or divergence across methods.

4. Significant variables should be examined from a conceptual perspective to identify logical patterns of relationships and meanings among findings from the application of different methods, with an eye toward generating new questions or hypotheses to be examined by later measurement efforts.
5. Data from the varied methods should be combined and analyzed for convergence using an appropriate procedure, such as confirmatory factor analysis, bivariate or multiple correlation and/or regression, path analysis, a linear structural relations (LISREL) approach, cross-classification analysis, and/or multiple analysis of variance (MANOVA).

Triangulation is an approach that may not be appropriate in all measurement situations. Because of the need to employ multiple methods, investigator and/or administrative costs may be a factor in some situations in deciding whether or not to use the approach. Because of the challenges in regard to the analysis of data, the approach is best employed in those situations where appropriate resources are available for designing complex analyses, handling large data sets, and/or obtaining the necessary variable-to-subject ratio required for the use of multivariate procedures. Similarly, triangulation may only be undertaken in those instances in which it is possible to identify a common unit of analysis for the design, data collection, and analysis. Mitchell (1986) notes that such a common focus of the data is critical for data from different sources or methods to be combined, and must be part of all aspects of the triangulation.

REFERENCES

Allalouf, A., Hambleton, R. K., & Sireci, S. G. (1999). Identifying the causes of DIF in translated verbal items. *Journal of Educational Measurement, 36*(3), 185–198.

Anastasi, A. (1976). *Psychological testing* (4th ed.). New York: Macmillan.

Angoff, W. H., & Cook, L. L. (1988). *Equating*

the scores of the *Prueba de Aptitud Academica and the Scholastic Aptitude Test* (College Board Report No. 88-2). New York: College Entrance Examination Board.

Aquillino, W. S., Wright, D. L., & Supple, A. J. (2000). Response effects due to bystander presence in CASI and paper and pencil surveys of drug use and alcohol use. *Substance Use and Misuse, 35*(6–8), 845–867.

Atwood, J. R. (1980). A research perspective. *Nursing Research, 29*(2), 104–108.

Babad, E. (1979). Personality correlates of susceptibility to biasing information. *Journal of Personality and Social Psychology, 37*(2), 195–202.

Baker-Ward, L., & Rankin, M. E. (1994, July). *Children's and parents' anxiety at first dental visits: Evidence for mutual influences.* Poster session presented at the annual meetings of the American Psychological Society, Washington, DC.

Bandura, A. (1969). *Principles of behavior modification.* New York: Holt, Rinehart & Winston.

Banik, B. J. (1993). Applying triangulation in nursing research. *Applied Nursing Research, 6*(1), 47–52.

Banville, D., Desrosiers, P., & Genet-Valet, V. (2000). Research note: Translating questionnaires and inventories using a cross-cultural translation technique. *Journal of Teaching in Physical Education, 19*(3), 374–387.

Barbour, R. S. (1998). Mixing qualitative methods: Quality assurance or qualitative quagmire? *Qualitative Health Research, 8*(3), 352–361.

Bargar, R. R., & Duncan, J. K. (1990). Creative endeavor in Ph.D. research. *Journal of Creative Behavior, 24*(1), 50–71.

Beck, C. T. (1997). Developing a research program using qualitative and quantitative approaches. *Nursing Outlook, 45*(6), 265–269.

Becker, W. (1976). Biasing effects of respondents' identification on responses to a social desirability scale: A warning to researchers. *Psychological Reports, 39*(3, Pt. 1), 756–758.

Beller, M. (1995). Translated versions of Israel's inter-university Psychometric Entrance Test (PET). In T. Oakland & R. K. Hambleton (Eds.) *International perspective of academic assessment* (pp. 207–217). Boston, MA: Kluwer Academic Publishers.

Bentler, P., Jackson, D., & Messick, S. (1971). Identification of content and style: A two-dimensional interpretation of acquiescence. *Psychological Bulletin, 76*(3), 186–204.

Berg, I. A. (1961). Measuring deviant behavior by means of deviant response sets. In I. A. Berg & B. M. Bass (Eds.), *Conforming and deviation* (pp. 328–379). New York: Harper & Row.

Bernal, H., Wooley, S., & Schensul, J. J. (1997). The challenge of using Likert-type scales with low-literate ethnic populations. *Nursing Research, 46*(3), 179–181.

Bloch, D. (1980). Interrelated issues in evaluation and evaluation research: A researcher's perspective. *Nursing Research, 29*(1), 69–73.

Bochner, S., & Van Zyl, T. (1987). Desirability rating of 110 personality-trait words. *The Journal of Social Psychology, 125*(4), 459–465.

Boeije, H. R., & Lensvelt-Mulders, G. L. M. (2002). Honest by chance: A qualitative interview study to clarify respondents' non-compliance with computer assisted randomized response. *Bulletin Methodologie Sociologique, 75*, 24–39.

Bontempo, R. (1993). Translation fidelity of psychological scales: An item response theory analysis of an individualism-collectivism scale. *Journal of Cross-Cultural Psychology, 24*(2), 149–166.

Bouchard, T. J. (1976). Unobtrusive measures: An inventory of nurses. *Sociological Methods and Research, 4*(3), 267–300.

Boyd, C. O. (2000). Combining qualitative and quantitative approaches. In P. L. Munhall & C. O. Boyd (Eds.), *Nursing research: A qualitative perspective* (2nd ed., pp. 454–475). Boston: Jones and Bartlett.

Breitmayer, B. J., Ayres, L., & Knafl, K. A. (1993). Triangulation in qualitative research in evaluation of completeness and confirmation purposes. *Image: Journal of Nursing Scholarship, 25*(3), 237–243.

Brislin, R. W., Lonner, W. J., & Thorndike, R. M. (1973). *Cross-cultural research method.* New York: John Wiley and Sons.

Brown, S. J. (2002). Nursing intervention studies: A descriptive analysis of issues important to clinicians. *Research in Nursing & Health, 25*(4), 317–327.

Browne, M. W. (1984). The decomposition of multitrait-multimethod matrices. *British Journal of Mathematical and Statistical Psychology, 37*(1), 1–21.

Bullinger, M., Anderson, R., Cella, D., & Aaronson, N. (1993). Developing and evaluating cross-cultural instruments from minimum requirements to optimal models. *Quality-of-Life Research, 2*(6), 451–459.

Burns, N., & Grove, S. K. (2001). *The practice of nursing research: Conduct, critique, & utilization* (4th ed.). New York: W. B. Saunders Company.

Burr, G. (1998). Contextualizing critical care family needs through triangulation: An Australian study. *Intensive and Critical Care Nursing, 14*(4), 161–169.

Byrne, B. M., & Campbell, T. L. (1999). Cross-cultural comparisons and the presumption of equivalent measurement and theoretical structure: A look beneath the surface. *Journal of Cross-Cultural Psychology, 30*(5), 555–574.

Campbell, D. T., & Fiske, D. W. (1959). Convergent and discriminate validation by the multitrait-multimethod matrix. *Psychological Bulletin, 56*, 81–105.

Carlson, E. D. (2000). A case study in translation methodology using the Health Promotion Lifestyle Profile II. *Public Health Nursing, 17*(1), 61–70.

Carstensen, L., & Cone, J. (1983). Social desirability and the measurement of psychological well-being in elderly persons. *Journal of Gerontology, 38*(6), 713–715.

Chamberlin, T. C. (1965). The method of multiple working hypotheses. *Scientific Monthly, 59*(1944), 357–362.

Chen, C., Lee, S., & Stevenson, H. W. (1995). Response style and cross-cultural comparisons of rating scales among east Asian and North American students. *Psychological Science, 6*(3), 170–175.

Chen, H., Horner, S. D., & Percy, M. S. (2002). Validation of the smoking self-efficacy survey for Taiwanese children. *Journal of Nursing Scholarship, 34*(1), 33–37.

Chinn, P. L., & Kramer, M. K. (1999). *Theory and nursing: Integrated knowledge development* (5th ed.). Philadelphia: Mosby.

Conn, V. S., Rantz, M. J., Wipke-Tevis, D. D., &

Maas, M. L. (2001). Designing effective nursing interventions. *Research in Nursing & Health, 24*(5), 433–442.

Connelly, L. M., Bott, M., Hoffart, N., & Taunton, R. L. (1997). Methodological triangulation in a study of nurse retention. *Nursing Research, 46*(5), 299–302.

Constantine, M. G., & Ladany, N. (2000). Self-report multicultural counseling competence scales: Their relation to social desirability attitudes and multicultural case conceptualization ability. *Journal of Counseling Psychology, 47*(2), 155–164.

Constantine, M. G., & Ladany, N. (2001). New visions for defining and assessing multicultural counseling competence. In J. G. Ponterotto, J. M. Casas, L. A. Suzuki, & C. M. Alexander (Eds.), *Handbook of multicultural counseling* (2nd ed., pp. 482–498). Thousand Oaks, CA: Sage.

Corcoran, S. A. (1986). Task complexity and nursing expertise as factors in decision making. *Nursing Research, 35*(2), 107–112.

Corless, I. B., Nicholas, P. K., & Nokes, K. M. (2001). Issues in cross-cultural quality of life research. *Journal of Nursing Scholarship, 33*(1), 15–20.

Couper, M. P., & Nicholls II, W. L. (1998). The history and development of computer assisted survey information collection methods. In M. P. Couper, R. P. Baker, C. Bethlehem, Z. F. Clark, J. Martin, J., W. L. Nicholls II, & O'Reilly (Eds.), *Computer assisted survey information collection* (pp. 1–21). New York: John Wiley and Sons.

Cronbach, L. J. (1949). *Essentials of psychological testing.* New York: Harper & Row.

Cronbach, L. J. (1970). *Essentials of psychological testing* (3rd ed.). New York: Harper & Row.

Crowne, D., & Marlowe, D. (1964). *The approval motive: Studies in evaluative dependence.* New York: Wiley & Sons.

Denzin, N. (1970). Strategies of multiple triangulation. In N. Denzin (Ed.), *The research act* (pp. 297–313). New York: McGraw-Hill.

Dillman, D. (1978). *Mail and telephone surveys.* New York: John Wiley & Sons.

Dillman, D. A., Phelps, G., Tortora, R., Swift, K., Kohrell, J., & Berck, J. (2001). *Response rate and measurement differences in mixed mode surveys using mail, telephone, interactive voice response and the internet.* Retrieved from http://survey. sesrc. wsu. edu/dillman/papers. htm

Donabedian, A. (1970). Patient care evaluation. *Hospitals, 44,* 131.

Duffy, M. E. (1987). Methodological triangulation: A vehicle for merging quantitative and qualitative research methods. *Image: Journal of Nursing Scholarship, 19*(3), 130–132.

Edwards, A. (1957). *The social desirability variable in personality assessment and research.* New York: Holt, Rinehart & Winston.

Edwards, A. (1970). *The measurement of personality traits by scales and inventories.* New York: Holt, Rinehart & Winston.

Eid, M., Lischetzke, T., Nussbeck, F. W., & Trierweiler, L. I. (2003). Separating trait effects from trait-specific method effects in multi-trait-multimethod models: A multiple indicator CT-C (M-1) model. *Psychological Methods, 8*(1), 38–60.

Ellis, T. (1985). The hopelessness scale and social desirability: More data and a contribution from the irrational beliefs test. *Journal of Clinical Psychology, 41*(5), 635–639.

Estrada, C. A., Hryniewicz, M. M., Higgs, V. B., Collins, C., & Byrd, J. C. (2002). Anticoagulant patient information material is written at high readability levels. *Stroke, 31*(12), 2966–2970.

Ethier, R. G., Poe, G. L., Schulze, W. D., & Clark, J. (2000). A comparison of hypothetical phone and mail contingent valuation responses for green-pricing electricity programs. *Land Economics, 76*(1), 54–67.

Fielding, N. G., & Fielding, J. L. (1986). *Linking data* (vol. 4). Beverly Hills, CA: Sage.

Floyd, J. A. (1993). The use of across-method triangulation in the study of sleep concerns in healthy older adults. *Advances in Nursing Science, 16*(2), 70–80.

Fogg, B. J., & Nass, C. (1997). Silicon sycophants: The effects of computers that flatter. *International Journal of Human-Computer Studies, 46*(5, May), 551–561.

Foster, R. L. (1997). Addressing epistemologic and practical issues in multimethod research: A procedure for conceptual triangulation. *Advances in Nursing Science, 20*(2), 1–12.

Fowler, F. (1984). *Survey research methods.* Beverly Hills: Sage Publications.

Furnham, A. (1986). The social desirability of the type A behavior pattern. *Psychological Medicine, 16*(4), 805–811.

Gafni, N., & Canaan-Yehoshafat, Z. (1993). *An examination of differential item functioning for Hebrew and Russian speaking examinees in Israel.* Paper presented at the Conference of the Israeli Psychological Association, Ramat-Gan.

Geisinger, K. F. (1994). Cross-cultural normative assessment: Translation and adaptation issues influencing the normative interpretation of assessment instruments. *Psychological Assessment, 6*(4), 304–312.

Gibson, D., Wermuth, L., Sorensen, J., Manicucci, L., & Bernal, G. (1987). Approval need in self-reports of addicts and family members. *The International Journal of the Addictions, 22*(9), 895–903.

Gillis, A., & Jackson, W. (2002). *Research for nurses methods and interpretation.* Philadelphia: F. A. Davis Co.

Goldfried, M. R., & Kent, R. N. (1972). Traditional versus behavioral personality assessment: A comparison of methodological and theoretical assumptions. *Psychological Bulletin, 77*(4), 409–420.

Good, M., Stiller, C., Zauszniewski, J. A., Anderson, J. C., Stanton-Hicks, M., & Grass, J. A. (2001). Sensation and distress of pain scales: Reliability, validity, and sensitivity. *Journal of Nursing Measurement, 9*(3), 219–238.

Goodwin, L. D., & Goodwin, W. I. (1984). Qualitative vs. quantitative research or qualitative and quantitative research? *Nursing Research, 33*(6), 378–380.

Greene, J. C., & Caracelli, V. J. (1997). *Advances in mixed-method evaluation: The challenges and benefits of integrating diverse paradigms.* San Francisco: Jossey-Bass.

Grimm, P. M. (1989). *Hope, affect, psychological status, and the cancer experience.* Dissertation, School of Nursing, University of Maryland, Baltimore.

Guillemin, F., Bombardier, C., & Beaton, D. (1993). Cross-cultural adaptation of health-related quality of life measures: Literature review and proposed guidelines. *Journal of Clinical Epidemiology, 46*(12), 1417–1532.

Gupta, S. (2002, December 21–23). *Circumventing social desirability response bias using randomized response techniques.* Paper presented at Ninth International Conference of Forum for Interdisciplinary Mathematics on Statistics Combinatorics and Related Areas. Allahabad, India.

Haase, J. E., & Myers, S. T. (1988). Reconciling paradigm assumptions of qualitative and quantitative research. *Western Journal of Nursing Research, 10*(2), 128–137.

Haddad, L. G., & Hoeman, S. P. (2001). Development of the Arabic language readiness to stop smoking questionnaire A-RSSQ. *Journal of Nursing Scholarship, 33*(4), 355–359.

Hambleton, R. K. (1994). Guidelines for adapting educational and psychological tests: A progress report. *European Journal of Psychological Assessment, 10*(3), 229–234.

Hays, R., & Ware, J. (1986). My medical care is better than yours. *Medical Care, 24*(6), 519–523.

Helmes, E., & Holden, R. (1986). Response styles and faking on the basic personality inventory. *Journal of Consulting and Clinical Psychology, 54*(6), 853–859.

Herrera, R. S., DelCampo, R. L., & Ames, M. H. (1993). A serial approach for translating family science instrumentation. *Family Relations, 42*(3), 357–360.

Hilton, A., & Skrutkowski, M. (2002). Translating instruments into other languages: Development and testing processes. *Cancer Nursing, 25*(1), 1–7.

Hinds, P. S. (1988). Adolescent hopefulness in illness and health. *Advances in Nursing Science, 10*(3), 79–88.

Hinds, P. S. (1989). Method triangulation to index change in clinical phenomena. *Western Journal of Nursing Research, 11*(4), 440–447.

Hogan, H., & Mookherjee, H. (1980). A multitrait test of social desirability. *The Journal of Social Psychology, 111*(2), 307–308.

Hogan, R., & Nicholson, R. (1988). The meaning of personality test scores. *American Psychologist, 43*(8), 621–626.

Holden, R., & Mendonca, J. (1984). Hopelessness, social desirability, and suicidal behav-

ior: A need for conceptual and empirical disentanglement. *Journal of Clinical Psychology, 40*(6), 1342–1344.

Hui, C. H., & Triandus, H. C. (1989). Effects of culture and response format on extreme response style. *Journal of Cross-Culture Psychology, 20*(3), 296–309.

Hwang, C., Yan, W., & Scherer, R. (1996). Understanding managerial behavior in different cultures: A review of instrument translation methodology. *International Journal of Management, 13*(3), 332–339.

Iwata, N., Roberts, C. R., & Kawakami, N. (1995). Japan–U. S. comparison of responses to depression scale items among adult workers. *Psychiatry Research, 58*(2), 237–245.

Jacobson, L. Berger, S., & Millham, J. (1970). Individual differences in cheating during a temptation period when confronting failure. *Journal of Personality and Social Psychology, 15*(1), 48–56.

Jacobson, L., Brown, R., & Ariza, M. (1983). A revised multidimensional social desirability inventory. *Bulletin of the Psychonomic Society, 21*(5), 391–392.

Jacobson, L., Kellogg, R., Cauce, A., & Slavin, R. (1977). A multidimensional social desirability inventory. *Bulletin of the Psychonomic Society, 9*(2), 109–110.

Jick, T. D. (1979). Mixing qualitative and quantitative methods: Triangulation in action. *Administrative Science Quarterly, 24*(4), 602–611.

Johnson, T. P., & Fendrich, M. (2002). *A validation of the Crowne-Marlowe Social Desirability Scale.* Presented at the Annual Meeting of the American Association for Public Opinion Research. St. Petersburg, Florida, May 2002.

Jones, E., & Kay, M. (1992). Instrumentation in cross-cultural research. *Nursing Research, 41*(3), 186–188.

Jones, E., & Sigall, H. (1971). The bogus pipeline: A new paradigm for measuring affect and attitude. *Psychological Bulletin, 76*(5), 349–364.

Kenny, D. A., & Kashy, D. A. (1992). Analysis of the multitrait-multimethod matrix by confirmatory factor analysis. *Psychological Bulletin, 112*, 165–172.

Kimchi, J., Polivka, B., & Stevenson, J. S.

(1991). Triangulation: Operational definitions. *Nursing Research, 40*(6), 364–366.

Klockars, A. (1975). Evaluative confounding in the choice of bipolar scales. *Psychological Reports, 45,* 771–775.

Knafl, K. A., & Breitmayer, B. J. (1991). Triangulation in qualitative research: Issues of conceptual clarity and purpose. In J. M. Morse (Ed.), *Qualitative research: A contemporary dialogue* (pp. 226–239). Newbury Park, CA: Sage.

Knafl, K., Breitmayer, B., Gallo, A., & Zoeller, L. (1996). Family response to childhood chronic illness: Description of management styles. *Journal of Pediatric Nursing: Nursing Care of Children and Families, 11*(5), 315–326.

Knapp, T. R., Kimble, L. P., & Dunbar, S. B. (1998). Distinguishing between the stability of a construct and the stability of an instrument in trait/state measurement. *Nursing Research, 47*(1), 60–62.

Knowles, E. (1988). Item context effects on personality scales: Measuring changes the measure. *Journal of Personality and Social Psychology, 55*(2), 312–320.

Kral, M. (1986). Item, person, and situation models of social desirability in personality measurement. *Dissertation Abstracts International, 46*(08), 2814B.

Krause, N. (1985). Stress, control beliefs, and psychological distress: The problem of response bias. *Journal of Human Stress, 11*(1), 11–19.

Krosnick, J. A. (1999). Surveys research. *Annual Review of Psychology, 50,* 537–567.

Krosnick, J. A., & Chang, L. (2001). *A comparison of the random digit dialing telephone survey methodology with internet survey methodology as implemented by Knowledge Networks and Harris Interactive.* Retrieved from http://www. psy. ohio-state. edu/social/kronick. htm

Kulik, J. A., Mahler, H. I. M., & Earnest, A. (1994). Social comparison and affiliation under threat: Going beyond the affiliate-choice paradigm. *Journal of Personality and Social Psychology, 66*(2), 301–309.

Lauver, D. R., Ward, S. E., Heidrich, S. M., Keller, M. L., Bowers, B. J., Brennan, P. F., et al. (2002). Patient-centered interventions. *Research in Nursing & Health, 25*(4), 246–255.

Lee, J. W., Jones, P. S., Mineyama, Y., & Zhang, X. E. (2002). Cultural difference in responses to a Likert scale. *Research in Nursing and Health, 25*(4), 295–306.

Leeuw, E. D., Hox, J. J., & Snijkers, G. (1998). The effect of computer assisted interviewing on data quality. In B. Blyth (Ed.), *Market research and information technology* (pp. 173–198). Amsterdam: Esomar.

Lincoln, Y. S., & Guba, E. G. (1985). *Naturalistic inquiry.* Newbury Park, CA: Sage.

Maddala, G. S. (1983). *Limited dependent and qualitative variables in econometrics.* Cambridge: Cambridge University Press.

Marin, G., & Marin, B. (1991). *Research with Hispanic populations.* Newbury Park, CA: Sage Publications.

McCrae, R. (1986). Well-being scales do not measure social desirability. *Journal of Gerontology, 41*(3), 390–392.

McGovern, F., & Nevid, J. (1986). Evaluation apprehension on psychological inventories in a prison-based setting. *Journal of Consulting and Clinical Psychology, 54*(4), 576–578.

Millham, J., & Kellogg, R. (1980). Need for social approval: Impression management or self-deception? *Journal of Research in Personality, 14*(4), 445–457.

Millsap, R. E. (1995). The statistical analysis of method effects in multitrait-multimethod data: A review. In P. E. Shrout & S. T. Fiske (Eds.), *Personality research methods, and theory: A Festschrift honoring D. W. Fiske* (pp. 93–109). Hillsdale, NJ: Erlbaum.

Mischel, W. (1969). Continuity and change in personality. *American Psychologist, 24*(11), 1012–1018.

Mischel, W. (1973). Toward a cognitive social learning reconceptualization of personality. *Psychological Review, 80*(4), 252–283.

Mitchell, E. S. (1986). Multiple triangulation: A methodology for nursing science. *Advances in Nursing Science, 8*(3), 18–26.

Nass, C., Fogg, B. J., & Moon, Y. (1996). Can computers be teammates? *International Journal of Human-Computer Studies, 45*(6), 669–678.

Nass, C., Moon, Y., & Carney, P. (1999). Are respondents polite to computers? Social desirability and direct response to computers.

Journal of Applied Social Psychology, 29(5), 1093–1110.

Nunnally, J. C., & Bernstein, I. H. (1994). *Psychometric theory* (3rd ed). New York: McGraw-Hill.

O'Grady, K. (1988). The Marlowe-Crowne and Edwards social desirability scales: A psychometric perspective. *Multivariate Behavioral Research, 23*(1), 87–101.

Otto, R., Lang, A., Magargee, E., & Rosenblatt, A. (1988). Ability of alcoholics to escape detection by the MMPI. *Journal of Consulting and Clinical Psychology, 56*(3), 452–457.

Owens, L., Johnson, T. P., & O'Rourke, D. (1999). *Culture and item nonresponse in health surveys.* Paper presented at the meeting of the 7th Conference on Health Survey Research Methods. Williamsburg, VA.

Phillips, D. (1972). Some effects of "social desirability" in survey studies. *American Journal of Sociology, 77*(5), 921–940.

Piantadosi, S. (1997). *Clinical trials: A methodologic approach.* New York: Wiley.

Polit, D. F., & Hungler, B. P. (1995). *Nursing research: Principles and methods* (6th ed.). Philadelphia: Lippincott.

Ponterotto, J. G., Rieger, B. P., Barrett, A., Harris, G., Sparks, R., Sanchez, C. M., & Magids, D. (1996). Development and initial validation of the multicultural counseling awareness scale. In G. R. Sodowsky & J. C. Impara (Eds.), *Multicultural assessment in counseling and clinical psychology* (pp. 247–282). Lincoln, NE: Burns Institute of Mental Measurements.

Pope-Davis, D. B., & Dings, J. G. (1995). The assessment of multicultural counseling competencies. In J. G. Ponterotto, J. M. Casas, L. A. Suzuki, & C. M. Alexander (Eds.), *Handbook of multicultural counseling* (pp. 287–311). Thousand Oaks, CA: Sage.

Ray, J. (1984). The reliability of short social desirability scales. *The Journal of Social Psychology, 123*(1), 133–134.

Reynolds, W. (1982). Development of reliable and valid short forms of the Marlowe-Crowne social desirability scale. *Journal of Clinical Psychology, 38*(1), 119–125.

Risjord, M. W., Dunbar, S. B., & Moloney, M. F. (2002). A new foundation for methodological triangulation. *Journal of Nursing Scholarship, 34*(3), 269–275.

Rohner, R. P. (1977). Advantages of the comparative method of anthropology. *Behavior Science Research, 12*(2), 117–144.

Rorer, L. (1965). The great response-style myth. *Psychological Bulletin, 63*(3), 129–156.

Rossman, G. B., & Wilson, B. L. (1985). Numbers and words: Combining quantitative and qualitative methods in a single large-scale evaluation study. *Evaluation Review, 9*(5), 627–643.

Rothert, M., Homes-Rovner, D., Rovener, D., Kroll, J., Breer, L., Talarcqyk, G., et al. (1997). An educational intervention as decision support for menopausal women. *Research in Nursing & Health, 20*(5), 377–387.

Scheers, N. J., & Dayton, C. M. (1987). Improved estimation of academic cheating behaviors using the randomized response technique. *Research in Higher Education, 26*(1), 61–69.

Serpell, R. (1993). *The significance of schooling: Life-journeys in an African society.* Cambridge, UK: Cambridge University Press.

Shih, F. J. (1998). Triangulation in nursing research: Issues of conceptual clarity and purpose. *Journal of Advanced Nursing, 28*(3), 631–641.

Sidani, S., & Braden, C. P. (1998). *Evaluating nursing interventions: A theory-driven approach.* Thousand Oaks, CA: Sage Publications.

Silverstein, A. (1983). Validity of random short forms: II. The Marlowe-Crowne social desirability scale. *Journal of Clinical Psychology, 39*(4), 582–584.

Sireci, G. (1997). Problems and issues in linking assessments across languages. *Educational Measurement: Issues and Practice, 16*(1), 12–19.

Sodowsky, G. R., Kuo-Jackson, P. Y., Richardson, M. F., & Corey, A. T. (1998). Correlates of self-reported multicultural competencies: Counselor multicultural social desirability, race, social inadequacy, locus of control, racial ideology, and multicultural training. *Journal of Counseling Psychology, 45*(3), 256–264.

Sohier, R. (1988). Multiple triangulation and

contemporary nursing research. *Western Journal of Nursing Research, 10*(6), 732–742.

Speilberger, C. D., et al. (1983). *Manual for the State-Trait Anxiety Inventory.* Palo Alto, CA: Consulting Psychologists Press.

Strickland, O. L. (1995). Assessment of perinatal indicators for the measurement of programmatic effectiveness. *Journal of Neonatal Nursing, 9*(1), 52–67.

Strickland, O. L. (1997). Challenges in measuring patient outcomes. *Nursing Clinics of North America, 32*(3), 495–512.

Strickland, O. L., & DiIorio, C. (Eds.). (2003a). *Measurement of nursing outcomes: Client outcomes and quality of care* (2nd ed., vol. 2). New York: Springer Publishing.

Strickland, O. L., & DiIorio, C. (Eds.). (2003b). *Measurement of nursing outcomes: Self care and coping* (2nd ed., vol. 3). New York: Springer Publishing.

Strosahl, K., Linehan, M., & Chiles, J. (1984). Will the real social desirability please stand up? Hopelessness, depression, social desirability, and the prediction of suicidal behavior. *Journal of Consulting and Clinical Psychology, 52*(3), 449–457.

Taylor, H. (2000). Does internet research work? Comparing online survey results with telephone survey. *International Journal of Market Research, 42*(1), 51–63.

Thurmond, V. A. (2001). The point of triangulation. *Journal of Nursing Scholarship, 33*(3), 253–258.

Tourangeau, R., Rips, L. J., & Rasinski, K. A. (2000). *The psychology of survey response.* Cambridge, NY: Cambridge University Press.

Tourangeau, R., & Smith, T. (1998). Collecting sensitive information with different modes of data collection. In M. P. Couper, R. P. Baker, C. Bethlehem, Z. F. Clark, J. Martin, J., W. L. Nicholls II, & O'Reilly (Eds.), *Computer assisted survey information collection* (pp. 431–453). New York: John Wiley and Sons.

Turner, C. F., Forsyth, B. H., O'Reilly, J. M., Cooley, P. C., Smith, T. R., Rogers, S. M., & Miller, H. G. (1998a). Automated self-interviewing and the survey measurement of sensitive behaviors. In M. P. Couper, R. P.

Baker, C. Bethlehem, Z. F. Clark, J. Martin, J., W. L. Nicholls II, & O'Reilly (Eds.), *Computer assisted survey information collection* (pp. 455–473). New York: John Wiley and Sons.

Turner, C. F., Ku, L., Rogers, S. M., Lindberg, L. D., Pleck, J. H., & Sonenstein, F. L. (1998b). Adolescent sexual behavior, drug use and violence: Increased reporting with computer survey technology. *Science, 280*(5365), 867–873.

Twinn, S. (1997). An exploratory study examining the influence of translation on the validity and reliability of qualitative data in nursing research. *Journal of Advanced Nursing, 26*(2), 418–423.

Van der Heijden, P. G. M., & Van Gils, G. (1996). Some logistic regression models for randomized response data. In A. Forcina, G. M. Marcheti, R. Hotzinger, & G. Salmatti (Eds.), *Statistical modeling: Proceedings of the 11th international workshop on statistical modeling.* Ormeto, Italy.

Van de Vijver, F. J. R., & Leung, K. (1997). *Methods and data analysis for cross-culture research.* Beverly Hills, CA: Sage.

Van de Vijver, F. J. R., & Poortinga, Y. H. (1992). Testing in culturally heterogeneous populations: When are cultural loadings undesirable? *European Journal of Psychological Assessment, 8*(1), 17–24.

Van de Vijver, F. J. R., & Poortinga, Y. H. (1997). Towards an integrated analysis of bias in cross-cultural assessment. *European Journal of Psychological Assessment, 13*(1), 21–29.

Waltz, C. F., & Jenkins, L. S. (Eds.) (2001). *Measurement of nursing outcomes: Measuring nursing performance in practice, education, and research* (2nd ed., vol. 1). New York: Springer Publishing.

Warner, S. L. (1965). The linear randomized response model. *Journal of the American Statistical Association, 66,* 884–888.

Watson, J. (2000). *Assessing and measuring caring in nursing and health science.* New York: Springer Publishing.

Webb, E. J., Campbell, D. T., Schwartz, R. D., & Sechrest, L. (1966). *Unobtrusive measures: Nonreactive research in the social sciences.* Chicago: Rand McNally.

Weiss, R. S. (1968). Issues in holistic research. In H. S. Becker et al. (Eds.), *Institutions and the person* (pp. 342–350). Chicago: Aldine Publishers.

Werner, O., & Campbell, D. T. (1970). Translating, working through interpreters and the problem of decentering. In R. Naroll & R. Cohen (Eds.), *A handbook of method in cultural anthropology* (pp. 398–422). New York: American Museum of Natural History.

Wilson, H. S., & Hutchinson, S. A. (1991). Triangulation of qualitative methods: Heideggerian hermeneutics and grounded theory. *Qualitative Health Research, 1*(2), 263–276.

Wilson, H. S., Hutchinson, S., & Holzemer, W. L. (1997). Salvaging quality of life in ethnically diverse patients with advanced HIV/AIDS. *Qualitative Health Research, 75*(1), 75–97.

Wothke, W. (1995). Covariance components analysis of the multitrait-multimethod matrix. In P. E. Shrout & S. T. Fiske (Eds.), *Personality research, methods, and theory: A Festschrift honoring D. W. Fiske* (pp. 125–144). Hillsdale, NJ: Erlbaum.

Wothke, W. (1996). Models for multitrait-multimethod matrix analysis. In G. A. Marcoulides & R. E. Schumacker (Eds.), *Advanced structural equation modeling: Issues and techniques.* Mahwah, NJ: Erlbaum.

Zuckerman, M., & Lubin, B. (1985). *Manual for the Multiple Affect Adjective Check List—Revised Manual.* San Diego, CA: Educational and Industrial Testing Service.

Appendix A

Measurement Resources

Nola Stair

This appendix provides a compilation of print, electronic, and internet resources for use within the nursing field and/or other related disciplines. Each section provides an introduction, key resources useful for measuring variables, and alternative methods for access. However, it is important to note that the resources identified within this appendix do not constitute or imply an endorsement of the content, products, or services.

JOURNALS

There are a variety of nursing journals that often report original research studies, expand or refine measurement theory, or discuss the application and validity of specific tests. A growing number of these journals are also available over the Internet. Online access to journals is typically included in the cost of a regular institutional subscription. However, electronic access may or may not include the ability to access articles from previous volumes or the right to download articles or make copies without paying additional fees or seeking permission.

Other online options include freely available electronic journals, such as the Directory of Open Access Journals (http://www.doaj.org) or the Free Medical Journals (http://www.freemedicaljournals.com). In addition, the Web of Science, also known as the ISI Citation Database (http://isi5.isi-knowledge.com) indexes more than 8,000 peer-reviewed journals and provides bibliographic data, abstracts, and cited references.

Journals Specific to Nursing

Advances in Nursing Science—each issue features one research topic with implications for patient care and peer-reviewed articles.
  • ISSN: 0161-9268 or Website: http://ans-info.net/

American Journal of Nursing—provides a variety of clinical articles, clinical, nursing and healthcare news, and research (including practice errors and research for practice).
  • ISSN: 0002-936X or Website: http://www.ajnonline.com/

International Journal of Nursing Studies—provides original papers that report research findings and research-based reviews and analysis of interest in all areas of nursing and caring sciences.
  • Website: http://www.elsevier.com/locate/ijnurstu

Journal of Nursing Administration—provides information on the latest developments and advances in patient care leadership (including research and innovations, health care policy, economics and legislation, and legal, ethical, and political issues)
  • ISSN: 0002-0443 or Website: http://www.jonajournal.com/

Journal of Advanced Nursing—provides access to scholarly papers covering a broad range of nursing care issues, and nursing education, management and research.
- ISSN: 0309-2402 or Website: http://www.journalofadvancednursing.com/

Journal of Nursing Education—provides access to original articles and new ideas for nursing educators that enhance the teaching-learning process, promote curriculum development, and stimulate creative innovation and research in nursing education.
- ISSN: 0148-4834 or Website: http://www.journalofnursingeducation.com/

Journal of Professional Nursing—a bi-monthly 2 scholarly journal that provides updates on legislative, regulatory, ethical, and professional standards that affect nursing careers.
- ISSN: 8755-7223 or Website: http://www.us.elsevierhealth.com

The Internet Journal of Advanced Nursing Practice—a peer-reviewed online journal consisting of review articles, original papers, case reports, letters to the editor, and multimedia material.
- Website: http://www.ispub.com

Journals Specific to Nursing Research

Clinical Nursing Research—International refereed journal which meets the increasing demand for an international forum of scholarly research focused on clinical practice.
- ISSN: 1054-7738, Electronic ISSN: 1054-7738 or Website: http://www.sagepub.co.uk/

Canadian Journal of Nursing Research—a peer-reviewed, quarterly journal published by the McGill University School of Nursing. The focus is to publish original nursing research that develops basic knowledge for the discipline and examines the application of the knowledge in practice. Also included are research articles related to education and history, as well as methodological, theoretical, and review papers that advance nursing science.
- Website: http://www.cjnr.nursing.mcgill.ca

Nursing Research—each issue highlights the latest research, qualitative and quantitative studies, state-of-the-art methodology, strategies, new computer techniques, commentaries, and briefs.
- ISSN: 0029-6562 or Website: http://www.nursingresearchonline.com/

Outcomes Management—covers outcomes research, measurement/management of patient outcomes, evaluation of clinical protocols/programs, selection of instruments and nursing tests for measuring interventions/outcomes, and utilization of data for performance improvement.
- ISSN: 1535-2765 or Website: http://www.outcomesmanagement.com/

Qualitative Health Research—provides an international, interdisciplinary forum to enhance health care and further the development and understanding of qualitative research in health-care settings.
  Website: http://www.sagepub.co.uk/home.aspx

Research in Nursing & Health—a general, peer-reviewed, research journal devoted to the publication of a wide range of research and theory that will inform the practice of nursing and other health disciplines.
- ISSN: 0160-6891 or Electronic ISSN: 1098-240X

Western Journal of Nursing Research—a forum for scholarly debate (commentaries and rebuttals), which also provides theoretical papers examining current issues in nursing research.
- ISSN: 0193-9459, Electronic ISSN: 0193-9459 or Website: http://www.sagepub.co.uk/

Journals Specific to Measurement in Nursing and Related Disciplines

Applied Psychological Measurement—provides cutting-edge methodologies and related empirical research in educational, organizational, industrial, social, or clinical settings (including techniques to address measurement problems in the behavioral and social sciences).
- ISSN: 0146-6216, Electronic ISSN: 0146-6216 or Website: http://www.sagepub.co.uk/

Educational and Psychological Measurement—provides data-based studies in educational measurement, as well as theoretical papers in the measurement field.
- ISSN: 0013-1644, Electronic ISSN: 0013-1644 or Website: http://www.sagepub.co.uk/

Journal of Applied Measurement—publishes refereed scholarly work from all academic disciplines that relates to measurement theory and its application to developing variables.
- ISSN: 1529-7713 or Website: http://home.att.net/~rsmith.arm/index.htm

Journal of Nursing Measurement—provides information on instruments, tools, approaches, and procedures developed or utilized to measure variables in nursing, and spanning practice, research, and education.
- ISSN: 1061-3749 or Website: http://www.springerpub.com/journals/nursing/nursing_measurement.html

Measurement and Evaluation in Counseling & Development—provides articles dealing with the theoretical problems of the measurement in schools and colleges, public and private agencies, business, industry, or government.
- ISSN: 0748-1756 or Website: http://www.counseling.org/publications/journals.htm

Measurement in Physical Education & Exercise Science—offers suggestions for better understanding of humans by measuring their physical performance.
- ISSN: 1091-367X or Website: http://www.erlbaum.com/Journals/journals/MPEE/mpee.htm

Journals Specific to Evaluation in Health and Related Disciplines

Educational Evaluation and Policy Analysis—publishes scholarly articles about important issues in the formulation, implementation, and evaluation of education policy.
- Website: http://www.aera.net/pubs/eepa/

Evaluation and the Health Professions—examines applications of evaluation in health care programs and interventions.
- Website: http://www.sagepub.co.uk/Journalhome.aspx

Evaluation: International Journal of Theory, Research & Practice—publishes original theoretical and empirical evaluation research, as well as literature reviews and developments in evaluation policy and practice.
- Website: http://www.sagepub.co.uk/Journalhome.aspx

Evaluation Review: Journal of Applied Social Research—provides methodological and conceptual approaches to evaluation for the development, implementation, and utilization of evaluation studies.
- Website: http://www.sagepub.co.uk/Journalhome.aspx

Practical Assessment, Research, and Evaluation (PARE)—on-line journal published by edresearch.org and the Department of Measurement, Statistics, and Evaluation at the University of Maryland, College Park, which provides refereed articles on assessment, research, evaluation, and teaching practice.
  • Website: http://edresearch.org/pare/

INSTRUMENT COMPENDIA

The following section provides a listing of measurement instruments in use by the nursing field and other related disciplines. Each resource is headed by the bibliographical citation and either a brief description or website address. Reproductions of instruments are not included.

Instruments Specific to Nursing

Fischer, J., & Corcoran, K. (2000). *Measures For Clinical Practice* (2nd ed., Vol. I). New York: Free Press.
Fischer, J., & Corcoran, K. (2000). *Measures For Clinical Practice* (2nd ed., Vol. II). New York: Free Press
  • Provide direct practice workers with assessment instruments for use in monitoring and evaluating client progress and the effectiveness of social work intervention.

Frank-Stromberg, M. (1997). *Instruments For Clinical Health Care Research.* Boston: Jones and Bartlett Publishers.
  • Reviews clinical research instruments and provides a description of each tool's psychometric properties, selected studies using the tool, strengths and weaknesses of the tool, and nursing relevance.

Hart, S. E., & Waltz, C. F. (1998). *Educational Outcomes: Assessment of Quality—State of the Art and Future Directions.* New York: National League for Nursing Publications
  • Three compendia and a directory of student outcome measurements were compiled as a result of this project's assessment of program outcomes to evaluate the educational quality of nursing programs:

    ° Waltz, C. F., & Miller, C. (Eds.). (1988). *Educational Outcomes: Assessment of Quality—A Compendium of Measurement Tools for Baccalaureate Nursing Programs.* New York: National League for Nursing Publications.
    ° Waltz, C. F., & Neuman, L. (Eds.). (1988). *Educational Outcomes: Assessment of Quality—A Compendium of Measurement Tools for Associate Degree Nursing Programs.* New York: National League for Nursing Publications.
    ° Waltz, C. F., & Sylvia, B. (Eds.). (1988). *Educational Outcomes: Assessment of Quality—A Compendium of Measurement Tools for Diploma Nursing Programs.* New York: National League for Nursing Publications.
    ° National League for Nursing. (1987). *Educational Outcomes: Assessment of Quality—A Directory of Student Outcome Measurements Utilized by Nursing Programs in the United State.* New York: National League for Nursing Publications.

Redman, B. (2002). *Measurement Tools in Patient Education* (2nd ed.). New York: Springer Publishing.
  • Provides descriptive review and critique, as well as information on administration, scoring, and psychometric properties of 52 instruments.
  • Website: http://www.springerpub.com

Salek, S. (1999). *The Compendium of Quality of Life Instruments.* Chichester, NY: Wiley, RA.
- This five-volume set (also available on CD-ROM) contains over 150 questionnaires and translations covering a wide range of disorders.
- Website: http://www.wiley.com/legacy/products/subject/reference/salek_toc.html

Sawin, K. J. (1995). *Measures Of Family Functioning For Research And Practice.* New York : Springer Publishing.
- Website: http://www.springerpub.com

Waltz, C. F., & Strickland, O. L. (1998). *Measurement of Nursing Outcomes* (Vol. I): *Measuring Client Outcomes.* New York: Springer Publishing.
- Website: http://www.springerpub.com/

Strickland, O. L., & Waltz, C. F. (1998). *Measurement of Nursing Outcomes* (Vol. II): *Measuring Nursing Performance.* New York: Springer Publishing.
- Website: http://www.springerpub.com/

Waltz, C. F., & Strickland, O. L. (1990). *Measurement of Nursing Outcomes* (Vol. III): *Measuring Clinical Skills & Professional Development in Education and Practice.* New York: Springer Publishing.
- Website: http://www.springerpub.com/

Strickland, O. L., & Waltz, C. F. (1990). *Measurement of Nursing Outcomes* (Vol. IV): *Measuring Clinical Skills & Professional Development in Education and Practice.* New York: Springer Publishing.
- Website: http://www.springerpub.com/

Waltz, C. F., & Jenkins, L. S. (2001). *Measurement of Nursing Outcomes* (2nd ed., Vol. I): *Measuring Nursing Performance in Practice, Education, and Research.* New York: Springer Publishing.
- Website: http://www.springerpub.com/

Strickland, O. L., & Dilorios, C. (Eds.). (2003). *Measurement of Nursing Outcomes* (2nd ed., Vol. II): *Client Outcomes and Quality Care.* New York: Springer Publishing.
- Website: http://www.springerpub.com/

Strickland, O. L., & Dilorios, C. (Eds.). (2003). *Measurement of Nursing Outcomes (2nd ed., Vol. III): Self-Care and Coping.* New York: Springer Publishing.
- Website: http://www.springerpub.com/

Waltz, C. F., & Jenkins, L. (2001). *Measurement of Nursing Outcomes—Volume 1: Measuring Nursing Performance in Practice, Education & Research* (2nd ed.). New York: Springer Publishing.
- Volume I contains over thirty tools for the measurement of professional and education outcomes in nursing.
- Website: http://www.springerpub.com/

Ward, M. J., & Lindeman, C. A. (Eds.). (1979). *Instruments for Measuring Nursing Practice and Other Health Care Variables.* Hyattsville, MD: U.S. Department of Health, Education, and Welfare.
- Relating directly to nursing practice, this compilation contains 138 psychosocial instruments and 19 instruments to measure physiologic variables.

Instruments in Related Disciplines

Plake, B., Impara, J., & Spies, R. (Eds.). (2003). *The Fifteenth Mental Measurements Yearbook.* Highland Park, NJ: Gryphon Press.
- Website: http://www.unl.edu/buros
- Internet Index: http://buros.unl.edu/buros/jsp/search.jsp

Murphy L., Plake, B., Impara, J., & Spies, R. (Eds.). (2002). *Tests in Print VI: An Index to Tests, Test Reviews, and the Literature on Specific Tests.* Lincoln, NE: Buros Institute of Mental Measurements
- Website: http://www.unl.edu/buros
- Internet index: http://buros.unl.edu/buros/jsp/search.jsp (Tests in Print)

INTERNET WEBSITES

The Internet is a vast system of computers that are linked together to exchange information, which makes it extremely easy for worldwide communication and sharing. For example, the National Institute of Nursing Research's website (http://www.nih.gov/ninr/) is able to reach a worldwide audience to support its mission of clinical and basic research.

This section provides a variety Web sites, search engines, academic guides, online tools, and organizations, that can assist with locating appropriate measurement resources.

While it might take less time to find references to published instruments on the Internet than a traditional literature database search, please note that some instruments found on the Internet may not have been submitted for review and found acceptable.

Search Engines

Search engines can be very useful for finding available measurement instruments and resources, locating information on the Internet by browsing through millions of interconnected Web pages, and/or providing an internal collection of reviewed Web pages for key words and/or phrases. The following table summarizes key distinctions of the most popular search engines:

Search Engines	Website	Usefulness
AllTheWeb	http://www.alltheweb.com	Detailed search for any keywords, phrases, quotes, and information buried in full-text web pages
Altavista	http://www.altavista.com	
Google	http://www.google.com	
Visisimo	http://vivisimo.com/	Quick Searches or Unique Terms
Yahoo	http://www.yahoo.com	Human-Compiled Directory

Academic Guides to Tests and Measurement Instruments

University libraries play an important role in reviewing and organizing the vast amount of knowledge/information that is available on the Internet:

University of Maryland Baltimore's Health Sciences and Human Services Library
- Website: http://www.hshsl.umaryland.edu/resources/measurements.html

University of Michigan's Taubman Medical Library
- Website: http://www.lib.umich.edu/taubman/info/testsandmeasurement.htm

University of Texas at Arlington's Health Sciences Library
  • Website: http://libraries.uta.edu/helen/test&meas/testmainframe.htm
University of Washington's Health Science Library's online tutorial
  • Website: http://healthlinks.washington.edu/help/measure.html

Online Tools

Agency for Healthcare Research and Quality (AHRQ)—provides evidence-based information on health care outcomes, quality, and cost, use, and access, including a specific section on quality assessment and measurement tools.
  • Website: http://www.ahcpr.gov/qual/measurix.htm

Evaluation Primer on Health Risk Communication Programs and Outcomes Sponsor—provided by the U.S. Department of Health and Human Services Environmental Health Policy Committee, the evaluation primer assists with the planning and execution of evaluating health risk communication programs and materials.
  • Website: http://www.atsdr.cdc.gov/HEC/evalprmr.html

Measuring the Difference: Guide to Planning and Evaluating Health Information Outreach—various phases of evaluation are integrated into the process of planning and implementing outreach activities.
  • Website: http://nnlm.gov/evaluation/guide/

Neurophysiology Functional Tests and Disease Assessment—provides various links for epilepsy, and other neuromuscular, movement, autonomic function, and sleep disorders.
  • Website: http://www.neurophys.com/diagnostics.html

Performance Assessment Network—a Web-based system for the distribution, administration, and analysis of professional assessments, tests, and surveys.
  • Website: http://www.pantesting.com/

Research Randomizer—a free Web-based program that permits instant online random sampling and random assignment.
  • Website: http://www.randomizer.org/

Nonprofit and/or Professional Organizations

Academy for Health and Productivity Management—provides health/productivity measurement resources for a variety of health care settings.
  • Website: http://www.ahpm.org

American Evaluation Association—international professional association devoted to the application and exploration of various forms of evaluation.
  • Website: http://www.eval.org/

American Psychological Association's FAQ/Finding Information About Psychological Tests—provides answers to frequently-asked questions for locating and using available psychological tests.
  • Website: http://www.apa.org/science/faq-findtests.html

Association of Test Publishers—a nonprofit organization representing providers of tests and assessment tools and/or services related to assessment, selection, screening, certification, licensing, educational, or clinical uses.
  • Website: http://www.testpublishers.org/

Measure Gateway—funded by the U.S. Agency for International Development (USAID), MEASURE provides information on population, health, and nutrition in developing countries, as well as advice on using data for monitoring and evaluation.
  • Website: http://www.measureprogram.org/

Measurement Excellence Initiative (MEI)—a resource for improving the overall quality of measurement in the health services research community.
  • Website: http://www.measurementexperts.org/site_evals.asp

National Association of Health Data Organizations (NAHDO)—a not-for-profit national membership organization dedicated to improving health care through the collection, analysis, dissemination, public availability, and use of health data.
  • Website: http://www.nahdo.org/

National Council on Measurement in Education (NCME)—a professional organization for individuals involved in assessment, evaluation, testing, and other aspects of educational measurement.
  • Website: http://www.ncme.org/

The Urban Institute—a multiyear research project that analyzes social programs (including health care) and measures effects, compares options, and reveals trends.
  • Website: http://www.urban.org/Content/Research/NewFederalism/AboutANF/AboutANF.htm

Evaluation and Research-Related Resources

Center for Mental Health Policy—housed within Vanderbilt University, this site focuses on the evaluation of child, adolescent, and family mental health services research.
  • Website: http://www.vanderbilt.edu/VIPPS/CMHP

Digital Resources For Evaluators—a compilation of associations, discussion groups, data sources, educational resources, government agencies, instruments, statistics, and surveys.
  • Website: http://www.resources4evaluators.info

ERIC Clearinghouse on Assessment and Evaluation—a comprehensive list of educational evaluation resources containing over 10,000 indexed and searchable instruments.
  • Website: http://ericae.net

Health Communication Unit, Center for Health Promotion, University of Toronto—aims to increase the capacity of community and public health agencies to plan, conduct and evaluate health promotion programs.
  • Website: http://www.thcu.ca/infoandresources/evaluation_resources.htm

Measurement Group—funded by the Health Resources and Services Administration, this website provides evaluation assistance and dissemination activities to national HIV/AIDS treatment programs.
  • Website: http://www.tmg-web.com/edc.htm

Government-Related Resources

Centers for Disease Control and Prevention (CDC) Evaluation Working Group—promotes evaluation activities related to public health and prevention initiatives.
- Website: http://www.cdc.gov/eval/

Federal Committee on Statistical Methodology—an interagency committee dedicated to improving the quality of federal statistics and providing access to methodology reports and statistical agendas/policies.
- Website: http://www.fcsm.gov

Substance Abuse and Mental Health Services Administration (SAMHSA)—provides technical assistance to states and nonprofit public organizations for improving the planning, development, and operation of adult mental health services.
- Website: http://www.samhsa.gov/

U.S. Department of Health and Human Services (DHHS), Administration for Children and Families, Office—provides evaluation of programs effecting children and families.
- Website: http://www.acf.dhhs.gov/programs/opre/

U.S. Department of Health and Human Services (DHHS), Office of the Assistant Secretary for Planning and Evaluation—coordinates and conducts congressionally mandated evaluation of Department of Health and Human Services programs.
- Website: http://aspe.os.dhhs.gov/

COMPUTER SOFTWARE

Technology can effectively enable the collection, storage, analysis, and reporting of clinical and other-health related data.

General Statistical and Graphical Analysis Packages

The following statistical software packages offer a full range of tools (and add-on modules) to uncover facts, patterns, and trends for decision-making purposes, display results in graphical format, and produce and share research results using a variety of reporting methods.

Statistical Software Packages	Website
Mini-Tab	http://www.minitab.com
NCSS (Number Cruncher Statistical System)	http://www.ncss.com
SPSS (Statistical Package for the Social Sciences)	http://www.spss.com
SAS/STAT	http://www.sas.com

Other Data Analysis Software

Ethnograph—a software package that imports text-based qualitative data for the analysis of data collected during qualitative research.
- Website: http://www.qualisresearch.com

NUD*IST N6—a software package that imports, organizes, and analyzes complex qualitative data.
- Website: http://www.qsr.com.au/products/n6.html

Public Domain Software

This section provides a listing of software programs that are free and downloadable from the Internet or function as fully Web-based applications. Reviews of many statistical programs are available at http://www.stats.gla.ac.uk/cti/activities/reviews/alphabet.html and a large repository of freeware and demonstration versions is available at http://www.statistics.com

AnSWR (Analysis Software for Word-based Records)—a free software system from the Centers for Disease Control and Prevention for coordinating and conducting large-scale, team-based analysis projects that integrate qualitative and quantitative techniques.
  • Website: http://www.cdc.gov/hiv/software/answr.htm

CONQUEST 2.0 (COmputerized Needs-Oriented QUality Measurement Evaluation SysTem for collecting and evaluating clinical performance measures)—a free public-domain software system used for collecting and evaluating clinical performance measures.
  • Website: http://www.ahcpr.gov/qual/conquest/conqcopy.htm

CSPro (Census and Survey Processing System)—a public-domain software package for entering, tabulating, and mapping census and survey data.
  • Website: http://www.census.gov/ipc/www/cspro/index.html

EZ-Text—a free software program from the Centers for Disease Control and Prevention developed to assist researchers create, manage, and analyze semistructured qualitative databases.
  • Website: http://www.cdc.gov/hiv/software/ez-text.htm

PQMethod—statistical program tailored to the requirements of Q-sort technique.
  • Website: http://www.rz.unibw-muenchen.de/~p41bsmk/qmethod/

SignStream—developed as part of the American Sign Language Linguistic Research Project and supported by the National Science Foundation, this tool analyzes linguistic data captured on video for noncommercial use only.
  • Website: http://www.bu.edu/asllrp/SignStream/index.html

STATS—a free statistical analysis program that provides commonly needed statistical functions for researchers, such as calculating sample sizes needed for surveys.
  • Website: http://www.decisionanalyst.com/download.asp

WebStat—a free Java-based statistical computing environment.
  • Website: http://www.webstatsoftware.com/

WebQ—a free Java-based statistical application used to analyze Q-Sort method data.
  • Website: http://www.rz.unibw-muenchen.de/~p41bsmk/qmethod/webq/index.html

DATABASES

Databases are organized collections of information. There are many different types of databases, which are available in print, online, or CD-ROM. This section will focus on:
  • **Fee-Based Indexes**—containing literature and measurement instruments.
  • **Numeric Information**—statistics or demographic information.

Fee-Based Indexes

CINAHL—an index of the literature of nursing and allied health professions for locating descriptions and/or reprints of test and survey instruments.
- Website: http://www.cinahl.com/

HAPI (Health and Psychosocial Instruments)—a subscription database for evaluation and measurement tools, questionnaires, and test instruments in the health fields, psychosocial sciences, organizational behavior, and library and information science.
- Vendor: Behavioral Measurement Database Services

ETS Test Collection—provides access to standardized tests and research instruments from a variety of U.S. publishers and individual test authors. Foreign tests from Canada, Great Britain, and Australia are also included.
- Website: http://www.ets.org/testcoll/index.html

PSYCLIT/PSYCINFO—an index of psychologically relevant materials (psychological journals, books, book chapters, dissertations, and technical reports) as well as assessment instruments.
- Website: http://www.apa.org/psycinfo/

Numberic Information

Agency for Healthcare Policy and Research—provides abstracts, data sets, and surveys.
- Website: http://www.ahcpr.gov/data/

Centers for Disease Control (CDC) Data Warehouse—compilation of statistical information to guide actions and policies to improve health conditions.
- Website: http://www.cdc.gov/nchs/products.htm

Community Health Status Indicators Project—developed by the U.S. Department of Health and Human Services, Health Resources and Services Administration, provides access to health assessment information at the local level.
- Website: http://www.communityhealth.hrsa.gov/

Demographic and Health Surveys—provides a variety of data from and about surveys (i.e., status /content of ongoing/past surveys) and data on key indicators of population and health.
- Website: http://www.measuredhs.com/

General Social Survey Data and Information Retrieval System—annual personal interview survey of U.S. households conducted by the National Opinion Research Center.
- Website: http://www.icpsr.umich.edu:8080/GSS/homepage.htm

International Archive of Educational Data—provides access to data collected by national, state, provincial, local, and private organizations, pertaining to all levels of education.
- Website: http://www.icpsr.umich.edu/IAED/

Library of Congress (Federal Research Division, Country Studies)—provides description and analysis of the historical setting and the social, economic, political, and national security systems and institutions of countries throughout the world.
- Website: http://lcweb2.loc.gov/frd/cs/cshome.html

National Quality Measures Clearinghouse—sponsored by the Agency for Healthcare Research and Quality (AHRQ), U.S. Department of Health and Human Services, is a database and Web site for information on specific evidence-based health care quality measures and measure sets.
  • Website: http://www.qualitymeasures.ahrq.gov/

UNICEF—provides worldwide statistics on maternity, vital statistics, and mortality.
  • Website: http://www.unicef.org/statis/

U.S. Census Bureau—provides a complete overview and description of topics, geographic entities, and data.
  • Website: http://www.census.gov/prod/2001pubs/mso-01icdp.pdf

World Health Organization Stats—provides health and health-related epidemiological and statistical information.
  • Website: http://www3.who.int/whosis/menu.cfm

Appendix B

Selected Health Data Sources

Meg Johantgen

Summarized below is information about selected data used in health services research. Data sources are grouped into 3 broad categories: clinical/epidemiology, administrative, and sociodemographic. This list of data sources and measures is illustrative rather than exhaustive.

	Description	Examples of Measures or Research
CLINICAL/EPIDEMIOLOGY **Disease Registries** Surveillance, Epidemiology, and End Results Program (SEER) NIH, NCI	Data collected from selected geographic areas based on their ability to operate and maintain a high-quality population-based cancer reporting system and for their epidemiological significant population subgroups. Provides information on cancer incidence and survival in the United States.	Diagnosis-specific national estimates of incidence, treatment, and outcomes including stage at diagnosis, course of treatment, mortality, etc.
National Nosocomial Infection Surveillance Systems CDC	Selected hospitals elect to provide indicators in four areas: hospital-wide component, adult and pediatric intensive care, high-risk nursery, and surgical patient surveillance.	Multiple types of infections including urinary tract infections, central line-associated blood stream infections, ventilator associated pneumonia, surgical site infection, etc.
Epidemiological Surveys **National Health Interview Survey** NCHS, CDC Special surveys: Access to Care Survey, Disability, Second Supplement on Aging, Second Longitudinal Study of Aging	Population-based survey of U.S. noninstitutionalized population that provides national estimates on the incidence of acute illness and injuries, the prevalence of chronic conditions and impairments, the extent of disability, the utilization of health services, and other health-related topics.	Incidence, prevalence, access, usual source of care, delays in care, utilization, injuries, satisfaction, routine check-up, blood pressure, hormone replacement therapy, usual source of care, immunization data, etc.
Medical Expenditure Panel Survey AHRQ	A nationally representative survey of health care use, expenditures, sources of payment, and insurance coverage for the U.S. civilian noninstitutionalized population. Consists of four component surveys:1) household component, 2) medical provider survey, 3) insurance component, and 4) nursing home component.	Incidence, prevalence, access, utilization, satisfaction, prevention and screening services, medical expenditures, and insurance coverage in the U.S. Nursing home component collects information on utilization, expenditures, insurance coverage, health status, prevalence, medications, and mortality.

	Description	Examples of Measures or Research
National Immunization Survey NCHS, CDC	Telephone survey of national household sample of children age 18–35 months. Data from immunization providers are used to validate the child's immunization history reported by the household respondent.	Estimates of vaccine coverage for 6 recommended vaccines by demographic and socioeconomic characteristics.
State and Local Area Integrated Telephone Survey (SLAITS) NCHS, CDC	Special purpose survey, piggyback to National Immunization Survey sample. Designed for state based estimation of health insurance coverage, utilization and barriers, performance partnership initiatives, and impact of welfare-related reforms. Includes special survey efforts: Families with young children Children with special needs HIV testing and STD risk behaviors.	Health insurance coverage, access to care, health status, utilization of services, basic demographic information.
National Survey of Family Growth NCHS, CDC	Survey based on personal interviews with a sample of women aged 15–44. Survey includes items on factors affecting birth and pregnancy, including sexual activity, infertility, sterilization, use of family planning services, and contraceptive use.	Use of care for family planning and reproductive health, risk for STDs, risk for pregnancy, and infertility services
National Health and Nutrition Examination Survey NCHS, CDC	Survey using home interviews and direct physical examinations to collect information on the health and diet.	Estimates of medically defined prevalence of specific diseases and the distribution in the population with respect to physical, physiological, and psychological characteristics.
National Household Survey on Drug Abuse (NHSDA) SAMHSA	Cross-sectional telephone survey collects information on the prevalence, patterns and consequences of drug and alcohol use and abuse in the U.S. civilian noninstitutionalized population, age 12 and older.	Prevalence, demographics, perceived harmfulness, and other measures of alcohol, tobacco, nonmedical use of psychotherapies, and illicit drug use.
Drug Abuse Warning Network (DAWN) SAMHSA	A national surveillance system that monitors trends in drug-related emergency visits and deaths from a sample of hospital emergency departments.	Number of episodes of drug abuse by type of drug, characteristics of medical problems, and demographic characteristics. Estimates of drug use by location are made.
Youth Risk Behavior Surveillance System (YRBSS) CDC	National, state, and school-based surveys of representative samples of 9th–12th graders in public and private schools. behaviors, etc.	Health risk behaviors including tobacco use, unhealthy dietary behaviors, physical activity, alcohol and drug use, sexual

	Description	Examples of Measures or Research
National Hospital Discharge Survey NCHS	Data abstracted from hospital inpatient records are aggregated to national sample. Includes information on hospital characteristics, diagnoses, surgical procedures, length of stay, expected source of payment, and patient characteristics.	Avoidable hospitalizations, mortality, complications, procedure rates, some quality indicators, etc.
National Ambulatory Medical Care Survey NCHS, CDC	Data collected on visits to physician's offices including patient characteristics, procedures, diagnoses, medications, disposition, and causes of injury, where applicable.	Prevention, screening, counseling, medication use, frequency of diagnoses, procedures, etc.
National Hospital Ambulatory Medical Care Survey NCHS, CDC	Data collected on visits to hospital outpatient departments and emergency department including patient characteristics, procedures, diagnoses, medications, disposition, and cause of injury, where applicable. An emergency department component also includes information on patient characteristics, patient complaint (ED), and types of providers seen.	Prevention, screening, counseling, medication use, frequency of diagnoses, procedures, etc. Emergency data includes time to see physician, presenting level of pain, diagnoses, and chief complaints.
National Nursing Home Survey NCHS, CDC	Series of national sample surveys of nursing homes, residents, and staff. Provides facility-level and patient information on current and discharged residents.	Utilization, diagnoses, procedures, functional status, continence, hearing or sight impairments, activities of daily living, pressure sores, etc.
National Home and Hospice Care Survey NCHS, CDC	Survey of agencies that are licensed or certified (Medicare of Medicaid) to provide home and hospice care. Data reflect information on current patients and discharges and include referral, length of service, diagnoses, number of visits, patient characteristics, health status, reason for discharge, and type of services provided.	Utilization, diagnoses, number of visits, length of service, patient charges, health status, reason for discharge, and type of equipment and services.
National Mortality Follow-Back Survey CDC	Follow-back from state death records. Uses telephone and/or personal interviews with informants. Includes use of hospital medical records and medical examiner/coroner records.	Mortality due to diabetes, associated with alcohol, functional status and use of home care, cancer, AIDS, substance abuse, suicide, quality of life in last year of life, effect of smoking.
AIDS Cost and Services Utilization Survey AHRQ	Longitudinal study of persons with HIV-related disease that uses a combination of personal interviews and record abstraction of medical and billing records.	Patterns of service use, expenditures for medical and nonmedical services, socioeconomic factors, changes over course of treatment, etc.

	Description	Examples of Measures or Research
ADMINISTRATIVE **Claims/Encounter** **Medicare Claims** CMS — Medicare Provider and Analyses Review (MEDPAR) — Standard Analytic Files	Beneficiary data collected by CMS in its administration of the Medicare fee-for-service program. Data represent care provided related to inpatient, outpatient, hospice, skilled nursing facility, home health, durable medical equipment, and physician services.	Examination of most services provided to Medicare population. Episodes of care can be created and varied outcomes can be examined.
Healthcare Cost and **Utilization Project** AHRQ — Nationwide Inpatient Sample — State Inpatient Database	Aggregates hospital discharge data from multiple state data organizations. Data represent information on hospital discharge abstract with some variation across states.	Patterns of hospitalization including avoidable hospitalizations, complications, in-hospital mortality, some quality indicators, diagnoses, and procedures.
Providers of services **Provider Specific Record** CMS	Hospital-level data used to estimate payments for hospitals operating and capital costs. Data are taken from various sources and include: average daily census, number of beds, case-mix index, medical resident to bed ratios, geographic location, and type of hospital.	Hospital characteristics that relate to cost (e.g., type of hospital, teaching, size, case mix, etc.) and change over time.
American Hospital **Association Annual** **Survey Database** AHA	Data derived from the AHA annual survey of health care providers. Variables represent services and characteristics as reported by the hospital.	A broad range of hospital characteristics that reflect hospital attributes, services, programs, and affiliations.
Certification and Survey **Medicare Current** **Beneficiary Survey** CMS	Continuous survey of national sample drawn from Medicare enrollment files, to examine expenditures, sources of payment, and changes in health status. Includes community interview and long-term care protocol for those institutionalized.	Access, utilization, health status, limitation of activity, health care coverage, usual source of care, medication use, satisfaction, wait time.
Online Survey Certification **and Reporting (OSCAR)** CMS	Data collected from institution survey and certification process. Program compliance records for the current survey and three preceding surveys are maintained along with descriptive information on provider characteristics.	Trends in organizational characteristics, deficiencies, and services.
Resident Assessment **Instrument (RAI) captured** **in the Minimum Data** **Set (MDS)** CMS	Data from nursing home resident assessment includes items on daily events, cognitive patterns, communication/hearing, vision, mood & behavior, psychosocial	Trends in resident characteristics, quality indicators (e.g., falls, bed sores, multiple medications, etc.).

	Description	Examples of Measures or Research
	well being, physical function, continence, disease diagnoses, and health conditions, oral/nutritional status, skin condition, activity pursuit patterns, medications, and special treatments and procedures. All certified long-term care facilities are required to transmit their MDS records.	
SOCIODEMOGRAPHIC **Vital Statistics and** **Census Data** **Vital Statistics** States and CDC	Annual data on births, deaths (including infant deaths), and fetal deaths. Variables include cause of death, demographics, and place of occurrence.	Teen births, access to prenatal care, maternal risk factors, causes of death, and life expectancy.
National Vital Statistics System (NVSS) NCHS, CDC	Provides the nation's official vital statistics through state-operated registration systems. These include births, deaths, marriages, and divorces.	Allows examination of variation in incidence, change over time, influence of policies, etc.
Linked Birth/Infant Death Program NCHS, CDC	Linked data from birth and death certificates facilitates analysis of infant mortality trends.	Data on infant mortality by birthweight, gestational age, prenatal care utilization, cause of death, and maternal characteristics such as age, education, marital status, and smoking and alcohol use during pregnancy.
National Death Index NCHS, CDC	Central computerized index of death record information compiled from data files submitted by state vital statistics offices.	Linkage for assessment of mortality.
Health Resource Data **National Sample Survey of Registered Nurses** HRSA	Comprehensive source of statistics on all those with current licenses to practice in the United States, whether or not they are employed in nursing.	Trends in licensed nurses including number, background, location, employment status, etc.
Area Resource File (ARF) HRSA	County-level database containing over 6,000 variables for each county in the U.S. obtained from multiple data sources, including number of hospitals, nursing homes, etc.	Data on geographic characteristics can be used to examine health service utilization and variation, changes over time based on policies, and other geographically based activities.

AHA = American Hospital Association

AHRQ = Agency for Healthcare Research and Quality

CDC = Centers for Disease Control

CMS = Centers for Medicaid and Medicare Services

HRSA = Health Resources Services Administration

NCHS = National Center for Health Statistics

SAMHSA = Substance Abuse and Mental Health Services Administration

Index

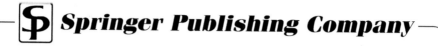

Springer Publishing Company

Self-Efficacy in Nursing
Research and Measurement Perspectives

Elizabeth R. Lenz, PhD, FAAN
Lillie M. Shortridge-Baggett, EdD, RN, FAAN, Editors

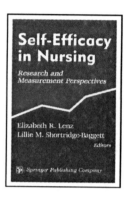

Self-efficacy, or the belief that one can self-manage one's own health, is an important goal of health care providers, particularly in chronic illness. This book explores the concept of self-efficacy from theory, research, measurement, and practice perspectives. The core of the book is an international collaboration of nurses from the U.S. and the Netherlands who have developed tools for promoting and measuring self-efficacy in diabetes management. Originally developed as a special issue of the journal *Scholarly Inquiry for Nursing Practice,* the book addresses the importance of theory-based interventions in enhancing self-efficacy.

Partial Contents:

Part I: Introduction

- Self-Efficacy: Measurement and Intervention in Nursing
  L.M. Shortridge-Baggett
- The Theory and Measurement of the Self-Efficacy Construct
  J.J. van der Bijl and *L.M. Shortridge-Baggett*

Part II: Self-Efficacy in Diabetes Management

- Self-Efficacy in Children with Diabetes Mellitus: Testing of a Measurement Instrument, *M.J. Kappen, et al.*
- Strategies Enhancing Self-Efficacy in Diabetes Education: A Review
  K.E.W. van der Laar and *J.J. van der Bijl*

Part III: Self-Efficacy and Other Clinical Conditions

- Self-Efficacy Targeted Treatments for Weight Loss in Postmenopausal Women, *K.E. Dennis, et al.*
- An Intervention to Increase Quality of Life and Self-Care Self-Efficacy and Decrease Symptoms in Breast Cancer Patients, *E.L. Lev, et al.*

2002   128pp   0-8261-1563-2   hard

11 West 42nd Street, New York, NY 10036-8002 • Fax: 212-941-7842
Order Toll-Free: 877-687-7476 • Order On-line: www.springerpub.com